Sustainable Practices in Biorefinery

Pradeep Verma
Editor

Sustainable Practices in Biorefinery

Springer

Editor
Pradeep Verma
Bioprocess and Bioenergy Laboratory,
Department of Microbiology
Central University of Rajasthan
Ajmer, Rajasthan, India

ISBN 978-981-95-6070-7 ISBN 978-981-95-6071-4 (eBook)
https://doi.org/10.1007/978-981-95-6071-4

This Springer imprint is published by the registered company Springer Nature Singapore Pte Ltd.
The registered company address is: 152 Beach Road, #21-01/04 Gateway East, Singapore 189721, Singapore

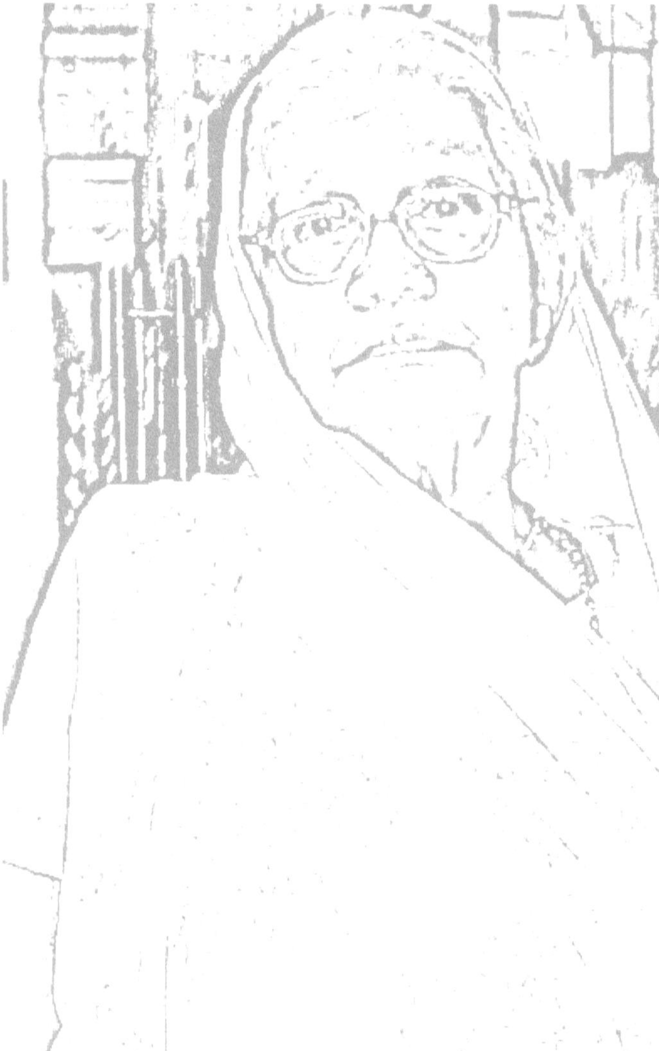

Dedicated to My Beloved Mother

Preface

The book aims to provide a comprehensive overview of the advances, applications, ethics, and policies related to biorefineries, while focusing on their production, utilization, and holistic applications in the light of human development. It is intended for academics, researchers, industry professionals, policymakers, and students in the fields of environmental science, renewable energy, and sustainable development, offering valuable insights into bioenergy and biofuels. While the biorefinery topic has a vast amount of literature, several aspects addressed in this book are not covered by other competitive texts. For instance, although existing literature discusses the use of lignocellulosic biomass for bioethanol and biofuel production, it often overlooks the agricultural and forestry techniques that can contribute to biorefinery success. Additionally, topics such as aviation biofuels and the role of nanotechnology in biorefineries are rarely discussed. This book aims to fill those gaps by covering less-explored subjects in the field.

The book encompasses a broad range of topics, including agricultural and forestry practices that enhance bioenergy efficiency, as well as complex ethical and policy-related decisions. It also examines technological and scientific developments, including innovations in wood pellet production, their environmental impacts, and market prospects, as well as the fundamentals of artificial photosynthesis and its applications, innovations in photobioreactor design, and the addressing of technical and economic challenges. Cellulosic ethanol is also examined in detail, with discussion on commercialization hurdles and strategies for cost reduction. Further, case studies demonstrating energy-efficient practices and their economic implications have also been discussed. The contents also discuss the harvesting of biogas from landfills, focusing on the processes for biogas extraction, advancements in technology, applications, and the environmental and economic benefits that arise from these practices. It highlights hydrothermal liquefaction, a novel biofuel production technology, along with its current research and future directions. The text also addresses the production of renewable natural gas (RNG) from biomethane processes, including its applications, benefits, recent market trends, and regulatory considerations. Furthermore, it covers sustainable aviation fuels (SAFs), examining their prospects, challenges in development and production, and their potential to reduce aviation emissions.

The role of nanotechnology in revolutionizing biofuel production is also discussed, highlighting innovations, applications, potential benefits, challenges, and future research directions. The ethical dimensions of bioenergy and biofuels are also explored, particularly their socio-economic and environmental impacts, bearing implications for policy and stakeholder perspectives. Finally, the text provides an overview of global biofuel policies and regulations. Together, these chapters provide a comprehensive understanding of the environmental, technological, and policy dimensions that shape biorefineries.

Ajmer, India Pradeep Verma

Acknowledgments

First and foremost, I would like to express my gratitude to Springer Nature for accepting my proposal to serve as editor for the current book proposal. The current book would not have been possible without the support of all the researchers and academicians who contributed to the book. Undeniably, the authors have made every possible attempt to overcome the existing limitations in the literature. I am grateful for their prompt response to my invitations and support throughout the revision stages. I am also thankful to the Central University of Rajasthan (CURAJ), Ajmer, India, for providing infrastructural support and a suitable teaching and research environment. The teaching experience for graduate, postgraduate, and young researchers at CURAJ provided the necessary understanding of the needs of academicians, students, and researchers, which was greatly helpful during the development of the book series. I am also thankful to the Department of Biotechnology for providing me with funds through sponsored projects (Grant No. BT/304/NE/TBP/2012, BT/PR7333/PBD/26/373/2012, and BT/PR54202/BSA/33/198/2024 for the establishment of my laboratory, "Bioprocess and Bioenergy Laboratory."

I am profoundly grateful to the Almighty and my parents for their boundless blessings and guidance. This book is affectionately dedicated to the most remarkable women in my life- my mother and wife. Their unwavering love, care, and faith have been my greatest source of strength and inspiration for pursuing knowledge and making meaningful contributions in the scientific world. I also extend my heartfelt gratitude to my lovely children, whose encouragement, patience, and joy have supported me through the making of this book and every chapter of my life.

Contents

Editor and Contributors

About the Editor

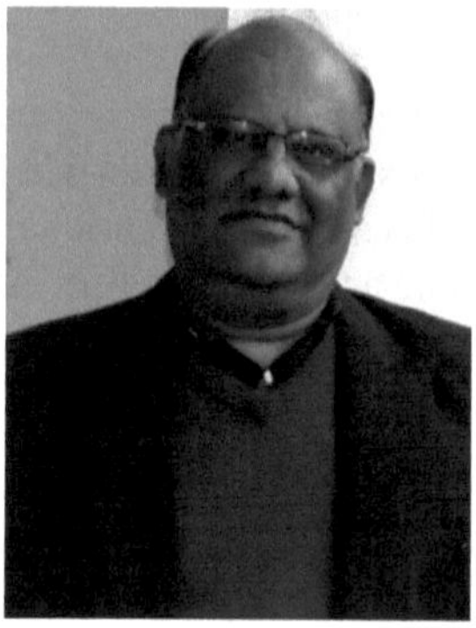

Prof. Pradeep Verma completed his Ph.D. at Sardar Patel University, Gujarat, India, in 2002. In the same year, he began his international research career as a UNESCO Fellow at the Czech Academy of Sciences, Prague, Czech Republic. His dedication to research soon led him to Charles University in Prague for a Postdoctoral Fellowship, followed by his tenure as a Visiting Scientist at the UFZ Centre for Environmental Research in Halle, Germany, in 2004. Recognizing his exceptional potential, Prof. Verma was awarded the prestigious DFG Fellowship, which facilitated his post-doctoral research at the University of Göttingen, Germany. In 2007, he returned to India and joined Reliance Life Sciences, Mumbai, where his pioneering work on biobutanol production resulted in several international patents. His scientific excellence further earned him the JSPS Post-Doctoral Fellowship, leading to a significant phase at the Laboratory of Biomass Conversion, Kyoto University, Japan.

Prof. Verma joined Assam University in 2009 as a Reader and the Founder Head of the Department. In 2011, he moved to Guru Ghasidas Vishwavidyalaya (a Central University) in Bilaspur as an Associate Professor. Since 2013, he has been serving as Professor at the School of Life Sciences, Department of Microbiology, Central University of Rajasthan (CURAJ), where he has also served as the Dean and Head. His areas of expertise include microbial diversity, bioremediation, bioprocess development, and biorefineries based on lignocellulosic and algal biomass. His contributions to fungal microbiology, industrial biotechnology, and environmental bioremediation have earned him numerous accolades, including the Fellow Award from the, International Academy of Wood Science (IAWS, 2024) Mycological Society of India (2020), the P.C. Jain Memorial Award (MSI), Fellowship of the Biotechnology Research Society of India (BRSI, 2020), and Fellowship of the Academy of Microbiological Sciences (AMI, 2021). He is also a recipient of Prof YSRK Sarma Mcmorial Award-2025 from the Society of Plant Research for his valuable contribution in microalgal research. He also received the JSPS Bridge Fellowship in 2022, which enabled further collaboration with Kyoto University in Japan.

Prof. Verma has nearly 200 publications, including research articles, book chapters, and proceedings in reputed journals, which have collectively received over 10165 citations, with an h-index of 52 and an i10-index of 138. In addition, he holds multiple patents, has edited over 30 books with leading academic publishers, and has successfully secured major national research grants amounting to INR 2.5 million. His outstanding contributions to microbial biotechnology and sustainable innovations, as reflected in globally acclaimed publications and a high citation impact, have earned him a place among the top 2% of scientists worldwide, as ranked by Stanford University, for three consecutive years. He also serves as an editorial board member of several journals. Additionally, he is affiliated with numerous national and international scientific societies and academies. His career exemplifies a lifelong commitment to advancing science and driving innovations in microbial biotechnology and environmental sustainability. e-mail: pradeepverma@curaj.ac.in

URL: pradeepverma@curaj.ac.in

Contributors

Komal Agrawal Department of Microbiology, School of Bio Engineering and Biosciences, Lovely Professional University, Phagwara, Punjab, India

Edayilam Anjana Department of Biosciences, Mangalore University, Mangalagangotri, Mangalore, Karnataka, India

Karan Arya Department of Biotechnology, Himachal Pradesh University, Shimla, India

Parul Bali Department of Microbiology, Himachal Pradesh University, Shimla, India

Anwesha Bandyopadhyay School of Biotechnology, Faculty of Applied Sciences & Biotechnology, Shoolini University, Solan, Himachal Pradesh, India

Khouloud M. Barakat National Institute of Oceanography and Fisheries (NIOF), Elanfoushy, Alexandria, Egypt

Ravi Kant Bhatia Department of Biotechnology, Himachal Pradesh University, Shimla, India

Emre Çolak Institute of Science, Department of Energy Systems Engineering, Giresun University, MSc Program, Giresun, Türkiye

Sayak Das Department of Life Science and Bioinformatics, Har Gobind Khurana School of Life Sciences, Assam University, Silchar, Assam, India

Suryasneha Deb Department of Life Science and Bioinformatics, Har Gobind Khurana School of Life Sciences, Assam University, Silchar, Assam, India

Deepshikha Department of Microbiology, School of Bio Engineering and Biosciences, Lovely Professional University, Phagwara, Punjab, India

Aseni.N. Ediriweera B-Hood Myco-Tropic Innovations, Matara, Sri Lanka

Ahmed El Nemr National Institute of Oceanography and Fisheries (NIOF), Elanfoushy, Alexandria, Egypt

Kandasamy Gajendiran PG and Research Department of Microbiology, M.G.R. College, Hosur, Tamil Nadu, India

Simant Giri Goswami Department of Biotechnology, Guru Ghasidas Vishwavidyalaya (A Central University), Bilaspur, Chhattisgarh, India

Abu Barkat Md. Gulzar Plant and Microbial Molecular Biology Laboratory, Department of Biotechnology, Assam University, Silchar, Assam, India

Niranjan Gunasekara Department of Export Agriculture, Faculty of Export Agriculture and Animal Science, Uva Wellassa University, Badulla, Sri Lanka

Rahul Gupta Amity Institute of Biotechnology, Amity University, Lucknow Campus, Lucknow, Uttar Pradesh, India

Mohamed A. Hassaan National Institute of Oceanography and Fisheries (NIOF), Kayet Bey, Elanfoushy, Alexandria, Egypt

Gaurishankar Jaiswal Department of Biotechnology, Guru Ghasidas Vishwavidyalaya (A Central University), Bilaspur, Chhattisgarh, India

Harit Jha Department of Biotechnology, Guru Ghasidas Vishwavidyalaya (A Central University), Bilaspur, Chhattisgarh, India

Samantha C. Karunarathna Center for Yunnan Plateau Biological Resources Protection and Utilization, College of Biology and Food Engineering, Qujing Normal University, Qujing, Yunnan, P.R. China

Vaishnavi Kashyap Department of Biotechnology, Himachal Pradesh University, Shimla, India

Aafreen Khan Department of Biotechnology, Guru Ghasidas Vishwavidyalaya (A Central University), Bilaspur, Chhattisgarh, India

Abhimanyu Kumar Department of Biological Sciences, Birla Institute of Technology and Science, Pilani, India

Priya Kumari Department of Microbiology, Himachal Pradesh University, Shimla, India

Mamta Department of Biological Sciences, Birla Institute of Technology and Science, Pilani, India

N. Mathiyazhagan Department of Biotechnology, Saveetha School of Engineering, Saveetha Institute of Medical and Technical Sciences, SIMATS, Thandalam, Chennai, Tamil Nadu, India

Pranab Behari Mazumder Plant and Microbial Molecular Biology Laboratory, Department of Biotechnology, Assam University, Silchar, Assam, India

Lakshana G. Nair Bioprocess and Bioenergy Laboratory (BPBEL), Department of Microbiology, Central University of Rajasthan, Kishangarh, Ajmer, Rajasthan, India

D. Natarajan Department of Biotechnology, Periyar University, Salem, Tamil Nadu, India

Priti Pal Amity Institute of Biotechnology, Amity University, Lucknow Campus, Lucknow, Uttar Pradesh, India

Tarun Pal School of Bioengineering and Food Technology, Faculty of Applied Sciences & Biotechnology, Shoolini University, Solan, Himachal Pradesh, India

Jitendra Panwar Department of Biological Sciences, Birla Institute of Technology and Science, Pilani, India

Ashna Parveen Department of Biotechnology and Microbiology, Meerut Institute of Engineering and Technology, Meerut, India

Minura peiris Department of Export Agriculture, Faculty of Export Agriculture and Animal Science, Uva Wellassa University, Badulla, Sri Lanka

Kaustav Purkayastha Department of Life Science and Bioinformatics, Har Gobind Khurana School of Life Sciences, Assam University, Silchar, Assam, India

Suchitra Rakesh Biofuel Research Laboratory, Department of Microbiology, Central University of Tamil Nadu, Thiruvarur, Tamil Nadu, India

Saurabh Singh Rathore Department of Biotechnology, School of Life Sciences, Mahatma Gandhi Central University, Motihari, Bihar, India

Bobita Ray Biofuel Research Laboratory, Department of Microbiology, Central University of Tamil Nadu, Thiruvarur, Tamil Nadu, India

Ritushree Roy Plant and Microbial Molecular Biology Laboratory, Department of Biotechnology, Assam University, Silchar, Assam, India

Uttam Kumar Sahoo Department of Forestry, Mizoram University, Aizawl, India

Tarek O. Said National Institute of Oceanography and Fisheries (NIOF), Alexandria, Egypt

Tarek O. Said National Institute of Oceanography and Fisheries (NIOF), Cairo, Egypt

Tarek O. Said National Institute of Oceanography and Fisheries (NIOF), Elanfoushy, Alexandria, Egypt

Prakash Kumar Sarangi College of Agriculture, Central Agricultural University, Imphal, India

Halil Şenol Faculty of Engineering, Department of Energy Systems Engineering, Giresun University, Giresun, Türkiye

Kodandoor Sharathchandra Department of Biosciences, Mangalore University, Mangalagangotri, Mangalore, Karnataka, India

Aditya Sharma Department of Biotechnology, Himachal Pradesh University, Shimla, India

Laxuman Sharma Department of Horticulture, Sikkim University, Gangtok, India

Shreya Sharma Department of Microbiology, School of Bio Engineering and Biosciences, Lovely Professional University, Phagwara, Punjab, India

Shobham Department of Biological Sciences, Birla Institute of Technology and Science, Pilani, India

Shristy Shreya Department of Biological Sciences, Birla Institute of Technology and Science, Pilani, India

Akhilesh Kumar Singh Department of Biotechnology, School of Life Sciences, Mahatma Gandhi Central University, Motihari, Bihar, India

Puneet Kumar Singh School of Biotechnology, Kalinga Institute of Industrial Technology (KIIT), Bhubaneswar, India

Kandikere Ramaiah Sridhar Department of Biosciences, Mangalore University, Mangalagangotri, Mangalore, Karnataka, India;
Central Research Laboratory, NITTE (Deemed to be University), KS Hegde Medical Academy (KSHEMA), Mangalore, Karnataka, India

Tanishq Department of Biotechnology, Himachal Pradesh University, Shimla, India

Pradeep Verma Bioprocess and Bioenergy Laboratory (BPBEL), Department of Microbiology, Central University of Rajasthan, Kishangarh, Ajmer, Rajasthan, India

Farhana Yasmin Plant and Microbial Molecular Biology Laboratory, Department of Biotechnology, Assam University, Silchar, Assam, India

Murat Yılmaz Bahçe Vocational School, Department of Chemistry and Chemical Processing Technologies, Osmaniye Korkut Ata University, Osmaniye, Türkiye

Chapter 1
Advances in Wood Pellet Technology: Emerging Trends, Market Dynamics, and Environmental Impacts

Lakshana G. Nair and Pradeep Verma

Abstract The vital role of the wood pellet industry in today's bioeconomy drives its transition towards sustainable and carbon-neutral systems. The current chapter examines recent developments in the wood pelletization sector, highlighting innovations in the process and technologies that have contributed to improvements in pellet durability, quality, and energy density. The integration of digitalization techniques in the pelletization process has also enabled predictive maintenance and adaptive process control. The environmental perspective emphasizes the importance of sustainable feedstock sourcing, waste valorization, and emission management in the production of pellets. The market dynamics, driven by shifts in international trade and policy guidelines across various countries, continue to influence the trajectory of the wood pellet industry. The remaining challenges in terms of economic viability and pollution control can be mitigated through further research, including process optimization, digitalization, the use of artificial intelligence, and machine learning, among others. The implementation of policy incentives, supply chain optimization, and integrated sustainability assessments may also help reinforce the wood pellet industry's role in achieving carbon neutrality.

Keywords Wood · Pelletization · Pollution · Process-optimization · Environmental impact

1.1 Introduction

The increase in energy demand, coupled with the depletion of fossil resources and the hike in waste generation, are all significant problems in the day-to-day world. The production of solid fuels like pellets from woody biomass, energy crops, sewage

L. G. Nair · P. Verma (✉)
Bioprocess and Bioenergy Laboratory (BPBEL), Department of Microbiology, Central University of Rajasthan, Kishangarh, Ajmer, Rajasthan, India
e-mail: pradeepverma@curaj.ac.in

P. Verma (ed.), *Sustainable Practices in Biorefinery*,
https://doi.org/10.1007/978-981-95-6071-4_1

sludge, etc., has been recognized as a potential solution for the reduction of environmental pollution (Siyal et al., 2021). Biomass has huge potential as a renewable energy source, as it does not contribute to additional carbon dioxide emissions in the atmosphere. The use of biomass as raw materials in energy production may also reduce the pollution from open burning and landfilling, and additionally becomes an energy source for the stakeholders (Cui et al., 2021). As the fourth-largest source of energy, biomass can be utilized to replace non-renewable energy sources through various approaches. However, impediments such as transportation, storage, its hygroscopic nature, lower grindability, lower bulk density, and spontaneous combustion limit the applications of biomass in bioconversion for energy. These issues can be addressed through biomass pelletization, which significantly reduces the costs associated with handling, transportation, and storage. Biomass pelletization also reduces the risk of dust emission during its handling and transportation (Ahmed et al., 2022). Wood pellets, also known as white pellets, are a densification product, synthesised from either lignocellulosic materials or residues from wood processing industries, by applying mechanical force for the compaction of biomass into the form of pellets (Chotikhun et al., 2022). Compared to coal, the wood pellets are a low-emission fuel alternative, with a calorific value of 4000–4600 kcal/kg, while that of coal is 6000 kcal/kg. Hence, to replace 1 ton of coal, approximately 1.3 tons of wood pellets are required. But the low pollution characteristics of the wood pellets support cleaner industrial applications (Lee & Hsu, 2025a) and sustainable goals.

The wood fibres, which are compressed to form pellets, have garnered attention as a commercially traded biofuel due to their attractive properties, such as high energy content, fibre malleability, and comparatively better combustion properties (Aguilar et al., 2020). Biomass pelletization produces solid fuels (E.g., pellets) with a uniform size, structure, and other desirable qualities, such as strength and high density. It also lowers the moisture content of the pellets to less than 10%, depending on the type of feedstock and its original moisture content (Ahmed et al., 2022). The biomass feedstocks or raw materials widely used in pellet production include softwood and hardwood species, depending on regional availability. The transition to lower fossil fuel dependency will lead to a higher demand for pelletized products. Hence, it is imperative to develop a pelletization process that is optimal for a variety of biomass sources, with varying chemical compositions, to accommodate different feedstocks as they become available (Berghel et al., 2022), which, to date, has not yet been fully developed. As conventional pellets are capable of absorbing moisture from their surroundings, they present difficulties in storage and transport, in addition to their low energy density. Hence, innovations in pelleting technology are imperative to improve its properties (Chotikhun et al., 2022).

The current chapter aims to discuss recent technological advancements in pelletization, focusing on enhanced production levels with low costs and minimal environmental impact. The challenges and economic and environmental impacts of pelletization are discussed in the context of life cycle and environmental analysis. Furthermore, the chapter also examines the various market trends associated with the wood pellet industry and the policy frameworks aimed at expanding the pellet industry.

1.2 Feedstocks and the Factors Associated with the Pellet Quality

Downed woody debris (DWD), including treetops, branches, pulpwood, and non-merchantable or defect stems, forms the main pellet feedstock. Coarse woody debris (CWD) (>7.62 cm) aids in nutrient retention, carbon storage, erosion control, and wildlife habitat. Fine woody debris (FWD) (<7.62 cm) supports carbon and nitrogen cycling and protects soil from erosion. Though small in volume, FWD holds about half of a tree's total macronutrients, making it ecologically vital. Feedstocks with elevated ash content are generally considered less efficient because they tend to perform poorly during combustion and generate greater amounts of residual waste. Materials derived mainly from tree tops and branches often exhibit higher ash levels, as their large proportion of bark contributes to exceeding the optimal ash content threshold (Bays et al., 2025). Pellets can also be produced from biomass feedstocks such as sawdust, corn stalks, sewage sludge, and furfural residues (Siyal et al., 2021). The low weight per volume of the biomass, including its irregular particle and chip sizes, as well as its bulk density, contributes to the difficulties in transport and management, resulting in high expenditures. In this light, the pelletization of the biomass results in uniform size and dry conditions, better mass volume dosage, minimised risk of mould/microbial growth, etc., enabling their easier handling (Berghel et al., 2022).

There are three phases in biomass pelletization, which include the compression, flow, and friction steps (Fig. 1.1). The biomass is initially compressed into a thin layer, which is then pushed down into an inlet cone and then subjected to friction in the die channel. The friction step generates the back pressure and temperature in the die, which further enables the rollers to create the pressure. The interaction between the energy requirements in the compression phase, flow step, temperature, back pressure, and other factors eventually results in the formation of pellets. As different feedstock materials result in varied friction, it is essential to adapt the die channel according to the type of raw material being used. Therefore, the length of the die channel of different species, also known as the die press length, may vary according to different biomass types. The total press way includes both the inlet cone and the die channel. To ensure the optimal bulk density, the press length is typically selected to be optimal for the chosen feedstock(s). The demerit is that this narrows down the applicability of the process to limited feedstocks and does not provide optimal results when the feedstock is varied (Berghel et al., 2022).

The quality of biomass-derived pellets depends mainly on the properties of the feedstock, which include the moisture content (MC), particle size, ash content in the biomass, binders used, and other process variables such as temperature, holding time, and pressure (Ahmed et al., 2022). The quality parameters of the biomass derived pellets, including the pellet strength, moisture content, the relaxed density, porosity, etc. are heavily dependent on the type of the biomass and other operating parameters like the pressure and temperature. The selection of optimal operating parameters is

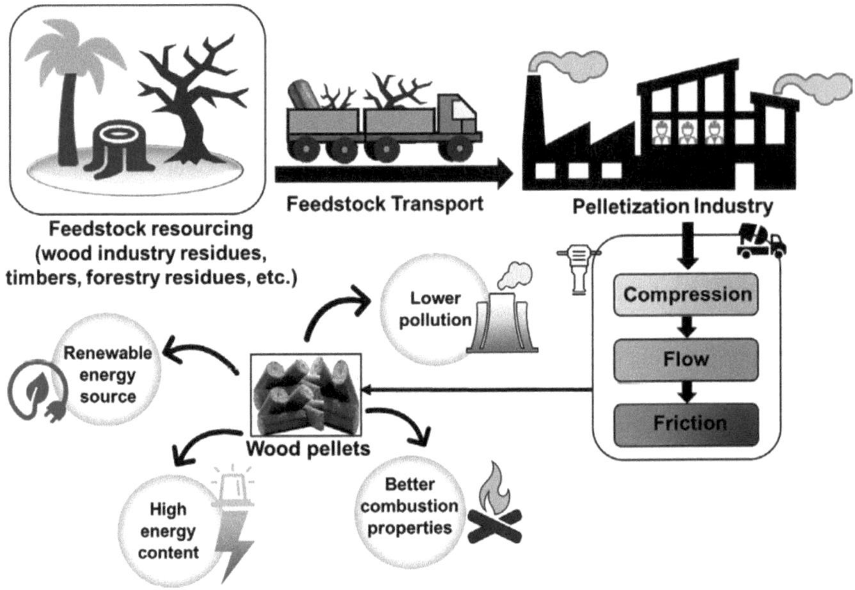

Fig. 1.1 Diagrammatic representation of the production and merits of wood pellets

essential for the activation of natural binders such as the lignin, cellulose, hemicellulose, and protein (Siyal et al., 2021). Particle size is one of the primary factors that holds significant importance in biomass pelletization, as it affects the total surface area, pore size, and inter-particle bonding of the pellets. These factors are all important for the improvement of pellet quality. During the process of compaction, the smaller particles fill in the voids between the larger particles, thereby increasing the packaging density and making the pellets more durable and stronger. The larger surface area of the smaller particles increases the rate of absorption of moisture content, leading to better heat absorption and ultimately better binding of the biomass during compaction. However, it is to be noted that the smaller particles also dry out quickly in arid seasons, which may cause difficulties during the pelletization process (Ahmed et al., 2022). The implementation of high pressure is known to substantially improve the pellet quality, provide a uniform pellet shape, and also minimize pellet dilation after extrusion. Although increasing pressure improves pellet quality, it reaches a limit after a certain point. However, the increase in pressure elevates process expenditures; hence, it is advisable to continue the process at lower pressure without compromising pellet quality (Siyal et al., 2021). Currently, many ISO standards are available for the industrial manufacture of biomass pellets, specifying the necessary criteria including moisture levels, sampling methods, particle size distribution, durability, ash content, and density (Berghel et al., 2022). Some of the available ISO standards relevant to the pelleting technology have been arranged in Table 1.1.

Table 1.1 Available ISO standards relevant to the industrial manufacture of pellets

ISO Standard number	Standard specifications
ISO 5370:2023	Solid biofuels - Determination of fines content in pellets
ISO 17225–1:2021	Solid biofuels - Fuel specifications and classes - Part 1: General requirements
ISO 17225–2:2021	Solid biofuels - Fuel specifications and classes - Part 2: Graded wood pellets
ISO 17225–7:2021	Solid biofuels - Fuel specifications and classes - Part 7: Graded non-woody briquettes
ISO 17225–8:2023	Solid biofuels - Fuel specifications and classes - Part 8: Graded thermally treated and densified biomass fuels for commercial and industrial use
ISO 17831–1:2025	Solid biofuels - Determination of mechanical durability of pellets and briquettes - Part 1: Pellets
ISO 18122:2022	Solid biofuels - Determination of ash content
ISO 18135:2017	Solid Biofuels - Sampling
ISO 18847:2024	Solid biofuels - Determination of particle density of pellets and briquettes
ISO 20023:2018	Solid biofuels - Safety of solid biofuel pellets - Safe handling and storage of wood pellets in residential and other small-scale applications
ISO 20024:2020	Solid biofuels - Safe handling and storage of solid biofuel pellets in commercial and industrial applications
ISO/TS 20,048–1:2020	Solid biofuels - Determination of off-gassing and oxygen depletion characteristics - Part 1: Laboratory method for the determination of off-gassing and oxygen depletion using closed containers
ISO 20049–1:2020	Solid biofuels - Determination of self-heating of pelletized biofuels - Part 1: Isothermal calorimetry
ISO/TS 21,596:2021	Solid biofuels - Determination of grindability - Hardgrove type method for thermally treated biomass fuels
ISO 21644:2021	Solid recovered fuels - Methods for the determination of biomass content
ISO 21645:2021	Solid recovered fuels - Methods for sampling
ISO 23343–1:2021	Solid biofuels - Determination of water sorption and its effect on durability of thermally treated biomass fuels - Part 1: Pellets
ISO/TR 25,078:2025	Wood and wood-based products - Examples of calculating displacement potentials for wood-based products and considerations for further analyses

Source International Organization for Standardization. https://www.iso.org

1.3 Technological Innovations in the Production of Wood Pellets

The production of wood pellets has evolved significantly in recent years, with increasing emphasis on efficiency, quality, and sustainability. Advancements in torrefaction, densification, binder optimization, and digital control systems have

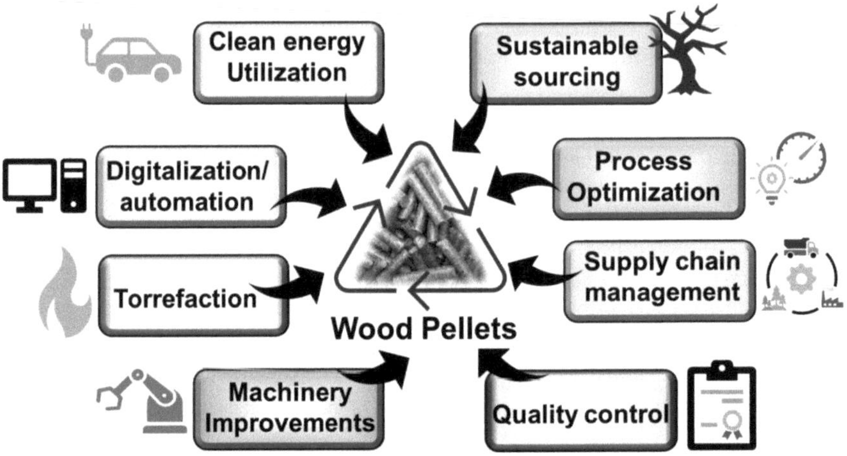

Fig. 1.2 Innovative approaches in the enhancement of wood pellet production

improved production efficiency while mitigating the challenges related to energy costs, mechanical reliability, and quality consistency across feedstocks. Figure 1.2 represents some of the innovative approaches in wood pellet production.

1.3.1 Material Variability and Quality Assurance

Different biomasses possess different compositions, leading to feedstock heterogeneity. The chemical composition of the biomass affects its calorific value (Kamperidou, 2022). The feedstocks can either be wastes from the processing of woodwork, logging, crop residues, or low-quality virgin woods (Kamperidou, 2022). The quality of the pellets determines the efficiency, service life, and combustion control of the heating devices, coupled with low emissions. The pellets should also have a clean and compact structure to avoid breaking and interrupting the automated fuel feeding systems in the machines. Further, the ash content in the pellets also plays a significant role as it forms a by-product after combustion, remaining either in the bottom of the device or floating in the air, ultimately leading to the corrosion and slagging phenomena. The bulk density, calorific value, etc., also determine the pellet's energy density. A high moisture content also negates their performance efficiency by reducing the net energy outputs and enhancing air pollution. The optimal moisture content of the feedstock for pelletization is generally 8–13% (Kamperidou, 2022). The selection of a suitable raw material and its processing before pelletization is necessary for optimal pellet production. Variations in the chemical compositions of the feedstock may heavily influence the pellet characteristics. The proximal and ultimate parameters of the pellets from different biomass feedstocks may vary depending on the compositional changes in them (Siyal et al., 2021).

1.3.2 Sustainable Sourcing of the Feedstock

The wood pellet technology in recent years has witnessed significant transformations in technological advancements, whilst aiming for the improvement of energy efficiency coupled with minimal environmental impact. From feedstock conditioning to densification and quality control, innovations have emerged in various stages, which reflect the ongoing industrial transitions towards smart and sustainable manufacturing systems. By integrating the total quality management principles (TQM), like process optimisation, supply chain management, and technological innovation, etc., the production efficiency can be enhanced with consistent pellet quality and reduced carbon emissions (Lee & Hsu, 2025a).

There are also concerns regarding the harvest of the feedstocks for the pellet production, and excessive debris removal includes reduced ground cover, higher erosion, loss of biodiversity, nutrient depletion, and poor water quality. The wood pellet production may lead to more intensive harvesting and reduce the downed woody debris (DWD) retained post-harvest, affecting the sustainability of the site. To tackle these challenges, several regions have introduced Biomass Harvesting Guidelines (BHGs) that recommend additional management practices alongside the traditional Best Management Practices (BMPs) for forestry and water quality. The adoption and implementation vary according to the physiographic conditions, being especially crucial in regions where biomass feedstock demand is particularly high (Bays et al., 2025). It was confirmed by a study by Bays et al. (2025) that wood pellet clearcuts, in this aspect, using the in-wood chipping reduces the DWD, with the remaining amounts within the acceptable ranges of the Biomass harvesting guidelines (Bays et al., 2025).

The use of waste or end-of-use products from various industries as feedstocks can also aid in the circularisation of the pellet production paradigms to reach a zero-waste approach. Vincevica-Gaile et al. (2025) utilised end-of-use products such as woody biomass ashes from energy production, coffee waste from food processing, and spruce needles from the forestry and chemical processing industries for pelletization. The pellets from the woody biomass ashes were found to have a comparatively high surface area, carbon framework density, and water adsorption properties. As a result, they can be used as a sorbent in wastewater treatment, for improving soil quality, and in sustainable agriculture (Vincevica-Gaile et al., 2025).

1.3.3 Process and Equipment Innovations

Drying of feedstock is also an energy-intensive process in biomass pellet manufacturing. In this light, a novel selective drying process was developed by Paczkowski et al. (2021) that separates raw material into fine and coarse fractions using sieving before drying only the finer portion, thereby saving large amounts of production costs. The improvements in pellet cooling after the press were also found to help in avoiding both the decrease in heating values and increase in the carbon emissions, by a post-production reduction in water content (Paczkowski et al., 2021). Ibrahim et al. (2025) designed and developed a pelleting machine suitable for crop residues, and it was found to be sustainable in the context of energy efficiency. The system also minimised the addition of synthetic additives, demonstrating its process efficiency (Ibrahim et al., 2025).

Mechanical optimization of pellet presses is also critical for the production of high-quality pellets. Żarczyński et al. (2025) evaluated the energy performance of biomass pelleting using both conventional stationary presses and mobile pelletizing systems such as the Krone Premos 5000. Their findings revealed that mobile presses achieved higher energy efficiency ratios (8.91–13.07) compared to the conventional stationary systems (4.87–8.91), highlighting the efficiency benefits of mobile pelleting technology. It also decentralizes the pellet production, lowering logistical emissions and increasing adaptability to distributed biomass resources like cereal straw, grasses, or low-quality hay. Sadeq et al. (2024) investigated the impact of press channel geometry on pellet microstructure and stability. By employing micro-computed tomography, they demonstrated that increasing the diameter-to-length (D/L) ratio of the die channel from 1:3 to 1:5 significantly leads to the production of pellets with uniform porosity, smoother surfaces (fewer cracks), and greater resistance to mechanistic degradation, under varying humidity conditions. These were shown to benefit both energy yield and product quality (Sadeq et al., 2024).

Biomass pellet combustion is beneficial compared to wood log combustion as it has improved reliability and reproducibility. Moreover, the possibility of automation, the ease of use, and combustion control add to its efficacy (Da Lio et al., 2025). There have been studies on the combustion interfaces of pellets. It was observed by Da Lio et al. (2025) that uneven fuel feeding in pellet stoves leads to variability in emission characteristics. Development of an improved screw feeder with 70% reduction in feed-flow variability, a reduction in CO (46%), and particulate-matter emission (52%) was observed at nominal (full) load. At partial load, the CO and particulate-matter emissions were found to have reduced by 37.5% and 44%, respectively (Da Lio et al., 2025).

1.3.4 Advances in Torrefaction-aided Pelletization

Torrefaction is a mild pretreatment process, performed under an inert or low oxygen environment to enable the thermal degradation of the biomass without combustion (Chandrasekharan Nair et al., 2025; Nair et al., 2022). The combination of torrefaction with pelletization is considered to be a promising technique for the production of solid fuels (pellets), for long-term storage as well as overseas transportation, without compromising their quality (Sarker et al., 2022). Torrefied pellets are the result of thermal pretreatment of the raw materials prior to or after pelletization. It produces stable pellets with improved energy density and hydrophobicity with low global warming impacts. The torrefied pellets (310 °C) produced from oil palm trunks as the raw materials also showed a 66.4% improvement in the heating value, as compared to non-torrefied pellets (Chotikhun et al., 2022).

It was observed in a study by Sarker et al. (2022) that the co-pelletization of torrefied biomass with raw biomass enhances the pellet quality, without the necessity for the use of external additives or severe operating conditions (high temperature and pressure). An increase in the heating values, energy density, and hydrophobicity was also found. The method was found to be suitable in terms of fuel pellet quality as well as energy consumption (Sarker et al., 2022). Compared to pyrolysis and gasification, torrefaction and hydrothermal carbonisation of biomass produce a relatively higher yield of solid products, suitable for pellet production (Seraj et al., 2025).

Torrefaction subsequent to pelletization was also found to be efficient to overcome the drawbacks of the wood pellets and also enhance their availability in different conversion processes. Torrefaction enhances the pellet grindability and reduces energy consumption for grinding by over 50% compared to untreated pellets. Ground torrefied pellets also exhibit smaller, more uniform particle sizes. Higher torrefaction severity enhances the pellet hydrophobicity, allowing them to resist water absorption and maintain integrity after immersion. Overall, torrefaction is known to enhance the grindability, uniformity, and suitability of wood pellets for pulverized fuel applications (Wang et al., 2020). The combined torrefaction with pelletization of the agricultural residues, with or without additives, was both found to be profitable in a techno-economic study by Sarker et al. (2023), with internal return rates of 25% and 22%, respectively (Sarker et al., 2023). Additionally, the optimization of the torrefaction process also ensures the pellets are resistant to weathering and biological degradation. This allows for the ease in outdoor storage and transport, similar to that of coal (Butler et al., 2023).

1.3.5 Enhancing Energy Efficiency and Additive Integration

The integration of additives and auxiliary materials can also enhance the pellet characteristics. In order to reduce energy consumption, during the process of pelletization, binders may also be employed, which include both organic and inorganic forms, depending on the cost, environmental affordability, and type of biomass involved in the pelletization process (Ahmed et al., 2022). Ståhl et al. (2016) examined the use of cornstarch and molasses as pellet-binding additives, finding that their inclusion improved pellet durability and reduced electricity consumption during pressing. However, the life-cycle assessment revealed that the use of additives slightly increased CO_2 equivalents per ton of pellets in countries with low-carbon electricity but decreased overall emissions where electricity generation remained fossil-fuel-intensive. Thus, it becomes necessary that the additive use must be regionally optimized according to grid carbon intensity and pellet durability requirements (Ståhl et al., 2016). Some of the quality improvement methods used in pelletization technology have been mentioned in Table 1.2.

Table 1.2 Pellet quality enhancement methods in different biomass and their outcomes

Feedstock	Quality enhancement method	Characteristics of the pellet formed	Remarks	References
Camelina straw Switchgrass	Biochar/HDPE addition Torrefaction	Improved pellet density, dimensional stability, tensile strength, and durability	Improved the effects of interparticle interaction on pellet properties	(Agu et al., 2025)
Sugarcane bagasse	Use of binders such as cow dung	Calorific value of 16.43 MJ kg $^{-1}$	84.2% durability index	(Akbar et al., 2021)
	Subsequent Torrefaction	10% improvement in the energy content of the biomass	Increased durability	
Shrub willow	Lignin additives	Significant increases in energy content, bulk density, and durability	Reduction in carbon monoxide emissions	(Elniski et al., 2023)
Sugarcane bagasse pith	Ozone pretreatment	Improved pellet density, mechanical properties, and stability	Enhanced combustion efficiency	(Nemati et al., 2025)
Spruce stem wood bark forest residues	Torrefaction	Improved grindability and uniformity of pellets	Lower energy requirements for grinding	(Wang et al., 2020)
Oil palm trunks	Torrefaction	Stable pellets with improved energy density and hydrophobicity	66.4% improvement in the heating value	(Chotikhun et al., 2022)

The durability and density of the pellets are indicators of process efficiency as well as end-use qualities. Although torrefaction is known to improve the pellet quality in many aspects, it may also result in the weakening of the natural binding ability of the lignin, which necessitates the addition of binders into the pellets to restore their strength during densification (Butler et al., 2023). The binders in use should also be cost-effective, in order to maintain the low-price levels of the solid fuel products, and their minimal addition quantity should be able to generate hydrophobic and strong, densified products. In a study by Butler et al. (2023), lignin by-products from the pulp and paper processing industries, biomass tar derived from the pyrolysis of biomass, lime, tall oil pitch, etc., were studied as potential binders (Butler et al., 2023).

1.3.6 Digitalization and Quality Management

Beyond process optimization and mechanistic innovations, the wood pellet industry has also embraced digitalization and quality management systems. A triadic Innovation Model integrating wood-pellet-based composites, IoT-enabled smart functions, and Total Quality Management (TQM) was studied for applications in sustainable smart furniture. The wood pellets were also observed to have high potential for smart applications, e.g., embedded IoT devices. The IoT integration in wood pellets was found to be excellent for modular design, easy to shape, cut, and integrate with embedded sensors or electronics (Lee & Hsu, 2025b).

TQM was also found to be effective in optimizing the pellet production efficiency and ensuring consistent quality across the supply chains. The Taiwanese wood pellet manufacturers use TQM to enhance the quality and stability of the wood pellets, in compliance with the environmental and market standards. Further, the use of smart technologies like Artificial Intelligence, IoT, automation, etc., was found to have significant impacts in improving production efficiency and reducing costs and carbon emissions. This lays the foundation of the competitiveness of the Taiwanese wood pellet industry, whilst also promoting the green energy development coupled with the global sustainability trends (Lee & Hsu, 2025a).

Machine learning models have also been integrated into the pellet manufacturing sector. You et al., (2022) used ensemble learning models for the prediction of the Pellet Durability Index (PDI) using different factors like the feed formulation, manufacturing parameters, and environmental data. Out of the various models used in the study, bagging was selected as the best model, with low Mean Square Prediction Error. This can be potentially applied in the feed mills for the prediction of pellet quality index for specific batches, and can be used as a key performance indicator for the management of the mill (2022). A vibration-based machine learning approach was applied by Nielsen et al. (2024) for the detection of roller gap during the production of biomass pellets. In the study, the variations in the roller gap of the rotary ring die pelleting technology were analysed using experimental testing, Response Surface Methodology (RSM), and Vibration-based ML, to optimise the operating conditions in the biomass pellet mill. Significant relationships were observed between the roller gap, feedstock layer mass, and the pelleting process matrices in the study (Nielsen et al., 2024).

1.3.7 Emission Dynamics and Product Quality

The pollution emission characteristics of the pellets are heavily dependent on their physical properties, like the ash yields, fines content, impurity levels, mechanical durability, etc. The wood pellets with lower nitrogen and bark content were observed to result in cleaner combustion (Drobniak et al., 2025). Hence, the quality control of the pellets can reduce the pollution levels, which can be directly translated to minimized hazards in the public health sector.

The addition of cardboard and straw to the wood pellets was found to increase their density from 3 to 15%. The straw component in the pellets also reduced the gas-phase ignition delays by 30%, compared to pellets without straw additives. The combustion of the composite pellets was also found to have lower contributions to the CO_2, CO, and SO emissions (Nyashina et al., 2025).

1.3.8 Supply Chain and Market Efficiency

A stochastic optimization model in the wood pellet supply chains, integrating the demand-driven supply planning and dynamic pricing strategies, was studied by Vazifeh and Mafakheri (2025). They implemented a Monte Carlo simulation approach with 10,000 iterations to study the correlation between the supply, demand, mechanism of pricing, and profitability of the supply chains, also including the seasonal demand fluctuations and the production capacity. It was revealed that there is a strong positive correlation between the price and the profit, whilst indicating that over 70% of the variance in profit can be explained by price changes. This not only underscores the need for smart pricing but also serves as a robust decision-support tool for strategic planning in the wood pellet industry by incorporating the market dynamics.

1.4 Environmental Impacts of Wood Pellet Production and Utilization

The environmental implications of wood pellet production and their utilization have become a central concern within global renewable energy discussions. While wood pellets are well promoted as a carbon-neutral alternative to fossil fuels, their full life-cycle impacts reveal a complex relationship between the benefits and trade-offs.

1.4.1 Life Cycle Environmental Performance

Life Cycle Assessment (LCA) is a valuable tool for evaluating the biomass conversion technologies, biomass characteristics (moisture content, grind size, etc.), and also for the management of waste (e.g., ash). The climate commitments made on the global level and the renewable energy policies, including the UN SDG 7, the European Green Deal, and the US Green New Deal, all lead to the generation of a steady biomass demand. (Żarczyński et al., 2025). Koido et al. (2025) studied the LCA and TEA of the wood pellet production and combined heat and power systems with different plant scales and sawdust drying processes. The drying process during the production of pellets is an energy-intensive step accounting for 35–39% of the total energy consumption, thereby significantly affecting the Primary Energy Demand (PED) and CO_2 emissions. Compared to the conventional grid-supplied drying, the systems employing wood-fired boilers and wood pellet-combined heat and power systems were observed to have reduced the PED by 12–26%, and CO_2 emissions by 14–31%. The scaling up was also observed to have enhanced the financial performance (up to 20%), with a reduced pay back period of 10 years in facilities that produce 2.5 tons of wood pellets every hour (Japan) (Koido et al., 2025). The optimisation of the drying process, scalability of the plant, efficient supply chains, etc., plays a significant role in the advancements of sustainable wood pellet-based bioenergy systems (Koido et al., 2025).

A comparative LCA for the pellet stoves with fireplaces and wood stoves revealed that the pellet stoves had relatively low impacts on the global warming potential as well as the ozone formation. However, it was found to add to eutrophication in marine and freshwater, and acidification (Quinteiro et al., 2019). Transportation also becomes a contributing factor during the determination of the LCA of wood pellet combustion. An increase in the transportation distance enhances the environmental impact, contributing to global warming, ozone formation, and fossil-fuel scarcity. Hence, it becomes imperative to design optimized supply chains to reduce such environmental impacts (Topić Božič et al., 2024). It was also observed that the decentralized production of pellets in sawmills and households had better environmental profiles as compared to the centralized industrial production of pellets. The high environmental impact of the industrial process may be due to the high electricity and diesel usage. However, the sustainability of the decentralized systems only extends to short distances and is not feasible for long distances (Quinteiro et al., 2020). The comparison of the environmental impact of pellet production using untreated mixed sawdust, torrefied sawdust, and steam-exploded sawdust revealed that the torrefied pellets were more environmentally friendly than the other methods. However, it was found to lead to aquatic eutrophication and ozone layer depletion. The utilization of torrefied pellets for the generation of electricity was found to be more beneficial in terms of resource depletion, climate change, ecosystem quality, etc. Also, considering the environmental footprints, the torrefied biomass was the cleanest option (Alizadeh et al., 2023).

1.4.2 Global and Regional Environmental Considerations

Beyond quantitative LCA results, there remain gaps in the social and ecological narratives surrounding the sustainability of wood pellet production. Etsuko Kinefuchi (2024) critiqued the largest wood pellet production company, Enviva, which frames itself as a sustainability leader, whilst it marginalizes the environmental injustices that are experienced by the communities in "shadow places", particularly where the feedstocks are sourced. Further, they point towards the accomplishment of greenwashing by the industry through the selective use of information, while leaving out the unfavourable outcomes. This reduces the transparency of the impacts and fails to recognize the affected localities (Kinefuchi, 2024).

Environmental outcomes vary geographically due to the differences in forest management regimes and policy frameworks. Saosee et al. (2022) studied the LCA for the wood pellet production for heat and power generation from fast-growing Leucaena and Acacia trees and para-rubber trees in Thailand and recommended a few policies to reduce the environmental impact and cost related to the pellet industries in Thailand. First, they recommended supporting the sustainable agricultural practices for para-rubber and fast-growing trees, which are some important raw materials in Thailand. Second, they suggested the switch to clean transportation, involving electric vehicles, cleaner fuels, or mobility models, to reduce pollution and fossil fuel dependency. Third, zoning of the pellet industries near the feedstock source to reduce the transportation costs, and finally, the consideration of external expenses of the pellet industries, for the polluter pays principle (Saosee et al., 2022). The LCA of wood pellet use in remote communities of Canada revealed that the pelletization and combustion of the wood pellets have significant environmental impacts, with non-carcinogenic effects from pelletization and respiratory effects from its combustion. The comparison of wood pellet combustion with diesel also revealed the former's performance superiority in non-carcinogenic effects. The role of long-distance transportation in adding to the environmental impacts was also discussed. The study also suggested the need for the reduction of energy consumption for pelletization and a shift to renewable energy sources during the process (Sadaghiani et al., 2023).

1.4.3 Forest Carbon and Biodiversity

The large-scale conversion of the natural forests to monoculture plantations for pellet feedstock can compromise the biodiversity of the forests. A study by Henderson et al. (2024) addressed the interaction of demand and land use change to change the mix of forest types in the US South, the total forest carbon, and the area of forests. The simulation of forest sector models also demonstrates that an increase in the forest product results in an increase in the forest land area, by increasing land rents or product prices (Henderson et al., 2024). Sperandio et al. (2024) approached the technological innovations in wood production from the viewpoint of feedstock rotation in poplar plantations, analysing their eco-efficiency. Through the life-cycle cost and environmental assessment framework, they found that three-year-old poplar stands produced pellets with a lower global warming potential (1.5×10^{-2} kg CO_2-eq MJ^{-1}) than six-year rotations, and the highest eco-efficiency index (EEI = 0.60 € kg CO_2-eq^{-1}). Short rotation of the crops can hence be deemed feasible for the efficient pelletization, as it reduces the life-cycle emissions substantially (Sperandio et al., 2024).

1.5 Market Trends and Policy Dynamics in the Global Wood Pellet Industry

The global wood pellet market has experienced dynamic growth over the past two decades, shaped by regional policy frameworks, shifting energy strategies, and evolving international trade dynamics. Policy remains the most significant driver shaping the global wood pellet trade. Government incentives and efforts towards standardisation are necessary for market development. There is a need for clear national and regional policy frameworks to set targets, reduce the uncertainty prevailing in the markets, and create demand pull to lower the commercial risk for investors and developers (Nair & Verma, 2025).

1.5.1 Policy Dynamics in the Promotion of Wood Pellet Industries

The European Union (EU), as well as many other governments, is increasingly adopting policies and measures for the promotion of sustainable use of natural resources for economic growth. The EU RED (Renewable Energy Directive), an important part of the EU bioeconomy strategy, aims to modernize energy production using natural resources. Although environmental sustainability has been central to the EU policy for a long time, the newly highlighted focus on bioresources may lead to the development of additional pressure on the ecosystems, countering its own environmental goals. The EU RED has significantly influenced the wood pelleting industry in the U.S. coastal southeast and other eastern regions, in response to both policy and domestic demands. About 18 million wood pellets were traded by the EU member nations, of which one-third were imported from the US. The trends in timberland pellet production align with the findings, suggesting that wood pellet production in the US may have contributed to enhanced tree growth and the expansion of carbon pools. These results align with the current EU RED biofuel trade requirements for preserving carbon content in the areas from which the biomass was sourced. However, it was also observed that the large or continuously operating mills showed a decline in soil carbon and fewer standing-dead trees, suggesting implications for wildlife and biodiversity. Although wood pellet production was shown to support the carbon content in live trees, the continued decline in soil carbon and forest structure may threaten the long-term sustainability of the forests (Aguilar et al., 2020). The Renewable Energy Directive (RED II), its successor, imposes minimum sustainability criteria for the import of wood pellets in the EU. The carbon constrained approach is considered to be a very strict interpretation of the EU RED II requirement that there exists a requirement for the management system at the level of the sourcing to maintain or improve the carbon stock as well as the sink levels (Visser et al., 2022). Indonesia has its own National Energy Policy (KEN/Kebijakan Energi Nasional) to ensure its renewable energy roadmaps are based on the principles of sustainability, justice, and environmental friendliness, among others, for the generation of independent energy and to ensure national energy security (Rimantho et al., 2023).

1.5.2 Existing Market Trends in the Wood Pellet Trade

North America has been observed as the major exporter of pellets, and a few European countries are the major importers. The USA and UK have also established trade relations for wood pellets, which may result in significant changes in the pellet trading sectors. The short-term demand for pellets may also arise in the near future from new market players like Japan and South Korea. The additional demand for the pellets is bound to cause a jump from a long/oversupply market to a short/undersupply market. In this light, Asia is expected to provide the largest growth opportunities in the medium to long run (Thrän et al., 2019).

The EU is one of the main importers of biomass-based products, especially wood pellets, and is also the global leader in the utilisation of biomass for energy. In Asian countries, a significant interest in the production and utilisation of wood pellets has been observed in countries such as South Korea, Japan, Vietnam, Malaysia, and Indonesia. The South Korean renewable portfolio standard, which became effective in 2012, has led to increased interest in wood pellets as a means to achieve its goal of renewably sourced energy generation within the timeframe of 2022 to 2027. The wood pellet imports by Japan are also expected to increase in the next five years. Indonesia experienced a nearly twofold increase in the production and export of wood pellets during the 2013 to 2014 period, while Thailand increased its production from 20,000 tons in 2013 to 115,000 tons in 2015. Vietnam is a country abundant in primary forest feedstock and by-product generation from the forest residues. This creates a promising environment for the development of the wood pellet market (Proskurina et al., 2019). In 2015, Vietnam was the fourth largest exporter of wood pellets in the world (7%) after the US (29%), Canada (10%), and Latvia (10%). However, in 2020, the Vietnamese enterprises were reported to have increased their exports to 3.2 million metric tons, thereby increasing their rank to the second largest exporter (Bui-Duy et al., 2023). The Southeast of the US has been considered to be the dominant producer in the export market, with a steady increase in export rates of 0.5 million tons in 2000 to 7 million tons in 2018 (Visser et al., 2022). Rodriguez Franco (2022) reviewed the forest biomass assessments for the production of wood pellets in the USA and hypothesized that the production of wood pellets from the Southeast USA in 2030 may vary from 74 to 95 million dry tons, depending on the price hike per dry ton. For 2050, this could range from 85 (low consumption) to 162 (high consumption) (Rodriguez Franco, 2022).

1.6 Conclusion and Future Prospects

The evolution of wood pellet technology reflects a broader global transition toward sustainable, circular, and intelligent energy systems. It is evident that the wood pellet industry has matured from a niche renewable option into a cornerstone of the modern bioeconomy, with high trade implementations between different countries. Advances in feedstock preparation, torrefaction, co-pelletization, and binder optimization have significantly improved the quality, stability, and energy performance of pellets, enabling their use in large-scale heating and power applications. These technological strides have been further supported by digitalization and smart manufacturing, which now allow real-time monitoring, predictive maintenance, and adaptive process optimization across production lines. However, the environmental assessments underscore the fact that true sustainability requires not only technological innovation but also responsible feedstock sourcing, waste valorization, and emissions control.

Globally, market and policy trends continue to shape the trajectory of the pellet industry. Supportive policy frameworks, such as renewable energy mandates and carbon pricing mechanisms, have spurred international trade and investment, while raising critical debates about land use, biodiversity, and the cascading use of biomass. The impediments to upscaling the industry, improving process efficiency, and reducing pollutant emissions call for focused research. Further incorporation of thermochemical treatments, AI-driven and ML approaches, and other relevant technologies can be applied in wood pellet research to develop sustainable systems. The convergence of AI, machine learning, and sensor technologies may transform pellet manufacturing into a smart, data-driven process. Reduction of transportation costs, achieved by switching to cleaner energy alternatives and shorter transport distances, may lower the production price point. Further policy incentives and encouragement for the use of biomass-based biofuels in these countries may motivate the industries and stakeholders to deepen their focus on the wood pellet industry. Design, monitoring, and optimisation of process parameters are necessary to ensure high energy efficiency from an economic perspective and a low pollution impact from an environmental perspective. Further research and market analysis are required to expand the wood pellet sector, ensuring its maximal production with minimised environmental impacts and carbon neutrality.

References

Agu, O. S., Tabil, L. G., Mupondwa, E., et al. (2025). Pelletization and quality evaluation of torrefied selected biomass with microwave absorber. *Results Eng, 25*, Article 104183. https://doi.org/10.1016/j.rineng.2025.104183

Aguilar, F. X., Mirzaee, A., McGarvey, R. G., et al. (2020). Expansion of US wood pellet industry points to positive trends but the need for continued monitoring. *Science and Reports, 10*, 1–17. https://doi.org/10.1038/s41598-020-75403-z

Ahmed, I., Ali, A., Ali, B., et al. (2022). Production of pellets from furfural residue and sawdust biomass: effect of moisture content, particle size and a binder on pellet quality and energy consumption. *Bioenergy Res, 15*, 1292–1303. https://doi.org/10.1007/s12155-021-10335-8

Akbar, A., Aslam, U., Asghar, A., & Aslam, Z. (2021). Effect of binding materials on physical and fuel characteristics of bagasse based pellets. *Biomass and Bioenergy, 150*, Article 106118. https://doi.org/10.1016/j.biombioe.2021.106118

Alizadeh, P., Mupondwa, E., Tabil, L. G., et al. (2023). Life cycle assessment of bioenergy production from wood sawdust. *Journal of Cleaner Product, 427*, Article 138936. https://doi.org/10.1016/j.jclepro.2023.138936

Bays, H. C. M., Bolding, M. C., Conrad, J. L., et al. (2025). Post-harvest assessment of downed woody debris and nutrient distribution following conventional pulpwood and wood pellet feedstock harvests in the southeastern US. *Journal Environmental Management, 386*, Article 125719. https://doi.org/10.1016/j.jenvman.2025.125719

Berghel, J., Ståhl, M., Frodeson, S., et al. (2022). A comparison of relevant data and results from single pellet press research is Mission Impossible: A review. *Bioresour Technol Reports, 18*, Article 101054. https://doi.org/10.1016/j.biteb.2022.101054

Bui-Duy, L., Le, L. T., Vu-Thi-Minh, N., et al. (2023). Economic and environmental analysis of biomass pellet supply chain using simulation-based approach. *Asia Pacific Manag Rev, 28*, 470–486. https://doi.org/10.1016/j.apmrv.2023.02.002

Butler, J. W., Skrivan, W., & Lotfi, S. (2023). Identification of optimal binders for torrefied biomass pellets. *Energies, 16*, 1–23. https://doi.org/10.3390/en16083390

Chandrasekharan Nair, S., John, V., Geetha Bai, R., & Kikas, T. (2025). Torrefaction of Lignocellulosic biomass: a pathway to renewable energy, circular economy, and sustainable agriculture. *Sustain, 17*, 1–28. https://doi.org/10.3390/su17177738

Chotikhun, A., Kittijaruwattana, J., & Pianroj, Y. (2022). Some properties of white and torrified pellets obtained from oil palm trunk as raw material. *BioResources 17*, 6818–6831. https://doi.org/10.15376/biores.17.4.6818-6831

Cui, X., Yang, J., Wang, Z., & Shi, X. (2021). Better use of bioenergy: a critical review of co-pelletizing for biofuel manufacturing. *Carbon Capture Sci Technol, 1*, Article 100005. https://doi.org/10.1016/j.ccst.2021.100005

Da Lio, L., Bortolus, M., & Canu, P. (2025). Emissions reduction from wood pellet stoves by uniform feeding. *Renewable Energy, 242*, Article 122273. https://doi.org/10.1016/j.renene.2024.122273

Drobniak, A., Jelonek, Z., & Widziewicz-Rzońca, K. (2025). Domestic combustion of biomass pellets: example from Poland. *International Journal Coal Geology 304*. https://doi.org/10.1016/j.coal.2025.104757

Elniski, A., Dongre, P., & Bujanovic, B. M. (2023). Lignin use in enhancing the properties of willow pellets. *Forests 14*. https://doi.org/10.3390/f14102041

Henderson, J. D., Abt, R. C., & Abt, K. L. (2024). Forest carbon under increasing product demand and land use change in the US Southeast. *For Policy Econ, 167*, Article 103296. https://doi.org/10.1016/j.forpol.2024.103296

Ibrahim, M. M., Younis, S. M., Taieb, A. E. A. Z., et al. (2025). Design and performance assessment of a pelleting machine for sustainable biomass pellet fuel production from plant residues. *Science and Reports, 15*, 1–21. https://doi.org/10.1038/s41598-025-93058-6

Kamperidou, V. (2022). Quality analysis of commercially available wood pellets and correlations between pellets characteristics. *Energies 15*. https://doi.org/10.3390/en15082865

Kinefuchi, E. (2024). Burning forests: The wood pellet industry's framing of sustainability and its shadow places. *Front Commun, 9*, 1–14. https://doi.org/10.3389/fcomm.2024.1237141

Koido, K., Konno, D., & Sato, M. (2025). Life cycle CO2 emissions and techno-economic analysis of wood pellet production and CHP with different plant scales and sawdust drying processes. *Sustain 17*. https://doi.org/10.3390/su17010140

Lee, H. H, & Hsu, C. M. (2025a). Total quality management enhances wood pellet utilization for sustainable energy. *Sustain 17*. https://doi.org/10.3390/su17041562

Lee, H. H, & Hsu, C. M. (2025b). Enhancing sustainable innovations in intelligent wood pellets through smart customized furniture and total quality management. *Sustain 17*, 1–35. https://doi.org/10.3390/su17146604

Nair, L. G., Agrawal, K., & Verma, P. (2022). An insight into the principles of lignocellulosic biomass-based zero-waste biorefineries: A green leap towards imperishable energy-based future. *Biotechnology & Genetic Engineering Reviews, 38*, 288–338. https://doi.org/10.1080/02648725.2022.2082223

Nair, L. G., & Verma, P. (2025). Harnessing carbon potential of lignocellulosic biomass: advances in pretreatments, applications, and the transformative role of machine learning in biorefineries. *Bioresour Bioprocess, 12*.

Nemati, Z., Kianmehr, M. H., & Arabhosseini, A. (2025). Ozone pretreatment and process optimization to improve fuel pellet production from sugarcane bagasse pith. *Bioresource Technology, 426*, Article 132321. https://doi.org/10.1016/j.biortech.2025.132321

Nielsen, M. K., Nielsen, S. K., & Tambo, T. (2024). A vibration-based machine learning approach for roller gap detection in biomass pellet production. *Biosystems Engineering, 248*, 283–296. https://doi.org/10.1016/j.biosystemseng.2024.11.007

Nyashina, G. S., Dorokhov, V. V., Shvedov, D. K., & Strizhak, P. A. (2025). Wood pellets with waste: Energy, environmental and mechanical aspects. *Renewable Energy, 250*, Article 123269. https://doi.org/10.1016/j.renene.2025.123269

Paczkowski, S., Labbé, R., & Sauer, C. (2021). A novel approach to improve the energy and cost efficiency of feedstock drying for pellet production. *Fuel, 290*. https://doi.org/10.1016/j.fuel.2020.119805

Proskurina, S., Junginger, M., & Heinimö J. (2019). Global biomass trade for energy—Part 2: production and trade streams of wood pellets, liquid biofuels, charcoal, industrial roundwood and emerging energy biomass. *Biofuels, Bioprod Biorefining 13*, 371–387. https://doi.org/10.1002/bbb.1858

Quinteiro, P., Greco, F., & da Cruz, Tarelho, L. A. (2020) A comparative life cycle assessment of centralised and decentralised wood pellets production for residential heating. *Science Total Environment 730*. https://doi.org/10.1016/j.scitotenv.2020.139162

Quinteiro, P., Tarelho, L., Marques, P., et al. (2019). Life cycle assessment of wood pellets and wood split logs for residential heating. *Science of the Total Environment, 689*, 580–589. https://doi.org/10.1016/j.scitotenv.2019.06.420

Rimantho, D., Hidayah, N. Y., Pratomo, V. A., et al. (2023). The strategy for developing wood pellets as sustainable renewable energy in Indonesia. *Heliyon, 9*, Article e14217. https://doi.org/10.1016/j.heliyon.2023.e14217

Rodriguez Franco, C. (2022). Forest biomass potential for wood pellets production in the United States of America for exportation: A review. *Biofuels, 13*, 983–994. https://doi.org/10.1080/17597269.2022.2059951

Sadaghiani, S., Mafakheri, F., & Chen, Z. (2023). Life cycle assessment of bioenergy production using wood pellets: A case study of remote communities in Canada. *Energies, 16*. https://doi.org/10.3390/en16155697

Sadeq, A., Pietsch-Braune, S., & Heinrich, S. (2024). Impact of press channel diameter-to-length ratio on the mechanical properties of biomass pellets during storage. *Fuel Processing Technology, 265*, Article 108149. https://doi.org/10.1016/j.fuproc.2024.108149

Saosee, P., Sajjakulnukit, B., & Gheewala, S. H. (2022). Environmental externalities of wood pellets from fast-growing and para-rubber trees for sustainable energy production: a case in Thailand. *Energy Convers Manag X, 14*, Article 100183. https://doi.org/10.1016/j.ecmx.2022.100183
Sarker, T. R., Azargohar, R., Stobbs, J., et al. (2022). Complementary effects of torrefaction and pelletization for the production of fuel pellets from agricultural residues: A comparative study. *Industrial Crops and Products, 181*, Article 114740. https://doi.org/10.1016/j.indcrop.2022.114740
Sarker, T. R., German, C. S., Borugadda, V. B., et al. (2023). Techno-economic analysis of torrefied fuel pellet production from agricultural residue via integrated torrefaction and pelletization process. *Heliyon, 9*, Article e16359. https://doi.org/10.1016/j.heliyon.2023.e16359
Seraj, S., Azargohar, R., & Dalai, A. K. (2025). Dry torrefaction and hydrothermal carbonization of biomass to fuel pellets. *Renewable and Sustainable Energy Reviews, 210*, Article 115186. https://doi.org/10.1016/j.rser.2024.115186
Siyal, A. A., Liu, Y., Mao, X., et al. (2021). Characterization and quality analysis of wood pellets: Effect of pelletization and torrefaction process variables on quality of pellets. *Biomass Convers Biorefinery, 11*, 2201–2217. https://doi.org/10.1007/s13399-020-01235-6
Sperandio, G., Suardi, A., Acampora, A., & Civitarese, V. (2024). Eco-efficiency of pellet production from dedicated poplar plantations. *Energies, 17*, 515–529. https://doi.org/10.3390/en17133137
Ståhl, M., Berghel, J., & Williams, H. (2016). Energy efficiency, greenhouse gas emissions and durability when using additives in the wood fuel pellet chain. *Fuel Processing Technology, 152*, 350–355. https://doi.org/10.1016/j.fuproc.2016.06.031
Thrän, D., Schaubach, K., Peetz, D., et al. (2019). The dynamics of the global wood pellet markets and trade – key regions, developments and impact factors. *Biofuels, Bioproducts & Biorefining, 13*, 267–280. https://doi.org/10.1002/bbb.1910
Topić Božič, J., Fric, U., Čikić, A., & Muhič, S. (2024). Life cycle assessment of using firewood and wood pellets in slovenia as two primary wood-based heating systems and their environmental impact. *Sustain, 16*. https://doi.org/10.3390/su16041687
Vazifeh, Z., & Mafakheri, F. (2025). Integrating dynamic pricing strategies and demand-driven supply planning in wood pellet supply chains: A stochastic optimization approach. *Energy Reports, 13*, 3869–3877. https://doi.org/10.1016/j.egyr.2025.03.038
Vincevica-Gaile, Z., Zhylina, M., Shishkin, A., et al. (2025). Selected residual biomass valorization into pellets as a circular economy-supported end-of-waste. *Clean Mater, 15*, Article 100295. https://doi.org/10.1016/j.clema.2025.100295
Visser, L., Latta, G., Pokharel, R., et al. (2022). Exploring the limits to sustainable pellet production for international markets: The impact of increasing pellet production in the US Southeast on feedstock use, production cost and carbon sequestration in forest areas. *GCB Bioenergy, 14*, 896–917. https://doi.org/10.1111/gcbb.12946
Wang, L., Riva, L., Skreiberg, Ø., et al. (2020). Effect of torrefaction on properties of pellets produced from woody biomass. *Energy and Fuels, 34*, 15343–15354. https://doi.org/10.1021/acs.energyfuels.0c02671
You, J., Tulpan, D., Malpass, M. C., & Ellis, J. L. (2022). Predicting pellet quality of pelleted feed using ensemble learning models. In *Animal science proceedings*, pp. 605–606.
Żarczyński, P. J., Krzebietke, S. J., Sienkiewicz, S., & Wierzbowska, J. (2025). Yield and energy efficiency of fallow biomass pelletized using different pelletizing technologies. *Ind Crops Prod 233*. https://doi.org/10.1016/j.indcrop.2025.121446
ISO 17831-1:2025(en), Solid biofuels—Determination of mechanical durability of pellets and briquettes—Part 1: Pellets.
ISO 18122:2022(en), Solid biofuels—Determination of ash content. Accessed 8 Oct 2025b. https://www.iso.org/obp/ui/#iso:std:iso:18122:ed-2:v1:en
ISO 20023:2018(en), Solid biofuels—Safety of solid biofuel pellets—Safe handling and storage of wood pellets in residential and other small-scale applications.

ISO 20049–1:2020(en), Solid biofuels—Determination of self-heating of pelletized biofuels—Part 1: Isothermal calorimetry. Accessed 8 Oct 2025d. https://www.iso.org/obp/ui/#iso:std:iso:20049:-1:ed-1:v1:en
ISO/TS 21596:2021(en), Solid biofuels—Determination of grindability—Hardgrove type method for thermally treated biomass fuels. Accessed 8 Oct 2025e. https://www.iso.org/obp/ui/#iso:std:iso:ts:21596:ed-1:v1:en
ISO 18847:2024(en), Solid biofuels—Determination of particle density of pellets and briquettes. Accessed 8 Oct 2025f. https://www.iso.org/obp/ui/#iso:std:iso:18847:ed-2:v1:en
ISO 5370:2023(en), Solid biofuels—Determination of fines content in pellets. Accessed 8 Oct 2025g. https://www.iso.org/obp/ui/#iso:std:iso:5370:ed-1:v1:en
ISO 21645:2021(en), Solid recovered fuels—Methods for sampling. Accessed 8 Oct 2025h. https://www.iso.org/obp/ui/#iso:std:iso:21645:ed-1:v1:en
ISO 21644:2021(en), Solid recovered fuels—Methods for the determination of biomass content. Accessed 8 Oct 2025i. https://www.iso.org/obp/ui/#iso:std:iso:21644:ed-1:v2:en
ISO/TR 25078:2025(en), Wood and wood-based products—Examples of calculating displacement potentials for wood-based products and considerations for further analyses. Accessed 8 Oct 2025j. https://www.iso.org/obp/ui/#iso:std:iso:tr:25078:ed-1:v1:en
ISO 18135:2017(en), Solid Biofuels—Sampling. Accessed 8 Oct 2025k. https://www.iso.org/obp/ui/#iso:std:iso:18135:ed-1:v1:en
ISO 17225–8:2023(en), Solid biofuels—Fuel specifications and classes—Part 8: Graded thermally treated and densified biomass fuels for commercial and industrial use. Accessed 8 Oct 2025l. https://www.iso.org/obp/ui/#iso:std:iso:17225:-8:ed-1:v1:en:term:3.1
ISO 20024:2020(en), Solid biofuels—Safe handling and storage of solid biofuel pellets in commercial and industrial applications. Accessed 8 Oct 2025m. https://www.iso.org/obp/ui/#iso:std:iso:20024:ed-1:v1:en
ISO 23343–1:2021(en), Solid biofuels—Determination of water sorption and its effect on durability of thermally treated biomass fuels—Part 1: Pellets. Accessed 8 Oct 2025n. https://www.iso.org/obp/ui/
ISO/TS 20048–1:2020–Solid biofuels—Determination of off-gassing and oxygen depletion characteristics—Part 1: Laboratory method for the determination of off-gassing and oxygen depletion using closed containers. Accessed 8 Oct 2025o. https://www.iso.org/standard/73235.html
ISO 17225–7:2021—Solid biofuels—Fuel specifications and classes—Part 7: Graded non-woody briquettes. Accessed 8 Oct 2025p. https://www.iso.org/standard/76094.html
ISO 17225–2:2021–Solid biofuels—Fuel specifications and classes—Part 2: Graded wood pellets. Accessed 8 Oct 2025q. https://www.iso.org/standard/76088.html
ISO 17225–1:2021—Solid biofuels—Fuel specifications and classes—Part 1: General requirements. Accessed 8 Oct 2025r. https://www.iso.org/standard/76087.html

Chapter 2
Artificial Photosynthesis: A Promising Clean Energy Source, Recent Breakthroughs and Challenges

Anwesha Bandyopadhyay, Tarun Pal, and Puneet Kumar Singh

Abstract Artificial photosynthesis is a clean and advanced energy production technology that mimics the natural process of photosynthesis to convert solar energy to chemical fuels such as hydrogen or hydrocarbons. Artificial photosynthesis aims to tackle sustainable global energy requirements by the integration of photochemistry, catalysis, and materials science. Recent advancements have led to the development of efficient photoelectrochemical cells, molecular catalysts, and hybrid systems that are capable of converting sunlight, water, and carbon dioxide (CO_2) into energy rich compounds. Despite these innovations the major challenges are in terms of circular economy, renewable fuel, system integration, and economic scalability. Overcoming these technical and commercial barriers is critical for transformation of artificial photosynthesis from laboratory research to practical and commercial applications.

Keywords Artificial photosynthesis · Photochemistry · Photo-electrochemical cell · Circular economy · Renewable fuel

2.1 Introduction

Concerns about climate change, depletion in the supply of fossil fuel and destruction of ecological systems are driving a shift in the global energy paradigm and increasing the demand for cleaner and sustainable alternatives. Artificial photosynthesis has become a feasible technological strategy for the production of renewable fuels. This approach aims to replicate and improve the photochemical conversion

A. Bandyopadhyay
School of Biotechnology, Faculty of Applied Sciences & Biotechnology, Shoolini University, Solan, Himachal Pradesh, India

T. Pal
School of Bioengineering and Food Technology, Faculty of Applied Sciences & Biotechnology, Shoolini University, Solan, Himachal Pradesh, India

P. K. Singh (✉)
School of Biotechnology, Kalinga Institute of Industrial Technology (KIIT), Bhubaneswar, India

P. Verma (ed.), *Sustainable Practices in Biorefinery*,
https://doi.org/10.1007/978-981-95-6071-4_2

of solar energy, water (H_2O), and carbon dioxide (CO_2) into energy rich chemical compounds. One of most significant applications of solar energy is the sustainable production of fuels, which offers a long-term solution to the expanding need of energy throughout the globe (Barber and Tran, 2013). During the natural photosynthesis plants convert solar energy into glucose, which serves as their primary energy source. However, when it comes to industrial energy production, lower production efficiency and reliance on biological growth cycles are two of the major disadvantages which come along with the natural photosynthesis (Hussain et al., 2021). With the development artificial photosynthesis, these drawbacks could be addressed. In order to generate fuels like hydrogen, methanol, or hydrocarbons, these systems often use semiconductors, photoelectrochemical cells and catalytic materials that can directly absorb sunlight and stimulate chemical processes. Artificial photosynthesis is an adaptable and scalable solution because these fuels can be utilised in combustion engines or as feedstock for other energy applications (Awogbemi et al., 2021). Low dependency on the land is one of the major benefits of artificial photosynthesis in comparison to traditional biofuel production because of the competition of food production and harvesting of corn, sugarcane and soy resulting in deforestation and loss of biodiversity (Liu et al., 2014). Further artificial photosynthesis uses carbon dioxide as a key substrate supporting global efforts to lower the level of greenhouse gases in the atmosphere converting a major pollutant into a valuable resource (Wang et al., 2022a, b, c). The tandem photoelectrochemical cells have been engineered in such a way that they can emulate the dual-step light reactions of natural photosynthesis, achieving comparatively high solar-to-fuel conversion efficiencies under laboratory conditions (Kim et al., 2019). Artificial photosynthesis systems need to compete with existing energy technologies regarding cost, reliability, and integration into infrastructure. Government support through research funding, tax incentives and regulatory frameworks will be crucial in speeding up the development and adoption of these technologies (Zhou et al., 2021). Moreover, partnerships between the public and private sectors, along with international collaboration, will be vital to overcome from the barriers of artificial photosynthesis (Solanki and Birman, 2024).

2.2 Natural Photosynthesis Versus Artificial Photosynthesis

Natural photosynthesis is a complex biochemical process in which the chloroplasts of green plants are involved (Machín et al., 2023). During this process, the plant uses sunlight, and converts carbon dioxide from the atmosphere, to glucose and oxygen (Udaypal et al., 2024). The chemical reaction can be explained as:

$$6CO_2 + 6H_2O + light\ energy \rightarrow C_6H_{12}O_6 + 6O_2$$

Photosynthesis provides the essential glucose needed for plant growth and metabolism. It also releases oxygen, which is crucial for the survival of nearly all aerobic organisms. Moreover, it forms the basis of the global food chain, as plants and other photosynthetic organisms act as primary producers. At the molecular level, photosynthesis has two distinct but interconnected stages. The first stage, called the light-dependent reactions, takes place in the thylakoid membranes. Here, chlorophyll pigments absorb solar energy. This energy splits water molecules, releasing oxygen as a by-product and generating high-energy molecules like ATP and NADPH. The second stage, the light-independent reactions or Calvin cycle, occurs in the stroma. In this stage, carbon dioxide is fixed and gradually converted into glucose molecules, driven by the energy carriers produced earlier (Rahman et al., 2025; Goswami et al., 2020).

In artificial photosynthesis, the goal is not to produce glucose but to create energy-rich chemicals such as hydrogen gas or carbon-based liquid fuels, which can directly meet human energy needs, including transportation and electricity generation. Like natural photosynthesis, the artificial process involves splitting water into hydrogen and oxygen and converting carbon dioxide into useful fuels. A detail pictorial presentation of artificial and natural photosynthesis is presented in Fig. 1. However, it includes technological and engineering changes to improve efficiency, scalability, and practicality for human use (Machín et al., 2023). The chlorophyll which acts as the light-absorbing pigment in the natural system and exactly the same mechanism is performed by some specialised materials like semiconductors in the artificial photosynthetic system (Das, 2020). These materials efficiently capture light and convert those into electrons which then go through some chemical transformation (Manzhos et al., 2021). Catalysis is essential in artificial photosynthesis, as reactions such as water oxidation and CO_2 reduction require catalysts to reduce activation energy, improve reaction kinetics, and enhance overall conversion efficiency (Zhao et al., 2024). Artificial photosynthesis has great potential to tackle energy shortages and reduce greenhouse gas emissions, helping to create a more sustainable and climate-resilient future. A comparative analysis of artificial and natural photosynthesis is further explained in Table 1.

2.3 Components of Artificial Photosynthetic System

Several essential elements come together in an artificial photosynthetic system which can be described as capture of light and separation of charges that can drive catalytic reactions which ultimately resulted in the production of fuel. For the system to work well, these elements must be carefully designed and put together in the right way. This will not only duplicate the efficiency of natural photosynthesis but also address practical problems like durability, affordability, and energy efficiency.

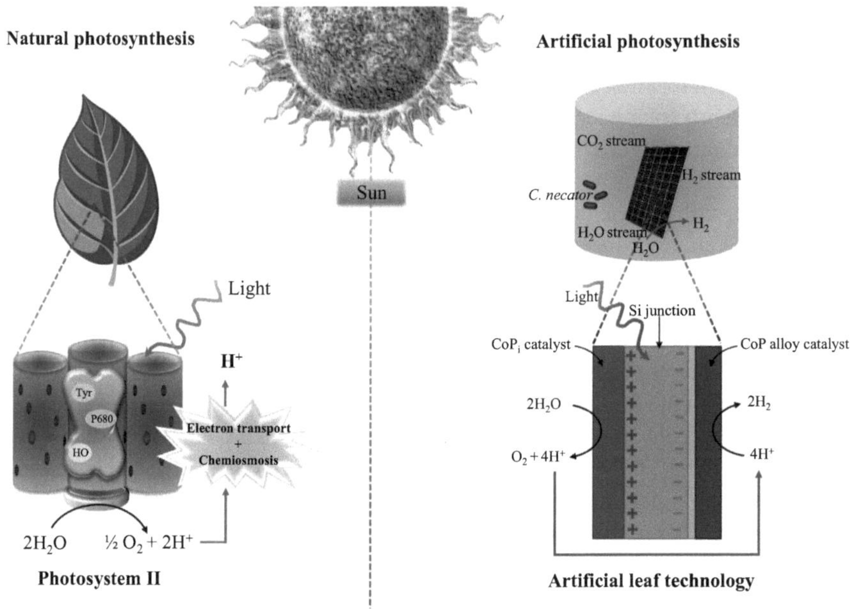

Fig. 1 Natural photosynthesis versus artificial photosynthesis

2.3.1 *Light Harvesting System*

The light harvesting unit is the system's starting point, where sunlight is collected and converted into charged carriers. For this function, silicon, titanium dioxide (TiO_2), and, more recently, perovskite semiconductors are the materials that are often utilised (Liu, 2016). The subsequent redox reactions are stimulated by the electron lone pairs produced by absorption of these photoactive materials of incoming photons. Hence choosing the right material is essential because it directly affects the quantity of solar spectrum that can be used and the energy conversion efficiency. Strong light absorption and long-term stability under illumination are two crucial variables that eventually define the system's overall performance.

2.3.2 *Photoelectrodes*

The conversion of solar energy into electrical energy is done by photoelectrodes which are basically conductive electrodes coated with light-absorbing materials (Thangamuthu et al., 2022). The performance of artificial photosynthesis is controlled by light absorption, transfer of charge, stability, and installation cost. Current research is focusing on the availability of earth-abundant metals and non-toxic materials to

Table 1 Comparative features of natural and artificial photosynthesis

Aspect	Natural photosynthesis	Artificial photosynthesis	Limitations/ challenges	References
Primary energy source & light harvesting	Pigments like chlorophyll absorb at ~400–700 nm; light harvesting in natural systems is tuned over evolution	Synthetic chromophores, semiconductors, MOFs etc. engineered to absorb visible / broader spectrum light; light harvesting optimised via nano-scale architectures	Artificial systems often suffer from less efficient light capture in full solar spectrum; losses due to non-ideal absorption, scattering, charge recombination	Blankenship et al. (2011)
Electron donor / oxidation reaction	Water is oxidised in photosystem II (Mn_4Ca cluster), producing O_2, protons and electrons.	Use of water oxidation catalysts (metal oxides, mixed metal catalysts, molecular catalysts) to achieve O_2 evolution, or other donor systems.	Catalyst stability, durability under illumination, cost of rare metals	McConnell et al. (2010)
Followed pathway and carbon fixation	CO_2 fixed via Calvin–Benson cycle into carbohydrates (glucose etc.); O_2 released; high specificity.	CO_2 is reduced to CO, methane, methanol, formate; H_2 produced via water splitting; sometimes hybrid bio-systems.	Lower selectivity, competing reactions (e.g. H_2 evolution vs CO_2 reduction), product separation, moderate yields	Navarro-Jaén et al. (2021)
Energy conversion efficiency	~1–2% solar-to-biomass in field crops; up to ~4.6% theoretical max in C_4 plants	Current lab devices: ~1–10% solar-to-fuel; hybrid photoelectrochemical systems up to ~19% demonstrated	Artificial efficiency often under non-practical lab conditions; natural efficiency constrained by photorespiration	Blankenship et al. (2011)
Stability/ durability	Natural photosynthesis has repair systems (e.g. PSII repair), long evolutionary optimization; organisms survive extended periods	Artificial catalysts and materials degrade (photocorrosion, catalyst poisoning, structural changes); need for protective layers, design for robustness.	Lack of natural repair mechanisms; high cost of durable catalysts	El-Khoulyet al. (2017)
Products	Carbohydrates, O_2, biomass (long-term energy storage in chemical bonds)	H_2, syngas, methanol, hydrocarbons (short-term fuels)	Artificial products need external storage/transport; not integrated into biology	Navarro-Jaén et al. (2021)

(continued)

Table 1 (continued)

Aspect	Natural photosynthesis	Artificial photosynthesis	Limitations/ challenges	References
Scalability	Naturally scaled globally in ecosystems (~100–130 TW captured biologically)	Lab-to-pilot scale reactors, PEC cells; large-scale still experimental	Limited by material cost, durability, and efficiency under real sunlight	Blankenship et al. (2011)
Selectivity & control	Enzyme-regulated, near 100% selectivity in CO_2 fixation pathways	Moderate selectivity; product distribution depends on catalyst surface/electrolytc	Side reactions (H_2 evolution versus CO_2 reduction)	Dogutan and Nocera (2019)

substitute costly, scarce ones for sustainable uses. Water oxidation to O_2 is driven by the photo-anode, and proton reduction to H_2 is facilitated by the photocathode.

2.3.3 *Catalysts*

In order to increase the system's efficiency, catalysts are essential for reducing the energy barriers of slow redox reactions. Strong catalysts, such as cobalt phosphate or iridium oxide, are employed for the oxygen evolution reaction because of their capacity to withstand severe oxidative conditions and high over potential. Platinum continues to be the standard catalyst for the hydrogen evolution reaction due to its exceptional efficiency. Nickel, molybdenum, copper, silver and molecular catalysts are being explored as cost-effective alternatives for this, though achieving selectivity, stability, and scalability remains the key challenge for commercialising artificial photosynthesis.

2.3.4 *Membranes or Separators*

Current research prioritises earth abundant, non-toxic materials to replace scarce, expensive ones for scalable applications. In artificial photosynthesis, the photo anode drives water oxidation to O_2 and the photocathode enables proton reduction to H_2. Performance is governed by light absorption, charge transfer, stability, and cost.

2.3.5 *Reaction Environment*

The reaction environment provides the medium for all photoelectrochemical processes. This can be a liquid electrolyte, usually aqueous solutions with supporting salts, or medium, which avoids issues such as evaporation and leakage. The reaction medium must allow efficient ion transport, maintain the stability of catalysts and photoelectrodes, and support long-term operation without degradation.

2.3.6 *Carbon Dioxide Capture Unit*

In artificial photosynthetic systems designed to produce fuels from carbon dioxide, an effective capture mechanism is a key requirement. This component works by concentrating CO_2either from the air, where it is highly diluted, or from emission streams such as industrial flue gases before channelling it into the reaction zone. Methods under active investigation include amine-based absorption, solid sorbent materials, and membrane separation technologies. Once captured, the CO_2 is delivered to catalytic surfaces, where sunlight drives its conversion into energy-rich fuels (Nwabueze and Leggett, 2024). By linking fuel generation with carbon capture and utilisation, this approach positions artificial photosynthesis as a promising strategy in the fight against climate change.

2.3.7 *Integrated Artificial Leaves*

The development of integrated artificial leaves is a new discovery in the field of artificial photosynthesis which are basically small devices that merge all the components into a single functional unit. Without the need for additional wiring, these artificial leaves are able to float on water surfaces and generate solar energy directly. While still in the experimental phase, integrated devices demonstrate how artificial photosynthesis could revolutionise energy harvesting by fusing cutting edge engineered materials with nature inspired design.

2.4 Recent Breakthroughs and Technological Advances

Recent developments in solar-driven water technologies build upon fundamental physicochemical processes that occur at multiple scales, including controlling energy conversion, activating water molecules, and driving liquids and vapours through a system (Wu et al., 2020). By combining nanoscale materials with large-scale design, researchers have generated advanced structures that better capture water, encounter

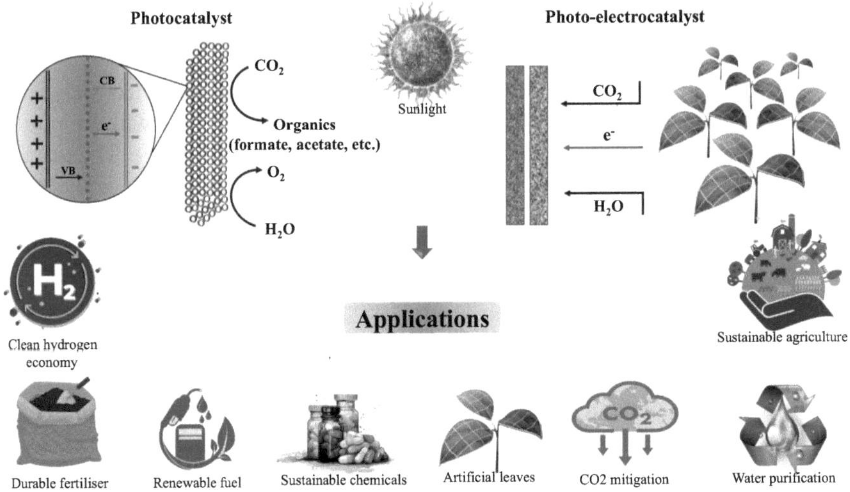

Fig. 2 Schematic representation of mechanistic insights and application of artificial photosynthesis

problems like fouling and salt accumulation hence converting solar energy into heat and vapor. This cross scale integration has significantly improved the resilience and sustainability of these systems which use sunlight to generate clean water (Jiang et al., 2025). The detailed mechanism of artificial photosynthesis and its uses are presented in Fig. 2.

2.4.1 *Recent Technological Advances in Artificial Photosynthesis*

In 2025 scientists have developed three dimensional solar evaporators that achieved huge amount of clean water (2.63 kg m^{-2} h^{-1}) with energy conversion efficiencies exceeding 90% in sunlight (Wu et al., 2020). These designs typically include bioinspired elements such as capillary patterns that resemble plant roots to effectively channelise water through sophisticated photothermal materials like carbon black cellulose sponges and graphene foams. The integration of these features at both nano and macroscale ensures rapid water transport and exceptional solar absorption making the systems resistant in handling high salinity water. One among the major short comings is salt accumulation which can clog systems and cut efficiency. Recent advances have introduced salt rejecting and self cleaning designs that actively prevent salt accumulation on sensitive surfaces. For example new evaporators with advanced structures and engineered surfaces can steadily evaporate highly salty water (10–25% salt) for several weeks without losing efficiency showing an unmatched durability level (Liu et al., 2023). Such resilience demonstrates the potential combination between environmental adaptability and system stability. According to recent research these systems can operate efficiently for more than a month in harsh conditions because of innovative designs that reduce energy waste by coordinating water delivery with sunlight-driven evaporation. When taken as a whole, these discoveries show how scientific innovation and useful engineering may come together effectively. The goal of easily accessible, cost effective, and durable clean water solutions is getting closer to reality as solar vapour generation achieves both high efficiency and long term durability (Wu et al., 2025).

2.4.2 Highly Efficient Water Splitting Systems

The energy-intensive process of splitting water into its constituent parts, such as hydrogen and oxygen, is one of the main aspects of artificial photosynthesis. Therefore, the development of effective photocatalysts and photoelectrochemical systems is essential. By optimising the materials utilised for the photoanode and photocathode, recent innovations have significantly increased the solar to hydrogen conversion efficiency (Machín et al., 2023). Innovations in semiconductor designing especially through the use of nanostructured materials like bismuth vanadate ($BiVO_4$) and tungsten trioxide (WO_3) have led to better light absorption and fast charge transport. These materials are often combined with O_2 releasing catalysts like cobalt phosphate ($Co_3(PO_4)_2$) and nickel-iron layered hydroxides to reduce the extra energy for water oxidation (Pihosh et al., 2015). On the cathode side photocathodes made from copper gallium selenide (CIGS), silicon and indium phosphide have shown improved performance in converting protons into hydrogen. These systems are typically coated with protective layers such as TiO_2 and nickel oxide to improve stability in harsh conditions (Hellstern et al., 2019). Systems without an external voltage input are also being developed. Water splitting efficiency of over 10% have been shown using dualphotoelectrode systems, which are capable of independently capturing and using sunlight at both electrodes. This accomplishment is seen as a significant step toward the commercial viability of these systems.

2.4.3 Integrated CO_2 Capture and Reduction Devices

Beyond the H_2 production direct conversion of CO_2 into value added fuels has become an important field of study. This approach addresses the issue of increasing atmospheric CO_2 levels while simultaneously promoting the production of renewable fuels. Recent developments streamline the process from CO_2 absorption to chemical conversion by combining carbon capture techniques with artificial photosynthesis. Ionic liquids and novel solid sorbents have been developed to concentrate CO_2 from industrial emissions and ambient air which is then fed into photocatalytic or electrochemical reduction devices (Machín et al., 2023). Catalytic platforms such as copper based nanostructures, silver nanoparticles, rhenium and cobalt containing molecular complexes have shown promising functionality in transforming CO_2 into carbon monoxide (CO), formic acid, methanol and higher forms hydrocarbons (Takeda et al., 2017).

Recent studies have focused on installing bioinspired catalytic devices to selectively reduce CO_2 in aqueous media. Improved selectivity and efficiency in turning CO_2 into fuel has been demonstrated for engineered metal organic frameworks (MOFs) that combine light harvesting and catalytic activities. CO_2 capture and reduction combined into a single modular platform is a step forward for self-sufficient and carbon neutral energy systems. In addition to helping the environment these systems make it possible to produce decentralized fuel which is especially important in isolated and off-grid areas (Jana et al., 2023).

2.4.4 *Tandem Cell Designs for Solar to Fuel Conversion*

Tandem cell designs have emerged as a key strategy to resolve the energy misbalance between the productions of chemical fuel and solar light. These systems include two or more light absorbing materials each of which is tuned to certain spectra of the solar light to optimise overall light utilisation and boost the driving power for redox reactions (Chen et al., 2015). A popular combination of narrow band gap photocathodes (silicon or perovskite) with a wide band gap photoanode ($BiVO_4$) are widely studied in CO_2 reduction while allowing more solar absorption (Chen et al., 2015; Lee et al., 2018).

Recent advancements have demonstrated solar to hydrogen conversion efficiencies exceeding 10% placing them in the same performance range as conventional photovoltaic systems. Further, tandem cells can be made for particular outputs based on the catalyst and reaction conditions enabling the selective synthesis of fuels such as hydrogen and methane (Hansora et al., 2025). Charge transmission between the tandem layers has been enhanced further by advancements in interfacial engineering. For instance, conductive inter layers and ultra-thin indirect coatings reduce recombination losses by facilitating the efficient space of electrons and holes (Liu et al., 2022). Overall, tandem cell architectures provide a flexible and scalable approach to solar fuel synthesis with the adaptability to meet diverse climatic conditions and energy demands.

2.4.5 *Artificial Leaves and Self-Healing Photocatalytic Systems*

Decades of work have gone into creating a small, effective and self-sustaining version of the fundamentals of natural photosynthesis which is reflected in the idea of an ‘artificial leaf’. These systems are frequently made to function directly in water and the open air combine the essential elements of artificial photosynthesis such as light harvesting catalysis and product separation in a single apparatus. The silicon-based artificial leaf developed at Harvard University is a seminal example in this context. This uses earth metal based catalysts to split water into H_2 and O_2 when exposed to sunlight. More sophisticated designs have expanded this capability to include CO_2 reduction making it possible to produce liquid fuels in addition to O_2 using the simple inputs of solar energy, water and air (Zhu et al., 2024). Table 2 extends detailed explanation of the many forms of artificial photosynthesis. Maintaining the stability and effectiveness of artificial leaf technology under prolonged exposure to sunshine, water, and reactive byproducts is a significant problem because these elements have a tendency to erode materials and diminish performance over time. To counteract this scientists have developed new photocatalytic materials capable of self-healing actively restoring their own light capturing and catalytic surfaces during operation. For example, certain cobalt-based catalysts used in water splitting can spontaneously reorganise into their active state while in use echoing the repair mechanisms observed in natural photosynthetic organisms. Water repellent films and specialised protective frameworks are being used to cover perovskite photocatalysts, another promising type making them more reliable and durable for long-term use in damp conditions. These developments bring artificial leaves that can repair themselves closer to real-world uses especially as decentralised clean fuel production systems in locations without conventional power grids and infrastructure (Dogutan and Nocera, 2019).

2.5 Effects of Artificial Photosynthesis on Flora and Fauna

Artificial photosynthesis is an innovative technology aimed for replicating the way plants convert sunlight, CO_2, and water into energy dense fuels. While the potential of this approach to reshape renewable energy systems is widely acknowledged, it is highly important to consider its peripheral impacts on living organisms and their environments as these systems move closer to commercial reality. Adopting artificial photosynthetic devices responsibly requires an understanding of how they may affect plants, animals, and the ecosystem as a whole. This chapter explores both the environmental benefits of artificial photosynthesis such as reducing greenhouse gas emissions and supporting sustainable fuel production (Machín et al., 2023). By offering a sustainable substitute for fossil fuels, artificial photosynthesis has the potential to reduce some of the stresses on natural ecosystems. For instance, these systems lessen the carbon footprint and aid in mitigating climate change, which endangers biodiversity and ecosystem stability globally, by efficiently capturing and converting CO_2 into useable fuels. Further applications related to agricultural could be made possible with the advancement of artificial photosynthesis. In order to grow food crops effectively in controlled environments or even in urban centres, researchers have shown the production of acetate through electrocatalytic artificial photosynthesis in the absence of sunlight. This could lessen the need for large agricultural land and the destruction of habitat (Mandad et al., 2025).

Table 2 Types, principles, materials utilised, advantages and challenges faced in artificial photosynthesis

System type	Working principle	Typical components/ materials	Key advantages	Challenges	References
Photoelectrochemical (PEC) cells (photoelectrodes)	Semiconductor photoanode/ photocathode absorbs light → generates charge carriers → drives O_2/H_2 (water splitting) or CO_2 reduction at electrodes	Inorganic semiconductors (TiO_2, $BiVO_4$, Fe_2O_3, Ta_3N_5), co-catalysts (Ni, co LDH), protective/ passivation layers; electrolytes and membranes.	Direct solar-to-fuel, modular (electrodes separated), potential for high STH if stability solved.	Photocorrosion, poor charge separation in many semiconductors, limited long-term stability and scaling.	Yu et al. (2020)
Photocatalytic particulate (suspension) systems	Powdered photocatalyst in suspension absorbs light; photogenerated electrons/holes reduce CO_2 or produce H_2 (often with sacrificial donors).	g-C_3N_4, TiO_2, doped oxides, MOFs, heterojunctions, co-catalyst nanoparticles (Pt, cu, etc.).	Easy to scale as slurries; simple reactors; many earth-abundant catalysts; good light absorption engineering.	Product separation, low selectivity for desired C-products, reliance on sacrificial agents for lab tests, charge recombination.	Kovacic et al. (2020)
Dye-sensitised systems (DSPEC / DSSC-derived for fuels)	Molecular/organic/inorganic dyes absorb light and inject charge into oxide semiconductor; chromophore–catalyst assemblies drive oxidation/ reduction (DSPECs for fuels).	Molecular dyes (Ru, organic dyes), TiO_2 / mesoporous oxide scaffolds, molecular catalysts immobilised on electrodes, redox mediators.	Molecular-level design (tuneable chromophores/ catalysts), modular DSPEC architectures, good photon capture at molecular scale	Dye/catalyst degradation, interfacial charge transfer losses, anchoring stability; currently modest solar-to-fuel efficiencies.	Brennaman et al. (2016)

(continued)

Table 2 (continued)

System type	Working principle	Typical components/ materials	Key advantages	Challenges	References
Molecular (homogeneous) photocatalysis/metal-complex systems	Soluble photosensitizer + molecular catalyst in solution: Light excites photosensitiser → electron transfer to catalyst → multi-electron CO_2 reduction or H_2 evolution (often with sacrificial donors)	Metal complexes (re, Ru, Ir, cu, co complexes), organic photosensitisers, homogeneous redox mediators, sacrificial electron donors (BIH, amines)	High mechanistic control; facile structure–function tuning; excellent selectivity in some homogeneous systems.	Requires sacrificial donors in many studies, challenges in coupling to water oxidation for overall artificial photosynthesis, separation/scalability issues.	Kumgai et al. (2023)
Biohybrid/semi-artificial systems (enzyme- or microbe-integrated)	Combine biological catalysts (enzymes, whole cells) with inorganic light-harvesters or electrodes to use biological selectivity for CO_2 reduction or fuel formation.	Photosensitising semiconductors or electrodes + enzymes (formate dehydrogenase, hydrogenase) or whole microbes; wiring (mediators or direct electron transfer).	Exceptional selectivity (enzymes), operate under mild conditions, potential for complex product formation and cascade reactions	Biocatalyst stability, interfacing efficiency, scale-up, and integration with robust light absorbers	Yang et al. (2023)
Photovoltaic-electrochemical (PV-EC)/tandem PV-electrolysis	High-efficiency PV cell(s) generate electricity which drives an external electrolyser (or electrocatalysts) for H_2 or CO_2 electroreduction, often combined as an integrated stack	High-efficiency PV (Si, III-V, perovskite) + PEM / alkaline / solid-oxide electrolysers or electrocatalysts; power electronics or direct coupling	Mature PV + electrolysertech allows high overall system engineering and independent optimisation of PV and catalysts; good scalability roadmap	Balance-of-system costs, coupling losses, electrolyser durability, need for decentralised/ storage solutions; not fully "single-device" artificial photosynthesis	Lee et al. (2022)

2.5.1 Potential Positive Effects

Artificial photosynthesis offers many benefits for the environment. Similar to natural photosynthesis and converting sunlight into storable chemical fuels with less waste, clean, renewable, and carbon neutral energy source. In lab setup the efficiency of solar to power conversion is 20% but the scalability in growing market is still a challenge (Mandad et al., 2025; Gust et al., 2009). Importantly, artificial photosynthesis integrates easily with existing energy systems and could operate in diverse environment. This versatility increases energy access along with supporting global decarbonisation efforts and biodiversity conservation. Sustained interdisciplinary research complemented by comprehensive environmental impact assessments (EIA) and robust policy frameworks is crucial for harnessing its full potential to achieve a greener and sustainable energy future. This directly supports the objectives of sustainable development as represented in the following positive impacts.

2.5.1.1 Reduction in Greenhouse Gases Emission

Artificial photosynthesis offers a powerful environmental advantage by passively reducing greenhouse gas emissions. This system captures CO_2 directly from the atmosphere and converts it into fuels thereby addressing one of the leading causes of climate change. Recent developments in the field have shown remarkable progress, with solar-powered catalytic systems achieving CO_2 reduction rates above 300 μmol g^{-1} h^{-1} and reaching nearly 100% efficiency in selectively producing valuable compounds such as carbon monoxide, even under diluted CO_2 conditions (Wang et al., 2024). Unlike natural photosynthesis, these engineered processes harness photocatalytic water splitting in tandem with CO_2 reduction, creating a more efficient pathway to recycle carbon in a sustainable manner (Machín et al., 2023). The downstream effects of such technology could be profound by curbing global warming, ecosystems and species that are highly sensitive to temperature fluctuations, such as polar wildlife and alpine plants, stand a better chance of survival. Moreover, stabilizing global temperatures would help preserve ecological balance, protecting migration routes, reproductive cycles, and food webs that are currently under threat from climate disruption.

2.5.1.2 Less Land Pressure

Artificial photosynthesis provides a distinct advantage over conventional biofuel production because it does not demand vast tracts of farmland. Instead, it could be implemented through compact and modular systems that operate independently for food crops and natural ecosystems. This reduces the dependency on the arable land and lowers pressure on habitats and help to limit deforestation. By moving energy production away from land intensive methods artificial photosynthesis contributes in the preservation of ecologically critical areas i.e., rainforests, wetlands, and grasslands (Machín et al., 2023). From an efficiency point of view these systems have the potential to overcome natural photosynthesis significantly. Plants convert solar energy into chemical energy at only 1–2% but on the other hand artificial systems could achieve much higher solar to fuel conversion efficiencies (Barber and Tran, 2013). This means that the equal amount of energy could be produced by using 90% less land area compared to biomass-based biofuels thereby easing agricultural land pressures (Hann et al., 2022). Further, because of their modular design these technologies can be installed in urban or industrial environments and generate clean fuel with minimal spatial requirements.

2.5.1.3 Reduced Water Pollution

Conventional fossil fuel mining and burning are major contributors to water pollution, releasing pollutants through oil spills, heavy metal discharge, and acid rain. Artificial photosynthesis, especially when based on water splitting avoids these issues altogether (Tachibana et al., 2012). Because it minimises toxic byproducts and eliminates the harmful solvents requirement, this approach lowers the risk of polluting rivers, lakes, and groundwater resources. Clean water directly benefits ecological health by improving plant health, supporting aquatic species, and reducing the toxins accumulation throughout food webs (House et al., 2015). Beyond the energy production research is advancing in artificial photosynthesis technologies for water purification. Systems that use visible light-based photocatalysts could break down organic pollutants and trap heavy metals without making secondary pollution. These systems are also adaptable with potential for decentralised low energy setups and provide safe water along with renewable fuel continuously in remote settings. Life cycle assessments suggest further benefits showing that such technologies can cut energy use by 30–60% compared to conventional water treatment methods by lowering both ecological and resource footprints (Eureka, 2025).

2.5.1.4 Habitat Preservation

By providing a decentralised energy source from artificial photosynthesis the requirement of big power stations and energy infrastructure reduces. This change could help to protect fragile ecosystems from the physical and chemical disruptions associated with regular energy facilities (Gust et al., 2009). For example, habitats that would be disrupted by mining and drilling could remain undisturbed and support biodiversity preservation and ecological health (Allakhverdiev, 2024).

2.5.1.5 Potential Anonymous Harmful Effects

Although artificial photosynthesis holds great potential, it also carries potential ecological risks. Like many emerging technologies, its large-scale deployment could lead to unintended consequences if not carefully managed. Without thorough EIA and proper regulatory frameworks, the extensive use of artificial photosynthetic systems may introduce unforeseen impacts on ecosystems and natural cycles (Mori et al., 2025).

2.5.1.6 Chemical Leaching of Catalysts

Several artificial photosynthesis systems use catalysts made up of transition metals and/or other synthetic materials. These catalysts may leach into soil and water if not contained properly. This contamination could alter soil chemistry, impacting plant growth and microbial communities that are important for nutrient cycling (Shiraishi et al., 2021). The aquatic life may also be harmed by heavy metals exposure thereby, disrupting physiological functions in fish and invertebrates.

2.5.1.7 Disruption of Local Microclimates

Large installations of artificial photosynthesis panels may impact local microclimates. As solar farms can change local air temperature and wind patterns, artificial leaves or panels could alter light penetration, humidity, and surface reflection (Barron-Gafford et al., 2016). These subtle changes could, in turn, affect plant transpiration rates, insect behaviour, and animal habitat preferences, especially in sensitive ecosystems like wetlands or alpine meadows.

2.5.1.8 Nanomaterials in Ecosystems

Some artificial photosynthesis designs involve using nanomaterials, such as quantum dots or carbon nanotubes, to improve efficiency. While these materials enhance performance, their environmental safety is mostly unknown. If nanoparticles enter ecosystems through runoff, wear, or improper disposal, they could pose risks to plants and animals. Studies indicate that some nanomaterials can penetrate cell membranes, potentially cause oxidative stress or interfere with biological processes in plants and animals (Klaine et al., 2008).

2.5.1.9 Habitat Displacement from Industrial Infrastructure

Scaling up artificial photosynthesis commercially may lead to building factories, processing units, and distribution networks. While smaller than traditional power plants, these facilities could still displace wildlife habitats and fragment ecosystems. The presence of infrastructure can disrupt animal migration paths, increase human-wildlife conflicts, and facilitate the introduction of invasive species (de Jonge et al., 2022).

2.5.2 Mitigation Strategies

2.5.2.1 Eco-Friendly Catalyst Development

Scientists should focus on creating non-toxic, abundant catalysts and explore the alternatives i.e., iron, cobalt, and manganese based materials by replacing harmful cadmium and platinum. Use of biodegradable and inert catalyst helps to lower the chance of chemical leaching. Recent advancements have shown that combining earth elements with nanomaterials increase the catalytic activity and more environmental friendly (Mori et al., 2025). Moreover, photocatalysts made up of carbon nitrides along with modified metal oxides have more stability and efficiency, offering better sustainable artificial photosynthesis systems. The rising green synthesis measures and recycling protocols in catalyst synthesis further minimise carbon footprints by ensuring overall well-being.

2.5.2.2 Environmental Rsk Assessments

An extensive EIA could be needed before large-scale installation of artificial photosynthesis systems. These assessments should investigate deeper into potential chemical, ecological and spatial impacts on local environment. A special attention needed for systems installation near protected and sensitive ecosystem zones. The advanced EIAs for artificial photosynthesis should consider potential life cycle assessments that evaluate the possible causes related to catalyst material supply, potential leaching, and end to end disposal impacts (Lazar, 2025). Moreover, monitoring frameworks using remote sensing and ecological modelling could help mitigating local environmental conflict before they become a serious burden (Mandad et al., 2025). Considering the stakeholder involvement along with relevant collaboration in the assessment ensures better understanding and acceptance of these technologies while protecting ecosystem health.

2.5.2.3 Containment and Recycling Systems

A closed loop system that could handle and recycle catalytic materials prevent environmental contamination. Engineers should consider protective coatings, leak proof housing, and recycling units to collect waste materials (Tachibana et al., 2012).

Consistent monitoring of neighbouring soil and water has to be carried out. Furthermore, combining sensor technologies for real time leakage detection and automated containment response systems could minimise risks associated with accidental catalyst release. Implement modular reactor design for easy catalyst retrieval and replacement for better operations. Collaboration with waste management sector to develop an efficient catalyst recycling method ensures resource recovery and reduced environmental burdens from disposal. These strategies collectively make a robust framework to safeguard ecosystems while enabling a sustainable system (Wang et al., 2022a, b, c).

2.5.2.4 Nanomaterial Regulation and Research

Advance research on the ecological effects of nanomaterials is needed before widely used in artificial photosynthesis. Regulatory frameworks should classify and monitor materials behaviour in the environment (Machín et al., 2023). When possible, biodegradable and inert alternatives should be considered. Strict measures and testing guidelines are essential to evaluate the toxicity, bioaccumulation, and presence of residual toxicity of nanomaterials in the environment. Continuous collaboration between researchers, policymakers, and industry stakeholders will be essential to develop adaptive regulations for advance technologies.

2.5.2.5 Minimal Footprint Infrastructure

To reduce the habitat disruption, artificial photosynthetic units may be built with a minimal spatial footprint. Rooftop setups, floating devices, or integration with existing structures could reduce the requirement for new construction. Buffer zones around installation sites could further reduce wildlife disturbance (Machín et al., 2023). Further, vertical and modular designs could minimise space utilisation by enabling energy production in urban or industrial environments. Using lightweight and flexible materials allow artificial photosynthetic systems to be setup on unconventional surfaces like building facades and water bodies. Strategic planning to align installations with existing infrastructure reduces the overall environmental footprints and supports coexistence with local flora and fauna while facilitating renewable energy integration on a bigger scale.

2.5.2.6 Microclimate Management

Installation practices should consider local climate conditions to prevent unwanted changes in temperature and humidity. Design choices like reflective coatings, vertical orientation, and partial canopy integration could help in keeping existed microclimates more secure (Barron-Gafford et al., 2016). Additionally, incorporating natural shading and using materials with high albedo can minimise heat absorption and prevent localised warming. Adjustable panel angles can optimise light and airflow that reduces impact on evaporation cum transpiration rates of neighbouring vegetation. Monitoring of microclimatic parameters after installation ensures early detection of any problem and allows adaptive management. Thoughtful integration ensures artificial photosynthesis installations coexist pleasantly with their surrounding environments while maximising energy production (Dogutan and Nocera, 2019).

2.6 Challenges in Scaling and Commercialisation

The laboratory experiments have shown that artificial photosynthesis could work, the road to commercialise its usage to overcome renewable dependency. These obstacles cover technological, economic, environmental, and social areas. This chapter discusses five main barriers such as economic viability, stability of photocatalytic systems, sustainability concerns, systems integration, and policy regulation (Machín et al., 2023).

2.6.1 Economic Viability and Techno-Economic Analysis

The economic competitiveness is a key challenge in bringing artificial photosynthesis to market. Even though the scientific advancements have been significant, the technology is still not as commercially viable as other sources such as solar power and wind turbines. Making synthetic fuels through artificial photosynthesis involves complex and energy consuming processes i.e., water splitting, CO_2 capture, and fuel production. These processes need highly efficient, durable materials and precise engineering systems. Techno-economic analysis (TEA) is important for evaluating commercial feasibility. The TEA includes capital expenditures, operational costs, system efficiency, and durability to estimate the average cost of fuel and energy requirement. Current TEA models suggest that artificial photosynthesis must significantly improve the solar to fuel efficiency and lower costs to compete with fossil fuels and other mainstream renewable resources (Atwater, 2023). Furthermore, it produces chemical fuels instead of electricity thus extra systems for storing, moving, and using these fuels will be needed that ultimately will raise the net cost. Bridging this economic gap may require ongoing research investment, targeted government subsidies, and regulatory incentives as carbon pricing (Jiao and Frei, 2014). Without these interventions, artificial photosynthesis could remain a promising but commercially unfeasible technology.

2.6.2 Stability and Longevity of Photocatalytic Systems

Another significant challenge is the long-term stability of photocatalytic systems. Many devices for artificial photosynthesis use semiconductors or catalysts that degrade over time due to exposure to sunlight, water, and reactive intermediates. This degradation lowers system efficiency and requires frequent component replacement, which is not suitable for large-scale industrial applications. The leaching or photodegradation observed in catalysts like CdS and TiO_2 (Chen et al., 2015). Co-catalysts made from new metals get deactivated due to oxidation and particle aggregation. These issues not only reduce durability but also create environmental hazard. To overcome these challenges, research could be more focused on anticorrosive materials, protective coatings, and self-healing systems. Even with these advancements, long shelf life of the system is still a big challenge before its commercialisation (Machínet al., 2023).

2.6.3 Materials Shortage and Sustainability Issues

Scaling up artificial photosynthesis depends on using materials that are both sustainable and readily available. Many high performing photocatalysts and electrocatalysts rely on rare and expensive elements like platinum, iridium, and ruthenium, limited and environmentally harmful in extraction (Wang et al., 2022a, b, c). Depending on these materials raise the economics and concerns about long term resource availability. Global production of these elements may not meet the needs for widespread use without causing supply issues or geopolitical dependencies. Extracting and processing these materials usually has a significant environmental impact, especially in developing countries where regulations may be weak (Machín et al., 2023). In response, researchers are looking for alternatives made from common elements like iron, cobalt, and nickel, which are less expensive and more sustainable. However, these materials often show lower catalytic performance, and closing the efficiency gap is a major research challenge (Maeda and Domen, 2010). Progress in this area is necessary to balance performance with environmental and economic sustainability.

2.6.4 Modular Design and Systems Integration

Artificial photosynthesis systems work by bringing together light absorbing materials, catalysts, membranes, and collection units, which all need to interact with each other. Lab experiments usually improve one part at a time, but the industry needs to design the complete system so that all the parts work well together in real world conditions. Modular design offers a practical way to standardise units for use in different places like rooftops, floating platforms, and industrial sites, but it also brings its own engineering challenges. For example, controlling how light spreads, managing heat, and keeping fluids flowing properly become harder for the larger systems (Wang et al., 2022a, b, c). This means synthetic fuels must work with current storage tanks, pipelines, and conversion units, even though many are not designed for them. Solving these issues is a key in making large-scale use possible (Ardo et al., 2018).

2.6.5 Regulatory Pathways and Community Involvement

Besides the technical issues artificial photosynthesis meets major challenges from unclear Government regulations and public acceptance for this technology. This creates ambiguity about environmental hazard, safe disposal and emission standards (MacFarlane et al., 2020). If this regulatory problem not addressed properly, it could slow down extensive commercial use along with public acceptance that is equally critical for the success. Unawareness in technology could cause health risks, landing in problems, misleading information on rare materials use similar to nuclear power and genetically modified organisms. To overcome these situations policymakers must establish clear guidelines including environmental monitoring, safety standards and EIAs. Additionally, education campaigns and advertisement strategies will play vital roles in raising public awareness. Bringing relevant stakeholders such as scientists, industrialists, policymakers and local communities for discussion to foster regulatory guidelines for sustainable installation of this technology (Ardo et al., 2018).

2.7 Conclusion

Artificial photosynthesis is a leading scientific breakthrough that offers a new way to solve global problems like energy reliance, climate change and sustainable growth. This field is inspired by photosynthesis works, materials science, light chemistry, catalysts and engineering. Advanced designs like photoelectrochemical cells, tandem cells, biohybrid and molecular systems use solar energy to make efficient chemical fuels. This chapter has clearly explained the basic ideas and recent breakthroughs in artificial photosynthesis on our environment and society. It works well with recycling carbon and has exciting possibilities for use in space, showing its potential to change the way we think about energy and the environment. However, moving from small-scale lab tests to real world commercial application faces many difficult challenges. Mainly, these are long-term issues of system stability, resource sustainability, cost competitiveness, and policy making. Addressing these hurdles will require continued scientific and engineering creativity along with visionary leadership in government, investment and public communication. Catalyst development and R&D in cost effective material select could make a mile stone of the future. This technology also can create a carbon neutral fuel for our future rising energy demands. As the world moves faster toward renewable energy, artificial photosynthesis stands out not just as a new option, but also as a powerful example of what could be made when combine nature's designs with human creativity.

References

Allakhverdiev, S. I. (2024). Artificial photosynthesis: Powering a green new deal for sustainable energy. *International Journal of Hydrogen Energy, 90*, 199–209.

Ardo, S., Rivas, D. F., Modestino, M. A., Greiving, V. S., Abdi, F. F., Llado, E. A., Artero, V., Ayers, K., Battaglia, C., Becker, J. P., & Bederak, D. (2018). Pathways to electrochemical solar-hydrogen technologies. *Energy & Environmental Science, 11*(10), 2768–2783.

Atwater, H. A. (2023). Artificial photosynthesis: A pathway to solar fuels. *Physics Today, 76*(12), 32–39.

Awogbemi, O., Kallon, D. V. V., Onuh, E. I., & Aigbodion, V. S. (2021). An overview of the classification, production and utilization of biofuels for internal combustion engine applications. *Energies, 14*(18), 5687.

Barber, J., & Tran, P. D. (2013). From natural to artificial photosynthesis. *Journal of the Royal Society Interface, 10*(81), 20120984.

Barron-Gafford, G. A., Minor, R. L., Allen, N. A., Cronin, A. D., Brooks, A. E., & Pavao-Zuckerman, M. A. (2016). The photovoltaic heat Island effect: Larger solar power plants increase local temperatures. *Scientific Reports, 6*(1), 35070.

Blankenship, R. E., Tiede, D. M., Barber, J., Brudvig, G. W., Fleming, G., Ghirardi, M., Gunner, M. R., Junge, W., Kramer, D. M., Melis, A., & Moore, T. A. (2011). Comparing photosynthetic and photovoltaic efficiencies and recognizing the potential for improvement. *Science, 332*(6031), 805–809.

Brennaman, M. K., Dillon, R. J., Alibabaei, L., Gish, M. K., Dares, C. J., Ashford, D. L., House, R. L., Meyer, G. J., Papanikolas, J. M., & Meyer, T. J. (2016). Finding the way to solar fuels with dye-sensitized photoelectrosynthesis cells. *Journal of the American Chemical Society, 138*(40), 13085–13102.

Chen, Y. S., Manser, J. S., & Kamat, P. V. (2015). All solution-processed lead halide perovskite-BiVO4 tandem assembly for photolytic solar fuels production. *Journal of the American Chemical Society, 137*(2), 974–981.

Das, R. (2020). Artificial photosynthesis. In *Handbook of Nanomaterials and Nanocomposites for energy and environmental applications* (pp. 1–19). Springer International Publishing.

de Jonge, M. M., Gallego-Zamorano, J., Huijbregts, M. A., Schipper, A. M., & Benítez-López, A. (2022). The impacts of linear infrastructure on terrestrial vertebrate populations: A trait-based approach. *Global Change Biology, 28*(24), 7217–7233.

Dincer, I., Zamfirescu, C., & Vezina, G. (2018). Modular and integrated artificial hotosynthesis systems. *Journal of Cleaner Production, 180*, 543–556.

Dogutan, D. K., & Nocera, D. G. (2019). Artificial photosynthesis at efficiencies greatly exceeding that of natural photosynthesis. *Accounts of Chemical Research, 52*(11), 3143–3148.

El-Khouly, M. E., El-Mohsnawy, E., & Fukuzumi, S. (2017). Solar energy conversion: From natural to artificial photosynthesis. *Journal of Photochemistry and Photobiology C: Photochemistry Reviews, 31*, 36–83.

Eureka. (2025). Artificial photosynthesis and its treatment in clean water process. Accessed on 21 Sep 2025. https://eureka.patsnap.com/report-artificial-photosynthesis-and-its-treatment-in-clean-water-processes.

Goswami, R. K., Agrawal, K., Mehariya, S., Molino, A., Musmarra, D., & Verma, P. (2020). Microalgae-based biorefinery for utilization of carbon dioxide for production of valuable bioproducts. In *Chemo-biological systems for CO_2 utilization* (pp. 203–228). CRC Press.

Gust, D., Moore, T. A., & Moore, A. L. (2009). Solar fuels via artificial photosynthesis. *Accounts of Chemical Research, 42*(12), 1890–1898.

Hann, E. C., Overa, S., Harland-Dunaway, M., Narvaez, A. F., Le, D. N., Orozco-Cárdenas, M. L., Jiao, F., & Jinkerson, R. E. (2022). A hybrid inorganic–biological artificial photosynthesis system for energy-efficient food production. *Nature Food, 3*(6), 461–471.

Hansora, D., Mehrotra, R., Noh, E., Yoo, J. W., Kim, M., Byun, W. J., Park, J., Jang, J. W., Seok, S. I., & Lee, J. S. (2025). Scalable and durable module-sized artificial leaf with a solar-to-hydrogen efficiency over 10%. *Nature Communications, 16*(1), 4186.

Hellstern, T. R., Nielander, A. C., Chakthranont, P., King, L. A., Willis, J. J., Xu, S., MacIsaac, C., Hahn, C., Bent, S. F., Prinz, F. B., & Jaramillo, T. F. (2019). Nanostructuring strategies to increase the photoelectrochemical water splitting activity of silicon photocathodes. *ACS Applied Nano Materials, 2*(1), 6–11.

House, R. L., Iha, N. Y. M., Coppo, R. L., Alibabaei, L., Sherman, B. D., Kang, P., Brennaman, M. K., Hoertz, P. G., & Meyer, T. J. (2015). Artificial photosynthesis: Where are we now? Where can we go? *Journal of Photochemistry and Photobiology C: Photochemistry Reviews, 25*, 32–45.

Hussain, S., Ulhassan, Z., Brestic, M., Zivcak, M., Zhou, W., Allakhverdiev, S. I., Yang, X., Safdar, M. E., Yang, W., & Liu, W. (2021). Photosynthesis research under climate change. *Photosynthesis Research, 150*(1), 5–19.

Jana, A., Snyder, S. W., Crumlin, E. J., & Qian, J. (2023). Integrated carbon capture and conversion: A review on C2+ product mechanisms and mechanism-guided strategies. *Frontiers in Chemistry, 11*, 1135829.

Jiang, J., Zhao, H., Li, S., Jin, B., Wang, R., Wei, Y., Li, H. & Dai, Y. (2025). Nano-to-macroscale insights into solar evaporation: Bridging fundamental principles to intelligent systems. *ACS nano.*

Jiao, F., & Frei, H. (2009). Nanostructured cobalt oxide clusters in mesoporous silica as efficient oxygen-evolving catalysts. *Angewandte Chemie, 121*(10), 1873–1876.

Kim, J. H., Hansora, D., Sharma, P., Jang, J. W., & Lee, J. S. (2019). Toward practical solar hydrogen production–an artificial photosynthetic leaf-to-farm challenge. *Chemical Society Reviews, 48*(7), 1908–1971.

Klaine, S. J., Alvarez, P. J. J., Batley, G. E., Fernandes, T. F., Handy, R. D., Lyon, D. Y., Mahendra, S., McLaughlin, M. J., & Lead, J. R. (2008). Nanomaterials in the environment: Behavior, fate, bioavailability, and effects. *Environmental Toxicology and Chemistry, 27*(9), 1825–1851.

Kovacic, Z., Likozar, B., & Hus, M. (2020). Photocatalytic CO2 reduction: A review of ab initio mechanism, kinetics, and multiscale modeling simulations. *ACS Catalysis, 10*(24), 14984–15007.

Kumagai, H., Tamaki, Y., & Ishitani, O. (2022). Photocatalytic systems for CO2 reduction: Metal-complex photocatalysts and their hybrids with photofunctional solid materials. *Accounts of Chemical Research, 55*(7), 978–990.

Lazar, L. (2025). Prospective life cycle assessment of early-stage CO_2-removing artificial photosynthesis producing synthesis gas, hydrogen peroxide, and methane. *Energy Technology, 2402224.*

Lee, M., Haas, S., Smirnov, V., Merdzhanova, T., & Rau, U. (2022). Scalable photovoltaic-electrochemical cells for hydrogen production from water-recent advances. *ChemElectroChem, 9*(24), e202200838.

Lee, Y. W., Boonmongkolras, P., Son, E. J., Kim, J., Lee, S. H., Kuk, S. K., Ko, J. W., Shin, B., & Park, C. B. (2018). Unbiased biocatalytic solar-to-chemical conversion by FeOOH/BiVO4/perovskite tandem structure. *Nature Communications, 9*(1), 4208.

Liu, J. (2016). Advanced materials for solar energy harnessing and conversion. In *Design, fabrication, properties and applications of smart and advanced materials* (pp. 413–459). CRC Press.

Liu, J., De Bastiani, M., Aydin, E., Harrison, G. T., Gao, Y., Pradhan, R. R., Eswaran, M. K., Mandal, M., Yan, W., Seitkhan, A., & Babics, M. (2022). Efficient and stable perovskite-silicon tandem solar cells through contact displacement by MgF x. *Science, 377*(6603), 302–306.

Liu, Y., Xu, Y., Zhang, F., Yun, J., & Shen, Z. (2014). The impact of biofuel plantation on biodiversity: A review. *Chinese Science Bulletin, 59*(34), 4639–4651.

Liu, Z., Ding, R., Xue, F., Zhao, X., Chen, Z., Zheng, H., Li, P., Yan, Q., Xu, L., Xiong, J., & Peng, Q. (2023). MXene-reduced graphene oxide sponge-based solar evaporators with integrated water-thermal management by anisotropic design. *Communications Materials, 4*(1), 70.

MacFarlane, D. R., Cherepanov, P. V., Choi, J., Suryanto, B. H., Hodgetts, R. Y., Bakker, J. M., Vallana, F. M. F., & Simonov, A. N. (2020). A roadmap to the ammonia economy. *Joule, 4*(6), 1186–1205.

Machín, A., Cotto, M., Ducongé, J., & Márquez, F. (2023). Artificial photosynthesis: Current advancements and future prospects. *Biomimetics, 8*(3), 298.

Maeda, K., & Domen, K. (2010). Photocatalytic water splitting: Recent progress and future challenges. *The Journal of Physical Chemistry Letters, 1*(18), 2655–2661.

Mandad, T., Chaubey, S., & Chaubey, V. (2025). Eco-friendly conversion of carbon dioxide into solar fuels via artificial photosynthetic routes: A review. *Main Group Chemistry, 24*(1), 3–16.

Manzhos, S., Chueh, C. C., Giorgi, G., Kubo, T., Saianand, G., Luder, J., Sonar, P., & Ihara, M. (2021). Materials design and optimization for next-generation solar cell and light-emitting technologies. *The Journal of Physical Chemistry Letters, 12*(19), 4638–4657.

McConnell, I., Li, G., & Brudvig, G. W. (2010). Energy conversion in natural and artificial photosynthesis. *Chemistry & Biology, 17*(5), 434–447.

Mori, S., Hashimoto, R., Hisatomi, T., Domen, K., & Saito, S. (2025). Artificial photosynthesis directed toward organic synthesis. *Nature Communications, 16*(1), 1797.

Navarro-Jaén, S., Virginie, M., Bonin, J., Robert, M., Wojcieszak, R., & Khodakov, A. Y. (2021). Highlights and challenges in the selective reduction of carbon dioxide to methanol. *Nature Reviews Chemistry, 5*(8), 564–579.

Nocera, D. G. (2012). The artificial leaf. *Accounts of Chemical Research, 45*(5), 767–776.

Nwabueze, Q. A., & Leggett, S. (2024). Advancements in the application of CO2 capture and utilization technologies-a comprehensive review. *Fuels, 5*(3), 508–532.

Pihosh, Y., Turkevych, I., Mawatari, K., Uemura, J., Kazoe, Y., Kosar, S., Makita, K., Sugaya, T., Matsui, T., Fujita, D., & Tosa, M. (2015). Photocatalytic generation of hydrogen by core-shell WO3/BiVO4 nanorods with ultimate water splitting efficiency. *Scientific Reports, 5*(1), 11141.

Rahman, S. R., Eng, N. E., Ashraf, M. A., Pang, W. L., Tan, K. B., Singh, A. K., & Chan, K. Y. (2025). Energy harvesting from living plant: A review on past research and way forward. *Energy Reports, 14*, 268–281.

Shiraishi, Y., Matsumoto, M., Ichikawa, S., Tanaka, S., & Hirai, T. (2021). Polythiophene-doped resorcinol–formaldehyde resin photocatalysts for solar-to-hydrogen peroxide energy conversion. *Journal of the American Chemical Society, 143*(32), 12590–12599.

Solanki, V., & Birman, S. (2024). Nature-driven renewable energy systems for sustainable development. In *Nature-based solutions in achieving sustainable development goals: Harmonizing nature and Progress* (pp. 131–166). Cham.

Tachibana, Y., Vayssieres, L., & Durrant, J. R. (2012). Artificial photosynthesis for solar water-splitting. *Nature Photonics, 6*(8), 511–518.

Takeda, H., Cometto, C., Ishitani, O., & Robert, M. (2017). Electrons, photons, protons and earth-abundant metal complexes for molecular catalysis of CO2 reduction. *ACS Catalysis, 7*(1), 70–88.

Thangamuthu, M., Ruan, Q., Ohemeng, P. O., Luo, B., Jing, D., Godin, R., & Tang, J. (2022). Polymer photoelectrodes for solar fuel production: Progress and challenges. *Chemical Reviews, 122*(13), 11778–11829.

Udaypal, G., & R. K., Mehariya, S. & Verma, P. (2024). Advances in microalgae-based carbon sequestration: Current status and future perspectives. *Environmental Research, 249*, 118397.

Wang, Y., Wei, J. X., Tang, H. L., Shao, L. H., Dong, L. Z., Chu, X. Y., Jiang, Y. X., Zhang, G. L., Zhang, F. M., & Lan, Y. Q. (2024). Artificial photosynthetic system for diluted CO2 reduction in gas-solid phase. *Nature Communications, 15*(1), 8818.

Wang, Z., Hu, Y., Zhang, S., & Sun, Y. (2022a). Artificial photosynthesis systems for solar energy conversion and storage: Platforms and their realities. *Chemical Society Reviews, 51*(15), 6704–6737.

Wang, Z., Hu, Y., Zhang, S., & Sun, Y. (2022b). Artificial photosynthesis systems for solar energy conversion and storage: Platforms and their realities. *Chemical Society Reviews, 51*(15), 6704–6737.

Wang, Z., Hu, Y., Zhang, S., & Sun, Y. (2022c). Artificial photosynthesis systems for solar energy conversion and storage: Platforms and their realities. *Chemical Society Reviews, 51*(15), 6704–6737.

Wu, B., Fan, X., Xue, C., Chang, Q., Yang, J., Hu, S., & Xu, H. (2025). High-performing clean water production by rational design of functional solar evaporator and vapor condensation. *Advanced. Science, e05008.*

Wu, L., Dong, Z., Cai, Z., Ganapathy, T., Fang, N. X., Li, C., Yu, C., Zhang, Y., & Song, Y. (2020). Highly efficient three-dimensional solar evaporator for high salinity desalination by localized crystallization. *Nature Communications, 11*(1), 521.

Yang, Y., Liu, L. N., Tian, H., Cooper, A. I., & Sprick, R. S. (2023). Making the connections: Physical and electric interactions in biohybrid photosynthetic systems. *Energy & Environmental Science, 16*(10), 4305–4319.

Yu, J. M., Lee, J., Kim, Y. S., Song, J., Oh, J., Lee, S. M., Jeong, M., Kim, Y., Kwak, J. H., Cho, S., & Yang, C. (2020). High-performance and stable photoelectrochemical water splitting cell with organic-photoactive-layer-based photoanode. *Nature Communications, 11*(1), 5509.

Zhao, H., Sun, J., Kumar, S., Li, P., Thalluri, S. M., Wang, Z. M., & Thumu, U. (2024). Recent advances in metal halide perovskite based photocatalysts for artificial photosynthesis and organic transformations. *Chemical Communications, 60*(46), 5890–5911.

Zhou, X., Zeng, Y., Lv, F., Bai, H., & Wang, S. (2021). Organic semiconductor–organism interfaces for augmenting natural and artificial photosynthesis. *Accounts of Chemical Research, 55*(2), 156–170.

Chapter 3
Progress and Challenges in Photo-Bioreactors: Development of Photo-Bioreactor Technology and Its Applications in Biofuel Production—Technical and Economical Challenges

Bobita Ray and Suchitra Rakesh

Abstract Photobioreactors are closed cultivation systems that grow photosynthetic microorganisms like microalgae and cyanobacteria in a controlled environment. The PBR facilitates controlled conditions, viz., carbon dioxide supply, nutrient level, pH, temperature, etc., for higher product purity growth rates. Various construction designs are used for PBRs, such as flat panels, tubular, vertical-column, etc. PBRs produce valuable products like biofuels, pharmaceuticals, pigments and food ingredients. The chapter provides detailed insight into various modes and systems of microalgae cultivation. The chapter also dealt with various photobioreactors with advantages and limitations of each model, mechanism of gas–liquid flow, enhancement of co-transfer and biomass productivity in PBRs, strategies for effective light transfer and nutrient utilization, Scale-up strategies and applications of PBRS. Finally, it discusses the technical and economic challenges with future perspectives.

Keywords Microalgae cultivation · Photobioreactors · Open cultivation · Biofuels · Limitations

3.1 Introduction

Microalgae cultivation for biofuel production has recently gained significant attention, and future research is projecting towards its commercial applications. With rising global energy demand and the environmental drawbacks of fossil fuel dependence, alternative renewable energy sources are being actively explored. Fossil fuels,

B. Ray · S. Rakesh (✉)
Biofuel Research Laboratory, Department of Microbiology, Central University of Tamil Nadu, Thiruvarur, Tamil Nadu, India
e-mail: suchitrar@cutn.ac.in

P. Verma (ed.), *Sustainable Practices in Biorefinery*,
https://doi.org/10.1007/978-981-95-6071-4_3

formed over geological time scales through fossilization, are finite and contribute significantly to greenhouse gas emissions. In contrast, biofuels are derived from biomass through biochemical and thermochemical processes, providing a more sustainable pathway for energy generation (Vaniyankandy et al., 2022). Microalgae comprises of rapid growth rate and high photosynthetic efficiency out of all sources for biofuel and other value-added products (Ray et al., 2023). The biomass generated from microalgae is 10–50 times higher than terrestrial plants (Vassilev et al., 2016). In addition, a crucial role in CO_2 sequestration by microalgae offers dual benefits of energy production and climate mitigation (Udaypal et al., 2024a). However, microalgaemass cultivation for biofuel commercialization involves open systems (open pond and raceways) and closed system (photobioreactors). Each system offers unique advantages and limitations, influencing their suitability for commercial biofuel production (Vassilev et al., 2016; Dhanvanti et al., 2024).

Among the various microalgae cultivation systems, the photobioreactor is the most preferred for large-scale biomass production, as it ensures purity of the culture without contamination (Razzak et al., 2024). These photobioreactors are usually used to grow photosynthetic organisms like microalgae, cyanobacteria, etc. The photobioreactor provides a controlled environment, viz., light availability, pH, temperature, carbon supply, and nutrients for the optimal growth and productivity of the microorganism (Chanquia et al., 2021; Fu et al., 2019). Since the PBRs have a closed configuration, chances of getting contamination will be nil as there is no direct contact between the culture and the outside environment (Tan et al., 2020). Based on the purpose for growth, scale and cost consideration, various PBRs are designed with distinct principles and operational features (Fu et al., 2019). This chapter discusses the fundamental aspects of photobioreactors and their types. Further, the chapter focuses on scale-up strategies and applications. Finally, the technical and economic challenges with future perspectives are discussed.

3.2 Various Modes of Microalgae Cultivation

The rapid growth rate and potential to generate high biomass make microalgae the most desired candidate for biofuel production. Hence, much global attention has been paid to large-scale cultivation for commercial applications. However, efficient cultivation requires the growth parameters like pH, temperature, etc., to be carefully regulated as they directly influence algal growth and biochemical productivity. The algae can be grown in various modes of cultivation, viz., phototrophic, heterotrophic, mixotrophic and photoheterotrophic. Each cultivation mode offers certain benefits and limitations, mainly concerning biomass yield, biochemical composition, and suitability for biofuel production (Ray et al., 2022; Udayan et al., 2022). The principal modes of microalgae cultivation are discussed below:

I. *Phototrophic Cultivation*

The phototrophic mode of microalgae cultivation is the primary and most widely used cultivation strategy, where CO_2 and sunlight are the primary sources of carbon and energy, respectively. Like plants, microalgae and cyanobacteria perform photosynthesis as the growth mode (Ganesan et al., 2020).

The microalgae under phototrophic mode of cultivation primarily depend on light intensity, wavelength and spectrum, to achieve high photosynthetic efficiency and biochemical composition. In phototrophic systems, CO_2 is fixed through photosynthesis, generating organic compounds essential for cell metabolism and growth. It is pointed out for phototrophic growth the microalgal strains that consists of high light dependent reactions, microalgal growth rate and biomass yield are much more desired (Zhang et al., 2012). Strains such as *Calothrix sp.*, *Chlorella sp.*, and certain green non-sulphur bacteria are widely used in phototrophic cultivation to produce pigments, proteins, and secondary metabolites (Amadu et al., 2021).

II. *Heterotrophic Cultivation*

In heterotrophic cultivation, microalgae are grown without light, utilizing organic substrates as a source of energy and carbon. This approach is relevant to the biofuel industry, as it often results in higher biomass productivity and lipid accumulation than phototrophic cultivation (Ganesan et al., 2020). Studies have reported that heterotrophic cultivation enhances growth and lipid production by 40% in *Chlorella protothecoides* (Xu et al., 2006). Although this method shortens cultivation time and enhances yields, it is associated with high costs of yield due to the requirement for biomass. Hence to overcome the cost of production, recently many studies are projecting towards cultivation of microalgae in wastewater that is enrich with nutrients like rice mill waste water (Venkata Kong et al., 2021; Mohan et al., 2015; Zhan et al., 2017) have been explored to reduce costs. Strains commonly grown under this mode include *C. vulgaris*, *C. protothecoides*, *Crypthecodiniumcohnii*, and *Schizochytriumlimacinum* (Vuppaladadiyam et al., 2018).

III. *Mixotrophic Cultivation*

Mixotrophic cultivation integrates features of both phototrophic and heterotrophic systems, allowing microalgae to utilize sunlight, inorganic CO_2, and organic carbon sources simultaneously (Udaypal et al., 2025b). Compared to purely autotrophic conditions, mixotrophic systems exhibit enhanced respiration and photosynthetic rates, with net photosynthetic activity reported to be nearly 1.5 times higher (Benavente-Valdes et al., 2016). Moreover, the algal strain and the type of organic substrate supplied can influence pigment concentration and photosystem activity. This mode offers the dual advantage of reducing CO_2 emissions through photosynthetic assimilation while maintaining pigment stability, such as β-carotene, under illuminated conditions. Despite lower energy conversion efficiency due to photosynthetic losses, mixotrophy has emerged as a promising strategy for enhancing biomass and metabolite production (Alkhamis & Qin, 2016; Udaypal et al., 2025c).

IV. *Photoheterotrophic Cultivation*

Photoheterotrophic cultivation involves the simultaneous requirement of light and organic carbon sources, but unlike mixotrophy, it does not rely on inorganic CO_2 assimilation. Instead, organic compounds serve as the sole carbon source, while light is primarily utilized for energy and nitrogen fixation. Although this mode has theoretical potential for producing value-added products, it is rarely employed at large scales, mainly due to its dependency on expensive organic substrates and relatively limited productivity outcomes compared to the other modes (Chen et al., 2011; Udayan et al., 2022).

3.3 Various Systems of Microalgal Cultivation

I. *Open Cultivation Systems*

Since the beginning of microalgal cultivation, open pond cultivation system is known to be the most primeval and easiest methods for mass production. These systems can be natural (ponds, lagoons, lakes, shallow water bodies) or artificial (open-raceway ponds, circular ponds) (Goswami et al., 2023). Their main advantages include low construction and operational costs, minimal energy input, and ease of scale-up, making them attractive for industrial applications (Rogers et al., 2014; Udayan et al., 2022).

In artificial circular ponds, the depth generally ranges within 30–70 cm, and approximate width of 45 cm with a centrally positioned rotating agitator that prevents sedimentation of algal biomass. Raceway ponds, constructed from concrete or earth, are among the most widely adopted open pond designs in commercial operations. These systems consist of closed-loop, shallow channels equipped with paddle wheels to maintain circulation and prevent cell settling. Raceway systems are considered cost-effective and energy-efficient options for producing large volumes of biomass (Ummalyma et al., 2023).

Despite these advantages, open cultivation systems face several limitations. Low cell densities, weak light penetration, and inadequate mass and heat transfer often constrain biomass productivity. Environmental fluctuations, such as rainfall, can alter key parameters like salinity and pH, while turbidity from soil erosion further reduces light availability (Fu et al., 2019). Open ponds are also highly susceptible to contamination by bacteria or other microorganisms, which can compromise biomass quality and stability. Significant diurnal temperature variations also present challenges for maintaining consistent growth conditions, further limiting large-scale productivity (Khan et al., 2018).

II. *Closed Cultivation Systems*

Photobioreactors represent closed-loop systems that provide a controlled environment for microalgal growth, requiring less land area and offering higher-quality biomass than open ponds. Several PBR configurations have been developed, including tubular, flat plate, airlift, stirred-tank, membrane, and biofilm-based systems (Mishra et al., 2019).

The tubular PBR is among the most common designs for large-scale applications. It consists of long transparent tubes (glass or plastic) arranged vertically or horizontally to maximise sunlight capture (Goswami et al., 2022). Gas exchange is achieved through spargers, which generate fine bubbles for effective CO_2 distribution and oxygen removal. These systems offer relatively low energy demand and ease of operation. However, their drawbacks include cleaning difficulties, reduced light penetration due to geometry, and decreased photosynthetic efficiency at scale (Huang et al., 2017a, 2017b). Vertical columns provide better gas exchange but have a low surface-to-volume ratio, while horizontal layouts allow greater light exposure but suffer from limited mass transfer and heat accumulation (Ganesan et al., 2020).

The airlift PBR improves culture circulation, preventing sedimentation and maintaining uniform mixing. However, its efficiency decreases with long tube lengths, which may lead to uneven substrate concentrations and reduced yields. Compared to bubble column PBR, random cell flow patterns often limit the performance, which can lead to uneven light exposure and increased cell sedimentation. Moreover, these columns exhibit lower productivity than tubular systems, though they remain attractive for applications where ease of operation and scalability outweigh maximum yield (Deprá et al., 2024). Flat plate PBRs, constructed from transparent rectangular panels (1–5 cm depth), provide high surface area-to-volume ratios, minimise oxygen accumulation, and enhance photosynthetic efficiency. Their main limitation is shear stress from aeration, which can damage sensitive cells (Gupta et al., 2015).

Stirred-tank PBRs are widely applied for heterotrophic and mixotrophic cultivation, offering efficient nutrient distribution and gas exchange. These systems are especially suitable for unicellular strains, though filamentous microalgae may suffer shear-related damage. Self-shading often limits light penetration, but internal light sources can improve illumination. Effective sparging ensures sufficient CO_2 supply, supporting photosynthetic performance (Erband et al., 2020).

Innovations such as membrane PBRs integrate separation technologies that enable biofilm formation on membrane surfaces. This approach improves nutrient uptake, gas exchange, and biomass productivity, while allowing customization of membrane properties to suit different strains (Roopashri & Makam, 2022). Similarly, biofilm PBRs enhance light penetration and reduce land footprint. Recent advances include 3D-printed porous biofilm reactors, which support biofilm growth and channel light directly into cultures, boosting productivity (Zeng et al., 2023).

While closed systems provide better control, reduced contamination, and higher productivity, they are constrained by high capital and operational costs and technical challenges in cleaning and scalability. For better understanding about the prospects and limitations of open and various closed systems, those are briefly mentioned in Table 3.1.

Table 3.1 Table showing the prospects and limitations of microalgae cultivation in various systems

Culture systems	Prospects	Limitations	References
Open ponds	Simple set up system Easy to construct and scale up Microalgae cultures are uniformly exposed to sunlight Operational cost is low Widely used for mass cultivation	Requires huge acres of land for cultivation Contamination from other microorganisms reducing culture stability Regulating environmental factors such as light intensity, temperature and pH Seasonal variations influences productivity	(Fu et al., 2019; Udayan et al., 2022)
Horizontal column tubular PBR	Maximizes light exposure over larger area Scalable for outdoor use Well approachable for continuous operation	Heat accumulation along tubes Reduced mass transfer efficiency Cleaning and fouling challenge	(Mishra et al., 2019; Huang et al., 2017a, 2017b)
Vertical column tubular PBR	Better gas exchange and mixing Reduces heat build up compared to horizontal	Less light capture efficiency Limited scalability	(Mishra et al., 2019; Ganesan et al., 2020)
Flat plate PBR	Better light utilization Low O_2 accumulation High photosynthetic efficiency	Shear stress damages sensitive cells Scale up challenges Materials are expensive	(Gupta et al., 2015)
Airlift PBR	Improved mixing and circulation Reduced sedimentation More uniform environment than bubble	Efficiency declines with long tubes Uneven substrate distribution Biomass yields still lower than tubular	(Deprá et al., 2024)
Bubble column PBR	Simple design, low cost Good gas–liquid mixing Scalable for certain applications	Occurs random cell flow with uneven light High cell sedimentation Lower productivity than tubular PBRs	(Deprá et al., 2024)

(continued)

Table 3.1 (continued)

Culture systems	Prospects	Limitations	References
Stirred tank PBR	Efficient nutrient distribution and gas exchange Suitable for heterotrophic and mixotrophic cultures Well established in fermentation industries	Shear stress damages filamentous strain Self shading reduces light Maintenance is quiet expensive	(Erband et al., 2020)
Membrane PBR	Promotes biofilm formation Enhance nutrient uptake and gas exchange Customizable membrane properties	High operational and material costs Membrane fouling and cleaning challenge	(Roopashri & Makam, 2022)
Biofilm PBR	Reduced land footprint Enhanced light penetration 3D printed reactors improve light distribution and biofilm growth	Limited to biofilm forming strains Scale up complexity High initial set up cost	(Zeng et al., 2023)

3.4 Mechanism of Gas–Liquid Flow in Photobioreactors

The gas–liquid interactions within PBR facilitates effective mixing and mass transfer, both of which are essential for cell growth. Aeration of PBR with CO_2-enriched gas bubbles allows mixing that leads to the internal circulation of culture suspension, and also prevents the microalgal cells from adhering to the walls and settling to the bottom of the PBR (Ye et al., 2018a, 2018b). The flow within the internal system not only promotes mixing between nutrients and microalgal cells but also guarantees their even distribution, thereby supporting improved growth rates (Carvalho et al., 2006). Mixing also ensures the uniform light exposure to all the microalgal cells, hence ensuring the transfer of CO_2 molecules from bubbles to microalgal cells. Hence, this gas–liquid flow removes the oxygen and heat produced during photosynthesis, thereby requiring pH and temperature in the PBR to be maintained for microalgal growth (Pires et al., 2017). Every high aeration leads to excessive mixing, which may damage the cells; hence, biomass production for *C. vulgaris* is decreased when cultivated in a bubble column PBR (Khoo et al., 2016; Wang & Lan, 2018). Elevated aeration rates generate intense shear forces as air bubbles rupture, which can damage microalgal cells, hinder growth, and ultimately lead to cell death (Lopez-Rosales et al., 2015). Therefore, maintaining an optimal gas–liquid two phase flow is crucial for sustaining microalgal growth and maximizing CO_2 fixation efficiency in PBRs (Table 3.2).

In recent years, increasing attention has been given to understanding gas–liquid flow and mass transfer in different PBRs through both experimental studies and numerical simulations. Simulation of two-phase flow in open raceway ponds revealed inefficient mixing of algal suspensions, often leading to cell settling at the bottom. In contrast, improved circulation and mixing were observed in the curved sections of the ponds (Prussi et al., 2014). Nauha and Alopaeus (2013) modeled microalgal growth kinetics, gas–liquid flow, and mass transfer in a column PBR, demonstrating that alternating movement of cells between illuminated and shaded regions can significantly improve biomass productivity. Similarly, computational fluid dynamics simulations of gas–liquid flow in tubular PBRs showed that incorporating spiral spoilers enhanced culture mixing and circulation, thereby promoting more efficient light–dark cycling and boosting microalgal growth (Zhang et al., 2013a, b). In bubble column PBRs, particle image velocimetry has been employed to visualize gas–liquid flow patterns with bottom gas injection. The findings indicated that the incorporation of internal baffles enhances mixing efficiency and prevents biomass accumulation by promoting more uniform gas–liquid distribution (Bitog et al., 2014). Hence, efficient mixing of multiphase flows within PBRs are crucial for their optimal design and reliable operation (Yang et al., 2014). Few studies treated PBR with a three-phase system, i.e., liquid (culture medium), solid (algal cells) and gas phase (CO_2 bubbles). Coupling all three phases to the biochemical interactions is the work that needs to be done in the future.

Table 3.2 Recent Advances in photobioreactors for microalgae cultivation

Type of PBR	Microalgal species	Objective	Biomass productivity	References
Flat panel PBR	*Chlorella sorokiniana* IPPAS C-1	CO_2 utilization efficiency	7.1 ± 0.4 g DW L^{-1}	(Groff et al., 2025)
Vertical column PBR	*Chlorella* spp. (FAUBA-17)	High value biomass	1.07 ± 0.1 g/L	(Gabrielyan et al., 2025)
Tubular PBR	*Scenedesmus obliquus UTEX 393*	Microalgal growth and biomass productivity	0.65 $g{\cdot}L^{-1}d^{-1}$	(Buscaglia et al., 2025)
Vertical Tubular PBR	*Arthrospira platensis*	Protein	52.64 ± 2.51 $g{\cdot}100\ g^{-1}$ dry weight	(Milia et al., 2025)
Hybrid PBR	*Arthrospira platensis*	CO_2 fixation	3 g L^{-1}	(Kubar et al., 2025)
Flat plate PBR	*Arthrospira platensis*	Biomass growth	0.126 g $L^{-1}.d^{-1}$	(Amanna et al., 2025)

3.5 Enhancement of CO_2 Transfer and Biomass Productivity in Photobioreactors

The photoautotrophic growth of microalgae in the photobioreactor will be improved by injecting CO_2 in bubbles form through gas aerator. CO_2 faces dissolution, transfer, absorption and biofixation processes and bubble rising. Since microalgae can only assimilate CO_2 dissolved in the liquid phase, bubble dynamics play a key role in determining mass transfer efficiency within PBRs by altering the gas–liquid flow patterns (Ding et al., 2016). Hence, bubble dissolution and kinetic properties are important parameters for enhanced microalgal growth and CO_2 biofixation capability.

CO_2 dissolving rate is an important parameter that decides microalgae growth in PBRs. The rate of CO_2 dissolution from bubble to microalgae suspension will be decided by the gas–liquid contacting area, bubble diameter, retention time of bubble and aeration (Fernandez et al., 2013). The strategies of effective CO_2 transfer for enhanced biomass productivity are mentioned below:

I. *Bubble Diameter and Gas–Liquid Contacting Area*

The bubble's diameter will generate within PBR influenced by factors such as aerator's diameter, the spacing of its perforations and effective contact area with the liquid medium. Among the various gas aerators commercially available, the multihole rubber pipe aerator is preferred for microalgae cultivation, as it provides tiny bubbles with the required diameter and hole spacing (Xia et al., 2018). Small gas aerators are more efficient for mixing and transferring mass amount in PBRs. The round stomata plate gas aerator is an advanced aerator with an inner pore diameter of 0.5 mm and a pore spacing of 1.5 mm (Huang et al., 2017a, b). This aerator provides more gas–liquid contacting area and facilitates mass transfer of 11.72 per hour in a cylindrical PBR. Hence, a higher biomass concentration of 2.88 g per L was obtained compared to the commercial rubber pipe aerator (1.57 g per L) reported by Huang et al., (2017a, 2017b). In a raceway pond, the CO_2 transfer rate is enhanced using a microporous fibrous diaphragm aerator with gradient micropores of 6–126 μm (Cheng et al., 2019). Falinski et al. (2018) utilized a minute-pore air stone diffuser for an efficient CO_2 mass transfer coefficient. The membrane module, viz., hollow fibre membrane that provides more gas–liquid contacting area, is highly efficient in reducing the bubble's diameter and improving the mass transfer efficiency of CO_2 (Zheng et al., 2016). As result of their enhanced surface availability, the hollow fibre membranes also improve the utilisation of CO_2 in microalgae suspension (Kim et al., 2016). Hence, for efficient gas–liquid mass transfer, the design of a gas aerator with a suitable pore size is a must.

II. *Bubble Retention Time*

The CO_2 dissolution in the PBR can be enhanced by rising bubble retention time. The photobioreactor's velocity and bubble rising pathway usually determine the bubble retention time. The CO_2 bubble generated from the gas aerator at the bottom of the airlift-driven raceway path increases the bubble retention time by 200% (Ketheesan &

Nirmalakhandan, 2012). This will further improve the CO_2 utilization efficiency and biomass productivity. The reduced pressure on the surface of the raceway pond facilitates rapid release of the CO_2 bubble. Hence, open raceway ponds are covered with a transparent sheet to raise the gas pressure. Thereby, the bubble rising velocity will be reduced and thus, bubble retention time within PBR will be increased (Li et al., 2013). Li et al. (2013) presented an advanced demonstration of closed raceway pond for enhanced CO_2 fixation efficiency. Hence, many advanced models of closed PBRs, like gas-lift circumflex column PBRs with serial lantern-shaped draft tubes, have been developed to increase the bubble retention time (Ye et al., 2018a, 2018b). In a liquid foam-bed PBR, bubbles with prolonged retention time, improved both mass transfer and biomass productivity. The presence of the surfactant Pluronic F68 helps stabilize the foam, allowing microalgal cells to adhere to its surface as it rises toward the top of the reactor. Because the foam rises more slowly than free bubbles, a greater number of cells attach to it, thereby extending the retention period and enhancing the CO_2 mass transfer coefficient (Janoska et al., 2018). The foam's high retention time allows microalgal cells to receive full light exposure. Biomass productivity will be enhanced; however, using pumps during commercialization involves huge operating costs for liquid foam-bed PBR. Hence, the expenses associated with gas transfer must be carefully evaluated for economical PBR commercialization design. The PBR with proper internal setup will be a good option not only from an economic point of view, but also for significant gas transfer and CO_2 utilization efficiency.

III. *Other Factors Influencing CO_2 Transfer in PBRs*

The mode of operation of gas aerators is an important factor that affects CO_2 dissolution and its transfer. For example, the swing gas aerator with a rubber pipe is more efficient for the CO_2 mass transfer coefficient than the oscillating gas aerator with an oscillating baffle (Yang et al., 2016a, 2016b). The intermittent aeration is also an important parameter for enhancing the CO_2 fixation rate in PBRs. The PIAT (Perforated Inverted Arc Trough) static mixer with pores on the surface in flat-plate PBR facilitates intermittent aeration (Xia et al., 2018). In the PIAT system, CO_2 gas tends to accumulate within the internal structures, leading to elevated pressure in the gas zone and thereby enhancing its solubilization and transport. Additionally, intermittent aeration provided by the PIAT static mixer promotes higher biomass concentration and improves the overall CO_2 fixation rate.

3.6 Strategies for Effective Light Transfer and Nutrients Utilization for PBRs

The PBR is capable to harvest for more microalgal photosynthetic energy, which can be further utilized for biomass accumulation (Chen et al., 2011). Hence, PBRs are usually constructed using highly transparent material with a high surface-to-volume ratio with flat panel and tubular designs being the most preferred industrial-scale microalgal biomass yield (Wang et al., 2012). In PBRs, the light distribution is usually not uniform for several reasons, such as light attenuation due to absorption, light scattering by pigment-enriched microalgae and the self-shading effect (Jung et al., 2014). The PBRs are usually divided into three important regions based on the light availability and microalgal growth rate, i.e., 1. Photoinhibition region (this region suppresses cell growth due to light intensity exceeding optimal levels) 2. Photo-limited region (this region restricts cell growth, although the growth rate rises with increasing light absorption); 3. Stagnation region (cell growth in this region is very limited since the light intensity is insufficient to sustain it). The light attenuation effect on microalgal growth can be overcome using light guiding materials and periodic pre-harvesting of cells with recycled medium (Liu et al., 2018; Sun et al., 2016). Light can be effectively utilized by properly circulating microalgal cells between the light and dark areas at an appropriate frequency (Yang et al., 2016a, 2016b, 2016c).

Like light, efficient utilization of nutrients is also important for growth of photosynthetic organisms. The two major nutrients required for microalgal growth are nitrogen and phosphorus (Chang et al., 2019). The phototrophic cultivation of microalgae requires inorganic nitrogen like nitrate, nitrite and ammonia, of which nitrates are commonly preferred. The phosphorus sources commonly used for microalgae phototrophic cultivation are biphosphate and dihydric phosphate (Xu et al., 2010). In PBRs, if the nitrogen concentration is reduced, the total chlorophyll in cells and the demand for light and CO_2 will be reduced, affecting the microalgae's photosynthetic efficiency. The high nitrogen concentration will also hinder microalgae growth (Beuckels et al., 2015). The major role phosphorus plays is to act as a substrate involved in various aspects of photosynthesis, like light absorption, formation of assimilative force, key enzymes regulation and assimilated product transportation (Xin et al., 2010). The appropriate amount or supply of nitrogen and phosphorus to PBR is significant for microalgae growth (Chang et al., 2016). A high microalgal biomass concentration is achieved by continuously supplying N and P from the feeding medium to the microalgal suspension through a membrane in the novel PBR (Fig. 3.1 and Table 3.1).

3.7 Applications of Photobioreactors

Photobioreactors (PBRs) represent a flexible and controlled platform for large-scale microalgal cultivation, supporting applications that range from renewable energy to high-value bioproducts. The closed configuration of PBRs allows fine regulation of growth conditions such as light intensity, nutrient supply, carbon dioxide concentration, and mixing which enhances product yield and minimizes contamination compared to open systems. These advantages make PBRs particularly attractive for industries targeting biofuels, pharmaceuticals, pigments, and functional food ingredients.

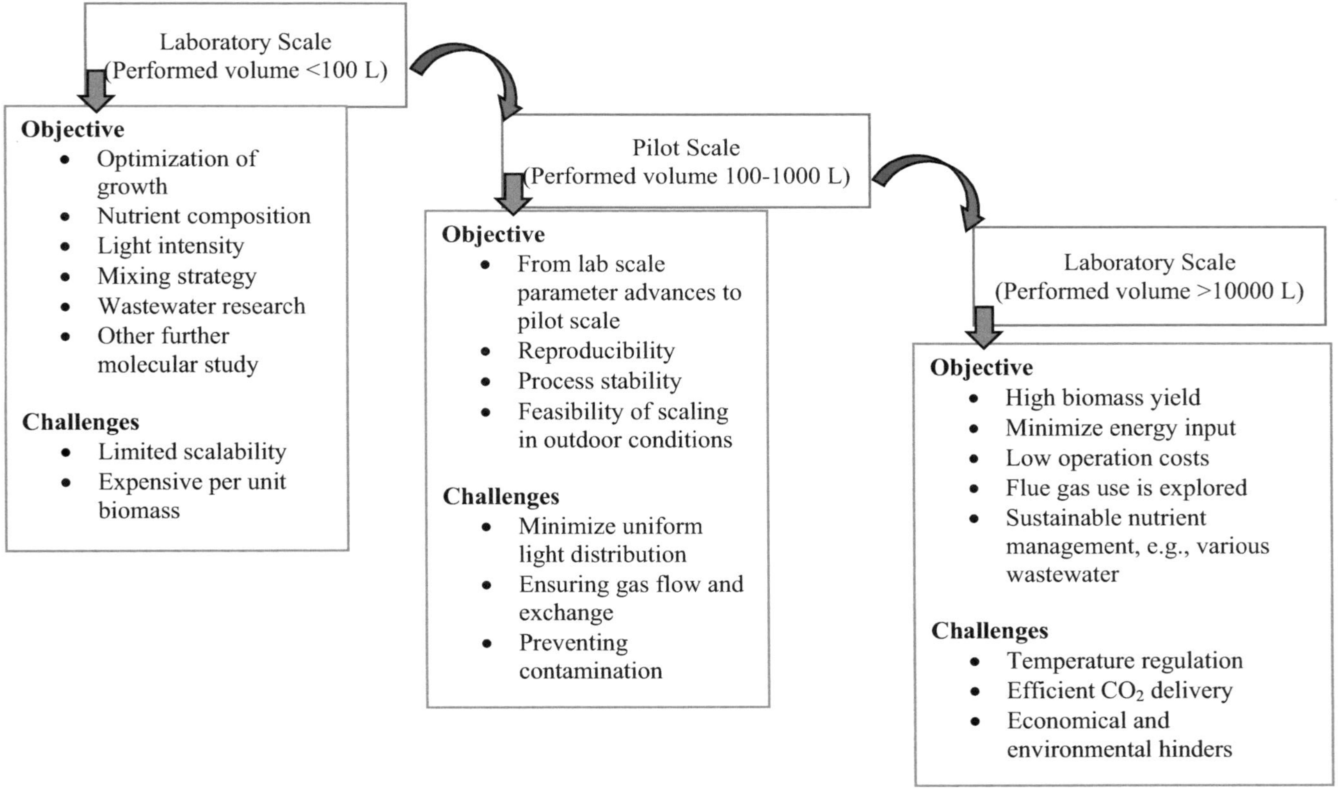

Fig. 3.1 Scale-up for photobioreactors: This flowchart represents calling-up strategies of photobioreactors (PBRs) from laboratory to pilot and industrial levels, highlighting key objectives and challenges at each stage. The diagram illustrates the progressive transition from small-scale experimental systems to large-scale commercial operations, emphasizing optimization of growth conditions, technical feasibility, and economic viability

Biofuels

Microalgae grown in PBRs are widely recognized as a potential feedstock for sustainable biofuel production. The ability of microalgae to accumulate substantial lipid and carbohydrate reserves under stress conditions, such as nutrient limitation or high light exposure, can be strategically exploited in PBRs. The controlled nature of these systems ensures uniform exposure to growth stressors, leading to higher yields of lipid and starch precursors suitable for biodiesel and bioethanol production. Comparative studies demonstrate that species like *Chlorella*, *Botryococcus*, and *Nannochloropsis* achieve significantly greater biomass and lipid productivity in PBRs than in open pond systems. However, despite the technical promise, large-scale cultivation is still hindered by challenges related to construction costs, energy demand, and downstream harvesting (Ganesan et al., 2020; Mazzei et al., 2017).

Pharmaceuticals

Microalgae are a valuable source of bioactive molecules with therapeutic and nutraceutical potential, including polyunsaturated fatty acids (PUFAs), carotenoids, flavonoids, and antioxidant compounds (Goswami et al., 2021). The pharmaceutical industry particularly benefits from PBR cultivation because the closed system ensures consistent metabolite profiles and reduces contamination risk, critical for compliance with regulatory standards. For instance, *Haematococcuspluvialis* cultured in PBRs is the major source of pharmaceutical-grade astaxanthin, while *Spirulina* is cultivated for bioactive peptides and immune-boosting metabolites. These compounds are explored for applications in anti-inflammatory, antimicrobial, anticancer, and cardiovascular health formulations (Deniz et al., 2020; Lee et al., 2023).

Pigments

Natural pigments produced by microalgae, such as carotenoids (β-carotene, lutein, astaxanthin), chlorophylls, and phycobiliproteins, are gaining industrial importance as natural colorants, antioxidants, and food additives (Udaypal et al., 2025a). PBRs provide the advantage of inducing pigment biosynthesis through controlled stress regimes, such as high light intensity or nitrogen starvation, while maintaining culture stability. For example, *Dunaliella* and *Haematococcus* strains cultivated in optimized PBR systems have been shown to accumulate pigments at concentrations several folds higher than in unregulated open ponds. Additionally, the closed environment of PBRs facilitates improved pigment extraction and stabilization, preventing degradation from environmental fluctuations during biomass production (Lee et al., 2023; Udayan et al., 2022).

Food Ingredients

Microalgae cultivated in PBRs also serve as an excellent source of nutritional ingredients, including proteins, vitamins, minerals, essential fatty acids, and dietary fibre. Species such as *Chlorella* and *Spirulina* are commonly grown in semi-closed or fully closed systems to produce protein powders, nutraceutical supplements, and functional food ingredients. PBR cultivation ensures higher product safety by lowering the risk of contamination with pathogens or toxins, while also improving the reproducibility of nutritional profiles. Beyond basic nutrition, PBR-derived microalgal biomass contributes to functional foods by enhancing flavor, texture, and color, and by supplying health-promoting compounds such as omega-3 fatty acids and antioxidants (Matos et al., 2017; Mazzei et al., 2017).

3.8 Challenges and Future Perspectives in Large-Scale Microalgal Cultivation

Despite the considerable potential of microalgae in biofuels and value-added products, large-scale cultivation continues to face significant hurdles. One of the foremost challenges is the demand for substantial quantities of water and nutrients to sustain mass production. To reduce freshwater dependency and improve cost efficiency, wastewater has been widely investigated as a culture medium. While wastewater not only supplements nutrients but also supports circular bioeconomy principles, its use introduces challenges such as contamination risks and the difficulty of sterilization. Even autoclaving, though effective for small-scale operations, is impractical at industrial scale due to its high energy requirements, creating barriers for sustainable large-volume cultivation (Ray et al., 2022; Ramsundar et al., 2017).

PBR-based cultivation has demonstrated promising results but remains at a relatively early stage of technological maturity. By contrast, large-scale open pond systems are already operational but encounter major drawbacks such as low productivity, contamination, and fluctuating environmental conditions. Although photobioreactors address some of these issues, their operation requires significant energy and capital inputs, with the balance between production cost and yield still under optimization (Liao et al., 2014).

Alternative cultivation modes, such as heterotrophic and mixotrophic systems, have been explored to overcome limitations of phototrophic growth. These systems allow microalgae to grow in low-light or dark environments with higher productivity, but they rely on supplementation with organic carbon sources. Glucose is often the preferred substrate, though its addition substantially increases production costs. Furthermore, in mixotrophic systems, elevated glucose concentrations may negatively impact lipid accumulation, thereby reducing biofuel potential (Cheirslip and Torpee, 2012). Membrane-based cultivation, such as hollow fiber photobioreactors, has also been trialed, though challenges remain due to clogging by algal cells, which limits their long-term functionality.

Advancing photobioreactor technologies from laboratory scale to commercial scale requires a comprehensive, multi-pronged strategy. This includes operational optimization, innovative engineering design, capacity building, infrastructure development, and rigorous evaluation of both economic and environmental feasibility. Strengthened collaboration among academic institutions, industries, and government agencies is essential to accelerate progress in photobioreactor development. Moreover, policy measures such as tax incentives and support for pilot-scale demonstrations are vital for assessing system performance under real-world conditions. Standardization of processes and optimization of cultivation protocols will help reduce operational costs and improve efficiency, paving the way for broader adoption of PBR technologies (Algavia, 2024).

To bridge the gap between open and closed systems, hybrid cultivation strategies are being investigated. These approaches aim to combine the advantages of both systems, such as initiating microalgal growth in closed PBRs under controlled conditions before transferring cultures to open ponds for large-scale biomass production (Narala et al., 2016). Similarly, efforts to improve photobioreactor performance have led to the development of advanced flat-plate systems, including twin-layer configurations that combine flat-plate and plastic photobioreactors, which enhance light capture and improve efficiency (Udayan et al., 2022; Vo et al., 2019). Commercial applications already provide evidence of success: for example, a company in the Czech Republic has achieved large-scale production of astaxanthin using flat-plate PBRs, demonstrating the potential of these technologies to move beyond research into viable industrial solutions.

3.9 Conclusions

The future of photobioreactors (PBRs) in microalgae cultivation is highly promising, with significant potential to advance biotechnology, environmental sustainability, and renewable energy production. A thorough understanding of the physical and biological parameters that govern algal growth, biomass yield, and metabolite synthesis is central to the effective design and operation of these systems. The ability to customize photobioreactor configurations for specific algal strains and desired bioproducts or biofuel production, further strengthens their industrial relevance.

Continued innovations aimed at reducing operational costs, enhancing energy efficiency, and improving productivity will be pivotal for the global integration of PBR technologies. Overcoming the current technological and economic challenges associated with large-scale cultivation will require both research-driven advancements and knowledge gained from practical applications of different PBR designs. As these systems progress from laboratory and pilot scales to full industrial production, they are expected to provide scalable and sustainable solutions for producing biofuels, pharmaceuticals, pigments, food ingredients, and other high-value products.

In this context, photobioreactors are poised to play a strategic role in the transition towards a bio-based economy, offering not only environmental benefits but also opportunities for innovation across multiple industrial sectors. With continued interdisciplinary collaboration and technological refinement, PBRs hold the potential to become a cornerstone of sustainable, green, and future-oriented industries.

References

Alkhamis, Y., & Qin, J. G. (2016). Comparison of pigment and proximate compositions of Tisochrysis lutea in phototrophic and mixotrophic cultures. *Journal of Applied Phycology, 28*(1), 35–42.

Amadu, A. A., Qiu, S., Ge, S., Addico, G. N. D., Ameka, G. K., Yu, Z., Xia, W., Abbew, A. W., Shao, D., Champagne, P., & Wang, S. (2021). A review of biopolymer (Poly- β-hydroxybutyrate) synthesis in microbes cultivated on wastewater. *Science of the Total Environment, 756*, Article 143729.

Amanna, B., Bahri, P. A., Zhang, G., & Moheimani, N. R. (2025). Enhancing Arthrospira platensis productivity by optimizing mixing rates in a self-cooling flat plate photobioreactor. *Algal Research, 88*, Article 104035.

Benavente-Valdes, J. R., Aguilar, C., Contreras-Esquivel, J. C., Mendez-Zavala, A., & Montanez, J. (2016). Strategies to enhance the production of photosynthetic pigments and lipids in chlorophycae species. *Biotechnology Reports, 10*, 117–125.

Beuckels, A., Smolders, E., & Muylaert, K. (2015). Nitrogen availability influences phosphorus removal in microalgae-based wastewater treatment. *Water Research, 77*, 98–106.

Bitog, J., Lee, I. B., Lee, C. G., Kim, K. S., Hwang, H. S., Hong, S. W., Seo, I. H., Kwon, K. S., & Mostafa, E. (2011). Application of computational fluid dynamics for modeling and designing photobioreactors for microalgae production: A review. *Computers and Electronics in Agriculture, 76*(2), 131–147.

Buscaglia, L., van den End, F., Janssen, M., & Barbosa, M. (2025). Real-time online monitoring of large-scale tubular photobioreactors through gas-phase composition analysis. *Algal Research*, 104172.

Carvalho, A. P., Meireles, L. A., & Malcata, F. X. (2006). Microalgal reactors: A review of en closed system designs and performances. *Biotechnology Progress, 22*(6), 1490–1506.

Chang, H. X., Fu, Q., Huang, Y., Xia, A., Liao, Q., Zhu, X., Zheng, Y. P., & Sun, C. H. (2016). An annular photobioreactor with ion-exchange-membrane for non-touch microalgae cultivation with wastewater. *Bioresource Technology, 219*, 668–676.

Chang, H., Fu, Q., Zhong, N., Yang, X., Quan, X., Li, S., Fu, J., & Xiao, C. (2019). Microalgal lipids production and nutrients recovery from landfill leachate using membrane photobioreactor. *Bioresource Technology, 277*, 18–26.

Chanquia, S. N., Vernet, G., & Kara, S. (2022). Photobioreactors for cultivation and synthesis: Specifications, challenges, and perspectives. *Engineering in Life Sciences, 22*(12), 712–724.

Cheirsilp, B., & Torpee, S. (2012). Enhanced growth and lipid production of microalgae under mixotrophic culture condition: Effect of light intensity, glucose concentration and fed-batch cultivation. *BioresourTechnol, 110*, 510–516.

Chen, C. Y., Yeh, K. L., Aisyah, R., Lee, D. J., & Chang, J. S. (2011). Cultivation, photo bioreactor design and harvesting of microalgae for biodiesel production: A critical review. *Bioresource Technology, 102*(1), 71–81.

Corbion-AlgaVia™ Culinary Algae Oils. https://www.corbion.com/products/algae-ingredients-products/ Algavia (accessed on 17 December 2024).

Deniz, I. (2020). Scaling-up of Haematococcuspluvialis production in stirred tank photobioreactor. *Bioresource Technology, 310*, Article 123434.

Deprá, M. C., Dias, R. R., Zepka, L. Q., & Jacob-Lopes, E. (2024). Tackling old challenges in microalgal biotechnology: The role of photobioreactors to advance the technology readiness level. *Processes, 13*(1), 51.

Dhanvanti, G. P., Tharunkumar, J., Bobita, R., & Rakesh, S. (2024). Bioconversion of waste to bioethanol production. In *Biotechnological Advances in Biorefinery* (pp. 249–265). Singapore: Springer Nature Singapore.

Ding, Y. D., Zhao, S., Liao, Q., Chen, R., Huang, Y., & Zhu, X. (2016). Effect of CO2 bubbles behaviors on microalgal cells distribution and growth in bubble column photo bioreactor. *International Journal of Hydrogen Energy, 41*(8), 4879–4887.

Erbland, P., Caron, S., Peterson, M., & Alyokhin, A. (2020). Design and performance of a low-cost, automated, large-scale photobioreactor for microalgae production. *Aquacultural Engineering, 90*, Article 102103.
Falinski, K. A., Timmons, M. B., Callan, C., & Laidley, C. (2018). Response of Tisochrysis lutea [Prymnesiophycidae] to aeration conditions in a bench-scale photobioreactor. *Journal of Applied Phycology, 30*(4), 2203–2214.
Fernández, F. A., Sevilla, J. F., & Grima, E. M. (2013). Photobioreactors for the production of microalgae. *Reviews in Environmental Science and Bio/Technology, 12*(2), 131–151.
Fu, J., Huang, Y., Liao, Q., Xia, A., Fu, Q., & Zhu, X. (2019). Photo-bioreactor design for microalgae: A review from the aspect of CO2 transfer and conversion. *Bioresource Technology, 292*, Article 121947.
Gabrielyan, D. A., Sinetova, M. A., Savinykh, G. A., Zadneprovskaya, E. V., Goncharova, M. A., Markelova, A. G., & Lobus, N. V. (2025). Productivity and carbon utilization of three green microalgae strains with high biotechnological potential cultivated in flat-panel photobioreactors. *Phycology, 5*(3), 43.
Ganesan, R., Manigandan, S., Samuel, M. S., Shanmuganathan, R., Brindhadevi, K., Chi, N. T. L., & Pugazhendhi, A. (2020). A review on prospective production of biofuel from microalgae. *Biotechnology Reports, 27*, Article e00509.
Goswami, R. K., Mehariya, S., Verma, P., Lavecchia, R., & Zuorro, A. (2021). Microalgae-based biorefineries for sustainable resource recovery from wastewater. *Journal of Water Process Engineering, 40*, Article 101747.
Goswami, R. K., Agrawal, K., Mehariya, S., & Verma, P. (2022). Current perspective on wastewater treatment using photobioreactor for *Tetraselmis* sp.: an emerging and foreseeable sustainable approach. *Environmental Science and Pollution Research, 29*(41), 61905–61937.
Goswami, R. K., Agrawal, K., & Verma, P. (2023). Multifaceted role of microalgae for municipal wastewater treatment: a futuristic outlook toward wastewater management. *CLEAN–Soil, Air, Water*, *51*(3), 2100286.
Groff, M. C., Puchol, C. F., Gil, R., Pedrozo, L. P., Albareti, S., Manzanares, A. B., & Scaglia, G. (2025). Integrated system of microalgae photobioreactor and wine fermenter: Growth kinetics for sustainable CO2 biocapture. *Fermentation, 11*(2), 58.
Gupta, P. L., Lee, S. M., & Choi, H. J. (2015). A mini review: Photobioreactors for large scale algal cultivation. *World J MicrobiolBiotechnol, 31*(9), 1409–1417.
Huang, Q., Jiang, F., Wang, L., & Yang, C. (2017a). Design of photobioreactors for mass cultivation of photosynthetic organisms. *Engineering, 3*(3), 318–329.
Huang, Y., Zhao, S., Ding, Y.-D., Liao, Q., Huang, Y., & Zhu, X. (2017b). Optimizing the gas distributor based on CO2 bubble dynamic behaviors to improve microalgal biomass production in an air-lift photo-bioreactor. *Bioresource Technology, 233*, 84–91.
Janoska, A., Barten, R., de Nooy, S., van Rijssel, P., Wijffels, R. H., & Janssen, M. (2018). Improved liquid foam-bed photobioreactor design for microalgae cultivation. *Algal Research, 33*, 55–70.
Jung, E. E., Jain, A., Voulis, N., Doud, D. F., Angenent, L. T., & Erickson, D. (2014). Stacked optical waveguide photobioreactor for high density algal cultures. *Bioresource Technology, 171*, 495–499.
Ketheesan, B., & Nirmalakhandan, N. (2012). Feasibility of microalgal cultivation in a pilot scale airlift-driven raceway reactor. *Bioresource Technology, 108*, 196–202.
Khan, M. I., Shin, J. H., & Kim, J. D. (2018). The promising future of microalgae: Current status, challenges, and optimization of a sustainable and renewable industry for biofuels, feed, and other products. *Microbial Cell Factories, 17*(1), 36.
Khoo, C. G., Lam, M. K., & Lee, K. T. (2016). Pilot-scale semi-continuous cultivation of mi croalgae Chlorella vulgaris in bubble column photobioreactor (BC-PBR): Hydro dynamics and gas–liquid mass transfer study. *Algal Research, 15*, 65–76.
Kim, H. W., Cheng, J., & Rittmann, B. E. (2016). Direct membrane-carbonation photo bioreactor producing photoautotrophic biomass via carbon dioxide transfer and nu trient removal. *Bioresource Technology, 204*, 32–37.

Kong, W., Shen, B., Lyu, H., Kong, J., Ma, J., Wang, Z., Feng, S. (2021). Review on carbon dioxide fixation coupled with nutrients removal from wastewater by microalgae. *Journal of Cleaner Production*, 125975.

Kubar, A. A., Mehmood, S., Schagerl, M., Kumar, S., Hu, X., Zhu, F., & Huo, S. (2025). Integrated hybrid Nested-bottled photobioreactor for enhanced mixing, mass transfer, and CO_2 fixation in Arthrospira platensis raceway pond cultivation systems. *Biotechnology for Biofuels and Bioproducts, 18*, 67.

Lee, J. Y., Yu, B. S., Chang, W. S., & Sim, S. J. (2023). A strategy to maximize astaxanthin production from Haematococcuspluvialis in a cost-effective process by utilizing a PBR-LGP-PBR array (PLPA) hybrid system using light guide panel (LGP) and solar cells. *Bioresource Technology, 376*, Article 128902.

Li, S., Luo, S., & Guo, R. (2013). Efficiency of CO2 fixation by microalgae in a closed raceway pond. *Bioresource Technology, 136*, 267–272.

Liao, Q., Li, L., Chen, R., & Zhu, X. (2014). A novel photobioreactor generating the light/dark cycle to improve microalgae cultivation. *Bioresource Technology, 161*, 186–191.

Liu, H., Chen, H., Wang, S., Liu, Q., Li, S., Song, X., Huang, J., Wang, X., & Jia, L. (2018). Optimizing light distribution and controlling biomass concentration by continuously pre-harvesting *Spirulina platensis* for improving the microalgae production. *Bioresource Technology, 252*, 14–19.

López-Rosales, L., García-Camacho, F., Sánchez-Mirón, A., Contreras-Gómez, A., & Molina Grima, E. (2015). An optimisation approach for culturing shear-sensitive dino f lagellate microalgae in bench-scale bubble column photobioreactors. *Bioresource Technology, 197*, 375–382.

Matos, J., Cardoso, C., Bandarra, N. M., & Afonso, C. (2017). Microalgae as healthy ingredients for functional food: A review. *Food & Function, 8*(8), 2672–2685.

Mazzei, R., Piacentini, E., Yihdego Gebreyohannes, A., & Giorno, L. (2017). Membrane bioreactors in food, pharmaceutical and biofuel applications: State of the art, progresses and perspectives. *Current Organic Chemistry, 21*(17), 1671–1701.

Milia, M., Andreotti, V., Giglioli, A., Pasquini, V., Addis, P., & Angioni, A. (2025). Use of enriched mine water to grow the cyanobacterium Arthrospira platensis in Photobioreactors. *Foods, 14*(10), 1665.

Mishra, A. K., Kaushik, M. S., Tiwari, D. 2019. Nitrogenase and hydrogenase: enzymes for nitrogen fixation and hydrogen production in cyanobacteria. In *Cyanobacteria* (pp. 173–191). Elsevier

Mohan, S. V., Rohit, M. V., Chiranjeevi, P., Chandra, R., & Navaneeth, B. (2015). Heterotrophic microalgae cultivation to synergize biodiesel production with waste remediation: Progress and perspectives. *Bioresource Technology, 184*, 169–178.

Narala, R. R., Garg, S., Sharma, K. K., Thomas-Hall, S. R., Deme, M., Li, Y., & Schenk, P. M. (2016). Comparison of microalgae cultivation in photobioreactor, open raceway pond, and a two-stage hybrid system. *Frontiers in Energy Research, 4*, 29.

Nauha, E. K., & Alopaeus, V. (2013). Modeling method for combining fluid dynamics and algal growth in a bubble column photobioreactor. *Chemical Engineering Journal, 229*, 559–568.

Pires, J. C. M., Alvim-Ferraz, M. C. M., & Martins, F. G. (2017). Photobioreactor design for microalgae production through computational fluid dynamics: A review. *Renewable and Sustainable Energy Reviews, 79*, 248–254.

Prussi, M., Buffi, M., Casini, D., Chiaramonti, D., Martelli, F., Carnevale, M., Tredici, M. R., & Rodolfi, L. (2014). Experimental and numerical investigations of mixing in raceway ponds for algae cultivation. *Biomass and Bioenergy, 67*, 390–400.

Ramsundar, P., Guldhe, A., Singh, P., & Bux, F. (2017). Assessment of municipal wastewaters at various stages of treatment process as potential growth media for Chlorella sorokiniana under different modes of cultivation. *BioresourTechnol, 227*, 82–92.

Ray, B., Jayakumar, T., & Rakesh, S. (2023). Comparative analysis of lipid content in mono and co-culture microalgae for potential biodiesel production using diverse cell disruption techniques. *Biomass Conversion and Biorefinery*, 1–9.

Ray, B., & Rakesh, S. (2022). Phycoremediation of aquaculture wastewater and algal lipid extraction for fuel conversion. *Highlights in BioScience, 5*, 1.

Razzak, S. A., Bahar, K., Islam, K. O., Haniffa, A. K., Faruque, M. O., Hossain, S. Z., & Hossain, M. M. (2024). Microalgae cultivation in photobioreactors: Sustainable solutions for a greener future. *Green Chemical Engineering, 5*(4), 418–439.

Rogers, J. N., Rosenberg, J. N., Guzman, B. J., Oh, V. H., Mimbela, L. E., Ghassemi, A., Betenbaugh, M. J., Oyler, G. A., & Donohue, M. D. (2014). A critical analysis of paddlewheel-driven raceway ponds for algal biofuel production at commercial scales. *Algal Research, 4*, 76–88.

Roopashri, A. N.; Makam, R. (2022). Development of operating process for continuous production of biomass by Tetradesmus obliquus (MT188616.1) in a hollow fiber membrane photobioreactor. *Journal of Biotechnology, 359*, 59–64.

Sun, Y., Huang, Y., Liao, Q., Fu, Q., & Zhu, X. (2016). Enhancement of microalgae production by embedding hollow light guides to a flat-plate photobioreactor. *Bioresource Technology, 207*, 31–38.

Tan, J. S., Lee, S. Y., Chew, K. W., Lam, M. K., Lim, J. W., Ho, S.-H., & Show, P. L. (2020). A review on microalgae cultivation and harvesting, and their biomass extraction processing using ionic liquids. *Bioengineered, 11*(1), 116–129.

Udayan, A., Sirohi, R., Sreekumar, N., Sang, B. I., & Sim, S. J. (2022). Mass cultivation and harvesting of microalgal biomass: Current trends and future perspectives. *Bioresource Technology, 344*, Article 126406.

Udaypal, Goswami, R. K., Mehariya, S., & Verma, P. (2024). Advances in microalgae-based carbon sequestration: Current status and future perspectives. *Environmental Research, 249*, 118397.

Udaypal, Goswami, R. K., & Verma, P. (2025b). Production of α-tocopherol biomolecules using various cultivation strategies of diverse microalgal species: Purification, characterization and assessment of antioxidant properties. *Biocatalysis and Agricultural Biotechnology*, 103635.

Udaypal, Goswami, R. K., & Verma, P. (2025c). Production of lutein from various microalgae species using different cultivation methods: Structural characterization and assessment of functional integrity. *Journal of Applied Phycology*, 1–16.

Udaypal, Goswami, R. K., & Verma, P. (2025a). Transforming dairy effluent into valuable resources: Harnessing microalgae for sustainable production of nutraceuticals and pharmaceuticals. *Process Biochemistry, 150*, 342–356.

Ummalyma, S. B., Sirohi, R., Udayan, A., Yadav, P., Raj, A., Sim, S. J., & Pandey, A. (2023). Sustainable microalgal biomass production in food industry wastewater for low-cost biorefinery products: A review. *Phytochemistry Reviews, 22*(4), 969–991.

Vaniyankandy, A., Ray, B., Karthikeyan, S., & Rakesh, S. (2022). Thermochemical conversion of algal based biorefinery for biofuel. In *Cyanobacteria-recent advances and new perspectives*. IntechOpen.

Vassilev, S. V., & Vassileva, C. G. (2016). Composition, properties and challenges of algae biomass for biofuel application: An overview. *Fuel, 181*, 1–33.

Vo, H. N. P., Ngo, H. H., Guo, W., Liu, Y., Chang, S. W., Nguyen, D. D., & Ren, J. (2019). Identification of the pollutants' removal and mechanism by microalgae in saline wastewater. *Bioresource Technology, 275*, 44–52.

Vuppaladadiyam, A. K., Prinsen, P., Raheem, A., Luque, R., Zhao, M. (2018). Microalgae cultivation and metabolites production: a comprehensive review. *Biofuels, Bioproducts and Biorefining, 12*(2), 304–324.

Wang, C., & Lan, C. Q. (2018). Effects of shear stress on microalgae–a review. *Biotechnology Advances, 36*(4), 986–1002.

Wang, B., Lan, C. Q., & Horsman, M. (2012). Closed photobioreactors for production of microalgal biomasses. *Biotechnology Advances, 30*(4), 904–912.

Xia, A., Hu, Z., Liao, Q., Huang, Y., Zhu, X., Ye, W., & Sun, Y. (2018). Enhancement of CO2 transfer and microalgae growth by perforated inverted arc trough internals in a flat plate photobioreactor. *Bioresource Technology, 269*, 292–299.

Xin, L., Hong-Ying, H., Ke, G., & Ying-Xue, S. (2010). Effects of different nitrogen and phosphorus concentrations on the growth, nutrient uptake, and lipid accumulation of a freshwater microalga *Scenedesmus sp. Bioresource Technology, 101*(14), 5494–5500.

Xu, H., Miao, X., & Wu, Q. (2006). High quality biodiesel production from a microalga Chlorella protothecoides by heterotrophic growth in fermenters. *Journal of Biotechnology, 126*(4), 499–507.

Xu, Z., Zou, D., & Gao, K. (2010). Effects of elevated CO2 and phosphorus supply on growth, photosynthesis and nutrient uptake in the marine macroalga *Gracilaria lemanei* formis (Rhodophyta). *Botanica Marina, 53*(2), 123–129.

Yang, Z., del Ninno, M., Wen, Z., & Hu, H. (2014). An experimental investigation on the multiphase flows and turbulent mixing in a flat-panel photobioreactor for algae cultivation. *Journal of Applied Phycology, 26*(5), 2097–2107.

Yang, Z., Cheng, J., Lin, R., Zhou, J., & Cen, K. (2016a). Improving microalgal growth with reduced diameters of aeration bubbles and enhanced mass transfer of solution in an oscillating flow field. *Bioresource Technology, 211*, 429–434.

Yang, Z., Cheng, J., Liu, J., Zhou, J., & Cen, K. (2016b). Improving microalgal growth with small bubbles in a raceway pond with swing gas aerators. *Bioresource Technology, 216*, 267–272.

Yang, Z., Cheng, J., Xu, X., Zhou, J., & Cen, K. (2016c). Enhanced solution velocity between dark and light areas with horizontal tubes and triangular prism baffles to improve microalgal growth in a flat-panel photo-bioreactor. *Bioresource Technology, 211*, 519–526.

Ye, Q., Cheng, J., Guo, W., Xu, J., Li, K., & Zhou, J. (2018a). Serial lantern-shaped draft tube enhanced flashing light effect for improving CO2 fixation with microalgae in a gas-lift circumflux column photobioreactor. *Bioresource Technology, 255*, 156–162.

Ye, Q., Cheng, J., Lai, X., An, Y., Chu, F., Zhou, J., & Cen, K. (2018b). Promoting photo chemical efficiency of chlorella PY-ZU1 with enhanced velocity field and turbulent kinetics in a novel tangential spiral-flow column photobioreactor. *ACS Sustainable Chemistry & Engineering, 7*(1), 384–393.

Zeng, W., Chen, K., Huang, Y., Xia, A., Zhu, X., Zhu, X., & Liao, Q. (2023). Three-dimensional porous biofilm photobioreactor with light-conducting frameworks for high-efficiency microalgal growth. *Algal Research, 69*, Article 102942.

Zhan, J., Rong, J., & Wang, Q. (2017). Mixotrophic cultivation, a preferable microalgae cultivation mode for biomass/bioenergy production, and bioremediation, advances and prospect. *International Journal of Hydrogen Energy, 42*(12), 8505–8517.

Zhang, Q., Wu, X., Xue, S., Liang, K., & Cong, W. (2013a). Study of hydrodynamic characteristics in tubular photobioreactors. *Bioprocess and Biosystems Engineering, 36*(2), 143–150.

Zhang, T. Y., Yu, Y., Wu, Y. H., & Hu, H. Y. (2013b). Inhibitory effects of soluble algae products (SAP) released by Scenedesmus sp. LX1 on its growth and lipid production. *BioresourTechnol, 146*, 643–648.

Zheng, Q., Martin, G. J., & Kentish, S. E. (2016). Energy efficient transfer of carbon dioxide from flue gases to microalgal systems. *Energy & Environmental Science, 9*(3), 1074–1082.

Chapter 4
Cellulosic Ethanol: Overcoming Hurdles in Commercialization, Production Processes for Cellulosic Ethanol: Technological and Economic Challenges, Strategies for Successful Commercialization

Murat Yılmaz, Mohamed A. Hassaan, and Ahmed El Nemr

Abstract Cellulosic ethanol is produced from non-food lignocellulosic biomass and is a sustainable alternative to fossil fuels and first-generation biofuels. Despite its potential to reduce greenhouse gas emissions and utilize abundant agricultural and forestry waste, commercialization is currently hindered by financial and technological barriers. This chapter examines the pretreatment, enzymatic hydrolysis, and fermentation processes involved in producing cellulosic ethanol while addressing significant challenges such as refractory biomass structure, high enzyme prices, and inhibitor formation during conversion. Alongside significant technological limitations like low conversion efficiency, scaling issues, and energy-intensive processes, economic barriers like high capital costs, feedstock logistics, and competitiveness with fossil fuels are also explored. Suggested approaches to successful commercialization that emphasize advancements in enzyme engineering, metabolic engineering of fermentative bacteria, integrated biorefinery models, and legislative incentives. Case studies of advanced technologies (e.g., CRISPR-edited yeast strains and centralized bioprocessing) and pilot-scale facilities demonstrate pathways to cost parity and scalability. This chapter provides a roadmap for reducing barriers to the widespread use of cellulosic ethanol and ultimately aiding the transition to a circular bioeconomy by integrating interdisciplinary techniques, such as supply chain optimization and technological developments.

M. Yılmaz
Bahçe Vocational School, Department of Chemistry and Chemical Processing Technologies, Osmaniye Korkut Ata University, Osmaniye, Türkiye
e-mail: muratyilmaz@osmaniye.edu.tr

M. A. Hassaan · A. El Nemr (✉)
National Institute of Oceanography and Fisheries (NIOF), Kayet Bey, Elanfoushy, Alexandria, Egypt
e-mail: ahmedmoustafaelnemr@yahoo.com; ahmed.m.elnemr@gmail.com

P. Verma (ed.), *Sustainable Practices in Biorefinery*,
https://doi.org/10.1007/978-981-95-6071-4_4

Keywords Cellulosic ethanol · Lignocellulosic biomass · Enzymatic hydrolysis · Biorefinery · Metabolic engineering · Commercialization

4.1 Introduction

The growing concerns over climate change and the depletion of fossil fuel reserves have significantly elevated the global interest in renewable and low-carbon energy sources (Olabi et al., 2023; Raihan & Mainul Bari, 2024). Among these alternatives, cellulosic ethanol stands out due to its notable potential to reduce carbon emissions in the transportation sector and support the advancement of a circular bioeconomy (Mujtaba et al., 2023; Sikiru et al., 2024). Derived from lignocellulosic materials such as agricultural residues, forestry by-products, and dedicated energy crops, cellulosic ethanol circumvents the food-versus-fuel dilemma associated with first-generation biofuels (Blaschek et al., 2010; Gupta & Verma, 2015; Blasi et al., 2023). Furthermore, depending on the type of biomass used and the specific production technology, it can achieve a reduction in greenhouse gas (GHG) emissions ranging from 60 to 90% when compared to conventional gasoline (Chowdhury et al., 2025; Yang et al., 2016).

Unlike ethanol derived from starches or sugars, cellulosic ethanol is produced using cellulose and hemicellulose, key structural components that make up a significant portion of terrestrial plant biomass (Ho et al., 2011; Liu et al., 2019; Zabed et al., 2016). This feedstock base supports a more sustainable and potentially scalable production system while mitigating land-use competition (Mattlar & Ekholm, 2025). Despite these advantages, the widespread commercialization of cellulosic ethanol remains limited (Liu et al., 2019). As of 2024, its global production is confined mainly to pilot and demonstration stages, with only a handful of commercial-scale plants operating below full capacity (Primrose, 2025). The slow pace of adoption can be attributed to a combination of technical challenges and economic constraints (Curry et al., 2021; Thirumal et al., 2024). However, recent advancements in bioconversion technologies, supportive policy frameworks, and improved system integration methods have renewed prospects for broader commercial deployment (Almomani et al., 2023; Makepa & Chihobo, 2024; Samoraj et al., 2024). This chapter examines production methodologies, prevailing challenges, and strategic approaches to overcome existing barriers.

4.2 Production Processes for Cellulosic Ethanol

Producing cellulosic ethanol involves several integrated stages, beginning with transforming lignocellulosic biomass into fermentable sugars, followed by fermentation into ethanol (Kumar et al., 2019). This pathway includes a series of interdependent processes such as feedstock pretreatment, enzymatic hydrolysis, and microbial fermentation. Each phase presents distinct technological challenges and opportunities for optimization that must be addressed to enhance process efficiency and support commercial-scale deployment (Richardd L Smith & Xinhuaa Qi, 2017).

4.2.1 Feedstock Preparation

The production of cellulosic ethanol begins with identifying and preparing lignocellulosic biomass (Bai et al., 2019; Liu et al., 2019; Shrivastava & Sharma, 2023). This biomass is composed of cellulose, hemicellulose, and lignin -each playing a distinct role in contributing to the structural complexity and resistance to degradation inherent in the feedstock (Lee et al., 2014; Mariana et al., 2021; Mujtaba et al., 2023).

4.2.1.1 Types of Biomass

As the primary raw material for producing cellulosic ethanol, lignocellulosic biomass includes a wide range of resources such as agricultural residues (e.g., wheat straw, maize stover), forestry waste (e.g., sawdust, wood chips), dedicated energy crops (e.g., miscanthus, switchgrass), and even municipal solid waste. Although these feedstocks are abundant and renewable, their complex and variable composition poses significant challenges for efficient conversion. Typically, lignocellulosic biomass consists of 35–50% cellulose, 20–35% hemicellulose, and 10–25% lignin, though these proportions can fluctuate depending on the biomass type and origin (Nair et al., 2022; Richardd L Smith & Xinhuaa Qi, 2017).

4.2.1.2 Pretreatment Methods

To facilitate enzymatic hydrolysis, biomass requires pretreatment that disrupts the lignin network and removes the hemicellulose barrier, thereby enhancing the accessibility of cellulose to enzymatic action (Chen et al., 2024; Novia et al., 2024).

4.2.1.3 Steam Explosion

This physical pretreatment involves exposing the biomass to high-pressure steam, which is then rapidly depressurized. The sudden drop in pressure causes the biomass structure to rupture, disrupting the lignin barrier and increasing the available surface area for subsequent processing. Although this method is efficient, it can also generate inhibitory byproducts, including furfural and hydroxymethylfurfural (HMF), which may hinder downstream biological conversions (Pielhop et al., 2016; Ziegler-Devin et al., 2021).

4.2.1.4 Acid/Alkali Treatment

Dilute acid pretreatment, often using sulfuric or hydrochloric acid, facilitates hemicellulose hydrolysis into its constituent monomeric sugars. In contrast, alkaline pretreatment -utilizing agents such as sodium hydroxide or ammonia- targets the removal of lignin to enhance the enzymatic accessibility of cellulose. Although both methods effectively improve biomass conversion, they frequently require extensive downstream processing, including pH neutralization and thorough washing, which can significantly increase operational expenses (Lorenci Woiciechowski et al., 2020; Sirohi et al., 2021).

4.2.1.5 Organosolv Process

The organosolv method employs organic solvents -such as ethanol, acetone, or an organic acid mixture under high temperature and pressure conditions to dissolve lignin and hemicellulose (Nair et al., 2023). This approach results in relatively pure cellulose, facilitates the recovery of lignin, and reduces the dependence on harsh chemical reagents (Mao et al., 2025; Wildschut et al., 2013). However, challenges related to solvent recovery and the overall cost of the process remain substantial barriers to widespread implementation (Behera et al., 2014; Preethi et al., 2021).

4.2.2 Enzymatic Hydrolysis

During enzymatic saccharification, complex polysaccharides are broken down into simple fermentable sugars (Saratale et al., 2022; Sharma & Horn, 2016).

4.2.2.1 Enzymes Involved

Enzymatic hydrolysis involves the conversion of cellulose and hemicellulose into fermentable sugars through the action of cellulase enzymes, which include *endoglucanases, exoglucanases* (also known as *cellobiohydrolases*), and *β*-glucosidases. Enzymes such as xylanases and mannanases are employed to break down hemicellulose. These enzymatic components operate synergistically to cleave glycosidic linkages, releasing simple sugars like glucose and xylose (Bhardwaj et al., 2021; Mojsov, 2016; Yi, 2021).

4.2.2.2 Challenges

Key challenges in enzymatic hydrolysis include inhibiting enzymes by reaction by-products, limited enzyme accessibility due to residual lignin, and the high production costs of enzyme formulations. Maintaining optimal pH and temperature conditions for enzymatic efficiency can also be particularly complex in large-scale operations (Klein-Marcuschamer et al., 2012; Ferreira et al., 2021).

4.2.2.3 Strategies for Improvement

- Strategies such as enzyme recycling and immobilization are employed to enhance enzyme stability and reduce overall costs (Woo et al., 2022).
- Efforts focus on engineering robust enzymes that maintain high catalytic activity under harsh industrial conditions (Ndochinwa et al., 2024).
- Production of tailored enzyme cocktails through microbial expression systems enables integrated and efficient bioconversion processes (Srivastava & Dafale, 2024).

4.2.3 Fermentation

Hydrolyzed carbohydrates are converted into ethanol through microbial fermentation (Moscoviz et al., 2021).

4.2.3.1 Key Microorganisms

- *Saccharomyces cerevisiae*: Highly efficient at fermenting glucose, yet limited in using pentose sugars (Nijland & Driessen, 2020).
- *Engineered Zymomonas mobilis* and *Escherichia coli*: Engineered to metabolize both five-carbon (C5) and six-carbon (C6) sugars (Yang et al., 2016).
- *Thermophilic bacteria* such as *Clostridium thermocellum* offer higher tolerance to process stressors (Mazzoli et al., 2022).

4.2.3.2 Advanced Techniques

Recent advancements in fermentation technologies include consolidated bioprocessing (CBP), in which a single microorganism or a consortium carries out enzyme production, biomass hydrolysis, and fermentation in one integrated step. This approach can reduce capital investment and operational expenses; however, it requires robust microbial strains capable of performing multiple functions. Other notable innovations involve the use of immobilized cell systems, co-culture strategies, and metabolic engineering techniques aimed at enhancing ethanol productivity, broadening substrate utilization, and increasing resistance to inhibitory compounds (Saxena et al., 2023; Stasiak-Różańska et al., 2025).

4.3 Technological Challenges

Despite the considerable promise of cellulosic ethanol as a sustainable biofuel, its large-scale commercialization faces numerous technological challenges. These obstacles span the production process, beginning with biomass pretreatment and extending to the final ethanol recovery stage. Overcoming these issues requires targeted progress in biotechnology, process engineering, and integrating complex system components.

4.3.1 Biomass Recalcitrance

A fundamental technological obstacle in cellulosic ethanol production is the inherent recalcitrance of lignocellulosic biomass. This resistance arises from plant cell walls' complex and rigid structure, where cellulose fibers are tightly bound to hemicellulose and encased within a lignin matrix. Such an arrangement limits enzyme accessibility, thereby reducing the efficiency of enzymatic hydrolysis. Although pretreatment processes aim to overcome these barriers, achieving thorough delignification and fiber disruption without compromising sugar yields or generating inhibitory compounds remains a significant challenge. Consequently, developing more efficient and selective pretreatment methods remains a critical area of research (Mujtaba et al., 2023; Nair & Verma, 2025).

4.3.2 Enzyme Cost and Stability

The high cost and limited operational stability of cellulolytic enzymes significantly impact the economic feasibility of producing cellulosic ethanol. Commercial enzyme preparations are often needed in large quantities because hydrolysis rates remain insufficient, especially when processing recalcitrant feedstocks. Additionally, enzyme activity frequently declines under industrial conditions due to factors such as shear forces, temperature fluctuations, and the presence of chemical inhibitors. To enhance enzyme performance and reduce associated costs, advancements in enzyme engineering, immobilization techniques, and microbial expression systems are critically needed (Ndochinwa et al., 2024).

4.3.3 Inhibitory Byproducts

Numerous inhibitory byproducts, such as furfural, 5-hydroxymethylfurfural (HMF), acetic acid, and phenolic compounds, are formed during the pretreatment and hydrolysis stages. These substances can hinder enzyme function and microbial fermentation by disrupting metabolic pathways or damaging cellular structures. Consequently, additional detoxification steps or robust, inhibitor-tolerant microbial strains become necessary. However, implementing these strategies often increases process complexity and operational challenges (Dessie et al., 2019).

4.3.4 Process Integration

Integrating the various stages of cellulosic ethanol production—such as pretreatment, enzymatic hydrolysis, fermentation, and product recovery—into a unified and efficient process remains a significant challenge. Factors such as the heterogeneity of feedstock composition, the differing optimal conditions required for each stage, and difficulties associated with scaling up operations complicate this integration. For example, enzymatic hydrolysis typically requires moderate temperatures, while fermentative microorganisms thrive within a range of pH and temperature conditions. Although approaches like simultaneous saccharification and fermentation (SSF) and consolidated bioprocessing (CBP) offer promising solutions, their widespread adoption is limited by inherent technical and biological constraints (Wo´zniak et al., 2025).

4.3.5 Waste Management

The production of cellulosic ethanol generates a variety of solid and liquid residues, including unconverted lignin, ash, and process water contaminated with organic and inorganic compounds. Poor handling of these byproducts can lead to environmental risks and diminish the overall sustainability of bioethanol production. Significant research efforts focus on lignin valorization, aiming to convert it into value-added chemicals, bioenergy, or composite materials. Additionally, implementing closed-loop water recycling systems and anaerobic digestion for wastewater treatment offers promising strategies to improve waste management and enhance the environmental performance of the process (Alam et al., 2024).

4.4 Economic Challenges

Transitioning from pilot-scale research to large-scale commercialization of cellulosic ethanol is hindered by significant technological barriers and considerable economic challenges. These issues impact the financial sustainability of production plants and weaken investor confidence regarding the long-term prospects of cellulosic biofuels. Therefore, a comprehensive understanding of these economic constraints is essential for formulating effective regulatory policies, investment frameworks, and sustainable business models.

4.4.1 High Capital Expenditure (CAPEX)

One significant economic barrier is the high capital investment required to build and operate cellulosic ethanol production plants. Second-generation plants demand more complex infrastructure than first-generation ethanol facilities to accommodate advanced pretreatment technologies, enzyme manufacturing, and integrated fermentation and purification processes. These substantial upfront costs pose significant financial risks, particularly without guaranteed market demand or government incentives. Additionally, long payback periods and the uncertainties linked to scaling emerging technologies further discourage private sector participation (Karimi et al., 2025; Patel et al., 2025).

4.4.2 Feedstock Supply Chain Issues

Although lignocellulosic biomass is widely available, establishing a reliable and consistent year-round supply chain remains a significant challenge. Variability in biomass availability caused by seasonal fluctuations, transportation logistics, land use competition, and regional differences in feedstock quality often leads to inconsistent supplies and fluctuating costs. Moreover, the costs associated with harvesting, collection, storage, and transport of bulky, low-energy–density biomass significantly impact the overall economic viability of the process. Addressing these issues through efficient supply chain management and developing decentralized processing facilities could mitigate some challenges but require coordinated investments and expanded infrastructure (Roni et al., 2016).

4.4.3 Market Competitiveness

Cellulosic ethanol faces intense competition from fossil fuels and first-generation biofuels, which benefit from well-established production infrastructures, lower costs, and mature distribution systems. The comparatively high production expenses associated with cellulosic ethanol -driven by the costs of enzymes, pretreatment chemicals, and energy inputs- reduce its attractiveness in current energy markets. Additionally, fluctuations in crude oil prices and shifts in renewable energy policies can further undermine its market competitiveness. Without supportive regulatory measures, such as carbon pricing mechanisms or mandated blending targets, reliance on market dynamics alone is unlikely to enable widespread adoption of cellulosic ethanol (Flavin et al., 2014; Pan et al., 2024).

4.4.4 Investor Uncertainty

Uncertainty regarding regulatory frameworks, technological progress, and anticipated returns on investment has led to investor reluctance in committing funds to cellulosic ethanol projects. Many early commercial-scale ventures have faced underperformance, budget overruns, and policy shifts, eroding investor confidence. This financial instability, compounded by the lack of long-term purchase agreements and the ongoing need for technological innovation, poses a significant barrier to securing steady capital inflows into the industry. To restore investor trust and stimulate investment, it is crucial to establish public–private partnerships, implement risk-sharing mechanisms, and develop transparent and stable regulatory policies (Egli, 2020).

4.5 Strategies for Successful Commercialization

The successful commercialization of cellulosic ethanol relies on the deliberate integration of technological advancements, regulatory frameworks, economic incentives, and efficient logistics. Addressing existing challenges through a holistic approach has the potential to transform cellulosic ethanol from a niche research focus into a sustainable and competitive component of the global bioenergy landscape. This section outlines key strategies within three main domains: technological innovation, enabling policies and financial support, and supply chain optimization.

4.5.1 *Technological Innovations*

4.5.1.1 CRISPR-Cas9 Genome Editing

Advances in genetic engineering, particularly through the CRISPR-Cas9 technology, hold transformative potential for enhancing cellulosic ethanol production. This precise genome-editing tool enables the optimization of microbial strains and enzyme-producing organisms. Modifying metabolic pathways in microorganisms such as *Saccharomyces cerevisiae* and *Zymomonas mobilis* can improve tolerance to inhibitors, increase ethanol output, and enable efficient co-fermentation of both pentose and hexose sugars. Similarly, genetic modification of cellulolytic fungi and bacteria can lead to the development of more efficient enzyme consortia, thereby reducing enzyme-related costs (Garg et al., 2023).

4.5.1.2 Consolidated Bioprocessing (CBP)

Consolidated bioprocessing (CBP) integrates enzyme synthesis, substrate hydrolysis, and fermentation into a single streamlined operation, eliminating the need for separate enzymatic and microbial stages. This integrated approach reduces operational complexity and capital costs, improving the process's overall economic feasibility. Current research in CBP focuses on engineered microbial consortia or specially designed strains capable of performing all three functions simultaneously. Although challenges remain, such as balancing enzyme production with ethanol output, CBP is a promising strategy to simplify production workflows and enhance scalability (De Oliveira Schmidt et al., 2025).

4.5.1.3 Hybrid Systems

Hybrid conversion systems that combine biochemical and thermochemical processes offer innovative avenues to maximize biomass utilization. By coupling gasification with fermentation, residual lignin and other non-fermentable fractions can be converted into synthesis gas (syngas), which is subsequently transformed into biofuels through catalytic processes. Such integrated approaches increase the total energy yield and support circular economy principles by minimizing waste generation. Additionally, incorporating anaerobic digestion to treat residual biomass can provide additional energy recovery and improve overall waste management efficiency (Liakakou et al., 2021).

4.5.2 *Policy and Economic Incentives*

4.5.2.1 Renewable Fuel Standards (RFS2)

Government policies, exemplified by the U.S. Renewable Fuel Standard (RFS2), play a pivotal role in promoting biofuel development. RFS2 designates cellulosic ethanol as an "advanced biofuel" subject to stringent greenhouse gas reduction targets. The system of compliance credits, known as Renewable Identification Numbers (RINs), offers financial motivation for producers; however, maintaining policy consistency is vital. Clear, long-term mandates combined with consistent enforcement mechanisms are essential to reduce investor uncertainty and stimulate economic growth in the sector (https://www.epa.gov/renewable-fuel-standard-program/renewable-fuel-standard-rfs2-final-rule, Accessed 13 June 2025).

4.5.2.2 Tax Credits and Carbon Pricing Mechanisms

Economic incentives, such as production and investment tax credits alongside carbon offset programs, help bridge the cost gap between cellulosic ethanol and conventional fossil fuels. Carbon pricing mechanisms -including cap-and-trade systems and carbon taxes- serve to internalize the environmental benefits of biofuels, thereby improving their competitiveness in the marketplace. To ensure fairness and avoid market imbalances, the implementation of these policies should be harmonized across different regulatory regions (Kiss & Popovics, 2021; Mengesha & Roy, 2025).

4.5.2.3 Public–Private Partnerships

Partnerships between government agencies, academic researchers, and industry stakeholders are crucial in accelerating technology adoption and reducing financial risks. Public–private partnerships (PPPs) enable joint investments in pilot plants, infrastructure development, and the widespread deployment of novel technologies. Cooperative research and development efforts can also drive innovation in key areas such as feedstock improvement, biocatalyst engineering, and process integration. The success of these collaborations depends on well-defined governance frameworks, aligned goals, and mutually beneficial arrangements (https://www.energy.gov/eere/bioenergy/bioenergy-technologies-office, Accessed 13 June 2025).

4.5.3 Supply Chain Optimization

4.5.3.1 Decentralized Pretreatment Hubs

Establishing decentralized pretreatment facilities close to biomass sources offers a promising solution to address logistical challenges associated with biomass transportation and storage. These regional hubs can process raw biomass into intermediate products, such as pretreated slurry or bio-oil, which are easier to store and transport. Modular pretreatment systems reduce transportation costs, enhance supply chain flexibility, and support local employment, thereby contributing positively to the regional bioeconomy (Kousar et al., 2023).

4.5.3.2 Valorization of Co-Products

Economic sustainability in cellulosic ethanol production can be significantly improved by valorizing co-products generated throughout the process. For instance, lignin can be converted into valuable chemicals, adhesives, resins, or carbon-based materials such as activated carbon. Process residues and waste can also be harnessed for energy recovery through heat and power generation or anaerobic digestion. By creating revenue streams from these co-products, producers can diversify their income and reduce overall production costs (Cao et al., 2019).

4.5.3.3 Digital Tools and AI

Integrating digital technologies -including artificial intelligence (AI), machine learning, and real-time monitoring systems- offers significant potential to optimize process efficiency and support informed decision-making. Predictive modelling can more effectively refine fermentation parameters, optimize enzyme dosing, and schedule maintenance activities. Furthermore, AI-powered supply chain analytics enable accurate forecasting of biomass availability, streamline logistics, and reduce operational downtime. As digital transformation progresses, leveraging data-driven approaches will become increasingly critical to maximizing the productivity and sustainability of cellulosic ethanol production (Arias et al., 2023).

4.6 Case Studies and Lessons Learned

The path toward commercializing cellulosic ethanol has involved notable progress alongside substantial challenges. Examining case studies of pioneering projects reveals valuable lessons regarding the technological, economic, and operational facets of scaling advanced biofuels. Such practical experiences yield critical knowledge that informs future research directions, investment decisions, and policy development. This section reviews successful and unsuccessful initiatives and emerging technologies to extract key insights that support the continued advancement of cellulosic ethanol.

4.6.1 Project LIBERTY (POET-DSM)

Project LIBERTY, a flagship collaboration between POET LLC and Royal DSM, is a leading effort to commercialize cellulosic ethanol in the United States. Located in Emmetsburg, Iowa, this facility was designed to produce 20 million gallons of ethanol annually from maize stover through enzymatic hydrolysis and fermentation. It showcased a sophisticated integration of proprietary enzyme technologies with advanced pretreatment methods. Despite initial setbacks and technical difficulties related to feedstock variability and process optimization, LIBERTY has a significantly advanced understanding of process dynamics and enzyme development. One of its key accomplishments includes progress in integrated biorefinery operations and implementing co-generation systems to meet on-site energy demands. However, the project's long-term sustainability has been challenged by fluctuating market conditions and shifts in policy support, underscoring the critical importance of stable regulatory frameworks and consistent market incentives for successful commercialization (Ward, 2015).

4.6.2 Clariant's Sunliquid® Technology

Clariant's Sunliquid® technology represents a significant European advancement in advanced biofuels. This versatile, feedstock-flexible process combines chemical-free pretreatment with enzymatic hydrolysis and fermentation, employing engineered microorganisms capable of co-fermenting C5 and C6 sugars. The flagship commercial-scale plant in Podari, Romania, began operations in 2022 and is designed to produce approximately 50,000 tons of ethanol annually from agricultural residues such as wheat straw. Key factors contributing to the success of the Sunliquid® platform include its modular design, energy-efficient operation, and proprietary enzyme production tailored to specific feedstocks. Clariant has emphasized sustainability by integrating residue valorization and striving for minimal greenhouse gas emissions. This project exemplifies the synergy of technological innovation, coordinated supply chain management, and strategic industrial partnerships in achieving commercial viability (Clariant, 2018).

4.6.3 Failures Such as Range Fuels

Not every venture within the cellulosic ethanol sector has achieved success. Range Fuels, once considered a pioneer in biomass thermochemical conversion, ultimately failed despite receiving significant government funding and facing intense public scrutiny. The Soperton, Georgia, facility was intended to convert woody biomass into ethanol through gasification followed by catalytic synthesis. However, the plant faced persistent technical challenges, particularly related to syngas quality and catalyst deactivation, which led to the unintended production of methanol instead of ethanol.

The collapse of Range Fuels highlights the risks associated with deploying emerging technologies at a commercial scale without sufficient pilot-scale validation and contingency planning. Additionally, the project suffered from cost overruns, management inefficiencies, and overly ambitious projections. This case serves as a cautionary example emphasizing the importance of phased development, transparent reporting, and comprehensive techno-economic assessments before scaling novel technologies (Range Fuels, 2008).

4.6.4 Emerging Technologies

LanzaTech utilizes gas fermentation to produce ethanol, complemented by AI-driven models that enable real-time optimization of process parameters, thereby offering innovative routes toward commercialization (Handler et al., 2016).

4.6.5 Lessons Learned

The collective experience gained from both past and ongoing projects highlights several critical lessons:

- A rigorous assessment of technological readiness at the pilot and demonstration stages is essential before scaling up to full commercial operations.
- Efficient management of feedstock logistics and the availability of local infrastructure plays a vital role in determining operational viability.
- Consistent policy frameworks combined with targeted incentives are key to bridging the gap between innovation and widespread commercialization.
- Partnerships between the public and private sectors facilitate knowledge exchange and risk mitigation, supporting long-term project sustainability.
- Incorporating adaptability into process designs and business models increases resilience amid market uncertainties.

Harnessing these insights can inform a more robust and sustainable path forward for the global cellulosic ethanol industry.

4.7 Future Directions and Conclusions

Achieving sustainable and cost-effective production of cellulosic ethanol requires coordinated advancements spanning biotechnology, logistics, and policy frameworks. Essential strategies encompass:

- **Modular biorefineries**: Modular and flexible units designed to utilize local feedstocks while minimizing risks associated with scale-up.
- **Integration with green hydrogen and CCUS (carbon capture, utilization, and storage)**: Aiming to establish a fuel cycle that achieves net negative greenhouse gas emissions.
- **International cooperation and standardization**: Essential for harmonizing regulations, promoting the exchange of best practices, and lowering barriers to market entry.

In conclusion, cellulosic ethanol represents a viable pathway for reducing transportation-related carbon emissions and enhancing energy security. While transitioning from pilot-scale demonstrations to full commercial deployment is underway, sustained innovation, targeted policy incentives, and collaborative stakeholder engagement remain essential to overcome existing challenges.

References

Alam, M. M., et al. (2024). Efficient and environmentally friendly techniques for extracting lignin from lignocellulose biomass and subsequent uses: A review. *Cleaner materials*. Elsevier Ltd. https://doi.org/10.1016/j.clema.2024.100253

Almomani, F., Abdelbar, A., & Ghanimeh, S. (2023). A review of the recent advancement of bioconversion of carbon dioxide to added value products: A state of the Art'. *Sustainability (Switzerland)*. Multidisciplinary Digital Publishing Institute (MDPI). https://doi.org/10.3390/su151310438

Arias, A., Feijoo, G., & Moreira, M. T. (2023). How could Artificial Intelligence be used to increase the potential of biorefineries in the near future? A review. *Environmental technology and innovation*. Elsevier B.V. https://doi.org/10.1016/j.eti.2023.103277

Bai, F. W., Yang, S., & Ho, N. W. Y. (2019). Fuel ethanol production from lignocellulosic biomass. In *Comprehensive biotechnology* (pp. 49–65). Elsevier. https://doi.org/10.1016/B978-0-444-64046-8.00150-6

Behera, S. et al. (2014). Importance of chemical pretreatment for bioconversion of lignocellulosic biomass. In *Renewable and sustainable energy reviews* (pp. 91–106). Elsevier Ltd. https://doi.org/10.1016/j.rser.2014.04.047

Bhardwaj, N. et al. (2021). Current perspective on production and applications of microbial cellulases: a review. *Bioresources and Bioprocessing, 8*(1). https://doi.org/10.1186/s40643-021-00447-6

Blaschek, H. P., Ezeji, T. C., & Scheffran, J. (2010). *Biofuels from agricultural wastes and byproducts*. Wiley-Blackwell.

Blasi, A. et al. (2023). Lignocellulosic agricultural waste valorization to obtain valuable products: An overview. In *Recycling*. Multidisciplinary Digital Publishing Institute (MDPI). https://doi.org/10.3390/recycling8040061

Cao, Y. et al. (2019). Advances in lignin valorization towards bio-based chemicals and fuels: Lignin biorefinery. In *Bioresource Technology*. Elsevier Ltd. https://doi.org/10.1016/j.biortech.2019.121878
Chen, J. et al. (2024). Physical–chemical–biological pretreatment for biomass degradation and industrial applications: A review. *Waste, 2*(4), 451–473. https://doi.org/10.3390/waste2040024
Chowdhury, P. et al. (2025). Biomass to biofuel: Impacts and mitigation of environmental, health, and socioeconomic challenges. *Energy Conversion and Management: X, 25*. https://doi.org/10.1016/j.ecmx.2025.100889
Clariant. (2018). Retrieved June 13, 2025, from https://www.clariant.com/en/Corporate/News/2018/09/Groundbreaking-for-Clariantrsquos-sunliquidreg-cellulosic-ethanol-plant-in-Romanianbsp
Curry, G. N. et al. (2021). Disruptive innovation in agriculture: Socio-cultural factors in technology adoption in the developing world. *Journal of Rural Studies, 88*, 422–431. https://doi.org/10.1016/j.jrurstud.2021.07.022
Dessie, W. et al. (2019). Inhibitory effects of lignocellulose pretreatment degradation products (hydroxymethylfurfural and furfural) on succinic acid producing Actinobacillus succinogenes. *Biochemical Engineering Journal, 150*. https://doi.org/10.1016/j.bej.2019.107263
De Oliveira Schmidt, V. K. et al. (2025). Clostridium sp.: A versatile microbial platform for advancing the consolidated bioprocessing of lignocellulosic residues. *Journal of Environmental Chemical Engineering*. Elsevier Ltd. https://doi.org/10.1016/j.jece.2025.116802
Egli, F. (2020). Renewable energy investment risk: An investigation of changes over time and the underlying drivers. *Energy Policy, 140*. https://doi.org/10.1016/j.enpol.2020.111428
Ferreira, R. G., Azzoni, A. R., & Freitas, S. (2021). On the production cost of lignocellulose-degrading enzymes. In *Biofuels, bioproducts and biorefining* (pp. 85–99). John Wiley and Sons Ltd. https://doi.org/10.1002/bbb.2142
Flavin, C. et al. (2014). *Study on the development of the renewable energy market in Latin America and the Caribbean. Study on the development of the renewable energy market in Latin America and the Caribbean under the IDB climate change evaluation.*
Garg, D. et al. (2023). Revolutionizing biofuel generation: unleashing the power of CRISPR-Cas mediated gene editing of extremophiles. In *Microbiological research*. Elsevier GmbH. https://doi.org/10.1016/j.micres.2023.127443
Gupta, A., & Verma, J. P. (2015). Sustainable bio-ethanol production from agro-residues: A review. In *Renewable and sustainable energy reviews* (pp. 550–567). Elsevier Ltd. https://doi.org/10.1016/j.rser.2014.08.032
Handler, R. M. et al. (2016). Life cycle assessments of ethanol production via gas fermentation: Anticipated greenhouse gas emissions for cellulosic and waste gas feedstocks. *Industrial and Engineering Chemistry Research, 55*(12), 3253–3261. https://doi.org/10.1021/acs.iecr.5b03215
Ho, N. et al. (2011). *3.06 Biofuels from cellulosic feedstocks.*
Kumar, B., Bhardwaj, N., & Verma, P. (2019). Pretreatment of rice straw using microwave assisted FeCl3-H3PO4 system for ethanol and oligosaccharides generation. *Bioresource Technology Reports, 7*, 100295. https://doi.org/10.1016/j.biteb.2019.100295
Karimi, M., Simsek, H., & Kheiralipour, K. (2025). Advanced biofuel production: A comprehensive techno-economic review of pathways and costs. In *Energy conversion and management: X*. Elsevier Ltd. https://doi.org/10.1016/j.ecmx.2024.100863
Kiss, T., & Popovics, S. (2021). Evaluation on the effectiveness of energy policies–Evidence from the carbon reductions in 25 countries. *Renewable and Sustainable Energy Reviews, 149*. https://doi.org/10.1016/j.rser.2021.111348
Klein-Marcuschamer, D., et al. (2012). The challenge of enzyme cost in the production of lignocellulosic biofuels. *Biotechnology and Bioengineering, 109*(4), 1083–1087. https://doi.org/10.1002/bit.24370
Kousar, S. et al. (2023). Optimizing transportation cost for biomass supply chain. *Thermal Science, 27*(Special Issue 1), S245–S251. https://doi.org/10.2298/TSCI23S1245K

Lee, H. V., Hamid, S. B. A., & Zain, S. K. (2014). Conversion of lignocellulosic biomass to nanocellulose: Structure and chemical process. *Scientific World Journal*. https://doi.org/10.1155/2014/631013

Liakakou, E. T., et al. (2021). Connecting gasification with syngas fermentation: Comparison of the performance of lignin and beech wood. *Fuel, 290*. https://doi.org/10.1016/j.fuel.2020.120054

Liu, C. G., et al. (2019). Cellulosic ethanol production: Progress, challenges and strategies for solutions. In *Biotechnology Advances* (pp. 491–504). Elsevier Inc. https://doi.org/10.1016/j.biotechadv.2019.03.002

Lorenci Woiciechowski, A., et al. (2020). Lignocellulosic biomass: Acid and alkaline pretreatments and their effects on biomass recalcitrance–Conventional processing and recent advances. In *Bioresource technology*. Elsevier Ltd. https://doi.org/10.1016/j.biortech.2020.122848

Makepa, D. C., & Chihobo, C. H. (2024). Barriers to commercial deployment of biorefineries: A multi-faceted review of obstacles across the innovation chain. In *Heliyon*. Elsevier Ltd. https://doi.org/10.1016/j.heliyon.2024.e32649

Mao, Y. et al. (2025). Comparisons of alkali, organosolv and deep eutectic solvent pre-treatments on the physiochemical changes and lignin recovery of oak and pine wood. *Industrial Crops and Products, 226*. https://doi.org/10.1016/j.indcrop.2025.120614

Mariana, M. et al. (2021). A current advancement on the role of lignin as sustainable reinforcement material in biopolymeric blends. *Journal of Materials Research and Technology*, 2287–2316. Elsevier Editora Ltda. https://doi.org/10.1016/j.jmrt.2021.08.139

Mattlar, T., & Ekholm, T. (2025). The impact of bioplastics production on climate change mitigation, fossil fuels and land-use. *Renewable and Sustainable Energy Reviews, 212*. https://doi.org/10.1016/j.rser.2024.115234

Mazzoli, R. et al. (2022). In vivo evolution of lactic acid hyper-tolerant Clostridium thermocellum. *New Biotechnology, 67*, 12–22. https://doi.org/10.1016/j.nbt.2021.12.003

Mengesha, I., & Roy, D. (2025). Carbon pricing drives critical transition to green growth. *Nature communications, 16*(1), 1321. https://doi.org/10.1038/s41467-025-56540-3

Mojsov, K. D. (2016). Aspergillus enzymes for food industries. In *New and future developments in microbial biotechnology and bioengineering: Aspergillus system properties and applications* (pp. 215–222). Elsevier Inc. https://doi.org/10.1016/B978-0-444-63505-1.00033-6

Moscoviz, R., Kleerebezem, R., & Rombouts, J. L. (2021). Directing carbohydrates toward ethanol using mesophilic microbial communities. In *Current opinion in biotechnology* (pp. 175–183). Elsevier Ltd. https://doi.org/10.1016/j.copbio.2021.01.016

Mujtaba, M., et al. (2023). Lignocellulosic biomass from agricultural waste to the circular economy: A review with focus on biofuels, biocomposites and bioplastics. *Journal of Cleaner Production*. Elsevier Ltd. https://doi.org/10.1016/j.jclepro.2023.136815

Nair, L. G., Agrawal, K., & Verma, P. (2022). An insight into the principles of lignocellulosic biomass-based zero-waste biorefineries: A green leap towards imperishable energy-based future. *Biotechnology and Genetic Engineering Reviews, 38*(2), 288–338. https://doi.org/10.1080/02648725.2022.2082223

Nair, L. G., Agrawal, K., & Verma, P. (2023). Organosolv pretreatment: an in-depth purview of mechanics of the system. *Bioresources and Bioprocessing, 10*(1), 50. https://doi.org/10.1186/s40643-023-00673-0

Nair, L. G., & Verma, P. (2025). Harnessing carbon potential of lignocellulosic biomass: advances in pretreatments, applications, and the transformative role of machine learning in biorefineries. In *Bioresources and Bioprocessing*. https://doi.org/10.1186/s40643-025-00935-z

Ndochinwa, O. G. et al. (2024). Current status and emerging frontiers in enzyme engineering: An industrial perspective. In *Heliyon*. Elsevier Ltd. https://doi.org/10.1016/j.heliyon.2024.e32673

Nijland, J. G., & Driessen, A. J. M. (2020). Engineering of pentose transport in saccharomyces cerevisiae for biotechnological applications. In *Frontiers in bioengineering and biotechnology*. Frontiers Media S.A. https://doi.org/10.3389/fbioe.2019.00464

Novia, N. et al. (2024). Delignification and enzymatic hydrolysis kinetics of KOH microwave-assisted pretreated banana stem for bioethanol production. *International Journal of Hydrogen Energy, 85*, 931–946. https://doi.org/10.1016/j.ijhydene.2024.08.279

Olabi, A. G. et al. (2023). Renewable energy systems: Comparisons, challenges and barriers, sustainability indicators, and the contribution to UN sustainable development goals. *International Journal of Thermofluids, 20*. https://doi.org/10.1016/j.ijft.2023.100498

Pan, A., Xu, S., & Zaidi, S. A. H. (2024). Environmental impact of energy imports: Natural resources income and natural gas production profitability in the Asia-Pacific economic cooperation Countries. *Geoscience Frontiers, 15*(2). https://doi.org/10.1016/j.gsf.2023.101756

Patel, R. et al. (2025). A review on techno-economic analysis of lignocellulosic biorefinery producing biofuels and high-value products. In *Results in chemistry*. Elsevier B.V. https://doi.org/10.1016/j.rechem.2025.102052

Pielhop, T. et al. (2016). Steam explosion pretreatment of softwood: The effect of the explosive decompression on enzymatic digestibility. *Biotechnology for Biofuels, 9*(1). https://doi.org/10.1186/s13068-016-0567-1

Preethi, et al. (2021). Lignocellulosic biomass as an optimistic feedstock for the production of biofuels as valuable energy source: Techno-economic analysis, environmental impact analysis, breakthrough and perspectives. In *Environmental technology and innovation*. Elsevier B.V. https://doi.org/10.1016/j.eti.2021.102080

Primrose, J. (2025). Retrieved June 13, 2025, from https://stillwaterassociates.com/cellulosic-ethanol-is-a-revival-underway/

Range Fuels. (2008). Retrieved June 13, 2025, from https://rangefuels.com/Range-Fuels-Raises-over-00-Million-in-Series-B-Financing

Retrieved June 13, 2025, from https://www.energy.gov/eere/bioenergy/bioenergy-technologies-office

Retrieved June 13, 2025, from https://www.epa.gov/renewable-fuel-standard-program/renewable-fuel-standard-rfs2-final-rule

Raihan, A., & Mainul Bari, A. B. M. (2024). Energy-economy-environment nexus in China: The role of renewable energies toward carbon neutrality. *Innovation and Green Development, 3*(3). https://doi.org/10.1016/j.igd.2024.100139

Richardd L Smith, Z., & Xinhuaa Qi Editors, J. (2017). *Biofuels and biorefi neries 7 production of platform chemicals from sustainable resources*. http://www.springer.com/series/11687

Roni, M. S. et al. (2016). Lignocellulosic crop supply chains (eg, Miscanthus, switchgrass, reed canary grass, rye, giant reed, etc.). In *Biomass supply chains for bioenergy and biorefining* (pp. 271–291). Elsevier Inc. https://doi.org/10.1016/B978-1-78242-366-9.00012-5

Samoraj, M., et al. (2024), Advancements in algal biorefineries for sustainable agriculture: Biofuels, high-value products, and environmental solutions. *Biocatalysis and Agricultural Biotechnology, 58*. https://doi.org/10.1016/j.bcab.2024.103224

Saratale, R. G., et al. (2022). A critical review on biomass-based sustainable biorefineries using nanobiocatalysts: Opportunities, challenges, and future perspectives. In *Bioresource technology*. Elsevier Ltd. https://doi.org/10.1016/j.biortech.2022.127926

Saxena, A., et al. (2023). Current status of metabolic engineering of microorganisms for bioethanol production by effective utilization of pentose sugars of lignocellulosic biomass. In *Microbiological research*. Elsevier GmbH. https://doi.org/10.1016/j.micres.2023.127478

Sharma, S., & Horn, S. J. (2016). Enzymatic saccharification of brown seaweed for production of fermentable sugars. *Bioresource Technology, 213*, 155–161. https://doi.org/10.1016/j.biortech.2016.02.090

Shrivastava, A., & Sharma, R. K. (2023). Conversion of lignocellulosic biomass: Production of bioethanol and bioelectricity using wheat straw hydrolysate in electrochemical bioreactor. *Heliyon, 9*(1). https://doi.org/10.1016/j.heliyon.2023.e12951

Sikiru, S., et al. (2024). Technology projection in biofuel production using agricultural waste materials as a source of energy sustainability: A comprehensive review. In *Renewable and sustainable energy reviews*. Elsevier Ltd. https://doi.org/10.1016/j.rser.2024.114535

Sirohi, R., et al. (2021). Harnessing fruit waste for poly-3-hydroxybutyrate production: A review. In *Bioresource technology*. Elsevier Ltd. https://doi.org/10.1016/j.biortech.2021.124734

Srivastava, S., & Dafale, N. A. (2024). Tailored microbial consortium producing hydrolytic enzyme cocktail for maximum saccharification of wheat straw. *Bioresource Technology, 399*. https://doi.org/10.1016/j.biortech.2024.130560

Stasiak-Różańska, L., et al. (2025). Co-fermentation and genomic insights into lactic acid bacteria for enhanced propionic acid production using a non-GMO approach. *Foods, 14*(9). https://doi.org/10.3390/foods14091573

Thirumal, S., et al. (2024). Barriers to adopting digital technologies to implement circular economy practices in the construction industry: A systematic literature review. In *Sustainability (Switzerland)*. Multidisciplinary Digital Publishing Institute (MDPI). https://doi.org/10.3390/su16083185

Ward, L. (2015). *2015 DOE bioenergy technologies office(BETO) IBR project peer review POET-DSM project LIBERTY 2015 DOE biomass platform peer review (BPR)*.

Wildschut, J., et al. (2013). Ethanol-based organosolv fractionation of wheat straw for the production of lignin and enzymatically digestible cellulose. *Bioresource Technology, 135*, 58–66. https://doi.org/10.1016/j.biortech.2012.10.050

Wo´zniak, A. W., et al. (2025). Review of lignocellulosic biomass pretreatment using physical, thermal and chemical methods for higher yields in bioethanol production. https://doi.org/10.3390/su17010287/Copyright

Woo, W. X., et al. (2022). An overview on cell and enzyme immobilization for enhanced biohydrogen production from lignocellulosic biomass. *International Journal of Hydrogen Energy, 47*(96), 40714–40730. https://doi.org/10.1016/j.ijhydene.2022.08.164

Yang, Q., et al. (2016). Greenhouse gas emissions of a biomass-based pyrolysis plant in China. In *Renewable and sustainable energy reviews* (pp. 1580–1590). Elsevier Ltd. https://doi.org/10.1016/j.rser.2015.09.049

Yang, S., et al. (2016). Metabolic engineering of Zymomonas mobilis for 2,3-butanediol production from lignocellulosic biomass sugars. *Biotechnology for Biofuels, 9*(1). https://doi.org/10.1186/s13068-016-0606-y

Yi, Y. (2021). Tiny bugs play big role. In *Advances in 2nd generation of bioethanol production* (pp. 113–136). Elsevier. https://doi.org/10.1016/B978-0-12-818862-0.00007-8

Zabed, H., et al. (2016). Fuel ethanol production from lignocellulosic biomass: An overview on feedstocks and technological approaches. In *Renewable and sustainable energy reviews* (pp. 751–774). Elsevier Ltd. https://doi.org/10.1016/j.rser.2016.08.038

Ziegler-Devin, I., Chrusciel, L., & Brosse, N. (2021). Steam explosion pretreatment of lignocellulosic biomass: A mini-review of theorical and experimental approaches. In *Frontiers in chemistry*. Frontiers Media S.A. https://doi.org/10.3389/fchem.2021.705358

Chapter 5
Strategies and Innovations Techniques in Bioenergy Production: A Case Study Demonstrating Energy-Efficient Practices

Priti Pal, Ashna Parveen, Akhilesh Kumar Singh, Prakash Kumar Sarangi, Rahul Gupta, Laxuman Sharma, Saurabh Singh Rathore, Uttam Kumar Sahoo, and Pradeep Verma

Abstract Bioenergy production, a critical renewable energy paradigm, is hindered by energy-intensive processes that challenge its techno-economic viability and environmental sustainability. This chapter investigates advanced strategies and cutting-edge innovations to enhance the net energy ratio (NER) in bioenergy systems, addressing the urgent need for energy efficiency in biomass conversion. Key techniques include process integration through integrated biorefineries, which co-produce biofuels, biopower, and biochemicals, and waste heat recovery systems leveraging organic Rankine cycles to capture thermal energy. Process intensification, such as microwave-assisted biomass pretreatment, reduces energy inputs while improving feedstock digestibility. Recent innovations in enzymatic hydrolysis, utilizing tailored

P. Pal · R. Gupta
Amity Institute of Biotechnology, Amity University, Lucknow Campus, Lucknow, Uttar Pradesh, India

A. Parveen
Department of Biotechnology and Microbiology, Meerut Institute of Engineering and Technology, Meerut, India

A. K. Singh (✉) · S. S. Rathore
Department of Biotechnology, School of Life Sciences, Mahatma Gandhi Central University, Motihari, Bihar, India
e-mail: akhiliit@gmail.com

P. K. Sarangi
College of Agriculture, Central Agricultural University, Imphal, India

L. Sharma
Department of Horticulture, Sikkim University, Gangtok, India

U. K. Sahoo
Department of Forestry, Mizoram University, Aizawl, India

P. Verma
Department of Microbiology, Central University of Rajasthan, Kishangarh, Rajasthan, India

P. Verma (ed.), *Sustainable Practices in Biorefinery*,
https://doi.org/10.1007/978-981-95-6071-4_5

enzyme cocktails, and genetically engineered microbial fermentation, including modified *Saccharomyces cerevisiae* strains, significantly boost bioethanol and biogas yields. Artificial intelligence (AI) driven digitalization, incorporating IoT sensors and predictive models, enables real-time biorefinery optimization, achieving energy savings of 10–22%. Supported by empirical data from 2023–2025, these advancements demonstrate NER improvements of 20–50%. Three case studies a bioethanol biorefinery in India, a biogas facility in Sweden, and a biomass combustion plant in Canada illustrate scalable, energy-efficient practices, integrating waste heat recovery, co-digestion, and flue gas condensation. Challenges, including high capital costs and feedstock variability, underscore the need for policy incentives, such as subsidies for integrated biorefineries and R&D grants for digitalization and thermochemical conversion. Cross-sector collaboration is essential to standardize energy efficiency metrics and scale innovations like nanocatalysts and high-selectivity membranes. This chapter highlights the transformative potential of these strategies to advance bioenergy's role in a sustainable energy future, emphasizing the synergy of biotechnology, digitalization, and process engineering in optimizing renewable energy systems.

Keywords Bioenergy · Energy efficiency · Integrated biorefineries · Waste heat recovery · Process intensification · Enzymatic hydrolysis · Microbial fermentation · Sustainability

5.1 Introduction

Bioenergy, derived from organic materials such as agricultural residues, forestry byproducts, energy crops, and organic waste, is a cornerstone of the global transition to renewable energy. As the world grapples with the dual challenges of rising energy demand and the urgent need to mitigate climate change, bioenergy offers a renewable, carbon–neutral alternative to fossil fuels. By 2023, bioenergy accounted for approximately 10% of global primary energy supply, with applications ranging from biofuels like ethanol and biodiesel to biogas and solid biomass for heat and power generation (Singh et al., 2025). However, the sustainability and economic viability of bioenergy depend heavily on the efficiency of its production processes. Energy efficiency, defined as the ratio of useful energy output to total energy input, is a critical metric in bioenergy systems, influencing both environmental impact and cost-effectiveness. The production of bioenergy involves multiple stages, including feedstock cultivation, harvesting, preprocessing, conversion, and energy distribution (Alazaiza et al., 2024). Each stage presents opportunities for energy losses, which can undermine the overall efficiency of the system. For instance, preprocessing steps like drying and grinding biomass are often energy-intensive, while conversion processes such as fermentation or combustion may yield suboptimal energy outputs due to inefficiencies in technology or feedstock quality. Inefficient bioenergy systems not only reduce the energy return on investment (EROI) but also increase greenhouse gas emissions, negating some of the environmental benefits of bioenergy. Consequently, improving energy efficiency is paramount to maximizing the potential of bioenergy as a sustainable energy source. The importance of energy efficiency in bioenergy production is underscored by the global push for net-zero emissions by 2070 (Chaturvedi et al., 2024). Bioenergy is projected to play a significant role in achieving this target, particularly in sectors like transportation and heating, where electrification is less feasible (Tian et al., 2023). However, inefficiencies in bioenergy production can lead to higher costs and resource demands, making it less competitive compared to other renewable energy sources like solar or wind. For example, the energy required to produce a liter of bioethanol from corn can be substantial, with some studies estimating that up to 40% of the total energy input is consumed during preprocessing and distillation (Assaf et al., 2024). Improving efficiency at each stage of the bioenergy value chain is therefore critical to reducing costs, minimizing environmental impacts, and enhancing the scalability of bioenergy systems. One illustrative example of the need for energy efficiency in bioenergy production is the case of corn-based ethanol in the United States. Corn ethanol is a widely used biofuelwith the U.S. producing over 15 billion gallons annually by 2021 (Strapasson et al., 2021). However, early ethanol production facilities were criticized for their low energy efficiency, with some studies suggesting that the energy input for growing, harvesting, and processing corn exceeded the energy content of the ethanol produced (Padhan et al., 2023). This led to debates about the sustainability of corn ethanol as a renewable fuel. In response, the industry adopted several energy-efficient practices, such as the use of combined heat and power (CHP) systems and advanced distillation technologies. For instance, a modern ethanol plant in Iowa implemented a CHP system to recover waste heat from the distillation process, reducing energy consumption by 25% and improving the EROI from 1.3 to 2.1 (Jamil et al., 2024). This example highlights how targeted improvements in energy efficiency can transform the sustainability and economic viability of bioenergy systems. The challenges to energy efficiency in bioenergy production are multifaceted. Feedstock variability, such as differences in moisture content or lignocellulosic composition, can affect the efficiency of conversion processes. For example, wet biomass requires energyintensive drying before combustion, while lignocellulosic biomass often necessitates pretreatment to break down complex structures, consuming significant energy (Prasad et al., 2023). Additionally, the choice of conversion technology whether fermentation, anaerobic digestion, gasification, or hydrothermal liquefaction plays a critical role in determining overall efficiency. Traditional technologies like direct combustion may have efficiencies as low as 20–30%, while advanced methods like gasification can achieve efficiencies exceeding 60% (Sivabalan et al., 2021). Furthermore, logistical challenges, such as the energy required for biomass transportation, add to the overall energy footprint of bioenergy systems. To address these challenges, a range of strategies and innovations have been developed to enhance energy efficiency in bioenergy production. These include optimizing feedstock pretreatment, integrating processes like CHP, improving anaerobic digestion systems, and adopting advanced conversion technologies (Huang, 2024). For example, enzymatic pretreatment methods have reduced the energy required for lignocellulosic biomass hydrolysis by 20–30%

compared to mechanical methods (Mustafa et al., 2022). Similarly, integrated biorefineries, which coproduce biofuels, biochemicals, and electricity, maximize resource utilization and achieve energy efficiencies of up to 85% (Kashif et al., 2025; Nair et al., 2022). These innovations not only improve energy efficiency but also enhance the environmental and economic performance of bioenergy systems. Real-world case studies provide valuable insights into the practical implementation of energy-efficient practices. For instance, in Brazil, sugarcane ethanol plants have leveraged bagasse (a byproduct of sugarcane processing) to fuel CHP systems, achieving energy self-sufficiency and generating surplus electricity for the grid (da Silva et al., 2025). In Europe, biogas facilities have adopted co-digestion and advanced control systems to boost methane yields and reduce energy consumption. The broader implications of improving energy efficiency in bioenergy production extend beyond technical and economic benefits. By reducing energy inputs, bioenergy systems can lower their carbon footprint, aligning with global climate goals. Moreover, energy efficient bioenergy production can enhance energy security by reducing reliance on fossil fuels and utilizing locally available biomass resources (Singh et al., 2025). In developing countries, where access to modern energy services is limited, efficient bioenergy systems can provide affordable and sustainable energy solutions, supporting rural development and poverty alleviation. However, achieving high energy efficiency in bioenergy production requires overcoming several barriers. High upfront costs for advanced technologies, such as hydrothermal liquefaction or integrated biorefineries, can deter investment, particularly in developing regions (Ranjbar & Malcata, 2023). Additionally, the heterogeneity of biomass feedstocks poses challenges for standardizing processes, necessitating tailored solutions for different feedstocks and regions. Policy support, such as subsidies for energy-efficient technologies and carbon pricing, can play a crucial role in accelerating adoption. Furthermore, continued research and development are needed to refine emerging technologies and reduce their costs, making them accessible to a wider range of bioenergy producers (Blay-Roger et al., 2024). This chapter aims to provide a comprehensive overview of strategies and innovations for enhancing energy efficiency in bioenergy production, with a focus on practical applications and real-world examples. The following sections explore key strategies, including feedstock pretreatment optimization, process integration, anaerobic digestion enhancements, and advanced conversion technologies. Innovations in process optimization, such as automation, waste heat recovery, and integrated biorefineries, are also discussed. Through case studies, we illustrate how these approaches are implemented in ethanol, biogas, and bio-oil production, highlighting their impact on energy efficiency and sustainability. By synthesizing current knowledge and practical examples, this article seeks to inform researchers, policymakers, and industry stakeholders about the opportunities and challenges in making bioenergy a cornerstone of the global renewable energy landscape. Figure 5.1 presents a bar chart illustrating energy efficiency percentages achieved through various strategies, innovations, and case studies in bioenergy production, including feedstock pretreatment (Denmark), CHP integration (Brazil), anaerobic digestion (Sweden), hydrothermal liquefaction (Netherlands), automation (Germany), waste heat recovery (USA), and integrated biorefinery (Italy), showcasing efficiencies ranging from 65 to 82%

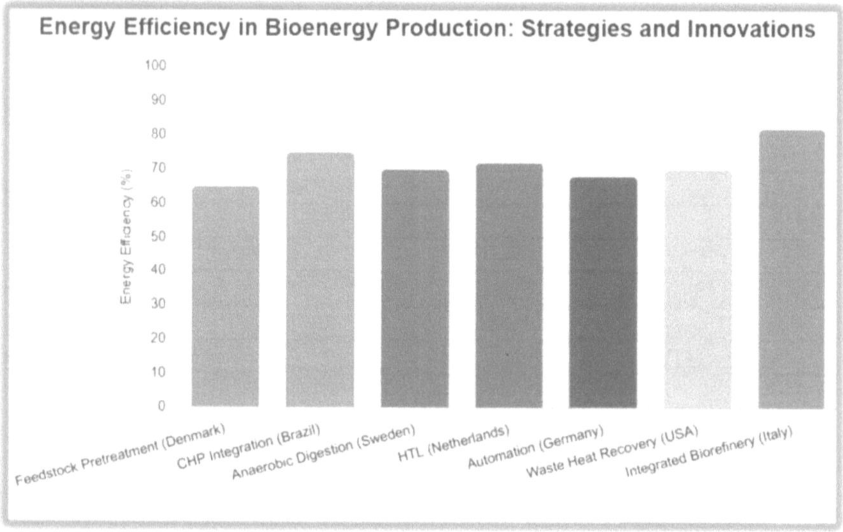

Fig. 5.1 Bar chart illustrating energy efficiency percentages achieved through various strategies, innovations, and case studies in bioenergy production, including feedstock pretreatment (Denmark), CHP integration (Brazil), anaerobic digestion (Sweden), hydrothermal liquefaction (Netherlands), automation (Germany), waste heat recovery (USA), and integrated biorefinery (Italy), showcasing efficiencies ranging from 65 to 82%

5.2 Strategies for Enhancing Energy Efficiency

Enhancing energy efficiency in bioenergy production is critical for maximizing energy output, reducing costs, and minimizing environmental impacts. The bioenergy value chain from feedstock cultivation to energy distribution presents multiple opportunities for efficiency improvements (Lai et al., 2022). Below, we discuss four key strategies: feedstock pretreatment optimization, process integration with combined heat and power (CHP) systems, anaerobic digestion enhancements, and advanced conversion technologies. Each strategy is accompanied by a detailed explanation and a practical example to illustrate its application. Figure 5.2 highlights these key strategies for enhancing energy efficiency in bioenergy systems, providing a visual summary of their core functions and benefits.

This figure illustrates four primary strategies to boost energy efficiency in bioenergy production: (1) *Feedstock Pretreatment Optimization* enhances biomass digestibility while reducing energy consumption; (2) *Process Integration and Combined Heat and Power (CHP)* recovers waste heat for simultaneous electricity and heat generation; (3) *Anaerobic Digestion Enhancements* focus on maximizing biogas yield with reduced energy input; and (4) *Advanced Conversion Technologies* employ efficient techniques such as hydrothermal liquefaction to improve overall energy conversion efficiency.

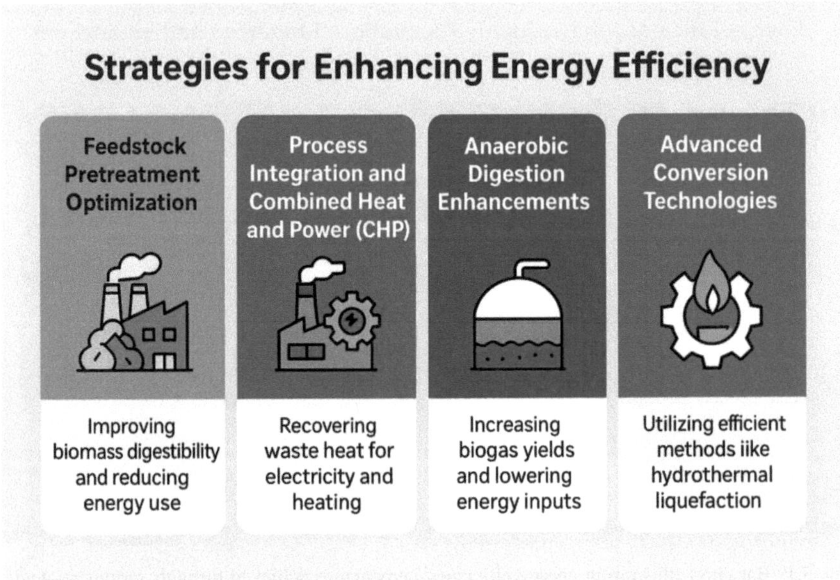

Fig. 5.2 Key strategies for enhancing energy efficiency in bioenergy systems

5.2.1 Feedstock Pretreatment Optimization

Feedstock pretreatment is often the most energy-intensive stage in bioenergy production, particularly for lignocellulosic biomass such as agricultural residues and woody materials. Lignocellulosic biomass consists of cellulose, hemicellulose, and lignin, which form a complex structure that resists breakdown. Traditional pretreatment methods, such as mechanical grinding or thermal drying, consume significant energy, often accounting for 20–30% of the total energy input in bioenergy processes (Kumar et al., 2020; Sitotaw et al., 2023). Innovations in pretreat ment aim to reduce energy consumption while improving biomass digestibility, thereby enhancing downstream conversion efficiency. One promising approach is steam explosion, which uses high-pressure steam to disrupt lignocellulosic structures, making cellulose more accessible for enzymatic hydrolysis. This method requires 20–30% less energy than mechanical grinding, as it relies on thermal and pressure gradients rather than physical force (Kishore et al., 2022). Another innovation is the use of ionic liquids, which dissolve lignin and hemicellulose at lower temperatures, reducing energy requirements by up to 40% compared to conventional acid or alkaline pretreatment (Roy & Chundawat, 2023). Additionally, biological pretreatment using fungi or enzymes can further reduce energy inputs by leveraging natural degradation processes, although these methods often require longer processing times. Cellulosic Ethanol Plant in Denmark A cellulosic ethanol plant operated by Inbicon in Kalundborg, Denmark, provides a practical example of feedstock pretreatment optimization. The facility processes wheat straw using a combination of steam explosion and enzymatic hydrolysis. By optimizing the steam explosion parameters (e.g., temperature and pressure), the plant reduced energy consumption for pretreatment by 25% compared to traditional methods (Erdoğan et al., 2023). The pretreated biomass is then subjected to enzymatic hydrolysis, which breaks down cellulose into fermentable sugars with minimal energy input. This approach has enabled the plant to achieve an overall energy efficiency of 65%, producing 5.4 million liters of ethanol annually while minimizing energy losses (Oke, 2023). The Inbicon plant demonstrates how advanced pretreatment methods can enhance energy efficiency and scalability in bioenergy production.

5.2.2 Process Integration and Combined Heat and Power (CHP)

Process integration involves combining multiple stages of bioenergy production to maximize resource utilization and minimize energy waste. Combined heat and power (CHP) systems are a prime example, as they capture waste heat generated during bioenergy production and repurpose it for electricity generation or heating. Traditional bioenergy systems, such as standalone combustion or fermentation plants, often lose 60–70% of their energy as waste heat (Ochieng et al., 2022). CHP systems can achieve overall energy efficiencies of up to 80% by recovering and reusing this thermal energy, compared to 30–40% for conventional systems. In bioenergy facilities, CHP systems are particularly effective when biomass residues, such as bagasse or wood chips, are used as fuel (Wijesekara et al., 2025). The heat generated from biomass combustion can power steam turbines for electricity production, while excess heat is used to meet process heating requirements, such as drying feedstocks or maintaining digester temperatures (Osman et al., 2023). CHP systems also reduce reliance on external energy sources, enhancing the energy self-sufficiency of bioenergy plants. Example: Sugarcane Ethanol Plant in Brazil A sugarcane ethanol plant in São Paulo, Brazil, illustrates the benefits of CHP integration. The plant uses bagasse, a byproduct of sugarcane processing, to fuel a CHP system that generates both electricity and process heat (Spyropoulos, 2024). By combusting bagasse in high-efficiency boilers, the plant produces 180 MW of electricity annually, meeting its own energy needs and supplying surplus power to the national grid (Kabeyi & Olanrewaju, 2023).The recovered heat is used to drive the distillation process, reducing the plant's external energy consumption by 30%. This integrated approach has resulted in an overall energy efficiency of 75%, demonstrating the transformative potential of CHP systems in bioenergy production.

5.2.3 Anaerobic Digestion Enhancements

Anaerobic digestion (AD) is a widely used process for producing biogas from organic waste, such as manure, food waste, and energy crops. However, traditional AD systems often suffer from low methane yields and high energy inputs for maintaining optimal conditions (e.g., temperature and pH). Innovations such as co-digestion, two-stage digestion, and advanced reactor designs have significantly improved the energy efficiency of AD systems. Co-digestion involves combining multiple feedstocks, such as manure and food waste, to optimize the carbon-to-nitrogen ratio and enhance methane production. This approach can increase biogas yields by 50–100% while reducing the energy required for mixing and heating (Feiz et al., 2022). Two-stage digestion separates the hydrolysis and methanogenesis phases, allowing for better control of microbial activity and higher methane content in the biogas. Additionally, advanced reactor designs, such as upflow anaerobic sludge blanket (UASB) reactors, improve biomass retention and reduce energy losses. Example: Biogas Facility in Sweden A biogas facility in Linköping, Sweden, provides a compelling example of AD enhancements (Senadheera et al., 2025). The plant employs co-digestion of food waste and sewage sludge, coupled with a two-stage digestion process. By optimizing the feedstock mix and digestion conditions, the facility increased its biogas yield by 70% and reduced energy consumption for heating and mixing by 15% (Obileke et al., 2024). The biogas is upgraded to biomethane and used as a vehicle fuel, while the digestate is applied as a fertilizer, creating a closed-loop system. This example highlights how AD enhancements can improve energy efficiency and support circular economy principles.

5.2.4 Advanced Conversion Technologies

Emerging conversion technologies, such as hydrothermal liquefaction (HTL) and gasification, offer significant improvements in energy efficiency compared to traditional methods like combustion or fermentation. HTL converts wet biomass into bio-oil under highpressure and high-temperature conditions, eliminating the need for energy-intensive drying. This process achieves energy efficiencies exceeding 70%, making it particularly suitable for feedstocks with high moisture content, such as algae or sewage sludge (Siddiqui et al., 2023). Gasification, on the other hand, converts biomass into syngas (a mixture of carbon monoxide and hydrogen), which can be used for electricity generation or biofuel synthesis. Gasification systems can achieve efficiencies of 60–70%, compared to 20–30% for direct combustion (Sivabalan et al., 2021). These technologies also enable the production of high-value products, such as bio-oils and synthetic fuels, which enhance the economic viability of bioenergy systems. Additionally, they can be integrated with other processes, such as CHP or biorefineries, to further improve overall efficiency. Example: Hydrothermal Liquefaction Pilot in the Netherlands A pilot-scale HTL facility in Rotterdam, Netherlands, demonstrates the potential of advanced conversion technologies (Ranjbar & Malcata, 2023). The facility processes wet organic waste, including food waste and sewage sludge, to produce bio-oil. By operating at high pressures (200–300 bar) and temperatures (300–350 °C), the plant converts 80% of the biomass energy into bio-oil, achieving an overall energy efficiency of 72% (Adeoye et al., 2024). Unlike traditional biofuel production methods, which require drying the feedstock, HTL processes wet biomass directly, saving up to 30% of the energy typically lost in drying. The bio-oil is used for industrial heating, while the aqueous byproduct is recycled for nutrient recovery. This example underscores the energy-saving potential of HTL for wet biomass feedstocks (Arias et al., 2023).

5.3 Innovations in Process Optimization

Process optimization is a cornerstone of improving energy efficiency in bioenergy production, focusing on minimizing energy waste and maximizing resource utilization across the production chain. Recent innovations leverage advanced technologies, data-driven approaches, and integrated systems to enhance the performance of bioenergy facilities (Alemde, 2025). Below, we discuss three key innovations in process optimization: automation and control systems, waste heat recovery, and integrated biorefineries. Each innovation is described in detail, supported by a practical example that illustrates its application in real-world bioenergy production. Figure 5.3 illustrates these innovations in process optimization for bioenergy systems, emphasizing their role in improving operational efficiency and sustainability outcomes.

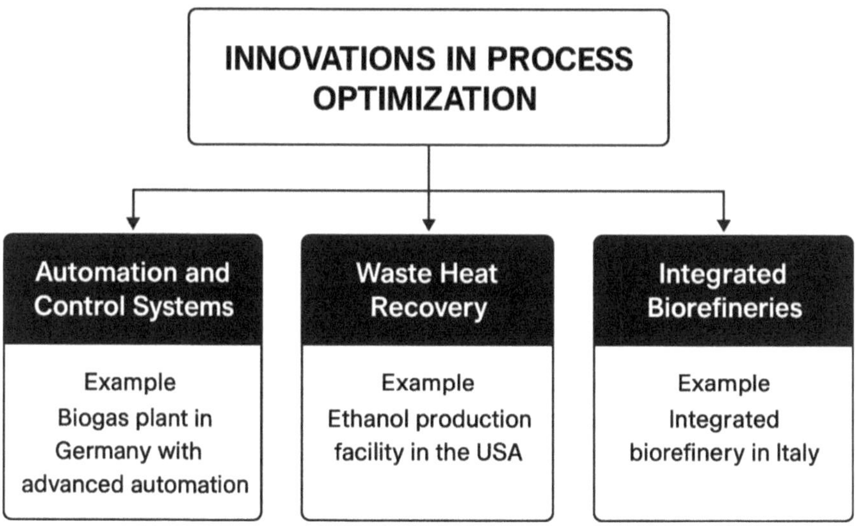

Fig. 5.3 Innovations in process optimization for bioenergy systems

The figure highlights three major innovations enhancing process efficiency in bioenergy production: (1) *Automation and Control Systems*, exemplified by an advanced biogas plant in Germany; (2) *Waste Heat Recovery*, as seen in ethanol production facilities in the USA; and (3) *Integrated Biorefineries*, demonstrated by a fully integrated biorefinery in Italy. These innovations contribute to improved resource utilization, operational efficiency, and sustainability.

5.3.1 Automation and Control Systems

Automation and control systems have transformed bioenergy production by enabling precise, real-time management of process parameters, significantly reducing energy losses and improving operational efficiency. These systems integrate sensors, actuators, and advanced algorithms often incorporating machine learning and artificial intelligence to monitor and adjust conditions such as temperature, pressure, pH, feedstock flow rates, and oxygen levels (Padhiary, 2023). In bioenergy processes like anaerobic digestion or ethanol fermentation, maintaining optimal conditions is critical for maximizing energy output. Manual control often leads to fluctuations that reduce yields and increase energy consumption, whereas automated systems can maintain stability, reducing energy use by 15–20% while enhancing product yields (Ghiasi et al., 2023). Machine learning algorithms play a pivotal role by analyzing real-time and historical data to predict and optimize process performance (Nair & Verma, 2025). For instance, in biogas production, machine learning can predict the optimal feedstock mix to maximize methane production while minimizing energy inputs for mixing and heating (Ling et al., 2024). These systems also enable predictive maintenance, identifying potential equipment failures such as pump malfunctions or heat exchanger fouling before they cause significant energy losses. Furthermore, automation reduces the need for on-site personnel, lowering operational costs and enabling remote monitoring, which is particularly beneficial for bioenergy facilities in remote locations (Pittalis et al., 2023). By integrating Internet of Things (IoT) technologies, automation systems can also provide real-time data dashboards, allowing operators to make informed decisions to further optimize energy use. Biogas Plant in Germany with Advanced Automation A biogas plant in Bavaria, Germany, exemplifies the impact of automation and control systems on energy efficiency (Tahir et al., 2025). The facility processes a mix of manure, energy crops, and food waste to produce biogas for electricity and heat generation. It implemented an advanced control system equipped with sensors for temperature, pH, volatile fatty acid levels, and gas composition, integrated with a machine learning algorithm (Feng et al., 2024). The system continuously monitors digester conditions and adjusts parameters in real time, such as reducing feedstock loading when pH drops to prevent microbial inhibition. This automation reduced energy consumption for heating and mixing by 18% and increased biogas yield by 20% compared to manual operation (Hanumanthakari et al., 2025). Additionally, the system's predictive maintenance module identifies potential equipment issues, such as pump inefficiencies, reducing downtime and energy losses by 10%. The plant's success highlights how automation can optimize bioenergy processes, improving both energy efficiency and operational reliability.

5.3.2 Waste Heat Recovery

Waste heat recovery is a critical innovation for enhancing energy efficiency in bioenergy production, as it captures and reuses thermal energy that would otherwise be lost to the environment. Bioenergy processes, such as combustion, distillation, and gasification, generate significant amounts of waste heat often 50–70% of the total energy input (Aboelela et al., 2023). Recovering this heat reduces the need for external energy sources, lowers operational costs, and decreases the carbon footprint of bioenergy facilities. Common waste heat recovery technologies include heat exchangers, organic Rankine cycles (ORC), and absorption chillers, each tailored to specific process requirements (Konur et al., 2022). Heat exchangers transfer heat from hot process streams, such as exhaust gases or distillation vapors, to colder streams, such as incoming feedstocks or water, reducing the energy required for heating. For example, in ethanol production, heat exchangers can recover up to 40% of the thermal energy used in distillation, significantly lowering energy costs (Botshekan et al., 2022). Organic Rankine cycles use organic fluids with low boiling points to generate electricity from low-grade waste heat, making them ideal for bioenergy plants with variable heat outputs. Absorption chillers, meanwhile, use waste heat to drive cooling systems, reducing the energy required for temperature control in processes like anaerobic digestion or fermentation (Hu et al., 2022). These technologies can be combined to maximize heat recovery, creating a cascade of energy reuse that enhances overall efficiency Example: Ethanol Production Facility in the USA An ethanol production facility in Nebraska, USA, demonstrates the effectiveness of waste heat recovery in bioenergy production (Ruffatto et al., 2022). The plant, which produces corn-based ethanol, installed a series of plate heat exchangers to capture waste heat from the distillation process, where high temperatures are used to separate ethanol from water. The recovered heat is used to preheat the mash (a mixture of corn and water) before fermentation, reducing the energy required for heating by 35% (Abo et al., 2024). Additionally, the facility implemented an organic Rankine cycle system to convert low-grade waste heat from the distillation column into electricity, generating 2 MW of additional power annually. This combined approach increased the plant's overall energy efficiency from 55 to 70% and reduced greenhouse gas emissions by 15% (Ahmed et al., 2022). The Nebraska facility illustrates how waste heat recovery can transform energy-intensive bioenergy processes into more sustainable and cost-effective operations.

5.3.3 Integrated Biorefineries

Integrated biorefineries represent a paradigm shift in bioenergy production, combining multiple processes within a single facility to maximize resource utilization, enhance energy efficiency, and produce a diverse range of products. Unlike traditional bioenergy plants that focus on a single output, such as ethanol or biogas, integrated biorefineries co-produce biofuels (e.g., ethanol, biodiesel, bio-oil), biochemicals (e.g., bioplastics, platform chemicals), and energy products (e.g., electricity, heat) from a variety of feedstocks, including lignocellulosic biomass, agricultural residues, energy crops, and organic waste (Kumar & Verma, 2021; Vasileiadou, 2024). By leveraging synergies between processes such as pretreatment, fermentation, anaerobic digestion, gasification, and combined heat and power (CHP) systems integrated biorefineries achieve energy efficiencies of up to 85%, compared to 50–60% for standalone facilities (Kashif et al., 2025).This holistic approach minimizes waste, optimizes energy flows, and enhances economic viability through diversified revenue streams. The core principle of an integrated biorefinery is the cascading utilization of biomass, where byproducts from one process become inputs for another, creating a closed-loop system. For example, lignocellulosic biomass can be fractionated into cellulose, hemicellulose, and lignin. Cellulose is used for ethanol production via enzymatic hydrolysis'. and fermentation, hemicellulose is converted into biochemicals like xylitol or furfural, and lignin is combusted in a CHP system to generate electricity and heat (Blasi et al., 2023). Residual biomass or process effluents can be processed in an anaerobic digester to produce biogas, with the digestate used as a biofertilizer for agriculture. This multi-product approach ensures that nearly all the energy content of the feedstock is extracted, significantly improving the energy return on investment (EROI). Integrated biorefineries also employ advanced technologies, such as automation and real-time process control, to optimize resource flows and minimize energy losses (Clauser et al., 2022). Integrated biorefineries can be classified into three main types: **lignocellulosic biorefineries**, which process woody or fibrous biomass; **green biorefineries**, which focus on wet biomass like grasses or algae; and **waste-based biorefineries**, which valorize organic waste streams. Each type is tailored to specific feedstocks and regional needs, enhancing flexibility and resilience. For instance, lignocellulosic biorefineries are ideal for regions with abundant agricultural residues, while waste-based biorefineries support urban areas with significant organic waste (Blasi et al., 2023). The integration of advanced conversion technologies, such as hydrothermal liquefaction (HTL) or pyrolysis, further enhances efficiency by processing challenging feedstocks like wet biomass or high-lignin materials without energy-intensive pretreatment steps. Recent advancements in integrated biorefineries include the development of **modular designs**, which allow for scalable and flexible operations, and **biocatalytic processes**, which use enzymes or microorganisms to produce high-value chemicals with lower energy inputs (John et al., 2025). Digital twins, which are virtual models of the biorefinery process, enable real-time simulation and optimization, thereby reducing energy waste and improving product yields. Additionally, carbon capture and utilization

(CCU) technologies are being integrated to capture CO_2 emissions from fermentation or combustion processes and convert them into value-added products such as methanol or polymers, further enhancing overall sustainability (Peres et al., 2022). These advancements address key challenges such as high capital costs, feedstock variability, and process complexity, thereby making integrated biorefineries more accessible and economically viable. The benefits of integrated biorefineries extend well beyond improved energy efficiency. By producing high-value biochemicals, these systems diversify revenue streams and reduce dependence on the often volatile biofuel markets. Their capacity to process a wide range of feedstocks enhances resilience to supply chain disruptions and supports local economies through the use of regionally available biomass. From an environmental perspective, integrated biorefineries contribute to significant reductions in greenhouse gas emissions by displacing fossil-based products and minimizing waste. Socially, they generate employment opportunities in rural areas and promote circular economy principles by valorizing agricultural and industrial waste streams. However, certain challenges persist. These include the need for substantial upfront investment often ranging between $100 million to $500 million for commercial scale facilities regulatory hurdles, and the technological complexity of integrating multiple effective processes with standardized operations (Bala et al., 2025). The Crescentino biorefinery in Piedmont, Italy, operated by Versalis (a subsidiary of Eni), stands as a pioneering example of an integrated biorefinery that optimizes both energy efficiency and product diversification. The facility processes approximately 270,000 tons of lignocellulosic biomass annually including wheat straw, corn stover, and energy crops like Arundo donax to produce cellulosic ethanol, electricity, biogas, and a range of biochemicals (Ray et al., 2022). The process begins with a steam explosion pretreatment at 200 °C and 1.5 MPa, which breaks down biomass into its main components: cellulose, hemicellulose, and lignin. The cellulose undergoes enzymatic hydrolysis and fermentation, yielding around 40,000 tons of ethanol per year (Igwebuike et al., 2024). Meanwhile, hemicellulose is converted into value-added biochemicals such as xylitol and furfural, which have applications in the food and chemical industries. Lignin is combusted in a high-efficiency Combined Heat and Power (CHP) system, producing 13 MW of electricity enough to meet 90% of the plant's energy requirements and supplying heat for the pretreatment and distillation processes, thereby reducing external energy consumption by 35% (Lackner et al., 2024).

Residual biomass and process effluents are treated in an anaerobic digester to generate approximately 1.5 million cubic meters of biogas annually (Abubakar, 2022). This biogas is upgraded to biomethane for use as a transportation fuel or injection into the national gas grid. The digestate is further processed into a nutrient-rich biofertilizer, which is used in local agriculture closing the loop in the resource cycle. The facility also features an advanced automation system equipped with IoT sensors and machine learning algorithms that optimize critical process parameters, such as enzyme dosing and digester performance. This digital integration reduces energy losses by an estimated 15% (Swami et al., 2023). Additionally, waste heat recovery systems, including heat exchangers, capture thermal energy from the CHP and fermentation processes, further improving overall efficiency. The Crescentino biorefinery achieves an impressive overall energy efficiency of 82%, compared to just 60% for conventional standalone ethanol plants. It also reduces greenhouse gas emissions by 25% relative to fossil-based alternatives (Kashif et al., 2025). By producing high-value biochemicals, the facility enhances economic resilience, while its use of locally sourced biomass supports regional agricultural communities. The Crescentino biorefinery exemplifies how integrated biorefineries can meet multiple sustainability objective maximizing energy efficiency, minimizing waste, and generating a diverse portfolio of bio-based products. Its success has inspired interest in replicating the model across Europe, supported by EU policies that promote the development of a sustainable bioeconomy (Skondras et al., 2024). Table 5.1 presents a comprehensive overview of techniques, innovations, and case studies for enhancing energy efficiency in bioenergy production, outlining strategies, real-world applications, and their measurable impacts.

5.4 Case Studies Demonstrating Energy-Efficient Practices

The following case studies demonstrate how energy-efficient practices are implemented in bioenergy production, highlighting measurable outcomes and lessons learned.

5.4.1 Case Study 1: Ethanol Production in Brazil

A sugarcane ethanol plant in São Paulo, Brazil, implemented a CHP system to utilize bagasse (a byproduct of sugarcane processing) for electricity and heat generation. By integrating CHP, the facility achieved an energy efficiency of 75%, producing 180 MW of electricity annually while meeting its own energy demands (Spyropoulos, 2024). The surplus electricity was sold to the grid, enhancing economic viability.

5.4.2 Case Study 2: Biogas Facility in Germany

A biogas plant in Bavaria, Germany, adopted co-digestion of manure and energy crops, coupled with an advanced control system. The facility increased its biogas yield by 60% and reduced energy consumption by 18% through optimized digestion parameters (Hidalgo-Sánchez et al., 2023). The use of waste heat to maintain digester temperatures further improved efficiency.

Table 5.1 Techniques, innovations, and case studies for enhancing energy efficiency in bioenergy production: strategies, applications, and measurable impacts

Category	Description	Key techniques	Case studies	Impact/outcpmes
Techniques for enhancing energy efficiency	Strategies to reduce energy inputs and maximize outputs across the bioenergy value chain	Feedstock pretreatment optimization: steam explosion, ionic liquids, biological pretreatment reduce energy use by 20–40%	Cellulosic Ethanol Plant, Denmark: Inbicon plant uses steam explosion and enzymatic hydrolysis, reducing pretreatment energy by 25%	Achieves 65% energy efficiency, producing 5.4 million liters of ethanol annually
		Process integration (CHP): combined heat and power systems recover waste heat, achieving up to 80% efficiency	Sugarcane Ethanol Plant, Brazil: uses bagasse for CHP, generating 180 MW electricity, meeting plant needs and supplying surplus to the grid	75% energy efficiency, 30% reduction in external energy consumption
		Anaerobic digestion enhancements: co-digestion and two-stage digestion increase biogas yields by 50–100% and reduce energy inputs	Biogas facility, Sweden: co-digestion of food waste and sewage sludge with two-stage digestion boosts biogas yield by 70%	15% reduction in energy for heating/mixing, supports circular economy principles
		Advanced conversion technologies: hydrothermal liquefaction (HTL) and gasification achieve efficiencies of 60–70%	HTL pilot, Netherlands: processes wet organic waste into bio-oil, achieving 72% efficiency without drying	Saves 30% energy typically lost in drying, produces bio-oil for industrial heating
Innovations in process optimization	Advanced technologies and data-driven approaches to minimize energy waste and enhance resource utilization	Automation and control systems: IoT sensors and machine learning optimize parameters, resulting in a 15–20% reduction in energy use	Biogas plant, Germany: advanced control system with machine learning increases biogas yield by 20% and reduces energy consumption by 18%	Enhances process stability, reduces downtime, and improves operational reliability

(continued)

Table 5.1 (continued)

Category	Description	Key techniques	Case studies	Impact/outcpmes
		Waste heat recovery: heat exchangers and organic Rankine cycles (ORC) recover 40–70% of waste heat	Ethanol Facility, USA: plate heat exchangers and ORC recover heat, reducing heating energy by 35% and generating 2 MW electricity	Increases efficiency from 55 to 70%, reduces GHG emissions by 15%
		Integrated biorefineries: Co-produce biofuels, biochemicals, and electricity, achieving up to 85% efficiency	Crescentino biorefinery, Italy: Processes lignocellulosic biomass for ethanol, electricity, and biochemicals, using CHP and anaerobic digestion	82% energy efficiency, 25% GHG reduction, supports local agriculture
Case studies demonstrating energy-efficient practices	Real-world applications showcasing measurable energy efficiency improvements	Brazil Ethanol production: CHP with bagasse achieves energy self-sufficiency and surplus power generation	Sugarcane Ethanol Plant, São Paulo: produces 180 MW electricity, meets plant needs, and supplies surplus to the grid	75% energy efficiency, enhances economic viability through grid sales
		Germany biogas facility: co-digestion and advanced controls optimize methane yields and reduce energy use	Biogas Plant, Bavaria: co-digestion and automation increase biogas yield by 60% and reduce energy use by 18%	Supports circular economy, reduces operational costs
		USA HTL Pilot: processes wet algae biomass, eliminating drying for high efficiency	HTL Facility, Iowa: Produces bio-oil with 72% efficiency, avoiding energy-intensive drying	Demonstrates scalability of HTL, significant energy savings for wet feedstocks

5.4.3 *Case Study 3: Hydrothermal Liquefaction Pilot in the USA*

A pilot-scale HTL facility in Iowa, USA, processed wet algae biomass to produce biooil. By eliminating the need for drying, the facility achieved an energy efficiency of 72%, compared to 50% for traditional lipid extraction methods (Chaudhary, 2024). The project demonstrated the scalability of HTL for wet feedstocks, reducing energy inputs significantly.

5.5 Key Challenges Hindering the Adoption of Energy-Efficient Bioenergy Technologies

One of the significant challenges in adopting energy-efficient technologies in bioenergy production is the high initial investment. Advanced systems such as Combined Heat and Power (CHP) units, gasifiers, and integrated biorefineries require costly equipment, sophisticated control systems, and skilled labor. For example, constructing a modern biogas CHP plant capable of processing 50,000 tons of organic waste per year may cost between $5 to $10 million (Kabeyi et al., 2024). Such financial demands are often unaffordable for small- and medium-scale operators, particularly in developing countries. In Southeast Asia, many small farmers, despite having abundant agricultural residues suitable for bioenergy production, are unable to invest in anaerobic digestion units with integrated CHP systems due to a lack of financial support or credit facilities (Beňová et al., 2021).

Another barrier is the variability in feedstock properties, including moisture content, composition, and biodegradability, which leads to fluctuations in energy yields and operational efficiency. This inconsistency creates challenges in maintaining stable reactor conditions, especially in biochemical processes like anaerobic digestion and fermentation. For instance, in Germany, co-digestion plants using mixtures of manure, crop residues, and food waste often encounter operational disruptions because of the fluctuating carbon-to-nitrogen (C:N) ratio in the feedstock (Schultz et al., 2025). Continuous monitoring and adjustment of the substrate mix are required to sustain optimal gas production. Furthermore, many innovative bioenergy technologies such as supercritical water gasification, bioelectrochemical systems, and thermochemical liquefaction remain confined to the pilot or laboratory scale, with limited commercial deployment. Technical challenges such as material corrosion, system fouling, and the complexity of operation, along with a shortage of skilled personnel, hinder the scalability of these systems. A pertinent example is microbial electrolysis cells (MECs), which can generate hydrogen from organic waste at high theoretical efficiencies but are rarely applied at a large scale due to technical and economic constraints (Guerrero-Sodric et al., 2023). In addition, the adoption of energy-efficient bioenergy systems often relies heavily on supportive policy frameworks, financial incentives, and carbon credit mechanisms. In many cases, inconsistent or weak policies fail to encourage private investment or technological innovation. A further complication is the absence of standardized methodologies for lifecycle energy accounting, which makes it difficult to accurately evaluate the true energy efficiency and environmental impact of bioenergy systems. For example, in several African countries, the lack of feed-in tariffs and government support for electricity generated from biomass has impeded the development of rural bioenergy projects, despite the availability of large quantities of agricultural waste (Uzoagba et al., 2024).

5.6 Future Directions for Advancing Energy Efficiency in Bioenergy Systems

The future of energy-efficient bioenergy lies in its integration with other renewable energy sources such as solar, wind, and green hydrogen, creating hybrid systems that enhance resource utilization and improve grid stability. This hybridization helps balance the intermittent supply from solar and wind with the continuous base-load capacity provided by bioenergy. For example, in Denmark, hybrid energy parks incorporate wind turbines, solar photovoltaic systems, and biogas-powered combined heat and power (CHP) units. Surplus electricity from wind and solar is used to produce hydrogen via electrolysis, which can then be blended into biogas pipelines or utilized in fuel cells (Panda et al., 2022). To address the limitations of centralized energy infrastructure, modular and decentralized bioenergy systems are gaining prominence. These systems are particularly well-suited for rural and remote areas where biomass is available but access to the national power grid is limited. In India, for instance, the Ministry of New and Renewable Energy (MNRE) has promoted the deployment of small-scale biomass gasifiers in villages. These units provide electricity and cooking fuel, reducing reliance on diesel and firewood. They are compact, require relatively low capital investment, and can be scaled up based on local demand (Pradhan et al., 2023). Improving the sustainability and reliability of bioenergy production also depends on establishing a stable feedstock supply chain. Precision agriculture utilizing technologies such as GPS-guided planting, remote sensing, and data analytics can significantly enhance the efficiency of feedstock production. This approach reduces input requirements like fertilizers and water while ensuring higher yields with more consistent quality, thereby addressing the problem of feedstock variability. In the United States, switchgrass is cultivated as a dedicated energy crop using precision farming techniques (Happs et al., 2024). This results in uniform biomass composition, which enhances the performance of biorefineries and reduces the energy required for pretreatment. Moreover, the development of energy-efficient bioenergy systems must be supported by strong policy frameworks and robust lifecycle energy accounting. Policymakers and investors can be guided by metrics such as Energy Return on Investment (EROI) and lifecycle greenhouse gas (GHG) assessments to identify the most efficient and sustainable options. A prime example is the

European Union's Renewable Energy Directive (RED II), which mandates lifecycle GHG accounting for biofuels and establishes minimum thresholds for emissions savings (Mizik, 2025). This incentivizes the adoption of bioenergy technologies that deliver higher energy efficiency and contribute meaningfully to climate goals.

5.7 Conclusion

Enhancing energy efficiency in bioenergy production is pivotal for its sustainability and economic viability, aligning with global goals for a low-carbon future. This chapter has explored strategies such as feedstock pretreatment optimization, process integration via combined heat and power (CHP) systems, anaerobic digestion enhancements, and advanced conversion technologies like hydrothermal liquefaction (HTL). Innovations in automation, waste heat recovery, and integrated biorefineries have further revolutionized the sector, achieving energy efficiencies of up to 85%, as demonstrated by case studies from Brazil, Germany, and the USA. For instance, Brazil's sugarcane ethanol plants leverage bagasse for CHP, achieving energy self-sufficiency, while Germany's biogas facilities optimize yields through co-digestion and digital controls. Despite these advancements, challenges like high capital costs and feedstock variability persist. Future progress hinges on scaling technologies like HTL and integrated biorefineries, supported by policy incentives and cross-sector collaboration to standardize efficiency metrics. By adopting these strategies and innovations, bioenergy can reduce its carbon footprint, enhance energy security, and support rural economies, solidifying its role as a cornerstone of the global renewable energy landscape and contributing significantly to net-zero emissions targets by 2050.

References

Abo, L. D., Hailegiorgis, S. M., Gindaba, G. T., Jayakumar, M., & Prabhu, S. V. (2024). A comprehensive review on fouling of heat transfer units in sugar factory ethanol plant: Mechanisms and mitigation methods. *Environmental Quality Management, 34*(2), Article e70003.

Aboelela, D., Saleh, H., Attia, A. M., Elhenawy, Y., Majozi, T., & Bassyouni, M. (2023). Recent advances in biomass pyrolysis processes for bioenergy production: Optimization of operating conditions. *Sustainability, 15*(14), 11238.

Abubakar, A. M. (2022). Biodigester and feedstock type: Characteristic, selection, and global biogas production. *Journal of Engineering Research and Sciences, 1*(3), 170–187.

Adeoye, A. O., Quadri, R. O., Lawal, O. S., Malomo, D., Emojevu, E. O., Omonije, O. O., & Saidu, A. U. (2024). Advanced techniques in upgrading crude bio-oil to biofuel. In *Intelligent transportation system and advanced technology* (pp. 321–353). Singapore: Springer Nature Singapore.

Ahmed, I., Rehan, M., Basit, A., & Hong, K. S. (2022). Greenhouse gases emission reduction for electric power generation sector by efficient dispatching of thermal plants integrated with renewable systems. *Scientific Reports, 12*(1), 12380.

Alazaiza, M. Y. D., Ahmad, Z., Albahnasawi, A., Nassani, D. E., & Alenezi, R. A. (2024). Biomass processing technologies for bioenergy production: Factors for future global market. *International Journal of Environmental Science and Technology, 21*(2), 2307–2324.
Alemde, V. O. (2025). Innovative process technologies: Advancing efficiency and sustainability through optimization and control.*International Journal of Research Publication and Reviews, 6*(2), 1941–1955.
Arias, D. M., García-Valladares, O., Besagni, G., & Markides, C. N. (2023). A vision of renewable thermal technologies for drying, biofuels production and industrial waste, gas or water recovery. *Applied Thermal Engineering, 223*, Article 120022.
Assaf, J. C., Mortada, Z., Rezzoug, S. A., Maache-Rezzoug, Z., Debs, E., & Louka, N. (2024). Comparative review on the production and purification of bioethanol from biomass: A focus on corn. *Processes, 12*(5), 1001.
Bala, R., Kaur, M., Thakur, H., Kashyap, P., Karnwal, A., & Malik, T. (2025). A sociotechnical review of carbon capture, utilization, and storage (CCUS) technologies for industrial decarbonization: Current challenges, emerging solution, and future directions. *International Journal of Chemical Engineering, 2025*(1), 7195300.
Beňová, D., Mareš, K., Hutla, P., Ivanova, T., Banout, J., & Kolaříková, M. (2021). Energy potential of agri residual biomass in Southeast Asia with the focus on Vietnam. *Agronomy, 11*(1), 169.
Blasi, A., Verardi, A., Lopresto, C. G., Siciliano, S., & Sangiorgio, P. (2023). Lignocellulosic agricultural waste valorization to obtain valuable products: An overview. *Recycling, 8*(4), 61.
Blay-Roger, R., Saif, M., Bobadilla, L. F., Ramirez-Reina, T., Nawaz, M. A., & Odriozola, J. A. (2024). Embracing the sustainable horizons through bioenergy innovations: A path to a sustainable energy future. *Frontiers in Chemistry, 12*, 1416102.
Botshekan, M., Moheb, A., Vatankhah, F., Karimi, K., & Shafiei, M. (2022). Energy saving alternatives for renewable ethanol production with the focus on separation/purification units: A techno-economic analysis. *Energy, 239*, Article 122363.
Chaturvedi, V., Ghosh, A., Garg, A., Avashia, V., Vishwanathan, S. S., Gupta, D., & Prasad, S. (2024). India's pathway to net zero by 2070: Status, challenges, and way forward. *Environmental Research Letters, 19*(11), Article 112501.
Chaudhary, V., Awadakkam, S., Borugadda, V. B., & Dalai, A. K. (2024). A critical review on the production and upgradation of sustainable biocrude from hydrothermal liquefaction of Canadian-grown agricultural biomass. *Sustainable Energy & Fuels, 8*(23), 5305–5328.
Clauser, N. M., Felissia, F. E., Area, M. C., & Vallejos, M. E. (2022). Integrating the new age of bioeconomy and industry 4.0 into biorefinery process design. *BioResources, 17*(3), 5510–5531.
da Silva, G. H. R., Nascimento, A., Nascimento, D., Hunt, J. D., & Mathias, M. H. (2025). Analysis of the sugarcane biomass use to produce green hydrogen: Brazilian case study.
Erdoğan, E. M., Karagöz, P., & Özkan, M. (2023). Bioethanol production from lignocellulosic wastes: Potentials and challenges. *Bioethanol: A Green Energy Substitute for Fossil Fuels*, 123–160.
Feiz, R., Johansson, M., Lindkvist, E., Moestedt, J., Påledal, S. N., & Ometto, F. (2022). The biogas yield, climate impact, energy balance, nutrient recovery, and resource cost of biogas production from household food waste—a comparison of multiple cases from Sweden. *Journal of Cleaner Production, 378*, Article 134536.
Feng, Y., Wang, Y., Beykal, B., Qiao, M., Xiao, Z., & Luo, Y. (2024). A mechanistic review on machine learning-supported detection and analysis of volatile organic compounds for food quality and safety. *Trends in Food Science & Technology, 143*, Article 104297.
Ghiasi, M., Wang, Z., Mehrandezh, M., & Paranjape, R. (2023). A systematic review of optimal and practical methods in design, construction, control, energy management and operation of smart greenhouses. *IEEE Access, 12*, 2830–2853.
Guerrero-Sodric, O., Baeza, J. A., & Guisasola, A. (2023). Exploring key operational factors for improving hydrogen production in a pilot-scale microbial electrolysis cell treating urban wastewater. *Chemical Engineering Journal, 469*, Article 144001.

Hanumanthakari, S., Kumar, R. V., Arputhabalan, J., Velmurugan, P., & Yalawar, M. S. (2025). Automated Electric Power Generation From Agricultural Resources. In *Integrating artificial intelligence into the energy sector* (pp. 185–210). IGI Global Scientific Publishing.

Happs, R. M., Hanes, R. J., Bartling, A. W., Field, J. L., Harman-Ware, A. E., Clark, R. J., & Davison, B. H. (2024). Economic and sustainability impacts of yield and composition variation in bioenergy crops: Switchgrass (Panicum virgatum L.). *ACS Sustainable Chemistry & Engineering, 12*(5), 1897–1910.

Hidalgo-Sánchez, V., Behmel, U., Hofmann, J., & Borges, M. E. (2023). Enhancing biogas production of co-digested cattle manure with grass silage from a local farm in Landshut, Bavaria, through chemical and mechanical pre-treatment and its impact on biogas reactor hydraulic retention time. *Sustainability, 15*(3), 2582.

Hu, T., Shen, Y., Kwan, T. H., & Pei, G. (2022). Absorption chiller waste heat utilization to the desiccant dehumidifier system for enhanced cooling–Energy and exergy analysis. *Energy, 239*, Article 121847.

Huang, X. (2024). The promotion of anaerobic digestion technology upgrades in waste stream treatment plants for circular economy in the context of "dual carbon": Global status, development trend, and future challenges. *Water, 16*(24), 3718.

Igwebuike, C. M., Awad, S., & Andrès, Y. (2024). Renewable energy potential: Second-generation biomass as feedstock for bioethanol production. *Molecules, 29*(7), 1619.

Jamil, F., Inayat, A., Hussain, M., Akhter, P., Abideen, Z., Ghenai, C., & Abdellatief, T. M. (2024). Valorization of waste biomass to biofuels for power production and transportation in optimized way: A comprehensive review. *Advanced Energy and Sustainability Research, 5*(10), 2400104.

John, S. U., Onu, C. E., Ezechukwu, C. M. J., Nwokedi, I. C., & Onyenanu, C. N. (2025). Multi-product biorefineries for biofuels and value-added products: Advances and future perspectives. *Academia Green Energy, 2*(1).

Kabeyi, M. J. B., & Olanrewaju, O. A. (2023). Bagasse electricity potential of conventional sugarcane factories. *Journal of Energy, 2023*(1), 5749122.

Kabeyi, M. J. B., Olanrewaju, O. A., & Akpan, J. (2024). Biogas production and process control improvements. In *From biomass to biobased products*. IntechOpen.

Kashif, M., Sabri, M. A., Aresta, M., Dibenedetto, A., & Dumeignil, F. (2025). Sustainable synergy: Unleashing the potential of biomass in integrated biorefineries. *Sustainable Energy & Fuels, 9*(2), 338–400.

Kishore, K., Sinha, M. K., Singh, A., Archana, Gupta, M. K., & Korkmaz, M. E. (2022). A comprehensive review on the grinding process: Advancements, applications and challenges. *Proceedings of the Institution of Mechanical Engineers, Part C: Journal of Mechanical Engineering Science, 236*(22), 10923–10952.

Konur, O., Colpan, C. O., & Saatcioglu, O. Y. (2022). A comprehensive review on organic Rankine cycle systems used as waste heat recovery technologies for marine applications. *Energy Sources, Part a: Recovery, Utilization, and Environmental Effects, 44*(2), 4083–4122.

Kumar, B., Bhardwaj, N., Agrawal, K., Chaturvedi, V., & Verma, P. (2020). Current perspective on pretreatment technologies using lignocellulosic biomass: An emerging biorefinery concept. *Fuel Processing Technology, 199*, Article 106244.

Kumar, B., & Verma, P. (2021). Life cycle assessment: Blazing a trail for bioresources management. *Energy Conversion and Management: X, 10*, Article 100063.

Lackner, M., Fei, Q., Guo, S., Yang, N., Guan, X., & Hu, P. (2024). Biomass gasification as a scalable, green route to combined heat and power (CHP) and synthesis gas for materials: A review. *Fuels, 5*(4), 625–649.

Lai, W., Qiao, Y., Zhang, J., Lin, Z., & Huang, H. (2022). Design strategies for markedly enhancing energy efficiency in the electrocatalytic CO 2 reduction reaction. *Energy & Environmental Science, 15*(9), 3603–3629.

Ling, J. Y. X., Chan, Y. J., Chen, J. W., Chong, D. J. S., Tan, A. L. L., Arumugasamy, S. K., & Lau, P. L. (2024). Machine learning methods for the modelling and optimisation of biogas production

from anaerobic digestion: A review. *Environmental Science and Pollution Research, 31*(13), 19085–19104.
Mizik, T. (2025). European Union guidelines for the production of different generations of biofuels. In *Biofuels and sustainability* (pp. 205–219). Elsevier Science Ltd.
Mustafa, A. H., Rashid, S. S., Rahim, M. H. A., Roslan, R., Musa, W. A. M., Sikder, B. H., & Sasi, A. A. (2022). Enzymatic pretreatment of lignocellulosic biomass: An overview. *Journal of Chemical Engineering and Industrial Biotechnology, 8*(1), 1–7.
Nair, L. G., & Verma, P. (2025). Harnessing carbon potential of lignocellulosic biomass: advances in pretreatments, applications, and the transformative role of machine learning in biorefineries. *Bioresources and Bioprocessing, 12*(1).
Nair, L. G., Agrawal, K., & Verma, P. (2022). An overview of sustainable approaches for bioenergy production from agro-industrial wastes. *Energy Nexus, 6*, Article 100086.
Nair, S. K., Emerson, R. M., & Solomon, J. R. (2024). Biomass supply chain risk: Towards a better understanding of feedstock availability, cost, variability, and uncertainty to catalyze and de-risk biobased investment. *Handbook of biorefinery research and technology: Biomass logistics to saccharification* (pp. 285–312). Springer, Netherlands.
Obileke, K., Makaka, G., Tangwe, S., & Mukumba, P. (2024). Improvement of biogas yields in an anaerobic digestion process via optimization technique. *Environment, Development and Sustainability*, 1–27.
Ochieng, R., Gebremedhin, A., & Sarker, S. (2022). Integration of waste to bioenergy conversion systems: A critical review. *Energies, 15*(7), 2697.
Oke, K. A. (2023). Assessing technology options to reduce the carbon intensity of bioethanol production.
Osman, A. I., Lai, Z. Y., Farghali, M., Yiin, C. L., Elgarahy, A. M., Hammad, A., & Yap, P. S. (2023). Optimizing biomass pathways to bioenergy and biochar application in electricity generation, biodiesel production, and biohydrogen production. *Environmental Chemistry Letters, 21*(5), 2639–2705.
Padhan, S. R., Jat, S. L., Mishra, P., Darjee, S., Saini, S., Padhan, S. R., & Ranjan, S. (2023). Corn for biofuel: Status, prospects and implications. *New Prospects of Maize.*
Padhiary, M. (2023). Bridging the gap: Sustainable automation and energy efficiency in food processing. *Agricultural Engineering Today, 47*(3), 47–50.
Panda, S., Mohanty, S., Rout, P. K., & Sahu, B. K. (2022). A conceptual review on transformation of micro-grid to virtual power plant: Issues, modeling, solutions, and future prospects. *International Journal of Energy Research, 46*(6), 7021–7054.
Peres, C. B., Resende, P. M., Nunes, L. J., & Morais, L. C. D. (2022). Advances in carbon capture and use (CCU) technologies: A comprehensive review and CO_2 mitigation potential analysis. *Clean Technologies, 4*(4), 1193–1207.
Pittalis, M., Sancho, A., Szabó, S., Lazopoulou, M., & Moner-Girona, M. (2023). Quantifying impacts and benefits of advanced remote monitoring solutions for the operation of mini grids in sub-Saharan Africa. *Energy for Sustainable Development, 77*, Article 101335.
Pradhan, P., Deore, S. P., Gadkari, P., Arora, A., & Mahajani, S. M. (2023). Field evaluation of biomass gasifier for bioenergy application: Case studies on institutional cooking in India. *Sustainable Energy Technologies and Assessments, 59*, Article 103409.
Prasad, B. R., Padhi, R. K., & Ghosh, G. (2023). A review on key pretreatment approaches for lignocellulosic biomass to produce biofuel and value-added products. *International Journal of Environmental Science and Technology, 20*(6), 6929–6944.
Ranjbar, S., & Malcata, F. X. (2023). Hydrothermal liquefaction: How the holistic approach by nature will help solve the environmental conundrum. *Molecules, 28*(24), 8127.
Ray, A., Yenumala, S. R., & Kumar, S. (2022). Bioenergy generation: Processes and technologies.
Roy, S., & Chundawat, S. P. (2023). Ionic liquid–based pretreatment of lignocellulosic biomass for bioconversion: A critical review. *BioEnergy Research, 16*(1), 263–278.

Ruffatto, K., Emaminejad, S. A., Juneja, A., Kurambhatti, C., Margenot, A., Singh, V., & Cusick, R. D. (2022). Mapping the national phosphorus recovery potential from centralized wastewater and corn ethanol infrastructure. *Environmental Science & Technology, 56*(12), 8691–8701.

Schultz, J., Scherzinger, M., Elbanhawy, A. Y., & Kaltschmitt, M. (2025). Long-term continuous anaerobic co-digestion of residual biomass—model validation and model-based investigation of different carbon-to-nitrogen ratios. *BioEnergy Research, 18*(1), 58.

Senadheera, U. E., Abeykoon, A. M. W. D. C. B., Sewmini, P. M. N., Weerasekara, W. M. R. B., Darshani, N. P., Jayasanka, J., & Jayawardena, T. U. (2025). Up-flow anaerobic sludge bed reactors for sustainable wastewater management: Challenges, innovations, and future directions. *Water, 17*(4), 476.

Siddiqui, M. I., Rameez, H., Farooqi, I. H., & Basheer, F. (2023). Recent advancement in commercial and other sustainable techniques for energy and material recovery from sewage sludge. *Water, 15*(5), 948.

Singh, R., Gaur, A., Soni, P., Jain, R., Pant, G., Kumar, D., & Ansari, K. (2025). A review of biofuels and bioenergy production as a sustainable alternative: Opportunities, challenges and future perspectives. *Journal of Environmental Health Science and Engineering, 23*(2), 23.

Sitotaw, Y. W., Habtu, N. G., Gebreyohannes, A. Y., Nunes, S. P., & Van Gerven, T. (2023). Ball milling as an important pretreatment technique in lignocellulose biorefineries: A review. *Biomass Conversion and Biorefinery, 13*(17), 15593–15616.

Sivabalan, K., Hassan, S., Ya, H., & Pasupuleti, J. (2021, March). A review on the characteristic of biomass and classification of bioenergy through direct combustion and gasification as an alternative power supply. In *Journal of physics: Conference series* (Vol. 1831, No. 1, p. 012033). IOP Publishing.

Skondras, A., Nastis, S. A., Skalidi, I., Theofilou, A., Bakousi, A., Mone, T., & Stylianidis, E. (2024). Governance strategies for sustainable circular bioeconomy development in Europe: Insights and typologies. *Sustainability, 16*(12), 5140.

Spyropoulos, G. (2024). *Bagasse utilization and management strategies in São Paulo Sugarcane Mills* (Master's thesis).

Strapasson, A., Lee, H., & Schnettler, J. (2021). Biofuels and the water-energy nexus: Perspectives for the United States.

Swami, S., Suthar, S., Singh, R., Thakur, A. K., Gupta, L. R., & Sikarwar, V. S. (2023). Integration of anaerobic digestion with artificial intelligence to optimise biogas plant operation. *Environment, Development and Sustainability*, 1–31.

Tahir, F., Rasheed, R., Fatima, M., Batool, F., & Nizami, A. S. (2025). Sustainability analysis of commercial-scale biogas plants in Pakistan vs. Germany: A Novel analytic hierarchy process—SMARTER approach. *Sustainability, 17*(5), 2168.

Tian, X., An, C., & Chen, Z. (2023). The role of clean energy in achieving decarbonization of electricity generation, transportation, and heating sectors by 2050: A meta-analysis review. *Renewable and Sustainable Energy Reviews, 182*, Article 113404.

Uzoagba, C., Onwualu, P. A., Okoroigwe, E., Kadivar, M., Oribu, W. S., Mguni, N. G., & Mozie, M. (2024). A review of biomass valorization for bioenergy and rural electricity generation in Nigeria. *Cureus, 1*(1), 1–16.

Vasileiadou, A. (2024). From organic wastes to bioenergy, biofuels, and value-added products for urban sustainability and circular economy: A review. *Urban Science, 8*(3), 121.

Wijesekara, D., Kularathna, L., Abesundara, P., Lankathilaka, U., Muhandiram, I., Amarasinghe, P., & Koswattage, K. (2025). Comparative energy and environmental analysis of combined cycle CHP combustion operations via simulation for biomass and industrial materials derived from waste. *Energies, 18*(12), 3062.

Chapter 6
Sustainable Unified Lignocellulosic Biorefinery for Cost-Effective Production of Value-Added Products in a Circular-Bioeconomy Framework

Mamta, Abhimanyu Kumar, Shristy Shreya, Shobham, and Jitendra Panwar

Abstract Lignocellulosic biorefineries are the most promising sustainable alternative to fossil-fuel based refineries for the production of various value-added products ranging from biofuels to bioplastics. Rice straw, an abundantly available lignocellulosic residue remains underutilized and is often burnt in open fields leading to environmental pollution. Value-added products sourced from rice straw biomass can potentially mitigate the environment pollution problems along with decreasing the reliability on fossil-fuel based non-renewable resources. Although, high availability and renewable nature makes rice straw a potential biomass feedstock for industrial applications, due to the highly recalcitrant nature, its efficient valorization remains a major obstacle. This chapter describes the major challenges and opportunities for efficient valorization of lignocellulosic biomass majorly focusing on rice straw as a key biomass feedstock for production of value-added products at industrial scale. The major obstacles and recent advances in various pre-treatment strategies for efficient valorization of rice straw have been examined. Strategies for low-cost enzyme cocktail production for saccharification of rice straw have been discussed. Furthermore, the chapter evaluates the environmental impact and economic viability of lignocellulosic biorefineries using techno-economic analysis framework, aiming to envision the cost-effective scale-up of lignocellulosic biomass based biorefineries towards establishment of circular bioeconomy.

Keywords Lignocellulosic biomass · Biorefinery · Rice straw · Pre-treatments · Enzymatic saccharification · Techno-economic analysis

Mamta · A. Kumar · S. Shreya · Shobham · J. Panwar (✉)
Department of Biological Sciences, Birla Institute of Technology and Science, Pilani, India
e-mail: jpanwar@pilani.bits-pilani.ac.in

P. Verma (ed.), *Sustainable Practices in Biorefinery*,
https://doi.org/10.1007/978-981-95-6071-4_6

6.1 Introduction

Rice is one of the most cultivated crops worldwide in more than 100 countries and predominately grown in Asia which accounts for more than 90% of the total global production. India, home to hundreds of millions of people, largely depends on rice as its main agricultural crop. The nation is not only the world's greatest consumer of rice, but the world's second-largest rice producer after China (Hassan et al., 2021). As per recent report, rice production has been estimated approximately 1378.25 lakh tonnes surpassing the previous five years average by 128.37 lakh tonnes (Ministry of Agriculture and Farmers Welfare Annual Report, 2024–2025). Nonetheless, this intensification in rice cultivation brings another major concern i.e. rice straw, a major agricultural residue. It has been estimated that each tonne of rice grain results in generation of around 1.5 tonnes of rice straw (Saini et al., 2023). This makes rice straw as one of the most prevalent lignocellulosic biomasses (LCBs) resource. Rice residue accounts for around 200 million tonnes (dry weight), representing 33 percent of the India's total annual residue biomass production, which is approximately 682.6 million tonnes on a dry weight basis.

Rice straw biomass is rich in cellulose, hemicellulose and lignin content, making it a potentially valuable biomass feedstock for the production of bio-based value-added products. Its high carbon content with a high calorific value, makes it a valuable energy source (Nath et al., 2025). Depending of the plant variety, around 700–1500 kg rice straw is generated for every ton of rice grain (Grisolia et al., 2022). Moreover, around 205 billion liters of bioethanol can be produced annually from rice straw, which is quite high in comparison to any other single biomass feedstock (Goodman, 2020; Mothe & Polisetty, 2021).

Given its higher abundance, availability, cost-effectiveness and renewable nature, rice straw can be an ideal substrate for bioprocessing in lignocellulosic biorefineries. Rice-straw based biorefineries are the future of sustainable biomass utilization which can operate similarly to petroleum refineries, where rice straw complex biomass can be converted to a wide range of bio-based materials using various process configurations. These biorefineries offers a circular and economically viable option while mitigating environmental pollution (Singh et al., 2024).

Despite its promising potential, rice straw remains underutilized. Hardly 20% of rice straw produced per year is utilized in manufacturing of bio-based products and other energy applications despite its higher energy content (10–14 MJ kg^{-1}) at 10% moisture level. A significant portion of rice straw ranging between 8–80% is burnt till date in open fields by farmers, especially in the north-western Indian states namely Punjab, Haryana and Uttar-Pradesh (Bhattacharyya et al., 2021; Kaur et al., 2022), which considerably worsens the air quality by adding fine and coarse dust particles (PM2.5) to the suspended particulate matter (PM10) and toxic gases like carbon monoxide (CO), carcinogenic polycyclic aromatic hydrocarbons (PAH), dioxins etc. to the environment. Moreover, burning of one kilogram of dried rice straw can lead to generation of 700–4100 mg of methane (CH_4) and 19–57 mg of nitrous oxide (N_2O), thereby increasing the greenhouse gas (GHG) emissions. These emissions not only intensify the climate change but also lead to substantial depletion of plant nutrients from the soil (Bhattacharyya et al., 2021).

In India various policies have been implemented and adopted to address the environmental pollution caused by rice straw burning. Based on the National Policy for Management of Crop Residue, the National Remote Sensing Agency and Centre of Pollution Control Board have taken multiple initiatives to control the crop residue burning. Moreover, research institutes such as the Indian Council for Agricultural Research (ICAR) and the Ministry of New and Renewable Energy (MNRE) have conducted extensive research to promote waste to energy bioconversion technologies using rice straw as an alternative and sustainable source (Bhuvaneshwari et al., 2019). However, despite the partial awareness of the ill effects of rice straw burning in India, many farmers still prefer burning over the other sustainable management practices. The main contributing causes are a very short span between harvesting and sowing of next crop, scarcity of labor during the crucial field operations and use of combine harvesters which leaves 20–30 cm of stubble on the ground, making it difficult for farmers to sow the next crop. Also, rice straw is not a preferred fodder for animals because of its high silica content, low amount of nutrients availability for animals, Deglana disease spread, and high oxalate content (Dutta et al., 2022).

Although rice straw holds immense potential as a renewable and abundant biomass resource, the highly recalcitrant nature of its complex lignocellulosic matrix poses significant challenges for its efficient valorization. High energy and chemical requirements for pretreatment of rice straw along with associated cost for enzymatic saccharification are major obstacles for its large-scale industrial applications. This chapter examines the challenges and opportunities associated with utilization of rice straw as a lignocellulosic biomass feedstock for production of bio-based value-added products. The focus is given on current challenges and recent advancements in the pretreatment strategies along with development of cost-effective enzyme cocktails aimed at addressing biomass recalcitrance. The economic viability of rice straw based biorefineries has also been discussed using techno-economic analysis framework.

6.2 Rice Straw as Lignocellulosic Biomass

6.2.1 Chemical Composition of Rice Straw

Rice straw, the left-over rice crop residue post-harvesting, is a valuable lignocellulosic biomass structure mainly composed of cellulose (25–48.88%), hemicellulose (18–31.6%) and lignin (5.6–31%) (Fig. 6.1; Table 6.1). Cellulose serves as the main structural element of the lignocellulosic biomass complex. It is a linear homopolymer composed of D-glucose monomer units interconnected by β-1,4 glycosidic bonds. Both inter- and intra-molecular hydrogen bonding among cellulose chains facilitates the formation of microfibrils. These microfibrils can reach several micrometers in length with diameter ranging from 12–35 nm and provide mechanical strength and integrity to the cell wall (Abe & Yano, 2009; Yang et al., 2011). Upon chemical or enzymatic hydrolysis, cellulose can be broken down into glucose which is a key fermentable sugar employed for the production of value-added products including biofuels (Haldar & Banerjee, 2022).

Hemicellulose is a branched and heterogenous group of polysaccharides. It is partially linked with cellulose via hydrogen bonding, and also partially connected to lignin through covalent bonding, forming a lignin-carbohydrate complex. Its structure is mainly composed of hexose (glucose, galactose, and mannose), pentose (xylose and arabinose) and acid sugars (Kululo et al., 2025). In rice straw, hemicelluloses exhibit relatively low molecular weight ranging from 18,800–48,700 Da with high degree of polydispersity, which makes it more prone to hydrolysis in comparison to cellulose (Satlewal et al., 2018). It also contributes in production of value-added products by proper hydrolysis which results in formation of fermentable sugars (Li et al., 2020).

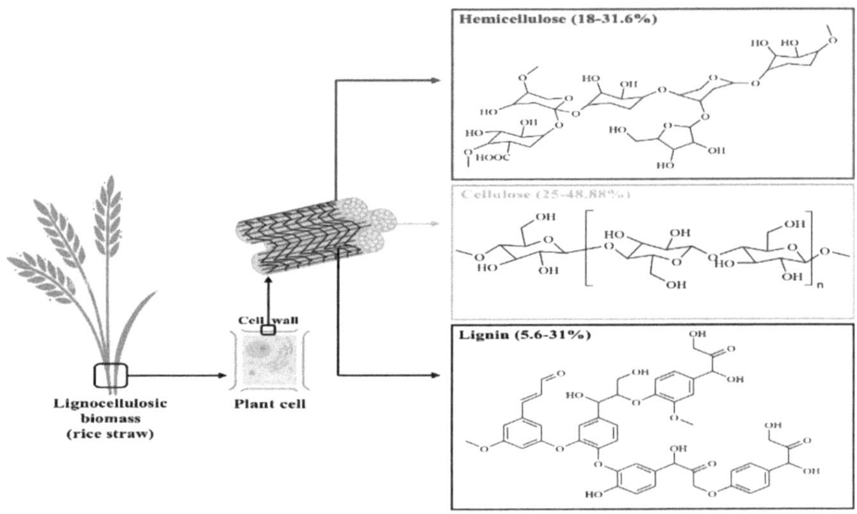

Fig. 6.1 Structural arrangement and composition of lignocellulosic biomass of rice straw

Table 6.1 Biochemical composition (weight %) of rice straw biomass reported in various studies

Cellulose	Hemicellulose	Lignin	References
30.3–38.2	19.8–31.6	7.2–12.8	Jin and Chen (2007)
36.21–48.88	9.98–23.70	11.59–26.70	Wang et al. (2020)
25–35	18–21	26–31	Kaniapan et al. (2022)
38.44	27.21	18.83	Alengebawy et al. (2023)
37.6–47.55	22.35–28.25	5.6–11.6	Malik et al. (2023)
29.7–41.1	21.5–29.27	13–24.4	Chakraborty et al. (2024)

Table 6.2 Elemental composition (weight %) of rice straw biomass reported in various studies

Carbon	Hydrogen	Oxygen	Nitrogen	References
38.8	6.7	38.8	0.2	Raj et al. (2015)
38.24	5.2	36.26	0.87	Mofijur et al. (2019)
37.40–46.12	4.39–8.46	33.56–44.53	0.13–1.58	Wang et al. (2020)
33.14–41.78	5.14–5.50	36.31–37.20	0.30–0.55	Kaniapan et al. (2022)
46.65	6.03	41.75	1.02	Alengebawy et al. (2023)
34.11–48.75	5.54–6.53	43.28–51.20	1.11–1.99	Chakraborty et al. (2024)

Lignin is primarily composed of three monomer units i.e. p-coumaryl alcohol, coniferyl alcohol, and sinapyl alcohol. These monomer units are interlinked via carbon-carbon and ether bonds. The β–O–4 linkage is the most prevalent ether bond, accounting for approximately 40–60% of rice straw lignin (Wang et al., 2017). Due to its highly recalcitrant structure, lignin has major processing challenges. However, technological advancements have facilitated its conversion into value-added products such as adhesives and aromatic compounds (Hu et al., 2022), which indicates the considerable potential of rice straw as a renewable energy source and an environmentally sustainable raw material for establishment of biorefineries.

In addition to biochemical composition, the elemental composition of rice straw, comprising carbon (C), hydrogen (H), oxygen (O) and nitrogen (N) provides valuable insights in accessing its suitability for various applications. C, H and O significantly influence the gross calorific value of straw materials. Carbon comprising 33.14–48.75% of rice straw biomass act as primary energy reservoir, contributing to high calorific value during combustion which makes the biomass a valuable heat source. Amount of hydrogen (4.39–8.46%) enhance the energy output of biomass by facilitating transformation into products like biofuels via processes such as gasification and liquefaction. Oxygen (33.56–51.20%) influence the combustion efficiency of biomass as it is crucial for processes like combustion, gasification and pyrolysis, facilitating the chemical reactions for synthesis of bio-based products. Nitrogen (0.13–1.99%), despite its lower concentration, essential for NOx formation which is responsible for biomass combustion (Nath et al., 2025; Satlewal et al., 2018) (Table 6.2). Overall, the biochemical and elemental composition of rice straw highlights its potential as a valuable lignocellulosic feedstock.

6.2.2 *Conversion of Rice Straw into Value-Added Products*

Thermochemical and biochemical are the two potential methods for conversion of rice-straw lignocellulosic biomass into bio-based products such as biofuels. Thermochemical methods convert the biomass feedstock into biofuels and other products by processes such as combustion, gasification, liquefaction and pyrolysis. Although thermochemical methods require lesser processing time but due to high energy consumption, utilization of catalysts and costly solvents, they are less preferred. In contrast, biochemical methods utilize microorganisms and their enzymes to convert biomass into bio-based products. Biochemical method involves three main steps i.e. pretreatment, hydrolysis and fermentation. Although productivity is often limited in biochemical conversion, yet it is widely accepted method due to its environment friendly, selective and energy-efficient nature. Despite its advantages, biochemical methods suffer from drawbacks such as high cost associated with pretreatment strategies of biomass and enzymes involved in the saccharification process (Poornima et al., 2024; Sukma et al., 2025). As the biochemical conversion methods offer sustainable benefits and aligns well with the circular economy models, it remains the most promising approach for the large scale biomass valorization. This chapter mainly discusses the current strategies, challenges and advances in biochemical conversion processes for production of bio-based value-added products by focusing on rice straw as feedstock.

6.3 Pretreatment Strategies for Lignocellulosic Biomass Saccharification

Lignocellulosic biomass is highly recalcitrant due to its complex structure consisting mainly of cellulose, hemicellulose and lignin. Although cellulose, consists of D-glucose units, which act as a key raw material for producing value-added products, its accessibility is significantly hindered due to the presence of lignin–hemicellulose complex. The major factors restricting the enzymatic hydrolysis of lignocellulosic biomass includes the presence of -1) crystalline cellulose microfibrils, exhibiting resistance towards enzymatic attack; 2) hemicellulose encasing cellulose fibers and thus restricting enzyme penetration; and 3) lignin, a rigid and complex phenolic polymer, recognized as the most recalcitrant component of the matrix (Kululo et al., 2025).

Although, using rice straw lignocellulosic biomass as a carbon source for production of value-added products is an innovative and sustainable idea, the complex structure of its lignin–hemicellulose complex, high content of lignin and crystalline structure of cellulose is holding it back for its direct utilization as substrate. Hence, in order to convert this complex lignocellulosic structure into utilizable monosaccharide forms, a pretreatment step is an essential requirement before saccharification of rice straw biomass into reducing sugars. Various categories of pretreatments include physical, chemical, physico-chemical and biological methods (Fig. 6.2). Their current status, challenges and advantages are discussed below.

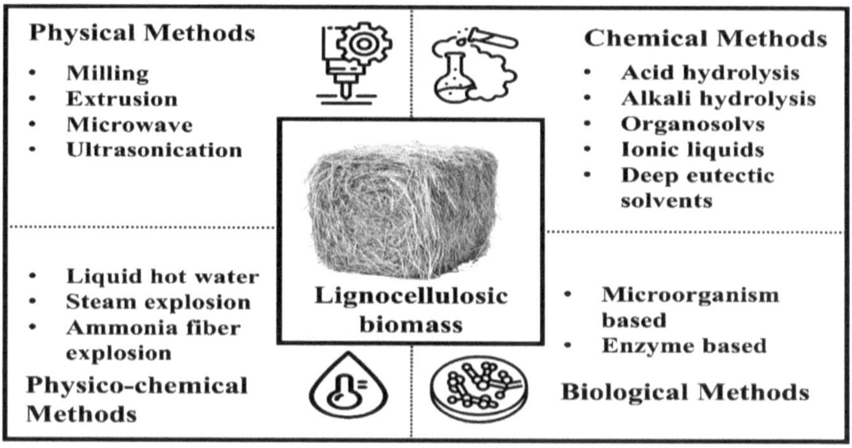

Fig. 6.2 A schematic representation of different types of pretreatment methods for lignocellulosic biomass

6.3.1 Current Status of Available Pretreatment Strategies: Pros and Cons

6.3.1.1 Physical Methods

Physical pretreatment methods utilize pressure, temperature, and mechanical forces to breakdown the complex lignocellulosic biomass into smaller sizes without any chemical modifications. Physical pretreatment methods lead to increase in porosity and surface area of biomass while decreasing the cellulose crystallinity (Jędrzejczyk et al., 2019). The most commonly used physical methods are milling, extrusion, microwave and ultrasonication which are discussed below.

Milling: It is a commonly used physical pretreatment method used to reduce the size of lignocellulosic biomass complex. Milling methods includes ball, rod, hammer, wet-disk milling etc. (Kumar et al., 2017). The efficiency of different milling methods is highly dependent on the biomass, time and processing method used. For example, rod-milling has been reported to show higher decrease in the crystallinity along with enhanced porosity and surface area in comparison to hammer-milling method while using wheat-straw as biomass feedstock. However, the major drawback is its high energy demand and the cost of mechanical equipment (Bai et al., 2018).

Extrusion: It is a thermo-mechanical pretreatment method which utilizes controlled heat and mixing within a temperature regulated barrel, resulting in structural disruption of lignocellulosic biomass, thereby enhancing the enzymatic digestibility. It offers advantages such as high shear, absence of effluent generation, lack of inhibitory compounds and moderate temperature (Kululo et al., 2025). Extrusion pretreatment of sugarcane bagasse under optimized conditions has been reported to produce 68.2%

glucose after enzymatic hydrolysis (Moro et al., 2017). Nonetheless, this process is energy intensive and requires high operational costs, making it unsuitable for scaling up at large industrial scale (Menon & Rao, 2012).

Microwave: The microwave assisted pretreatment is an effective method for lignocellulosic biomass due to its short reaction time, lower activation energy, and formation of minimum inhibitory compounds (Tayyab et al., 2018). The pretreatment of rice straw with microwave irradiation at 240 W enhanced the yield of total reducing sugar by 200% (Intanakul et al., 2003). In most of the studies, microwave pretreatment is generally employed as an additional method alongside other treatments such as alkali and/or acid pretreatment methods to enhance the degradation of lignocellulosic biomass (Ravindran et al., 2018; Tsegaye et al., 2019). Microwave assisted pretreatment of switchgrass combined with alkali pretreatment (0.05–0.3 g/g lignocellulosic biomass) has been reported to significantly enhance the reducing sugar yields up to 70–90% (Hu & Wen, 2008).

Ultrasonication: This pretreatment operates on the principle of cavitation facilitated by the ultrasonic radiations. Cavitation induces shear forces which disrupts the complex biomass structure and facilitate the extraction of simpler compounds (Ravindran & Jaiswal, 2016). Ultrasound based pretreatment methods operates on the principle of surface erosion and delignification. The implied benefits include reduced pretreatment time, reduced heating requirements, and utilization of fewer chemicals (Cheah et al., 2020). Ultrasound based methods when combined with chemical pretreatment methods enhances the overall efficiency of pretreatment. An ultrasound assisted alkali pretreated wheat straw has been reported to show 70% delignification efficiency along with higher reducing sugar yield (up to 90% glucose and 65% xylose) after enzymatic saccharification (Saratale et al., 2020).

6.3.1.2 Chemical Methods

Chemical pretreatment methods utilize a range of reagents such as acid, alkali, organosolvs, ionic liquids and deep eutectic solvents to disrupt the complex structure of lignocellulosic biomass. These methods are generally performed at ambient temperature and atmospheric pressure to break the intra and inter polymer linkages, which enable the delignification and improved enzymatic hydrolysis (Norrrahim et al., 2021). Chemical methods are preferred over other pretreatment methods owing to their higher efficiency in solubilizing complex biomass structure and their potential for scalability (Jose et al., 2022). Various chemical methods are discussed below.

Acid hydrolysis: It efficiently disrupts the lignocellulosic matrix through the cleavage of glycosidic bonds which results in conversion of polysaccharide biomass into oligomer and monomer sugars. Use of acids mainly hydrolyzes the hemicellulose fraction with partial solubilization of cellulose and lignin. Tang et al. (2021) reported 92.9% enzymatic hydrolysis efficiency with 96.2% hemicellulose removal and 40.6% delignification on acidic pretreatment of wheat straw. However, a significant limitation of acid pretreatment method is the production of inhibitory compounds including aldehyde, ketone and phenolics which hinders the further downstream processing (Solarte-Toro et al., 2019). As per estimates, these inhibitory compounds can increase the overall processing cost varying from 0.02 to 1.10 US dollars per kilogram (Preethi & Banu, 2023).

Alkali hydrolysis: It is a widely used efficient pretreatment method for the delignification of lignocellulosic biomass. It offers various advantages such as better performance at low temperature, reduced cellulose crystallinity and enhanced pore size (Behera et al., 2014; Kim et al., 2016). Shetty et al. (2017) reported 34% increase in the methane yield in case of alkali pretreated rice straw biomass in comparison to untreated biomass. This study showed significant reduction in the hemicellulose and lignin content with 1% NaOH pretreatment for 3 h. However, this method suffers from several disadvantages such as prolonged reaction time, elevated downstream processing cost for the recovery of added alkalis and reduced efficacy for high lignin feedstocks (Bali et al., 2015).

Organosolv: This pretreatment method has gained significant attention due to its ability to fractionate the lignocellulosic biomass into high purity cellulose, hemicellulose and lignin along with easy solvent recovery and reuse. This method utilizes organic/aqueous organic solvents (acetone, methanol, ethanol, butanol, ethylene glycol, formic acid, acetic acid) at elevated temperature ranging from 100 °C to over 200 °C (Rezania et al., 2020). Use of organosolv process dissolve the lignin and hemicellulose and separate them from the solid cellulose fraction which becomes more accessible for the further enzymatic hydrolysis. The purified lignin can be used for various applications. Asadi and Zilouei (2017) reported that the use of 75% ethanol at 180 °C for 90 min in rice straw pretreatment led to a 41% reduction in lignin and 62% reduction in hemicellulose content, while cellulose content was increased by 31%. Although organosolv pretreatment is an emerging method, it faces key limitations such as high cost and energy demands associated with the solvent recovery. Moreover, the volatile and flammable nature of solvents demands maintenance of stringent conditions (Baruah et al., 2018).

Ionic liquids: Due to their high thermal stability, recyclability, low-toxicity, high delignification efficiency, and substantial sugar yield, ionic liquids are recognized as effective solvents in lignocellulosic biorefinery. Ionic liquids are highly specific in removing hemicellulose and lignin part of the biomass complex, yielding pure cellulose which can be further used for downstream processing. However, it faces challenges such as complicated processing, pH compatibility issues and elevated costs (Chaudhary et al., 2024). Recently, a study has shown the higher efficiency and recyclability of ionic liquid pretreatment method highlighting it as a suitable pretreatment method in lignocellulosic biorefinery. 1-ethyl-3-methylimidazolium acetate pretreated rice straw showed 89% more ethanol production compared to the untreated rice straw (Chuetor et al., 2022).

Deep eutectic solvents: These solvents have emerged as a cost-effective and biodegradable green alternative to ionic liquids for the pretreatment of lignocellulosic biomass. Deep eutectic solvents consist of hydrogen bond donor such as urea and acceptors including quaternary ammonium salts. Its components form a low-melting mixtures via hydrogen bonding which disrupts the complex biomass structure. The fractionation of rice straw pretreatment utilizing oxalic acid dihydrate and choline chloride under optimized conditions achieved a delignification rate of 70% and a purity exceeding 82%, alongside a significant hemicellulose yield of 93%, with a substrate loading of 5% (Hou et al., 2018; Sheraz et al., 2025).

6.3.1.3 Physico-Chemical Methods

Physicochemical methods employs both the physical and chemical mechanisms of the pretreatment method involved. The most commonly used physico-chemical pretreatments includes liquid hot-water hydrothermal treatment, steam explosion method and ammonia fiber explosion methods.

Liquid hot water: This pretreatment involves use of water at elevated temperature (170 °C–230 °C) and high pressure (5 MPa) to hydrolyze the hemicellulose and remove lignin in order to increase the accessibility of cellulase. No inhibitory compounds are formed during this pretreatment process. The liquid hot water pretreatment is an eco-friendly method as there is no need of any chemical addition. Moreover, it reduces the waste generation by eliminating the need of subsequent washing and disposal. Nonetheless, it requires high energy, reportedly 3.5 times higher than the HCl pretreatment, which substantially increase the overall expenses. Additionally, the large amount of water requirement further contributes to high energy demand during this process (Kumar & Sharma, 2017; Yu et al., 2013).

Steam-explosion: This pretreatment is a hydrothermal process which involve subjecting the lignocellulosic biomass to elevated pressure (0.69–4.83 MPa) and temperature (160 °C–260 °C), followed by rapid depressurization. It results in fibril rupture that enhance the enzymatic accessibility of cellulose (Sarker et al., 2021; Zhang et al., 2022). The effectiveness of steam-explosion pretreatment is significantly influenced by factor including time, temperature and particle size. Therefore, addition of different chemicals like acid and alkali improves the steam-explosion pretreatment results. However, the major limitation is the extreme environmental conditions which results in production of inhibitors such as aromatic and furan derived compounds that can significantly affect the further downstream processing (Banu et al., 2021; Sarker et al., 2021).

Ammonia fiber explosion: This method involves the treatment of biomass at moderate temperature (60 °C–120 °C) and high pressure (1.72–2.06 MPa) followed by rapid depressurization. The rapid ammonia expansion disrupts the biomass fibers, thereby improving the enzymatic hydrolysis. In contrast to steam explosion method, it does not directly release sugars by hydrolyzing hemicellulose, instead this process enhances the surface area of polymers, thereby promoting enzymatic hydrolysis. Ammonia fiber explosion method has demonstrated enhanced biomass conversion rates across different lignocellulosic complexes such as rice straw. Although it is a potential pretreatment method, it has limited applicability due to utilization of ammonia which is highly corrosive and have significant environmental risks. Also, it is less effective for biomasses having higher lignin content (Baruah et al., 2018; Capolupo & Faraco, 2016; Flores-Gómez et al., 2018).

6.3.1.4 Biological Methods

Unlike chemical and physico-chemical methods, biological pretreatment is a chemical free, cost-effective and sustainable strategy to decompose the lignocellulosic biomass into accessible form prior to enzymatic hydrolysis for the production of value-added products (Mood et al., 2013). In this approach microorganisms i.e. fungi and bacteria are either directly used or their enzymes are used.

Various microorganisms have been explored for the pretreatment of lignocellulosic biomass. Among these, white rot fungi are commonly used microorganism for the pretreatment of lignocellulosic biomass and have up to 60% of delignification efficiency. However, it is also known to degrade the carbohydrate portion (~58%) of the biomass complex which can further affect the fermentable sugar production (Ghasemzadeh et al., 2018). Thus, the selection of appropriate fungal species for the pretreatment is quite essential. *Pleurotus ostreatus* producing lignolytic enzymes has shown up to 60% delignification while maintaining minimal loss of cellulose (3%) and hemicellulose (17%) after 30 days of incubation (25 °C) using rice straw as biomass feedstock (Datsomor et al., 2022). Moreover, filamentous fungi have also been reported for the pretreatment of rice straw biomass. *Aspergillus oryzae* showed 25% delignification with a 15% increase in the cellulose content of pretreated rice straw biomass (Anu et al., 2023). Additionally, various laccase-producing bacterial species have also been explored. Considering their high tolerance to alkaline conditions and various inhibitory compounds. *Bacillus ligniniphilus* is reported to show 4% delignification at 30 °C after 24 h in the pretreated rice straw biomass (Nazar et al., 2022). Although bacterial species requires lesser incubation time, fungi are preferred for the pretreatment studies due to their high delignification efficiency (Zhang et al., 2019). The lignin degrading enzymes produced by microorganisms have also been explored for the biological pretreatment. The key lignolytic enzymes playing an important role in biomass degradation are laccase, lignin peroxidase, versatile peroxidase and manganese peroxidase (Zámocký et al., 2014). Although biological pretreatment is a cost-effective and eco-friendly approach, it has key challenges such as longer reaction times, low sugar yield, and requirement of sterilization conditions, thereby limiting its utilization at industrial scale (Vasco-Correa & Shah, 2019).

6.3.2 Challenges and Recent Advances in Pretreatment Strategies

Although pretreatment strategies efficiently enhance the accessibility of biomass for its conversion to value-added products, the commercial feasibility of the available pretreatment methods is still limited. Pretreatment is considered as the second most expensive step in bioprocessing for conversion of lignocellulosic complex to value-added products. Around 40% of total processing costs comes from the employed pretreatment methods (Bhutto et al., 2017). Table 6.3 summarizes various pretreatment methods for lignocellulosic biomass along with their key benefits and challenges.

Physical methods such as milling requires high energy (~33% of total energy requirement for overall process) with no delignification, which is major barrier for further enzymatic saccharification (Mankar et al., 2021). Microwave irradiation also requires high energy consumption and provides uneven heating with limited scalability (Zhu et al., 2023). Hydrothermal pretreatment methods such as steam explosion and low hot water pretreatment often lead to production of inhibitory compounds and weak acids which further interferes with the fermentation process (Teixeira et al., 2014). Chemical methods such as acid and alkali treatments also face limitations due to generation of inhibitory compounds, cellulose degradation and recovery of used alkali resulting in wastewater generation. Although organosolv is an emerging pretreatment method, it is a highly energy-intensive and expensive process (Baruah et al., 2018). Green pretreatment methods such as ionic liquids are eco-friendly but are highly expensive and utilize non-biodegradable petroleum-based compounds. Deep eutectic solvents have been found to be one of the most effective pretreatment method for conversion of lignocellulosic biomass into value -added products due to high solubility and low-cost but still more research is needed to understand the interactions between deep eutectic solvents and lignocellulosic biomass (Chakraborty et al., 2024). Although biological pretreatment method is cost-effective, environment friendly and produces no inhibitory compounds during the process, it is not preferred at large scale due to low efficiency, more time requirement, limited lignin degradation and challenges in scalability (Baruah et al., 2018; Chakraborty et al., 2024).

The above-mentioned challenges highlight the need to develop a cost-effective, eco-friendly and sustainable processing method. For this, the pretreatment method should follow following prerequisites i.e. (1) low-cost; (2) production of more sugar; (3) minimum carbohydrate degradation; and (4) negligible inhibitory compounds formation (Sheraz et al., 2025). Recent advancements highlight the importance of integrated and hybrid pretreatment methods that merge the physicochemical and biological approaches in order to mitigate the challenges posed by individual pretreatment methods. This integration is mainly aimed at minimizing energy consumption, reducing time-consumption, and negligible inhibitor formation while enhancing the delignification efficiency. Vasco-Correa and Shah (2019), reported enhanced biomass conversion efficiency using combinational approach of pretreatment methods. This

Table 6.3 Comparative analysis of lignocellulosic biomass pretreatment methods: Key benefits and challenges

Pretreatment method	Technique used	Benefits	Challenges	References
Physical	Milling	Enhances porosity and surface area	Highly energy-intensive, higher equipment cost	Kumar et al. (2017), Bai et al. (2018)
	Extrusion	Zero effluent generation, no inhibitory compounds formation	High operational costs, highly energy -intensive	Menon and Rao, (2012), Kululo et al. (2025)
	Microwave	Shorter operation time, minimum inhibitors	Scalability, often used in combination to yield high sugar	Ravindran et al. (2018), Tayyab et al. (2018), Tsegaye et al. (2019)
	Ultrasonication	Low heat requirement, shorter reaction time	Requires combinational pretreatments for higher efficiency	Cheah et al. (2020), Saratale et al. (2020)
Chemical	Acid hydrolysis	High sugar yield	Formation of inhibitory compounds, corrosive nature, high cost	Solarte-Toro et al. (2019), Tang et al. (2021), Preethi and Banu, (2023)
	Alkali hydrolysis	Low-temperature requirements, increases pore size	High processing time, less effective for lignin rich feedstocks	Behera et al. (2014), Bali et al. (2015), Kim et al. (2016)
	Organosolv	High delignification efficiency, pure cellulose recovery	High cost associated with solvent recovery	Asadi and Zilouei (2017), Baruah et al. (2018)
	Ionic liquids	High thermal stability, low-toxicity, high sugar yields	Costly, processing complexity, pH sensitive	Chuetor et al. (2022), Chaudhary et al. (2024)
	Deep eutectic solvents	Environment friendly solvents, biodegradable, low-cost	Limited scalability data, optimization studies needed	Hou et al. (2018), Sheraz et al. (2025)

(continued)

Table 6.3 (continued)

Pretreatment method	Technique used	Benefits	Challenges	References
Physico-chemical	Liquid hot water	No chemical requirements, eco-friendly	High water consumption requirements, energy intensive	Yu et al. (2013), Kumar and Sharma (2017)
	Steam-explosion	Efficient processing	High energy requirements, formation of inhibitor compounds	Banu et al. (2021), Sarker et al. (2021)
	Ammonia fiber explosion	Moderate temperature requirements, enhance enzymatic hydrolysis	Highly corrosive, less effective for lignin rich feedstock	Capolupo and Faraco (2016), Baruah et al. (2018), Flores-Gómez et al. (2018)
Biological	Fungal	Eco-friendly, high delignification efficiency	Time-consuming, maintenance of sterilization conditions	Datsomor et al. (2022), Anu et al. (2023)
	Bacterial	Short time, eco-friendly	Less delignification efficiency than fungi, maintenance of sterilization conditions	Zhang et al. (2019), Nazar et al. (2022)
	Enzyme based	Specifically target lignin	High cost, low-sugar yield	Zámocký et al. (2014), Vasco-Correa and Shah (2019)

study showed a 75% increase in sugar generation rate with reduced processing time, indicating the synergistic benefits of combinational pretreatment methods over single pretreatment method. Another combined hydrothermal-mechanical pretreatment strategy for biofuel production has demonstrated high energy efficiency, enhanced sugar recovery and minimum waste generation (Phojaroen et al., 2022). Although integrated pretreatment strategies demonstrate significant potential for sustainable and economically viable valorization of biomass, further research is needed to develop a cost-effective, eco-friendly approach capable of whole biomass conversion to value-added products.

6.4 Enzymatic Saccharification of Lignocellulosic Biomass: Challenges and Advances

After pretreatment of lignocellulosic biomass enzymatic saccharification or hydrolysis is the next step which results in production of fermentable sugars that can be further converted into various bio-based value-added products. Enzymatic hydrolysis is a less energy requiring process that can be operated under mild conditions and thus promote environmental sustainability. However, at industrial scale, it proves to be an expensive and ineffective method (Lugani et al., 2020). Previous studies have shown that enzyme cost is a significant barrier in industrialization of lignocellulosic biomass-based refineries as cellulase alone constitutes 25–30% of the overall expenses in biorefineries (Valdivia et al., 2016). As lignocellulosic biomass is a complex heterogenous structure, a combination of synergistic enzymes (enzyme cocktails) such as cellulases (exoglucanases, endoglucanases and β-glucosidases) and hemicellulases are required for the efficient hydrolysis (Adsul et al., 2020). Commercially available enzyme cocktails possess various challenges such as low-specificity and undefined composition, which makes their use difficult in case of varied biomass feedstocks (Guo et al., 2018).

In view of above-mentioned challenges, on-site cellulase production has emerged as a cost-effective approach to reduce the enzyme cost for establishment of biorefineries at large scale, as it eliminates the need of expensive commercial enzymes. The on-site production of enzymes in biorefineries using same lignocellulosic biomass feedstock intended for hydrolysis, minimizes the raw-material cost and also eliminates the transportation and storage expenses. Furthermore, the on-site generated enzymes are highly substrate-specific, thereby improving the hydrolytic efficiency. Overall, the on-site enzyme production using lignocellulosic biomass as feedstock supports economic viability and scalability of value-added product generation (Siqueira et al., 2020).

6.5 Techno-Economic Analysis of Biomass Refineries

Techno-economic analysis is an essential framework for assessing the feasibility and scalability of lignocellulosic biomass refineries. This analysis integrates evaluation of technical process with economic modelling to assess the feasibility of biomass conversion into value-added products at large scale (Mungodla et al., 2019).

Biomass feedstock cost represents a significant amount of expenses, accounting for as much as 35–50% of total production cost, which includes collection, handling, pre-processing, transportation and storage (Fales et al., 2007; Sokhansanj & Hess, 2009). Although lignocellulosic biomass such as agricultural residues are accessible at very less prices, various challenges such as seasonal availability, transportation and storage affect their cost-effectiveness. In a recent study, it has been shown that wheat straw was collected from fields at a cost of 0.053 \$ kg^{-1} and utilized as feedstock for bioethanol production using steam-explosion as a pretreatment method. The final product cost analysis indicated market selling price of 1.03–1.23 $ kg^{-1} (Saini et al., 2020).

Pretreatment is also one of the significant cost components, which accounts for more than 40% of total processing cost (Bhutto et al., 2017). As mentioned above, various pretreatment methods such as steam-explosion, acid hydrolysis and ionic liquids etc. requires high energy, costly solvents, produces various inhibitory compounds which requires further expensive detoxification processes before fermentation. Among different reported pretreatment methods, very few methods such as ball milling, acid treatment and ammonium explosion are commercially accepted (Saini et al., 2020). Although these methods are commercially employed, high maintenance are needed for their operations at the industrial scale. For example, the expenses associated with dilute acid pretreatment followed by enzymatic hydrolysis of corn stover lignocellulosic biomass reached 6.05 $ per gallon of bioethanol, making it uncompetitive compared to the petroleum-based ethanol production (Zhao et al., 2015). Enzymatic hydrolysis has been reported to account for approximately 25% of total processing cost (Rocha-Martín et al., 2017). The total cost of lignocellulosic biomass processing from collection to hydrolysate formation has been estimated to be 65–67% of total processing cost (Huang et al., 2013; Rocha-Martín et al., 2017).

Capital investment remains a significant barrier for commercialization of biorefineries. Various companies such as Beta Renewable and Abengoa (known for biofuel production); and Metabolix (known for bioplastic production) could not compete the market price and faced failure due to the high capital investment and inadequate product output. These failure highlights the need of techno-economic analysis prior to the upscaling operations (Saini et al., 2020). Considering these facts, numerous studies have conducted economic potential analysis for lignocellulosic biomass refineries. Techno-economic analysis conducted by Zhao et al. (2015) for bioethanol production using corn stover as feedstock indicated the high cost of bioethanol production (6.05 $ gal^{-1}) which makes it uncompetitive in comparison to the ethanol derived from fossil fuels. In another study, the production cost of biofuel derived from different lignocellulosic biomasses was found be $ 1.11 L^{-1}, $ 1.19 L^{-1}, and $ 1.25 L^{-1} for spruce, corn stover and wheat straw, respectively (Patel et al., 2019). Gurgel et al. (2019) evaluated the efficiency of different pretreatment methods for corn stover and concluded dilute acid pretreatment as the most economical method for ethanol production with an estimated annual return of $ 39.2 million. These findings highlight the need and importance of techno-economic analysis for the selection of processing conditions in order to improve the commercial viability of value-added products.

6.6 Conclusion

Lignocellulosic biomass of rice straw serves as an abundant, renewable and sustainable feedstock source in biorefineries for production of value-added products. However, the bioconversion is majorly hindered by its structural recalcitrance and techno-economic challenges associated with biomass processing. Among various processing steps, pretreatment is one of the most crucial and expensive process which significantly affect the efficiency of downstream processing. Despite considerable advancements in various physical, chemical, physico-chemical and biological pretreatment methods, none of these methods when applied individually, have achieved the comprehensive criteria for their commercial implementation, which includes cost-effectiveness, scalability, high delignification efficiency and minimal environmental impact. Recent advancements in the pretreatment methods by integrating and combining different approaches has shown promising solutions to the limitations of individual pretreatment methods. However, the scalability and economic viability of these integrated systems are yet to be explored. Similarly, although enzymatic saccharification is a green and efficient method, its commercialization is limited due to the high cost of enzymes. On-site enzyme production utilizing lignocellulosic biomass as a substrate is becoming a viable and scalable option by enhancing the enzyme efficiency and lowering the operational costs. Techno-economic analysis of the cost associated with biomass processing indicates that more than two-thirds of total expenses are contributed by the feedstock availability, pretreatment and enzyme costs. Further, the failures of bio-based industries highlight the need of conducting a thorough techno-economic analysis before scaling up.

References

Abe, K., & Yano, H. (2009). Comparison of the characteristics of cellulose microfibril aggregates of wood, rice straw and potato tuber. *Cellulose, 16*, 1017–1023.

Adsul, M., Sandhu, S. K., Singhania, R. R., Gupta, R., Puri, S. K., & Mathur, A. (2020). Designing a cellulolytic enzyme cocktail for the efficient and economical conversion of lignocellulosic biomass to biofuels. *Enzyme and Microbial Technology, 133*, Article 109442.

Alengebawy, A., Ran, Y., Ghimire, N., Osman, A. I., & Ai, P. (2023). Rice straw for energy and value-added products in China: A review. *Environmental Chemistry Letters, 21*(5), 2729–2760.

Anu, K. V., Singh, D., & Singh, B. (2023). A greener, mild, and efficient bioprocess for the pretreatment and saccharification of rice straw. *Biomass Conversion and Biorefinery, 13*(5), 4121–4133.

Asadi, N., & Zilouei, H. (2017). Optimization of organosolv pretreatment of rice straw for enhanced biohydrogen production using Enterobacter aerogenes. *Bioresource Technology, 227*, 335–344.

Bai, X., Wang, G., Yu, Y., Wang, D., & Wang, Z. (2018). Changes in the physicochemical structure and pyrolysis characteristics of wheat straw after rod-milling pretreatment. *Bioresource Technology, 250*, 770–776.

Bali, G., Meng, X., Deneff, J. I., Sun, Q., & Ragauskas, A. J. (2015). The effect of alkaline pretreatment methods on cellulose structure and accessibility. *Chemsuschem, 8*(2), 275–279.

Banu, J. R., Kavitha, S., Tyagi, V. K., Gunasekaran, M., Karthikeyan, O. P., & Kumar, G. (2021). Lignocellulosic biomass based biorefinery: A successful platform towards circular bioeconomy. *Fuel, 302*, Article 121086.

Baruah, J., Nath, B. K., Sharma, R., Kumar, S., Deka, R. C., Baruah, D. C., & Kalita, E. (2018). Recent trends in the pretreatment of lignocellulosic biomass for value-added products. *Frontiers in Energy Research, 6*, 141.

Behera, S., Arora, R., Nandhagopal, N., & Kumar, S. (2014). Importance of chemical pretreatment for bioconversion of lignocellulosic biomass. *Renewable and Sustainable Energy Reviews, 36*, 91–106.

Bhattacharyya, P., Bisen, J., Bhaduri, D., Priyadarsini, S., Munda, S., Chakraborti, M., Adak, T., Panneerselvam, P., Mukherjee, A. K., Swain, S. L., Dash, P. K., Padhy, S. R., Nayak, A. K., Pathak, H., Kumar, S., & Nimbrayan, P. (2021). Turn the wheel from waste to wealth: Economic and environmental gain of sustainable rice straw management practices over field burning in reference to India. *Science of the Total Environment, 775*, Article 145896.

Bhutto, A. W., Qureshi, K., Harijan, K., Abro, R., Abbas, T., Bazmi, A. A., Karim, S., & Yu, G. (2017). Insight into progress in pre-treatment of lignocellulosic biomass. *Energy, 122*, 724–745.

Bhuvaneshwari, S., Hettiarachchi, H., & Meegoda, J. N. (2019). Crop residue burning in India: Policy challenges and potential solutions. *International Journal of Environmental Research and Public Health, 16*(5), 832.

Capolupo, L., & Faraco, V. (2016). Green methods of lignocellulose pretreatment for biorefinery development. *Applied Microbiology and Biotechnology, 100*, 9451–9467.

Chakraborty, P., Kumar, R., Chakrabortty, S., Saha, S., Chattaraj, S., Roy, S., Banerjee, A., Tripathy, S. K., Ghosh, A. K., & Jeon, B. H. (2024). Technological advancements in the pretreatment of lignocellulosic biomass for effective valorization: A review of challenges and prospects. *Journal of Industrial and Engineering Chemistry, 137*, 29–60.

Chaudhary, G., Chaudhary, N., Saini, S., Gupta, Y., Vivekanand, V., & Panghal, A. (2024). Assessment of pretreatment strategies for valorization of lignocellulosic biomass: Path forwarding towards lignocellulosic biorefinery. *Waste and Biomass Valorization, 15*(1), 1–36.

Cheah, W. Y., Sankaran, R., Show, P. L., Tg Ibrahim, T. N. B., Chew, K. W., Culaba, A., & Chang, J. S. (2020). Pretreatment methods for lignocellulosic biofuels production: Current advances, challenges and future prospects. *Biofuel Research Journal, 7*(1), 1115–1127.

Chuetor, S., Panakkal, E. J., Ruensodsai, T., Cheenkachorn, K., Kirdponpattara, S., Cheng, Y. S., & Sriariyanun, M. (2022). Improvement of enzymatic saccharification and ethanol production from rice straw using recycled ionic liquid: The effect of anti-solvent mixture. *Bioengineering, 9*(3), 115.

Datsomor, O., Gou-Qi, Z., & Miao, L. (2022). Effect of ligninolytic axenic and coculture white-rot fungi on rice straw chemical composition and *in vitro* fermentation characteristics. *Scientific Reports, 12*(1), 1129.

Dutta, A., Patra, A., Hazra, K. K., Nath, C. P., Kumar, N., & Rakshit, A. (2022). A state of the art review in crop residue burning in India: Previous knowledge, present circumstances and future strategies. *Environmental Challenges, 8*, Article 100581.

Fales, S. L., Hess, J. R., Wilhelm, W., Erbach, D., Provine, W. D., Vogel, K. P., Peterson, T. A., & Runge, E. C. (2007). Convergence of agriculture and energy: II. producing cellulosic biomass for biofuels. *Publications from USDA-ARS/UNL Faculty*, 291.

Flores-Gómez, C. A., Escamilla Silva, E. M., Zhong, C., Dale, B. E., da Costa Sousa, L., & Balan, V. (2018). Conversion of lignocellulosic agave residues into liquid biofuels using an AFEX™-based biorefinery. *Biotechnology for Biofuels, 11*, 1–18.

Ghasemzadeh, R., Mosavian, M. T. H., & Karimi, A. (2018). Analysis of biological pretreatment of rapeseed straw with white rot fungi for enzymatic hydrolysis. *Maderas. Ciencia y Tecnología, 20*(4), 725–736.

Goodman, B. A. (2020). Utilization of waste straw and husks from rice production: A review. *Journal of Bioresources and Bioproducts, 5*(3), 143–162.

Grisolia, G., Fino, D., & Lucia, U. (2022). Biomethanation of rice straw: A sustainable perspective for the valorisation of a field residue in the energy sector. *Sustainability, 14*, 5679.

Guo, H., Chang, Y., & Lee, D. J. (2018). Enzymatic saccharification of lignocellulosic biorefinery: Research focuses. *Bioresource Technology, 252*, 198–215.

Gurgel, R., da Silva, A., Giuliano, A., Errico, M., Rong, B. G., & Barletta, D. (2019). Economic value and environmental impact analysis of lignocellulosic ethanol production: Assessment of different pretreatment processes. *Clean Technologies and Environmental Policy, 21*, 637–654.

Haldar, S., & Banerjee, S. (2022). Enzyme technology for the degradation of lignocellulosic waste. *Biotechnology for Zero Waste: Emerging Waste Management Techniques*, 143–153.

Hassan, M. K., Chowdhury, R., Ghosh, S., Manna, D., Pappinen, A., & Kuittinen, S. (2021). Energy and environmental impact assessment of Indian rice straw for the production of second-generation bioethanol. *Sustainable Energy Technologies and Assessments, 47*, Article 101546.

Hou, X. D., Lin, K. P., Li, A. L., Yang, L. M., & Fu, M. H. (2018). Effect of constituents molar ratios of deep eutectic solvents on rice straw fractionation efficiency and the micro-mechanism investigation. *Industrial Crops and Products, 120*, 322–329.

Hu, S., Kamimura, N., Sakamoto, S., Nagano, S., Takata, N., Liu, S., Goeminne, G., Vanholme, R., Uesugi, M., Yamamoto, M., Hishiyama, S., Kim, H., Boerjan, W., Ralph, J., Masai, E., Mitsuda, N., & Kajita, S. (2022). Rerouting of the lignin biosynthetic pathway by inhibition of cytosolic shikimate recycling in transgenic hybrid aspen. *The Plant Journal, 110*(2), 358–376.

Hu, Z., & Wen, Z. (2008). Enhancing enzymatic digestibility of switchgrass by microwave-assisted alkali pretreatment. *Biochemical Engineering Journal, 38*(3), 369–378.

Huang, C., Chen, X. F., Xiong, L., Chen, X. D., Ma, L. L., & Chen, Y. (2013). Single cell oil production from low-cost substrates: The possibility and potential of its industrialization. *Biotechnology Advances, 31*(2), 129–139.

Intanakul, P., Krairiksh, M., & Kitchaiya, P. (2003). Enhancement of enzymatic hydrolysis of lignocellulosic wastes by microwave pretreatment under atmospheric pressure. *Journal of Wood Chemistry and Technology, 23*(2), 217–225.

Jędrzejczyk, M., Soszka, E., Czapnik, M., Ruppert, A. M., & Grams, J. (2019). Physical and chemical pretreatment of lignocellulosic biomass. In *Second and third generation of feedstocks*, pp. 143–196. Elsevier.

Jin, S., & Chen, H. (2007). Near-infrared analysis of the chemical composition of rice straw. *Industrial Crops and Products, 26*(2), 207–211.

Jose, D., Kitiborwornkul, N., Sriariyanun, M., & Keerthi, K. (2022). A review on chemical pretreatment methods of lignocellulosic biomass: Recent advances and progress. *Applied Science and Engineering Progress, 15*(4), 6210–6210.

Kaniapan, S., Pasupuleti, J., Patma Nesan, K., Abubackar, H. N., Umar, H. A., Oladosu, T. L., Bello, S. R., & Rene, E. R. (2022). A review of the sustainable utilization of rice residues for bioenergy conversion using different valorization techniques, their challenges, and techno-economic assessment. *International Journal of Environmental Research and Public Health, 19*(6), 3427.

Kaur, M., Malik, D. P., Malhi, G. S., Sardana, V., Bolan, N. S., Lal, R., & Siddique, K. H. (2022). Rice residue management in the Indo-Gangetic plains for climate and food security. A review. *Agronomy for Sustainable Development, 42*(5), 92.

Kim, J. S., Lee, Y. Y., & Kim, T. H. (2016). A review on alkaline pretreatment technology for bioconversion of lignocellulosic biomass. *Bioresource Technology, 199*, 42–48.

Kululo, W. W., Habtu, N. G., Abera, M. K., Sendekie, Z. B., Fanta, S. W., & Yemata, T. A. (2025). Advances in various pretreatment strategies of lignocellulosic substrates for the production of bioethanol: A comprehensive review. *Discover Applied Sciences, 7*(5), 1–24.

Kumar, A. K., & Sharma, S. (2017). Recent updates on different methods of pretreatment of lignocellulosic feedstocks: A review. *Bioresources and Bioprocessing, 4*(1), 7.

Kumar, R., Sharma, R. K., & Singh, A. P. (2017). Cellulose based grafted biosorbents-Journey from lignocellulose biomass to toxic metal ions sorption applications-A review. *Journal of Molecular Liquids, 232*, 62–93.
Li, X., Zhang, X., Yao, S., Chang, H., Wang, Y., & Zhang, Z. (2020). UV-blocking, transparent and hazy cellulose nanopaper with superior strength based on varied components of poplar mechanical pulp. *Cellulose, 27*, 6563–6576.
Lugani, Y., Rai, R., Prabhu, A. A., Maan, P., Hans, M., Kumar, V., Kumar, S., Chandel, A. K., & Sengar, R. S. (2020). Recent advances in bioethanol production from lignocelluloses: A comprehensive review with a focus on enzyme engineering and designer biocatalysts. *Biofuel Research Journal, 7*, 1267–1295.
Malik, K., Sharma, A., Harikarthik, D., Rani, V., Arya, N., Malik, A., Rani, S., Sangwan, P., & Bhatia, T. (2023). Deciphering the biochemical and functional characterization of rice straw cultivars for industrial applications. *Heliyon, 9*(6), Article e16339.
Mankar, A. R., Pandey, A., Modak, A., & Pant, K. K. (2021). Pretreatment of lignocellulosic biomass: A review on recent advances. *Bioresource Technology, 334*, Article 125235.
Menon, V., & Rao, M. (2012). Trends in bioconversion of lignocellulose: Biofuels, platform chemicals & biorefinery concept. *Progress in Energy and Combustion Science, 38*(4), 522–550.
Ministry of Agriculture and Framers Welfare. (2025). Annual report 24–25 Department of Agriculture, Cooperation and Framers Welfare. Ministry of Agriculture and Framers Welfare (Government of India).
Mofijur, M., Mahlia, T. M. I., Logeswaran, J., Anwar, M., Silitonga, A. S., Rahman, S. A., & Shamsuddin, A. H. (2019). Potential of rice industry biomass as a renewable energy source. *Energies, 12*(21), 4116.
Mood, S. H., Golfeshan, A. H., Tabatabaei, M., Jouzani, G. S., Najafi, G. H., Gholami, M., & Ardjmand, M. (2013). Lignocellulosic biomass to bioethanol, a comprehensive review with a focus on pretreatment. *Renewable and Sustainable Energy Reviews, 27*, 77–93.
Moro, M. K., Teixeira, R. S. S., da Silva, A. S. A., Fujimoto, M. D., Melo, P. A., Secchi, A. R., & da Silva Bon, E. P. (2017). Continuous pretreatment of sugarcane biomass using a twin-screw extruder. *Industrial Crops and Products, 97*, 509–517.
Mothe, S., & Polisetty, V. R. (2021). Review on anaerobic digestion of rice straw for biogas production. *Environmental Science and Pollution Research, 28*, 24455–24469.
Mungodla, S. G., Linganiso, L. Z., Mlambo, S., & Motaung, T. (2019). Economic and technical feasibility studies: Technologies for second generation biofuels. *Journal of Engineering, Design and Technology, 17*(4), 670–704.
Nath, B., Ahmmed, M. M., Paul, S., Huda, M. D., Hossain, M. A., & Islam, S. (2025). Unlocking the potential of rice straw: Sustainable utilization strategies for Bangladesh. *Circular Economy, 4*(1), Article 100126.
Nazar, M., Xu, L., Ullah, M. W., Moradian, J. M., Wang, Y., Sethupathy, S., Iqbal, B., Nawaz, M. Z., & Zhu, D. (2022). Biological delignification of rice straw using laccase from *Bacillus ligniniphilus* L1 for bioethanol production: A clean approach for agro-biomass utilization. *Journal of Cleaner Production, 360*, Article 132171.
Norrrahim, M. N. F., Ilyas, R. A., Nurazzi, N. M., Rani, M. S. A., Atikah, M. S. N., & Shazleen, S. S. (2021). Chemical pretreatment of lignocellulosic biomass for the production of bioproducts: An overview. *Applied Science and Engineering Progress, 14*(4), 588–605.
Patel, M., Oyedun, A. O., Kumar, A., & Gupta, R. (2019). What is the production cost of renewable diesel from woody biomass and agricultural residue based on experimentation? A comparative assessment. *Fuel Processing Technology, 191*, 79–92.
Phojaroen, J., Jiradechakorn, T., Kirdponpattara, S., Sriariyanun, M., Junthip, J., & Chuetor, S. (2022). Performance evaluation of combined hydrothermal-mechanical pretreatment of lignocellulosic biomass for enzymatic enhancement. *Polymers, 14*(12), 2313.
Poornima, S., Manikandan, S., Prakash, R., Deena, S. R., Subbaiya, R., Karmegam, N., Kim, W., & Govarthanan, M. (2024). Biofuel and biochemical production through biomass transformation using advanced thermochemical and biochemical processes–a review. *Fuel, 372*, Article 132204.

Preethi, & Banu. J. R. (2023). Indexing energy and cost of the pretreatment for economically efficient bioenergy generation. *Frontiers in Energy Research, 10*, 1060599.

Raj, T., Kapoor, M., Gaur, R., Christopher, J., Lamba, B., Tuli, D. K., & Kumar, R. (2015). Physical and chemical characterization of various Indian agriculture residues for biofuels production. *Energy & Fuels, 29*(5), 3111–3118.

Ravindran, R., & Jaiswal, A. K. (2016). A comprehensive review on pre-treatment strategy for lignocellulosic food industry waste: Challenges and opportunities. *Bioresource Technology, 199*, 92–102.

Ravindran, R., Jaiswal, S., Abu-Ghannam, N., & Jaiswal, A. K. (2018). A comparative analysis of pretreatment strategies on the properties and hydrolysis of brewers' spent grain. *Bioresource Technology, 248*, 272–279.

Rezania, S., Oryani, B., Cho, J., Talaiekhozani, A., Sabbagh, F., Hashemi, B., Rupani, P. F., & Mohammadi, A. A. (2020). Different pretreatment technologies of lignocellulosic biomass for bioethanol production: An overview. *Energy, 199*, Article 117457.

Rocha-Martín, J., Martinez-Bernal, C., Pérez-Cobas, Y., Reyes-Sosa, F. M., & García, B. D. (2017). Additives enhancing enzymatic hydrolysis of lignocellulosic biomass. *Bioresource Technology, 244*, 48–56.

Saini, R., Osorio-Gonzalez, C. S., Hegde, K., Brar, S. K., Magdouli, S., Vezina, P., & Avalos-Ramirez, A. (2020). Lignocellulosic biomass-based biorefinery: An insight into commercialization and economic standout. *Current Sustainable/Renewable Energy Reports, 7*, 122–136.

Saini, S., Kuhad, R. C., & Sharma, K. K. (2023). Valorization of rice straw biomass for co-production of bioethanol, biopesticide and biofertilizer following an eco-friendly biorefinery process. *Process Safety and Environmental Protection, 173*, 823–836.

Saratale, G. D., Saratale, R. G., Varjani, S., Cho, S. K., Ghodake, G. S., Kadam, A., Mulla, S. I., Bharagava, R. N., Kim, D. S., & Shin, H. S. (2020). Development of ultrasound aided chemical pretreatment methods to enrich saccharification of wheat waste biomass for polyhydroxybutyrate production and its characterization. *Industrial Crops and Products, 150*, Article 112425.

Sarker, T. R., Pattnaik, F., Nanda, S., Dalai, A. K., Meda, V., & Naik, S. (2021). Hydrothermal pretreatment technologies for lignocellulosic biomass: A review of steam explosion and subcritical water hydrolysis. *Chemosphere, 284*, Article 131372.

Satlewal, A., Agrawal, R., Bhagia, S., Das, P., & Ragauskas, A. J. (2018). Rice straw as a feedstock for biofuels: Availability, recalcitrance, and chemical properties. *Biofuels, Bioproducts and Biorefining, 12*(1), 83–107.

Sheraz, M., Cao, L., Zhao, S., Gao, H., Dansawad, P., Xue, C., Li, Y., & Li, W. (2025). Lignocellulosic biomass pretreatment methods and application of extracted fractions. *Arabian Journal for Science and Engineering, 50*(6), 3717–3736.

Shetty, D. J., Kshirsagar, P., Tapadia-Maheshwari, S., Lanjekar, V., Singh, S. K., & Dhakephalkar, P. K. (2017). Alkali pretreatment at ambient temperature: A promising method to enhance biomethanation of rice straw. *Bioresource Technology, 226*, 80–88.

Singh, S., Kaur, G., Singh, D. P., Arya, S. K., & Krishania, M. (2024). Exploring rice straw's potential from a sustainable biorefinery standpoint: Towards valorization and diverse product production. *Process Safety and Environmental Protection, 184*, 314–331.

Siqueira, J. G. W., Rodrigues, C., de Souza Vandenberghe, L. P., Woiciechowski, A. L., & Soccol, C. R. (2020). Current advances in on-site cellulase production and application on lignocellulosic biomass conversion to biofuels: A review. *Biomass and Bioenergy, 132*, Article 105419.

Sokhansanj, S., & Hess, J. R. (2009). Biomass supply logistics and infrastructure. *Biofuels: Methods and Protocols*, 581, 1–25.

Solarte-Toro, J. C., Romero-García, J. M., Martínez-Patiño, J. C., Ruiz-Ramos, E., Castro-Galiano, E., & Cardona-Alzate, C. A. (2019). Acid pretreatment of lignocellulosic biomass for energy vectors production: A review focused on operational conditions and techno-economic assessment for bioethanol production. *Renewable and Sustainable Energy Reviews, 107*, 587–601.

Sukma, A. C. T., Budiyono, B., & Al-Baarri, A. N. M. (2025). Recent advances in bioethanol production from rice straw: Strategies, new concepts, and challenges. *International Journal of Environmental Research, 19*(1), 1–36.
Tang, W., Wu, X., Huang, C., Ling, Z., Lai, C., & Yong, Q. (2021). Natural surfactant-aided dilute sulfuric acid pretreatment of waste wheat straw to enhance enzymatic hydrolysis efficiency. *Bioresource Technology, 324*, Article 124651.
Tayyab, M., Noman, A., Islam, W., Waheed, S., Arafat, Y., Ali, F., Zaynab, M., Lin, S., Zhang, H., & Lin, W. (2018). Bioethanol production from lignocellulosic biomass by environment-friendly pretreatment methods: A review. *Applied Ecology & Environmental Research, 16*(1), 225–249.
Teixeira, R. S., Silva, A. S., Moutta, R. O., Ferreira-Leitão, V. S., Barros, R. R., Ferrara, M. A., & Bon, E. P. (2014). Biomass pretreatment: a critical choice for biomass utilization via biotechnological routes. *BMC Proceedings, 8*, 1–3. BioMed Central.
Tsegaye, B., Balomajumder, C., & Roy, P. (2019). Optimization of microwave and NaOH pretreatments of wheat straw for enhancing biofuel yield. *Energy Conversion and Management, 186*, 82–92.
Valdivia, M., Galan, J. L., Laffarga, J., & Ramos, J. L. (2016). Biofuels 2020: Biorefineries based on lignocellulosic materials. *Microbial Biotechnology, 9*(5), 585–594.
Vasco-Correa, J., & Shah, A. (2019). Techno-economic bottlenecks of the fungal pretreatment of lignocellulosic biomass. *Fermentation, 5*(2), 30.
Wang, H., Ben, H., Ruan, H., Zhang, L., Pu, Y., Feng, M., Ragauskas, A. J., & Yang, B. (2017). Effects of lignin structure on hydrodeoxygenation reactivity of pine wood lignin to valuable chemicals. *ACS Sustainable Chemistry & Engineering, 5*(2), 1824–1830.
Wang, X., Yang, Z., Liu, X., Huang, G., Xiao, W., & Han, L. (2020). The composition characteristics of different crop straw types and their multivariate analysis and comparison. *Waste Management, 110*, 87–97.
Yang, B., Dai, Z., Ding, S. Y., & Wyman, C. E. (2011). Enzymatic hydrolysis of cellulosic biomass. *Biofuels, 2*(4), 421–449.
Yu, Q., Zhuang, X., Lv, S., He, M., Zhang, Y., Yuan, Z., Qi, W., Wang, Q., Wang, W., & Tan, X. (2013). Liquid hot water pretreatment of sugarcane bagasse and its comparison with chemical pretreatment methods for the sugar recovery and structural changes. *Bioresource Technology, 129*, 592–598.
Zámocký, M., Gasselhuber, B., Furtmüller, P. G., & Obinger, C. (2014). Turning points in the evolution of peroxidase–catalase superfamily: Molecular phylogeny of hybrid heme peroxidases. *Cellular and Molecular Life Sciences, 71*, 4681–4696.
Zhang, B., Li, H., Chen, L., Fu, T., Tang, B., Hao, Y., Li, J., Li, Z., Zhang, B., Chen, Q., Nie, C., You, Z. Y., Guan, C. Y., & Peng, Y. (2022). Recent advances in the bioconversion of waste straw biomass with steam explosion technique: A comprehensive review. *Processes, 10*(10), 1959.
Zhang, L., Cui, H., Zou, Z., Garakani, T. M., Novoa-Henriquez, C., Jooyeh, B., & Schwaneberg, U. (2019). Directed evolution of a bacterial laccase (CueO) for enzymatic biofuel cells. *Angewandte Chemie International Edition, 58*(14), 4562–4565.
Zhao, L., Zhang, X., Xu, J., Ou, X., Chang, S., & Wu, M. (2015). Techno-economic analysis of bioethanol production from lignocellulosic biomass in China: Dilute-acid pretreatment and enzymatic hydrolysis of corn stover. *Energies, 8*(5), 4096–4117.
Zhu, L., Liang, K., Wang, M., Xing, T., Chen, C., & Wang, Q. (2023). Microwave-assisted formic acid/cold caustic extraction for separation of cellulose and hemicellulose from biomass. *BioResources, 18*(4), Article p6896.

Chapter 7
Mushroom Technology: Large-Scale Cultivation and Its Life Cycle Assessment

Aseni.N. Ediriweera, Samantha C. Karunarathna, Niranjan Gunasekara, and Minura peiris

Abstract Large-scale farming of mushrooms calls for cultivating mushrooms in high volumes and counts on modern technology to optimize the growth conditions unique for different species of mushrooms and increase healthy yield. China, USA, Japan, South Korea, India, Canada and Germany play a significant role in large-scale mushroom production. Modern technologies involve precise control of environmental factors such as temperature, humidity and CO_2 levels, as well as automation of processes such as substrate preparation and sterilization. Modern techniques also employ automated irrigation and lightning systems, mycelium propagation technology, automated harvesting, packing and specialized technical applications such as bioreactors focusing large-scale mycelial production. For healthy and rich yield of mushrooms of large-scale production, further focus is on waste management, value addition and energy-efficient systems. Substrate preparation, climate-controlled cultivation, casing and harvesting are the major processes which drive the life cycle of mushroom production, while waste valorization, energy use, composting processes and resource efficiency are the other key environmental impact contributors for sustainable maintenance of large-scale mushroom cultivation.

Keywords Abundant harvest · Efficient · Environment · High-tech · Impact

Aseni.N. Ediriweera (✉)
B-Hood Myco-Tropic Innovations, Matara, Sri Lanka
e-mail: aseniediriweera@gmail.com

S. C. Karunarathna
Center for Yunnan Plateau Biological Resources Protection and Utilization, College of Biology and Food Engineering, Qujing Normal University, Qujing, Yunnan, P.R. China

N. Gunasekara · M. peiris
Department of Export Agriculture, Faculty of Export Agriculture and Animal Science, Uva Wellassa University, Badulla, Sri Lanka

P. Verma (ed.), *Sustainable Practices in Biorefinery*,
https://doi.org/10.1007/978-981-95-6071-4_7

7.1 Large-Scale Cultivation of Mushroom Technologies and Its Life Cycle Assessment

7.1.1 What is Large-Scale Mushroom Cultivation?

Mushroom cultivation, which dates back many decades, is still evolving, bridging the gap in the daily nutrient requirement of humans worldwide. While the evolution and rejuvenation of the global mushroom industry is being written in such a way, large-scale cultivation or farming of mushrooms comes into being with commercial production of mushrooms in quantities adequate for global market distribution as a response to the huge demand (Dey et al., 2020; Jayaraman et al., 2024; Veljović & Krstić, 2020). Massive levels of mushroom production unlock opportunities for consumers to experience a variety of flavours and dishes of this culinary wonder while facilitating consumers in obtaining a vast range of avenues to get their protein requirement fulfilled (Thakur, 2020). But, large-scale mushroom cultivation is still quite challenging for many countries due to the novel technological applications applied (Sangeeta et al., 2024, Muyal et al., 2018).

Large-scale mushroom cultivation implies optimized growing conditions, specialized facilities, and efficient management practices with the objectives of maximizing yields while minimizing costs. Further, the practices of large-scale mushroom farming generally include indoor cultivation using supplemented sawdust blocks, controlled environments, and year-round production capabilities (Leithäuser et al., 2025; Thakur, 2020).

7.2 Key Aspects of Large-Scale Mushroom Cultivation

- **Specialized Facilities with Controlled Environments**

Large-scale mushroom cultivation often requires dedicated adequate spaces for quality raw material reception, sorting and storage area, substrate preparation yard, substrate sterilization/pasteurization unit, inoculation area, incubation chambers, fruiting and post-harvest handling units (Bakratsas et al., 2021; Sangeeta et al., 2024). Depending on the species of mushrooms cultivated, the system should be equipped with instruments to assess the prepared substrate for its pH, EC (electric conductivity), consistency and moisture for best results. Precise and specific external factors such as temperature, humidity and air quality control are crucial for optimal growth and yield, especially for varieties requiring specific conditions (Sangeeta et al., 2024).

- **Optimized Substrates**

Supplemented sawdust blocks are one of the most common approaches in the large-scale farming of mushrooms, especially in large-scale cultivation of species such as *Lentinula edodes* (shiitake mushrooms). But some species, such as *Agaricus bisporus* (button mushrooms), *Pleurotus ostreatus* (oyster mushrooms), undergo large-scale cultivation and maintain themselves based on paddy or wheat straw under different sorting and chopping actions. Occasionally, depending on the availability and suitability, coffee hulls and corn cobs are applied in particular proportions to optimize the quality of substrates, increasing the yield and health of mushrooms (Geng et al., 2024, Desisa, 2023).

- **High-Throughput Processes**

Large-scale mushroom farming requires massive quantities of raw material to reach the expected high outcome of mushroom production. Therefore, starting from raw material handling to packaging and transportation, automated systems are often employed to increase efficiency. In the main, automated systems become crucial for substrate preparation, sterilization, inoculation, harvesting and packaging (Mishurov, 2021).

- **Strain Selection and Development**

Selecting the most appropriate strain of the selected species for cultivation is a vital concern in large-scale farming of mushrooms. Each particular strain holds common characteristics of a certain species but differs from each other at the level of strain with some characteristics such as yield, decreased tolerance and chemical properties (Raaman & Selvakumar 2024, Zied et al., 2016). Nevertheless, for large-scale farming, securitized assessments are crucial on characteristics such as yield, disease tolerance, appearance, flavour and odour to attract consumers. Occasionally, scientists modify different strains of mushroom species using genetic modifications in order to potentially develop new strains through selective breeding (Raaman & Selvakumar, 2024).

- **Marketing and Distribution**

Large-scale operations must consider marketing and distribution strategies to reach consumers and ensure a steady market for their produce. Marketing of the mushrooms comes from large-scale production lines mandatorily requiring an appropriate marketing plan and strategies to reach the targeted market and customer group. Through large-scale mushroom production facility, the quantity of yield produced is quite higher compared to the other farming systems (Luan et al., 2022; Mishurov et al., 2021). Therefore, the marketing strategies should be strong enough to address the perishability of mushrooms while boosting the brand recognition, promoting sales and revenue. Distribution of the product also has to reach consumers via the fastest path in order to secure the quality of the product. Unlike other products, the distribution of large quantities of mushrooms has to be handled and managed carefully to ensure the shelf life and the wastage of the product. Further, the distribution has to be well managed in order to meet the customer requirements in different markets (Mishurov et al., 2021).

7.3 Specific Examples of Large-Scale Cultivation Methods

- **Indoor Block Production**

Supplemented sawdust blocks, which are manufactured according to different formulas depending on the species cultivated, are a common method, permitting fast cropping cycles with better quality and high yields. Generally, this method is applied for the production of *Pleurotus* species, *Macrocybe* species, *Calocybe* species and some of the *Ganoderma* species (Nguyen et al., 2023). Each type of substrate in blocks for different species has to be optimized with required levels of nutrients, pH, EC and moisture for the best quality yield (Banfi et al., 2015).

- **Log Cultivation**

Log cultivation is mainly applied in farming mushrooms such as shiitake, lion's mane and some of the wood ear species. In the same way as block cultivation, mushrooms belonging to different species can be managed year-round with the environment-controlled techniques where temperature, relative humidity, carbon dioxide and ventilation are regulated (Contato & Conte-Junior, 2025; Desisa et al., 2023; Suntornmeth et al., 2025).

- **Field Cultivation**

Field farming methods are widely applied for mushroom species such as button mushrooms (*Agaricus bisporus*), paddy mushrooms (*Volvariella volvaceae*) and some *Ganoderma* varieties, where they are grown in pasteurized substrate/compost prepared either in crates or beds supported with a specific casing layer. This method has been identified as an efficient method for large-scale farming of mushrooms as it facilitates the use of huge quantities of compost as the substrate (Annepu & Gupta 2022, Pathak et al. 2022).

7.4 Challenges in Large-Scale Cultivation

- **High-Initial Investment**

Large-scale setting up of a mushroom facility requires a significant investment of capital and maintenance costs for infrastructure, machinery, equipment and technology. Especially, indoor facilities with intensive management equipped with automated systems, standard sterilization practices and other necessary equipment require a significant initial investment.

- **Management Intensive**

Besides, maintenance of optimal growth conditions, pest and disease management, and efficient operations management require expertise, as well as a dedicated management and controlling system for the whole large cultivation system.

Further, large-scale operations require close monitoring of environmental conditions, substrate preparation, sterilization, harvesting and post-harvest management processes.

- **Sustainability Concerns**

Large-scale mushroom cultivation is a very complex, sensitive and capital-intensive process that employs infrastructure, specialized knowledge, facilities and careful management practices to manufacture different species of mushrooms efficiently and sustainably to meet the market demand. Further, environmental influence, waste disposal and energy consumption have to be strictly addressed for maximum levels of yield. But, despite the well-maintained cultivation system, there is always a risk of disease outbreak arising due to contaminants which ultimately negatively affect yields and the product quality (Boukary et al. 2024, Moxley et al. 2022).

7.5 Importance of Large-Scale Mushroom Cultivation

Large-scale mushroom cultivation has become significant for many reasons. It brings a sustainable and nutritious food source, a source of medicines, utilizes agricultural waste, creates economic opportunities and can be integrated into sustainable agricultural practices. Therefore, it indirectly offers a way to address food security, especially in regions with land scarcity or limited resources (Jayaraman et al., 2024; Zhang et al., 2014).

Higher yields: Large-scale mushroom farming produces higher yields of mushrooms under optimized growing conditions for different species, paving the path to significantly higher, healthy yields of mushrooms compared to conventional methods. Besides, mushroom cultivation with advanced technologies is a year-round, constant production regardless of external weather conditions. A stable and constant production of mushrooms with higher yields is enhanced further by automated systems and AI applications, ensuring optimal conditions for healthy mushroom growth, leading to higher quality and more consistent yields (Zhang et al., 2014, Grimm & Wosten, 2018). In the facilitation of higher yields, automation significantly reduces the amount of manual labour required for cultivation and harvesting.

Higher yields of healthy mushrooms produced by large-scale farming, consistent quality and reduced labour costs increase the profitability of mushroom production. Generating economic opportunities, large-scale mushroom cultivation can be introduced as a lucrative source of income generation for individuals, families, investors and communities (Mukherjee et al., 2024). Further, the industry creates employment opportunities in various stages of production, from seed production, raw material supplying and cultivation to processing and marketing. Besides, the growth of the well-directed mushroom industry enhances local economies through increased trade and the development of related industries (Ojha and Shukla 2023, Lou et al., 2017).

Mushroom cultivation is an industry based on agricultural waste or agricultural by-products such as straw, cobs, husks, hulls, chips and dust. With the action of fungi/mushrooms, the by-products are converted effectively into a nutrient source or nutritious food. Large-scale mushroom farming can be integrated into agro-ecosystems where the system is incorporated into existing healthy agricultural systems, improving soil health and biodiversity of certain ecosystems.

Internationally, the global demand for mushrooms is steadily increasing due to their nutritional value, versatility and potential health benefits. Countries with well-established mushroom industries capitalize on export opportunities that support boosting the economies while contributing to global food safety and security (Rungjindamai et al., 2024). Nevertheless, large-scale mushroom cultivation depicts a multifaceted approach that stands for food security, sustainable agriculture and economic opportunities while converting the agricultural waste into nutritious food, unlocking job opportunities and making the industry a valuable and competent component of a sustainable and resilient food system (Akter et al. 2024, Kumla et al., 2020, Sardar et al., 2020).

7.6 Major Regions Involved in Large-Scale Mushroom Cultivation

Global production of mushrooms has grown at an 8.26% compound growth rate per annum (CAGR) over the past 20 years. This CAGR stands with the highest for the Asian continent (8.97%), followed by Africa (6.31%) (Bijla and Sharma 2024). For the present market, China, Japan, Poland, the United States and the Netherlands are the major countries engaged in large-scale mushroom cultivation. These nations lead the industry in global production of different mushrooms on a large scale, dominated by button and shiitake mushrooms. Currently, China is the largest mushroom producer for global requirements, accounting for a significant percentage. The CAGR of fresh mushroom production of China (9.23%) and India (8.58%) is comparable for the last 20 years, despite the advancements in China (Bijla and Sharma 2024). Production of button mushrooms is supported by the Netherlands and Poland to some extent, while the Chinese industry of mushrooms shows a rapid growth, with a wide range of varieties of mushrooms, including exotic species, being cultivated. But for shiitake mushrooms, Japan takes the lead. Nevertheless, the United States is also a major producer of mushrooms, with a substantial market for both white button and most of the other varieties. For oyster mushrooms and most of the tropical varieties, India is a notable producer. Besides, Canada and Spain contribute with large-scale production and consumption of mushrooms (Table 7.1). Nevertheless, majorly six mushrooms appear to be prominent (Fig. 7.1) in the global production and market, where shiitake mushroom (26%), oyster mushroom (21%), black ear mushroom (21%), button (11%), *Flammulina* (7%), paddy straw mushroom (1%) and other mushrooms (13%) (Bijla and Sharma 2024).

Table 7.1 Production trend & CAGR of top 10 countries for fresh mushrooms in the world (2000–2021) (million tonnes)

Year	China	Japan	Poland	USA	Netherlands	India	Spain	Canada	Russia	France
2000	6.644	0.424	0.109	0.384	0.265	0.024	0.063	0.080	0.006	0.204
2001	7.828	0.427	0.110	0.377	0.275	0.030	0.110	0.086	0.006	0.196
2002	8.774	0.430	0.120	0.377	0.270	0.040	0.135	0.075	0.007	0.175
2003	10.396	0.434	0.135	0.388	0.263	0.040	0.129	0.088	0.006	0.170
2004	11.610	0.406	0.150	0.388	0.260	0.040	0.139	0.085	0.006	0.165
2005	13.360	0.420	0.160	0.387	0.245	0.040	0.138	0.080	0.005	0.139
2006	14.749	0.430	0.169	0.383	0.235	0.035	0.135	0.089	0.006	0.116
2007	16.829	0.440	0.180	0.360	0.240	0.037	0.132	0.083	0.006	0.132
2008	18.278	0.450	0.185	0.369	0.255	0.037	0.134	0.116	0.006	0.139
2009	20.214	0.460	0.207	0.372	0.230	0.037	0.131	0.114	0.006	0.114
2010	22.020	0.470	0.230	0.359	0.266	0.041	0.133	0.115	0.005	0.119
2011	25.726	0.470	0.220	0.391	0.304	0.041	0.146	0.122	0.004	0.116
2012	28.289	0.460	0.230	0.403	0.307	0.030	0.147	0.125	0.005	0.117
2013	31.705	0.460	0.249	0.408	0.323	0.017	0.150	0.120	0.008	0.104
2014	32.708	0.460	0.263	0.432	0.310	0.028	0.150	0.122	0.008	0.109
2015	34.772	0.450	0.269	0.421	0.310	0.051	0.219	0.115	0.009	0.101
2016	35.979	0.460	0.280	0.428	0.300	0.076	0.148	0.119	0.010	0.100
2017	37.130	0.459	0.291	0.423	0.300	0.102	0.159	0.120	0.016	0.086
2018	37.901	0.467	0.200	0.416	0.300	0.134	0.166	0.126	0.031	0.083
2019	38.981	0.470	0.235	0.384	0.270	0.182	0.170	0.132	0.048	0.088
2020	40.008	0.471	0.320	0.370	0.260	0.211	0.166	0.133	0.086	0.080
2021	41.127	0.469	0.379	0.344	0.260	0.243	0.164	0.138	0.111	0.099
CAGR	9.23	0.57	5.04	0.22	0.63	8.58	2.54	2.81	11.70	-3.91

7.7 Mushroom Species that Are Being Cultivated in Large-Scale Mushroom Cultivation

According to the current status of international mushroom farming and market systems, the most popular mushroom species cultivated on a large scale are white button mushrooms (*Agaricus bisporus*), oyster mushrooms (*Pleurotus ostreatus*) and shiitake mushrooms (*Lentinula edodes*).

1. White Button Mushrooms (*Agaricus bisporus*): *Agaricus bisporus* is the most commonly cultivated mushroom globally on a larger scale. The market demand for button mushrooms arises from its mild flavour and versatility. They should be grown indoors under controlled environments, using pre-prepared compost as a substrate (Dimopoulou et al., 2025).

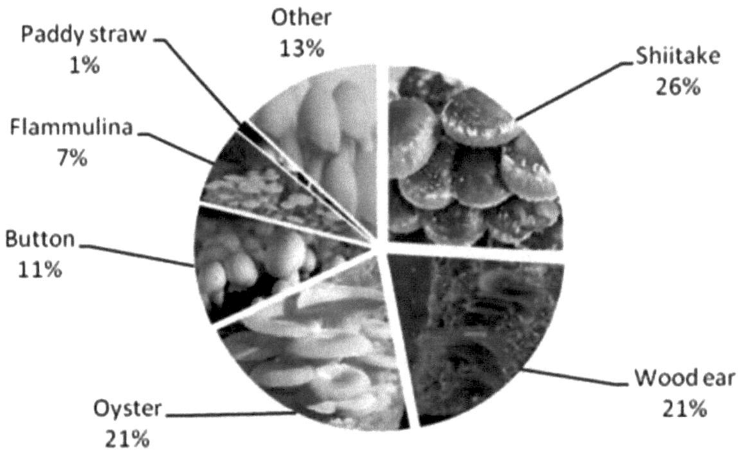

Fig. 7.1 Species-wise share of mushrooms in global production (Bijla and Sharma 2024)

2. Oyster Mushrooms (*Pleurotus ostreatus*): Oyster mushrooms are popular for their diverse flavours and ability to grow on most of the agricultural waste-based substrates. The easy cultivation methods have made them popular and valuable for both large-scale and small-scale farms. Oyster mushrooms come with variations, including grey oyster, king oyster and pink oyster (Deepalakshmi & Mirunalini, 2014).
3. Shiitake Mushrooms (*Lentinula edodes*): Shiitake mushrooms stand in line with button mushrooms, with a huge demand for its distinctive savoury flavour and are used in various dishes. Traditionally, they are grown on natural wood logs collected in large-scale commercial cultivations, but can also be grown on substrate made of sawdust and other materials. Globally, shiitake cultivation is well-established for many years, with both large- and small-scale farming systems (Atila, 2021).
4. Enoki Mushrooms (*Flammulina velutipes*): Another popular variety in countries like China, Japan, Korea, Thailand, the Philippines and Vietnam. This species is well recognized for its lengthy, thin stems and delicate flavour (Sengar et al., 2019).
5. Lion's Mane (*Hericium erinaceus*) is highly valued for its medicinal properties and unique appearance. Lion's mane mushrooms have been applied in the pharmaceutical industry for many years for its medicinal properties, and the industry requires them in larger quantities (Sokol et al., 2016a, 2016b).

7.8 Large-Scale Cultivation of Mushroom Technology

Large-scale mushroom farming utilizes advanced technologies to optimize environmental control, automate processes and manage the supply chain. Key technologies include automated growing systems, AI and machine learning for optimizing conditions and robotic harvesting and sorting, leading to increased efficiency, higher yields and reduced labour costs.

7.9 Technologies in Large-Scale Mushroom Farming

- **Automated Growing Systems**

Environmental control is one of the highly required applications in automated growing systems. Automated cultivation systems for mushrooms employ sensors and automated controllers to precisely manage environmental factors such as temperature, humidity and CO_2 levels, and ventilation, ensuring optimal growing conditions and expanding yields. Generally, all the environmental factors have to be controlled depending on the requirements of the desired species (Rehman & Sarwar, 2025). Poor management of the environment causes declined yields, deformed fruit bodies and increased risk of pest and disease attacks (Sujatanagarjuna et al. 2023).

- **AI and Machine Learning**

AI algorithms are applied to analyse data detection and feed from different sensors set for different parameters to identify patterns and forecast the best conditions for mushroom growth. This helps to conclude improved yields and quality while minimizing waste generation and energy consumption, while improving the efficiency of the process (Lu et al., 2019; Yin et al, 2022).

- **Robotic Harvesting and Sorting**

Modern farms make use of robotic hands/harvesters, automated conveyors and AI-powered sorters, depending on the quality of the mushrooms, to handle mushrooms gently. Such applications ensure consistency of size and quality (Ghahraei et al., 2023; Koirala et al., 2024).

- **Advanced Substrate Preparation**

In the large-scale mushroom industry, it is always recommended to empower the manufacturing process with specialized machinery for compost preparation, sterilization/pasteurization and mixing with humus, under controlled environments for optimal mycelial growth, which ultimately influences the yield of the production (Nandeha 2024).

- **Automated Packaging and Refrigeration**

After harvesting and sorting, mushrooms are packed whole or chopped and fresh or dehydrated. Then, it was sealed and cooled in a refrigerated storage facility. Automated loading systems and refrigerated transportation methods, such as trucks and containers, ensure speedy delivery to markets, preserving freshness and the quality of the product (Abed et al., 2024; Koirala et al., 2024).

- **Internet of Things (IoT)**

Modern farming systems use IoT sensors and data analytics, which are useful for remote monitoring and control of environmental conditions within the growing units. It provides valuable data acquisition and data storage for optimizing growth and identifying potential threats (Chong et al., 2023, Rukhiran et al. 2023).

- **Precision Farming Techniques**

These techniques help use data-driven insights and feedback in order to optimize resource allocation, resource assessments, including water and required nutrients, leading to more sustainable, effective and efficient farming practices (Nandeha 2024, Rukhiran et al. 2023).

- **Modular and Scalable Systems**

Modular and scalable systems are used in modern mushroom cultivation systems. Through the use of a modular and scalable system, the farming units or production levels can be adapted to desired scales. These kinds of systems allow for flexibility and growth (Yaeger et al., 2022).

- **Production of Healthy Spawns**

Healthy spawns are the foundation of a healthy farming system. The process of growing the mycelia of mushroom on sterile grains is a significant step in large-scale cultivation. The quality of spawns has a high impact on the yield as it is used to inoculate the growing substrate for fruiting (Aditya et al., 2024, Zhang et al., 2019).

- **Composting and Casing**

Mushroom species such as button mushrooms utilizes a two-step composting process as the nutrient-rich medium for the mushroom growth. Once the mycelial growth on the compost is completed, a layer of peat moss or other suitable material is often added/spread on top of the compost to stimulate or promote fruiting.

7.10 Benefits of Using Large-Scale Mushroom Cultivation Technologies

- Increased Yields:

Precisely controlled environmental conditions and optimized growth conditions pave the path to health and higher yields with improved mushroom quality.

- Reduced Labour Costs:

Application of automated systems supported with AI-supported applications and sensor systems reduces the need for manual labour in stages of the manufacturing processes, leading to cost savings.

- Improved Efficiency:

Automated systems, accurate protocols and effective management practices streamline the process, from raw material selection, substrate preparation and sterilization to harvesting and packaging, boosting the overall efficiency of manufacturing, distribution and marketing procedures.

- Enhanced Quality Control:

Robotic sorting, harvesting and AI-powered analysis systems ensure consistent quality and good health of mushrooms.

- Sustainable Practices:

Precise farming practices minimize waste of resource usage, maintain standards and are more sustainable and environmentally friendly.

7.11 Life Cycle Assessment in Mushroom Cultivation

7.11.1 Background and Rationale

Mushroom cultivation has become an important part of modern agriculture, especially as the world is moving towards more sustainable food systems. Compared to traditional crops, mushrooms can grow on agricultural residues, need less land and have high nutritional value. However, when produced on a large scale, especially under controlled environments, they still contribute to environmental problems like high-energy consumption, packaging waste and emissions from substrate processing (Robinson et al., 2019; Vinci et al., 2023). These impacts are not always visible when looking only at production or yield.

To properly understand the environmental effects of mushroom farming, a system-wide analysis is needed. Life Cycle Assessment (LCA) is a scientific method that can help assess these impacts by considering all stages of production, from raw material extraction to harvesting. LCA allows identifying which parts of the process have the most environmental impact, and also supports decisions for improving sustainability (Goglio et al., 2024; Leiva et al., 2017; Ta et al., 2024).

7.11.2 What is Life Cycle Assessment (LCA)

Life Cycle Assessment is a standardized tool for assessing the environmental performance of a product or process. It follows the ISO 14040 and 14,044 standards and is widely used in agriculture and food production (Goglio et al., 2024; Leiva et al., 2017). In mushroom farming, LCA typically starts from substrate preparation and ends at the farm gate, which includes harvesting and basic packaging. It usually does not cover transportation to the market or consumer use, mainly because of data limitations.

Using LCA, researchers can measure greenhouse gas emissions, energy use, water consumption, land use and other environmental factors (Dorr et al., 2021; Vinci et al., 2023). These assessments are useful for farmers, researchers and policymakers to improve efficiency and reduce negative impacts.

7.11.3 Why LCA is Important for Mushroom Sector

Life Cycle Assessment is a useful decision-making tool in mushroom production. It helps identify environmental hotspots in the production cycle and offers information on where resources are overused. For example, using LCA, it is possible to decide whether changing the substrate type, improving insulation or using renewable energy sources would have more impact on reducing emissions.

Farmers can use LCA to monitor their environmental performance, and companies can use it to meet sustainability standards or certifications. Researchers and designers can apply LCA results to improve production technologies, like designing energy-saving climate systems or better compost management practices. LCA data is also important for international markets where environmental labels or carbon footprint limits are being considered.

Moreover, LCA supports larger goals such as the Sustainable Development Goals (SDGs), especially in areas like responsible production, climate action and innovation. In future, LCA could also be combined with economic and social indicators to create more complete sustainability assessments for mushroom farms (Nabavi-Pelesaraei et al., 2023; Robinson et al., 2019; Vinci et al., 2023).

7.11.4 Methodology and Scope

- **Goal Definition**

Life Cycle Assessment studies usually begin by defining a clear goal. In the LCA of mushroom cultivation, the main goal is to evaluate the environmental performance of the production process and find out the most impactful stages. This can help to make decisions on how to reduce energy use, emissions or other environmental problems (Goglio et al., 2024). In some studies, different types of substrates or cultivation methods are compared to understand which one is more sustainable. In the present, researchers also try to understand how circular practices like reusing waste or co-products can improve the environmental profile of mushroom production.

The goal depends on the focus of the study. Some studies focus only on composting while others assess the whole production process until harvest. In this chapter, the goal is to summarize available studies and identify the common environmental hotspots in large-scale mushroom farming, especially for *Agaricus bisporus*, and compare with selected data from other species like *Pleurotus ostreatus* (Leiva et al., 2016; Robinson et al., 2019).

- **Functional Unit Selection**

The functional unit in LCA defines what is being measured. In mushroom LCA, the most common functional unit is 1 kg of fresh mushroom (Goglio et al., 2024; Leiva et al., 2015). This unit is used because it matches how mushrooms are sold in the market, and it helps to compare results between different systems or regions. Most of the reviewed studies used this unit to report greenhouse gas emissions, energy use or water consumption for each kilogram of mushroom produced.

In some cases, other functional units are also used. One alternative is per square metre of cultivation area, which helps to understand land use or spatial efficiency. Another emerging approach is per production cycle, especially useful when comparing systems that have different growing times or yields (Robinson et al., 2019; Ueawiwatsakul et al., 2014). In this chapter, the main focus will remain on 1 kg of fresh mushroom, as this is the most commonly used unit and gives more consistent results across the literature.

- **System Boundaries**

System boundaries define which parts of the production process are included in the LCA study. Most mushroom LCAs use a cradle-to-farm-gate approach (Leiva et al., 2015; Robinson et al., 2019). This means the analysis starts from the raw material extraction or preparation and ends when the mushrooms are harvested and packed at the farm. This boundary includes substrate preparation, composting, spawning, incubation, cropping, harvesting and initial packaging.

In many studies, post-farm stages like transport, retail or consumer use are not included. This is mostly due to a lack of reliable data. However, some studies discuss the possible impacts of cold storage or long-distance transport but do not include them in the actual assessment. So, the cradle-to-gate system is the most practical and widely used approach in mushroom LCA.

In some newer studies that follow circular economy principles, the system boundaries are extended to include reuse of spent mushroom substrate or other co-products (Dorr et al., 2021; Vinci et al., 2023). But these are still not common in the standard mushroom LCAs and are often treated as side systems.

- **Allocation and Data Challenges**

When the system produces more than one useful output, allocation is needed to divide the environmental impacts among the products. In mushroom systems, this is relevant when spent mushroom substrate is reused for compost or energy generation. The allocation can be done based on mass, economic value or energy content. Each method gives different results, and the choice depends on the study objective.

Some European studies use economic allocation, where more value is assigned to fresh mushrooms and less to by-products. Other studies prefer mass allocation, especially when outputs are similar in weight. A few researchers apply system expansion, where the co-product is treated as replacing another product (like SMS replacing chemical fertilizer), and the avoided impacts are subtracted from the total results (Dorr et al., 2021; Goglio et al., 2024; Vinci et al., 2023).

Another challenge is the availability and accuracy of data. Many small-to-medium farms do not keep detailed records on energy, water or substrate use. Even in commercial farms, conditions can change depending on species, season and location. For example, farms in Europe often use mechanical ventilation and insulation, while farms in Thailand or Iran use simpler systems. This affects the total energy and emission values and can make comparisons difficult (Nabavi-Pelesaraei et al., 2023; Ueawiwatsakul et al., 2014).

The data for climate control systems is also not always easy to collect. In some studies, the energy use is measured directly. In others, it is estimated based on machine ratings or electricity bills. Similarly, emissions from composting are sometimes calculated using emission factors from IPCC or national databases, instead of direct measurements (Leiva et al., 2016). These choices can lead to variation in the final results.

Because of these challenges, LCA results in mushroom studies should be interpreted carefully, especially when comparing across different countries or species.

7.11.5 Life Cycle Inventory

The life cycle inventory (LCI) is an important stage in LCA where all the materials and energy inputs and outputs are listed. It includes raw materials like straw or manure, energy for heating or lighting, water use and emissions during processes like composting or harvesting. A good inventory is very important because all the environmental impacts are calculated based on these inputs and outputs. However, in mushroom production, collecting reliable inventory data for all aspects is not easy.

- ***Agaricus bisporus* Systems**

The most detailed inventory data is available for *Agaricus bisporus*. Several European studies collected real production data from farms in Spain, Italy and Poland. These studies measured or estimated energy use, emissions, substrate composition and packaging materials during full production cycles.

Substrate preparation is a key part of the inventory. Most *A. bisporus* farms use a mix of wheat straw, horse or poultry manure, gypsum and sometimes water conditioning agents. For every 1 kg of fresh mushroom, about 7–10 kg of raw substrate materials are used, depending on yield and compost density. The composting phase involves mixing, watering and temperature control in tunnels, which consumes a large amount of diesel or electricity (Goglio et al., 2024; Leiva et al., 2015).

Climate control is another major input in the inventory. Growing rooms are maintained at specific temperature and humidity levels for several weeks. Energy is mainly used for heating, cooling, ventilation, fans and lighting. In some farms, energy use for HVAC systems accounts for 40–60% of the total energy input during the production stage (Robinson et al., 2019).

Water use in *A. bisporus* farms is also significant. Around 150–180 L of water is used per kilogram of mushrooms in some systems, mostly for compost wetting, humidification and cleaning processes (Goglio et al., 2024).

On the output side, the main product is fresh mushrooms, but there are also co-products like spent mushroom substrate (SMS), wastewater and packaging waste. Some studies try to account for these co-products either by allocation or system expansion. But often, the data for these outputs are limited or variable between farms.

- ***Pleurotus* Species Systems**

The inventory data for *Pleurotus ostreatus* and other oyster mushrooms is less complete compared to *A. bisporus*. However, a few studies from Thailand, Iran and urban farms in Europe have reported basic inputs and outputs for oyster mushroom production (Dorr et al., 2021; Nabavi-Pelesaraei et al., 2023; Ueawiwatsakul et al., 2014).

The main difference is in substrate materials. Oyster mushrooms are grown on a wide variety of agricultural wastes, such as rice straw, sawdust, cotton stalks, corn cobs and even paper waste. The substrate is usually sterilized by steam or boiling water, but in small farms, sun drying or simple fermentation is also practiced. These practices use less energy compared to tunnel composting in *A. bisporus* systems.

Energy use in oyster mushroom farms is lower in general because there is less need for tight climate control. However, if the farm is located in hot or dry regions, fans and humidifiers may still be required. Lighting is usually minimal. Outputs include the mushrooms and the leftover substrate, which is sometimes reused or sold as compost. However, many LCA studies do not include the benefits or environmental impacts of these downstream uses (Vinci et al., 2023).

- **Other Species**

Data for other species like *Lentinula edodes* (shiitake) and *Ganoderma lucidum* (reishi) is still very limited. In most cases, these mushrooms are grown on hardwood logs or sterilized sawdust in bags (Ta et al., 2024). These systems often have longer growing periods and different input structures.

The energy required for sterilizing sawdust can be high, especially if it is done using pressurized steam. Also, the use of plastic bags or bottles in log-based systems creates packaging waste that is not always considered in the inventory. So far, very few studies report full LCI data for these mushrooms in a standardized way. Some recent studies are starting to explore these systems as part of integrated biorefineries, but the details are still not sufficient for comparison (Ta et al., 2024; Zhu et al., 2024).

7.11.6 Infrastructure and Equipment

Infrastructure and equipment are usually excluded or estimated very roughly in mushroom LCA studies. For example, the lifespan of tunnels, growing shelves and machines is often not known or not recorded in farms. Some studies try to divide the total building material impact over the lifetime of the facility and assign a fraction to each production cycle. But this is not always consistent (Robinson et al., 2019).

Energy use for equipment like fans, pumps and sprayers is sometimes measured with electricity metres, but in many farms, these devices are connected to shared circuits, making it hard to separate the exact energy consumption. Because of this, energy use may be underestimated or generalized using published values or manufacturer data. Packaging materials like plastic trays or wrapping films are included in some studies, especially in Europe. But in others, packaging is not measured or assumed to be negligible. This is another area where more consistent data is needed (Goglio et al., 2024; Leiva et al., 2017).

7.11.7 Data Challenges

There are several common data challenges in mushroom LCA:

- Farms often do not keep detailed records of energy or water use.
- Substrate compositions vary by season and supplier.
- Emission factors for composting are often estimated, not measured.
- Co-product uses (like SMS reuse) are not always included.
- Infrastructure impacts are rarely documented in detail.

Because of these gaps, results from different studies may not be directly comparable. Researchers usually try to fill missing data with estimates from the literature or national databases, but this can introduce uncertainty. This is why LCA practitioners recommend more primary data collection and standard protocols for mushroom systems.

7.11.8 Environmental Impact Categories

After collecting inventory data, the next step in LCA is to assess the environmental impacts linked to those inputs and outputs. This step is known as Life Cycle Impact Assessment (LCIA). For mushroom production systems, several impact categories are commonly used. Some categories, like global warming potential and energy demand, are included in almost every study, while others, like water use or acidification, are less consistent. This section explains which impact categories are most important in mushroom LCA, based on available evidence.

- **Primary Impact Categories**

Global Warming Potential (GWP)

GWP is the most reported impact category in mushroom LCA. It measures the total greenhouse gas emissions from all stages of production, usually reported in kilograms of CO_2-equivalent per kilogram of mushroom.

For *Agaricus bisporus*, the reported GWP values range between 2.1 and 4.4 kg CO_2-eq per kg of fresh mushroom. These values depend on the energy source used for heating and the efficiency of composting systems. Most emissions come from diesel or electricity used for climate control, and methane or nitrous oxide released during composting. In systems using renewable energy or efficient composting, the GWP can be reduced significantly (Gunady et al., 2012; Leiva et al., 2015; Robinson et al., 2019). However, in most commercial farms, especially in Europe, fossil fuels are still the main source of energy.

Cumulative Energy Demand (CED)

Energy demand is another key impact category. This includes both direct energy (like electricity and diesel used in machinery) and indirect energy (like the energy needed to produce and transport raw materials).

Energy use in *A. bisporus* production is mainly from heating, ventilation and substrate preparation. In one study, energy use was found to be around 10.9 MJ per kg of mushroom when using a combined energy mix, while in others it went as high as 15.5 MJ/kg depending on the season and location (Dorr et al., 2021; Goglio et al., 2024).

Land Use Efficiency

Mushroom production is known for high land-use efficiency. This is because mushrooms can be grown in stacked beds inside tunnels or climate-controlled rooms. The land footprint per kg of mushroom is very low compared to many vegetables or animal products. Even though most studies do not calculate land-use impacts in detail, they still mention it as a benefit of mushroom farming (Goglio et al., 2024; Ueawiwatsakul et al., 2014).

- **Secondary Impact Categories**

Water Consumption

Water use is reported in some studies, but not always in the same way. In *A. bisporus* systems, water is used for composting, humidifying growing rooms and cleaning equipment. In one study from Italy, water use was around 168 L per kg of mushroom. For *Pleurotus* species, water use is usually lower, especially when using pre-treated dry substrates like straw or sawdust. But actual measurements are rare, and more studies are needed to confirm this (Goglio et al., 2024).

Eutrophication Potential

This impact category measures the potential for nutrient runoff (mainly nitrogen and phosphorus) to cause algal blooms in water bodies. It is usually linked to the use of manure in compost or wastewater from cleaning processes. Many studies do not measure it directly, yet it is relevant in areas where mushroom farms are close to rivers or other water bodies (Leiva et al., 2016).

Acidification Potential

Acidification is caused by gases like ammonia (NH_3), sulphur dioxide (SO_2) and nitrogen oxides (NO_x) released during composting or fuel combustion. This category is included in a few LCA studies, often using CML or TRACI methods. The values are generally low, but composting under poor aeration can increase ammonia emissions (Leiva et al., 2016).

7.11.9 Emerging and Less Reported Categories

- **Human Toxicity**

Human toxicity is rarely included in mushroom LCAs, mainly due to a lack of data. This category tracks the potential for chemical exposure to harm human health. It can be relevant when chemical pesticides or sterilizing agents are used, but these are not common in mushroom production. One or two studies that use ReCiPe or TRACI methods mention this category, but the results are uncertain because they are based on generic assumptions (Nabavi-Pelesaraei et al., 2023).

- **Biodiversity Impact**

Biodiversity is an important issue in agriculture, but very few mushroom LCA studies assess it. Some studies mention that mushroom farms use less land and do not require pesticides, which could be better for biodiversity. But actual biodiversity impact assessment needs detailed field data and is beyond the scope of most LCA studies reviewed (Ueawiwatsakul et al., 2014) (Table 7.2).

Table 7.2 Summary of impact categories in reviewed studies

Impact category	Commonly reported	Typical value range
Global warming Potential	Yes	2.1–4.4 kg CO_2-eq/kg mushroom
Energy demand	Yes	10–15 MJ/kg
Water use	Sometimes	120–180 L/kg
Eutrophication	Sometimes	Varies (low, but present)
Acidification	Sometimes	Varies (from NH_3 or NO_x emissions)
Human toxicity	Rarely	Not consistently reported
Biodiversity	Rarely	No standardized data

Sources Dorr et al., 2021; Goglio et al., 2024; Gunady et al., 2012; Leiva et al., 2015; Nabavi-Pelesaraei et al., 2023; Robinson et al., 2019; Ueawiwatsakul et al., 2014)

7.11.10 Critical Analysis of LCA Hotspots

When looking at the Life Cycle Assessment of mushroom cultivation, not all stages contribute equally to the overall environmental impacts. Some processes create more emissions, consume more energy or have a larger resource footprint. These processes are known as hotspots. Identifying these hotspots is very important because it helps to focus improvement efforts where they matter the most. Based on available LCA studies, most of the environmental burdens in mushroom production come from energy use, substrate processing and composting. Some impacts also come from packaging, transport and the scale of operation.

- **Energy Intensive Processes**

One of the biggest hotspots in mushroom production is the energy used for climate control systems. In large-scale *Agaricus bisporus* farms, the temperature and humidity inside growing rooms must be carefully maintained throughout the production cycle. Heating, ventilation, air conditioning (HVAC) and sometimes humidifiers and dehumidifiers are used depending on the climate. These systems consume a lot of electricity and, in some cases, diesel or gas. Studies from Spain and Italy show that climate control alone can account for 40–60% of the total energy used during the entire cultivation process (Goglio et al., 2024; Robinson et al., 2019).

Substrate sterilization is another energy-demanding step, especially in systems that grow mushrooms on sawdust or agricultural waste. In *Pleurotus* cultivation, sterilization is usually done with steam generated using firewood or liquefied petroleum gas (LPG). In small and medium farms in Thailand, this sterilization process caused significant emissions, especially when firewood was burned without proper controls (Ueawiwatsakul et al., 2014).

Post-harvest cooling and storage can also contribute to energy use, but they are not always included in system boundaries. In some systems, mushrooms are chilled immediately after harvest, and depending on the electricity source, this can raise the carbon footprint.

- **Substrate-Related Impacts**

Substrate production and composting are major contributors to emissions in *A. bisporus* systems. The compost is made using a mix of wheat straw, manure, gypsum and water. These materials are often transported over long distances, adding to fuel use and transport-related emissions. In some European farms, straw is transported from nearby regions, but manure may be brought in from commercial poultry farms located 100 km or more away. This transport can increase the overall emissions significantly, depending on the distance and fuel type used (Leiva et al., 2015).

During composting, especially in the early phases, emissions of methane (CH_4) and nitrous oxide (N_2O) are released due to microbial activity under warm and sometimes anaerobic conditions. These gases have a very high global warming potential. For example, nitrous oxide is around 298 times more potent than carbon dioxide. In most LCA studies, these emissions are estimated using IPCC emission factors, not measured directly. This means the actual impact could be even higher in poorly managed compost piles (Leiva et al., 2015).

Fresh substrates such as raw straw or manure require more processing and water compared to pre-composted or pelleted materials. Some studies suggest that using already processed or dried substrates can reduce emissions and save energy, but this depends on the local availability of such materials (Leiva et al., 2015).

- **Packaging and Post-farm Processes**

Packaging is sometimes included in the LCA, but not always in detail. Mushrooms are often packed in plastic trays, wrapped with film or placed in cardboard boxes for sale. These materials are mostly single-use and contribute to plastic waste. One study estimated that packaging could contribute up to 0.15 kg CO_2-equivalent per kg of mushroom, depending on the type and amount used (Goglio et al., 2024).

Post-farm transport is usually excluded from the core system boundary. But when included, it shows that long-distance cold-chain transport adds to the overall emissions. For example, mushrooms exported across regions or countries require refrigerated trucks, which use more fuel and energy (Leiva et al., 2015).

- **Scale Effects and Automation**

The size and automation level of the farm also affect environmental impacts. Large farms can benefit from economies of scale and use more efficient machinery and climate systems. But they also have higher total energy use and often depend more on fossil fuels. Small farms may use simpler methods, but because of lower yields and manual processes, their environmental impact per unit of mushroom can be higher.

A study from Thailand compared small, medium and large farms growing *Pleurotus sajor-caju*. It was found that medium farms had the highest emissions per kilogram of mushroom, due to less efficient energy use and poor waste management. The emissions ranged from 3.01 to 5.00 kg CO_2-equivalent per kg, with medium-sized farms being the worst performers (Ueawiwatsakul et al., 2014).

Automation can reduce labour but may increase electricity demand. For example, automated harvesting machines or climate monitoring systems may need constant power, which adds to energy demand unless renewable sources are used (Nabavi-Pelesaraei et al., 2023).

7.11.11 Regional and Technological Variations

The environmental impacts of mushroom cultivation are not the same everywhere. They change depending on the location, the size of the farm, the type of technology used, and how the process is managed. In different regions, farms use different substrates, energy sources and climate-control methods. Also, some countries are moving towards automation and renewable energy, while others still depend on traditional or manual systems. This section explains how these regional and technological differences affect Life Cycle Assessment results in mushroom production.

- **Documented Regional Studies**

Europe

Europe has some of the most detailed LCA studies on *Agaricus bisporus*. Farms in Spain, Italy, Poland and Serbia follow well-controlled systems with tunnel composting, HVAC systems and packaging standards. These farms often use a mix of wheat straw, horse or poultry manure and gypsum. The composting is usually done in controlled tunnels, which gives better quality but also uses more energy.

For example, a study from Spain found that compost preparation and climate control contributed the most to greenhouse gas emissions. Composting emissions came from the microbial breakdown of organic matter, and energy use was high during heating and pasteurization steps. However, the use of EU electricity mixes, which include some renewable energy, helped to reduce total emissions per kilogram of mushroom.

In Italy, the use of groundwater for irrigation and cleaning added to the water footprint. But efficient waste handling and use of SMS as fertilizer helped to improve the overall sustainability of the system (Goglio et al., 2024; Leiva et al., 2016).

Asia

In Asia, mushroom cultivation methods are more diverse. Large-scale production of *A. bisporus*, *Pleurotus* and *Lentinula edodes* is common in China, India, Thailand and South Korea. However, only a few studies from this region include full LCA data.

In Thailand, *Pleurotus sajor-caju* is grown using cotton waste and rice straw as substrate. Most farms are small to medium-sized and use firewood for steam sterilization. A study found that energy use and emissions were higher in medium farms due to less efficient fuel use and higher wastage rates. Transportation of substrates and lack of insulation also increased the environmental impacts. In Iran, studies looked at how to improve substrate formulation using machine learning. They tested different mixtures of paper waste and wheat straw to reduce environmental impacts. Using more paper waste helped to lower energy consumption and improve substrate reuse, which gave better LCA results. Data from China is more limited in terms of peer-reviewed LCAs, but some reports mention high use of coal-based energy and plastic packaging, which can increase emissions (Mesri Gundoshmian et al., 2022; Nabavi-Pelesaraei et al., 2023; Ueawiwatsakul et al., 2014; Zhu et al., 2024).

Urban Circular Farms

Some recent studies from Europe also focus on circular and urban mushroom farms. These farms use spent coffee grounds or brewery waste as substrates. One study in the Netherlands assessed an urban mushroom farm using circular principles. Although the substrate was based on waste, the results showed that electricity for climate control was still the biggest contributor to emissions. So, even in circular systems, energy efficiency is a key factor (Dorr et al., 2021).

- **Technology Integration Assessment**

Automation and Monitoring

Automation is becoming more common in modern mushroom farms. Climate sensors, irrigation timers and ventilation controls are used to maintain stable conditions. These technologies can improve yield and reduce labour, but they also require constant electricity supply. If renewable energy is not used, the total energy demand may increase, affecting the LCA results (Nabavi-Pelesaraei et al., 2023).

Some farms use smart control systems to reduce unnecessary use of energy. For example, using sensor-based ventilation instead of fixed timers can reduce fan running time and save energy. But the actual benefit depends on how well the system is managed and whether energy-efficient equipment is used (Mesri Gundoshmian et al., 2022).

Renewable Energy Integration

A few studies discuss the use of solar power or biogas to reduce the environmental footprint of mushroom farming. In theory, solar panels can supply electricity for fans, lights and small pumps. Biogas from SMS or organic waste can be used for heating. However, in practice, the adoption of these technologies is still limited due to cost and maintenance needs. LCA studies with detailed data on renewable energy in mushroom farms are still lacking.

In Italy, the idea of integrating mushroom production with wastewater and biofertilizer systems has been tested with the goal to create a circular system where resources are reused and waste is minimized. This approach showed promising results, especially when biogas was used for heating and SMS was turned into compost (Vinci et al., 2023).

IoT and Smart Farming

Some modern farms are beginning to use Internet of Things (IoT) systems to track temperature, CO_2 and humidity in real time. This can lead to better control of the microclimate and more efficient use of resources. However, these systems require infrastructure, training and a stable power supply. There are not many LCA studies yet that include these technologies, so their exact environmental impact is still not well known (Dorr et al., 2021).

7.11.12 Waste Valorization and Circular Economy

Mushroom farming produces not only mushrooms but also different types of waste. The most common one is spent mushroom substrate (SMS), which is the leftover material after harvesting. There are also smaller amounts of wastewater, plastic packaging and sometimes unused mushrooms. If these materials are properly managed, they can become useful resources instead of environmental burdens. This idea is part of the circular economy, where waste from one process is used as input for another. Several studies have looked at how to reuse mushroom waste and reduce the environmental footprint of the system. Some of these waste reuse options also help reduce emissions and improve overall sustainability.

- **Applications of Spent Mushroom Substrate (SMS)**

  Spent mushroom substrate is produced in large quantities. On average, 5 to 6 kg of SMS is generated for every 1 kg of *Agaricus bisporus* harvested (Goglio et al., 2024). Instead of sending this material to a landfill, many farms now try to reuse it in agriculture, energy production or even construction materials.

- **SMS as Organic Fertilizer**

  One of the most common uses of SMS is as a soil amendment or organic fertilizer. It contains leftover nutrients like nitrogen, phosphorus and potassium, and also improves soil structure. When SMS is applied to agricultural land, it can reduce the need for synthetic fertilizers. Some LCA studies have included this benefit using system expansion or avoided burden methods, where the avoided impact of producing chemical fertilizer is subtracted from the total emissions of the mushroom system (Dorr et al., 2021; Vinci et al., 2023).

  This approach can reduce the global warming potential of mushroom cultivation by a significant amount, depending on how much fertilizer is replaced and the transport distance of SMS to the fields.

- **SMS for Biogas and Energy Recovery**

  SMS can also be used to produce biogas through anaerobic digestion. In this process, the organic matter in SMS is broken down by bacteria to produce methane, which can be used for heating or electricity. This method has been tested in pilot studies, and the results show good energy recovery potential. Some studies calculated that biogas from SMS could replace up to 15–20% of the energy demand in a typical mushroom farm, especially for heating during cold months (Vinci et al., 2023; Zhu et al., 2024).

However, full-scale adoption is still limited due to technical and economic barriers. Infrastructure costs and maintenance are two main reasons why many small and medium farms do not adopt biogas systems. Also, proper moisture content and pre-treatment of SMS are needed to improve gas yields.

- **SMS in Construction Materials**

A newer and more experimental use of SMS is in building materials like bricks or insulation panels. Some studies explored mixing SMS with clay or other binders to make low-cost bricks. These materials have lower embodied energy and emissions compared to conventional bricks. While this is not yet common, it shows that SMS can have value beyond agriculture or energy (Zhu et al., 2024).

The inclusion of such reuse options in LCA is not yet standardized, but some circular economy studies have started exploring them as part of broader sustainability frameworks.

7.11.13 Co-Product Analysis

Besides SMS, mushroom farms may produce other co-products like bioethanol (from integrated biorefineries), mushroom powder or dried mushrooms. In these systems, the environmental impacts must be divided among different outputs and this is where allocation comes in.

Some studies use mass allocation, where the total impacts are divided based on the weight of the products. Others use economic allocation, which gives more weight to products with higher market value. In integrated systems like mushroom + bioethanol production, this becomes more complex. For example, a study showed that when herbal mushrooms and ethanol were produced together, the total emissions per unit could be reduced if energy recovery and co-product credits were included (Zhu et al., 2024).

There is no single best way to handle co-products, and the results can change depending on the chosen method. It is important for LCA practitioners to explain their allocation choices clearly and test how sensitive the results are to those choices.

7.11.14 Optimization Strategies

Once environmental hotspots are identified in a Life Cycle Assessment, the next important step is to find ways to reduce those impacts. In mushroom farming, several strategies have already been tested or suggested to make production more sustainable.

These strategies can be grouped into proven approaches that are supported by research and real-world use, and emerging technologies that are still under development or testing. This section presents both categories based on available evidence.

- **Proven Approaches**

Use of Agro-Waste for Substrate Optimization

Using agricultural and food industry wastes as substrate materials is one of the most effective ways to reduce environmental impact. Substrates like wheat straw, sawdust, paper waste and cotton stalks can replace more energy or resource-intensive materials. This also helps in managing regional waste streams.

In one study, mixing 20% waste paper with 80% wheat straw gave better mushroom yield and reduced the total environmental impact compared to using only straw or paper. These kinds of substrate improvements can reduce emissions, save water and lower costs at the same time.

Another benefit of agro-waste substrates is that they often require less sterilization or composting energy compared to raw manure-based materials. This directly reduces greenhouse gas emissions from the composting stage and avoids methane and nitrous oxide emissions (Mesri Gundoshmian et al., 2022; Ueawiwatsakul et al., 2014).

Energy Efficiency Improvements

Energy use is one of the main contributors to greenhouse gas (GHG) emissions in mushroom farming, especially for *Agaricus bisporus*. Improving energy efficiency in climate control systems is a key strategy. This includes:

- Installing better insulation to reduce heating/cooling needs
- Using energy-efficient fans and LED lights
- Optimizing HVAC system operation through timers and sensors
- Recovering heat from composting tunnels or exhaust air

Studies from Spain and Italy found that even small changes in fan-speed control and insulation can reduce total energy use by 10–20%, depending on the season. Also, regular maintenance of equipment and better layout of growing rooms can avoid unnecessary energy losses. These are low-cost measures that can be implemented even in small farms (Goglio et al., 2024; Leiva et al., 2017).

Water Recycling and Resource Management

Water is used in many parts of the production process, including wetting compost, humidifying air, cleaning rooms and sterilizing substrates. In some farms, wastewater from cleaning is collected and reused for non-sensitive steps like compost wetting. This helps to reduce water consumption and lower the water footprint of the farm. Some integrated farms also treat wastewater from mushroom cultivation and use it to irrigate vegetables or fruit trees, making the system more circular. These resource management strategies are often simple to apply but require proper hygiene control (Goglio et al., 2024; Vinci et al., 2023).

- **Emerging Technologies**

Bioreactor Systems for Spawn and Mycelium Production

Bioreactors are now being tested for producing mushroom spawn or liquid mycelium. This method can be more sterile and energy efficient than traditional grain-based spawn. It also reduces the need for large storage and reduces waste from unused spawn bags. Though this is still at a pilot scale in most places, the use of bioreactors could improve the overall environmental profile if powered by renewable energy or integrated into existing production systems (Nabavi-Pelesaraei et al., 2023).

Solar Energy Integration

Using solar panels for electricity or water heating is one way to reduce reliance on fossil fuels in mushroom farming. Solar energy can power lights, fans, pumps and even climate control systems during daytime hours. In circular or urban farms, rooftop solar panels are already used to offset energy use. The impact depends on the local solar potential and investment costs, but LCA modelling shows strong potential for emission reduction when solar replaces grid electricity (Vinci et al., 2023).

Advanced Packaging Materials

Packaging is a minor but consistent contributor to total emissions. Some farms are starting to test biodegradable trays, paper wraps or reusable containers to replace traditional plastic packaging. These materials have lower life-cycle emissions and reduce waste, especially in countries where recycling is not widely practiced. LCA studies are still limited in this area, but certified or organic mushroom brands show a positive trend towards using those (Goglio et al., 2024).

7.11.15 Comparative Assessment

Understanding the environmental performance of mushroom production systems becomes more meaningful when we compare different species, technologies and regions. Life Cycle Assessment results can vary depending on many factors such as species grown, type of substrate, energy source, scale of the farm and packaging. This section presents comparisons between *Agaricus bisporus* and other commonly cultivated species from different countries or systems.

- **Species Comparison**

Most LCA studies focus on *A. bisporus* because it is the most widely cultivated species globally. However, some data is available for *Pleurotus ostreatus* and a few other species, which allows limited comparisons.

Agaricus Bisporus versus Pleurotus Ostreatus

A. bisporus is usually grown on compost made from straw, manure and gypsum. This requires tunnel composting, pasteurization and strict climate control, which makes the process energy and emission-intensive (Leiva et al., 2015; Robinson et al., 2019). On the other hand, *P. ostreatus* is often grown on pasteurized agro-waste such as straw, sawdust or paper, and usually requires less energy for climate control (Mesri Gundoshmian et al., 2022; Ueawiwatsakul et al., 2014).

In different studies the GHG emissions for *A. bisporus* ranged from 2.1 to 4.4 kg CO_2-equivalent per kg of mushroom (Gunady et al., 2012; Leiva et al., 2015; Robinson et al., 2019). For *Pleurotus*, the range was lower, from 1.7 to 3.2 kg CO_2-equivalent, depending on the substrate and farm scale (Dorr et al., 2021; Ueawiwatsakul et al., 2014). However, the difference is not only due to species, but also the cultivation method.

Resource Efficiency Per Species

Mushrooms like *Pleurotus* spp. generally require less water and space, and the production cycle is shorter (about 25–30 days) compared to *A. bisporus*, which takes around 40–50 days. This improves throughput and reduces fixed energy use per cycle (Ueawiwatsakul et al., 2014). Also, *Pleurotus* can grow on a wider range of substrates, including some that are not suitable for *A. bisporus*. This flexibility allows for better use of local waste materials, which supports circular economy goals (Mesri Gundoshmian et al., 2022).

Limitations in Species Comparison

It is important to mention that data for other species like *Lentinula edodes* (shiitake) or *Ganoderma lucidum* (reishi) is very limited (Ta et al., 2024; Zhu et al., 2024). Also, different studies use different system boundaries, functional units and allocation methods. Because of this, results must be compared carefully.

- **International Benchmarking**

  LCA results also vary across regions due to differences in energy mix, climate and infrastructure. For example:

- In Spain, high energy use during composting and heating is the main impact contributor. But relatively modern facilities and EU electricity grids help reduce GHG emissions per unit.
- In Italy, water use and substrate transport were found to be important hotspots. Circular reuse of water and SMS improved performance, especially in integrated systems.
- In Thailand, small and medium Pleurotus farms using firewood for sterilization showed higher emissions per kg of mushroom due to inefficient fuel use.
- In Iran, changing substrate mixes (e.g. using more paper waste) helped reduce energy use and improve environmental outcomes.

- In urban farms in the Netherlands, circular systems using spent coffee grounds as substrate performed well in substrate-related emissions but still had high electricity use due to indoor climate control.

Benchmarking these systems shows that substrate type and energy efficiency are two of the most important factors in determining environmental impact. Farms with better insulation, renewable energy, and optimized substrate use perform better in almost all impact categories (Dorr et al., 2021; Goglio et al., 2024; Leiva et al., 2015; Mesri Gundoshmian et al., 2022; Nabavi-Pelesaraei et al., 2023; Ueawiwatsakul et al., 2014; Vinci et al., 2023).

7.11.16 Data Gaps, Challenges and Research Needs

- Although several Life Cycle Assessment studies have been done on mushroom cultivation, there are many gaps and challenges that exist. Some are related to data availability, while others come from methodological differences between studies. These limitations can affect the reliability of the results and make it hard to compare between systems or countries. This section summarizes the main issues and research needs that must be addressed for more accurate and useful LCA in mushroom farming.
- **Current Limitations**

Lack of Standardized LCA Databases

One major challenge is the lack of mushroom-specific data in LCA databases. Most studies use general agriculture or composting emission factors from tools like Ecoinvent or IPCC. These may not match the actual conditions in mushroom production, especially when composting is done under different aeration or temperature settings.

Because of this, researchers often estimate values or use data from unrelated systems, which can reduce the accuracy of the assessment. For example, the methane and nitrous oxide emissions during composting are usually not measured directly but taken from default factors (Leiva et al., 2016).

Variability in System Boundary Definitions

Different studies include different parts of the production system. Some stop at harvesting, while others include packaging or transport. A few go beyond and add waste valorization, bioethanol production or fertilizer credits from spent substrate. These differences make it difficult to compare environmental results across studies, even if they use the same functional unit (Dorr et al., 2021; Robinson et al., 2019; Zhu et al., 2024).

Limited Data on Medicinal Mushroom Processing

Most LCA studies focus on edible species like *Agaricus bisporus* and *Pleurotus ostreatus*. There is very little information on the environmental impacts of producing medicinal mushrooms such as *Ganoderma lucidum* or *Cordyceps militaris*. These mushrooms often involve additional processing steps like drying, extraction or encapsulation. Without LCA data on these processes, it is hard to know their true environmental footprint (Ta et al., 2024; Zhu et al., 2024).

Lack of Social LCA Integration

So far, almost all mushroom LCAs focus only on environmental indicators like CO_2 emissions, water use or energy demand. But mushroom farming also has social impacts like providing rural employment, improving food security or affecting worker health and safety. These are not included in current LCA studies. Including social indicators could give a more complete view of sustainability (Mesri Gundoshmian et al., 2022).

- **Methodological Challenges**

Allocation Methods for Co-Products

Many mushroom farms produce more than just mushrooms. They may generate spent substrate, biogas, compost or mushroom powder. Dividing environmental impacts among these products is not easy. Studies use different allocation methods; some use mass, others use economic value and a few use system expansion. Depending on the method, the results can vary significantly. For example, giving credit for SMS used as fertilizer can reduce overall emissions, but the benefit depends on how the SMS is used and how far it is transported (Dorr et al., 2021; Goglio et al., 2024; Vinci et al., 2023).

Infrastructure Impact Allocation

Very few studies include the impacts of building materials, growing tunnels or harvesting equipment. These are long-lasting assets, so their environmental impacts should be shared across many production cycles. But most LCA studies either ignore them or assume rough estimates. This can understate the environmental impact, especially in small or newly built farms (Robinson et al., 2019).

Regional Adaptation of Impact Factors

Impact factors such as emission coefficients or energy grid mix can vary between regions. Using European electricity data for a farm in Asia or Africa can distort the LCA results. Similarly, composting emissions may differ based on temperature and humidity, which are rarely considered in global LCA databases. More regionalized LCA models are needed to make results more accurate and context specific (Leiva et al., 2016; Nabavi-Pelesaraei et al., 2023).

7.11.17 Future Directions and Industry Applications

Mushroom cultivation plays an increasingly important role in sustainable agriculture, especially in urban and circular food systems. But for Life Cycle Assessment to remain relevant and useful, it must evolve along with new technologies, policies and market needs. This section presents the key research priorities and how LCA can be applied in the mushroom industry in the coming years.

- **Research Priorities**

Developing Mushroom-Specific LCA Databases

Most current mushroom LCAs rely on general agricultural or composting data from global databases like Ecoinvent. These datasets may not reflect real emissions from composting tunnels or substrate sterilization in mushroom farms. There is a clear need for developing mushroom-specific emission factors, energy-use data and inventory profiles that match actual production practices.

Detailed data collection from farms in different climate zones and production scales would improve the reliability of future LCAs. Having region-specific emission profiles for spent mushroom substrate, heating systems and packaging materials would allow more accurate comparisons between systems (Goglio et al., 2024; Leiva et al., 2016; Nabavi-Pelesaraei et al., 2023).

Integration with Carbon Accounting Systems

As countries and companies move towards carbon neutrality targets, carbon accounting is becoming a common requirement in agriculture and food systems. Mushroom producers, especially those exporting to environmentally conscious markets, may soon be required to report their carbon footprint.

LCA can serve as a base for carbon footprinting under ISO 14067 or GHG Protocol standards. If LCA tools are linked with carbon accounting software, farmers could get automated reports on their environmental performance. This would also support climate-smart agriculture programs (Dorr et al., 2021).

Social and Economic Impact of Inclusion

Mushroom farming contributes to employment, especially in rural and peri-urban areas. It also offers income opportunities for women and youth in many developing countries. However, these benefits are not captured in traditional environmental LCA.

In future, a more complete Life Cycle Sustainability Assessment (LCSA) could combine environmental, social and economic indicators. This would help stakeholders understand trade-offs between emissions, costs and livelihoods. Such integrated models are still rare in the mushroom sector but have strong potential (Mesri Gundoshmian et al., 2022).

Standardization of LCA Methods for Mushroom Cultivation

There is a need to harmonize how LCA is applied in mushroom farming. Studies use different system boundaries, functional units and impact categories. If standard guidelines are developed similar to what exists in dairy or grain production, results would become more comparable. This is especially important for researchers, policymakers and certification bodies (Robinson et al., 2019).

- **Policy and Industry Implications**

LCA-Based Sustainability Certification

As the mushroom market grows, especially for organic and speciality products, there is an increasing demand for environmental labelling. Including LCA results in sustainability certification could help farmers demonstrate their environmental responsibility and meet consumer expectations. Programs like Environmental Product Declarations (EPDs) or eco-labels for low-emission food products could be applied to mushrooms. This would also support marketing efforts, especially in export markets in Europe or North America (Goglio et al., 2024).

Integration into Corporate Sustainability Reporting

Mushroom farms that are part of larger food companies or cooperatives may be required to report environmental impacts under corporate sustainability frameworks like GRI or CSRD. LCA provides a scientific way to calculate and report these impacts.

Companies can also use LCA results to justify investments in energy-saving equipment, renewable energy or circular waste-handling systems. This strengthens their environmental, social and governance (ESG) credentials (Vinci et al., 2023).

Role in Sustainable Food System Planning

Governments and NGOs promoting sustainable agriculture can use LCA findings to support policy development. For example, subsidies or incentives could be given for farms that reduce emissions or adopt circular economy practices. LCA can also guide training programs for farmers on efficient resource use and waste management.

Urban planners may use mushroom LCA data to integrate mushroom farms into smart city designs or food waste recycling programs. Circular models using local agro-waste and rooftop mushroom farms can be evaluated using simplified LCA tools before implementation (Dorr et al., 2021).

7.12 Conclusion

Large-scale farming of mushrooms stands for the production in high volumes with modern technology optimizing the growth conditions for different species. Modern and latest technologies are involved in controlling environmental factors such as humidity, temperature, CO2 and Oxygen levels for the healthy growth, while automation processes support substrate preparation, log/block production and sterilization. Currently, China, USA, Japan, South Korea, India, Canada and Germany play a vital role in large-scale mushroom production. Modern techniques are also applied in automated irrigation and lighting systems, mycelium propagation technology, automated harvesting, packing and specialized technical applications such as bioreactors focusing on large-scale mycelial production. For a healthy and rich yield of mushrooms of large-scale production, further focus on waste management, value addition and energy-efficient systems.

Life Cycle Assessment has become a valuable tool to understand the environmental impacts of mushroom cultivation. From substrate preparation to harvesting and packaging, different stages of production contribute differently to energy use, emissions, water consumption and waste generation. This chapter reviewed the current knowledge and data available on LCA for mushroom production, mainly focusing on *Agaricus bisporus*, while also including comparisons with *Pleurotus ostreatus* and selected alternative systems.

LCA studies show that the biggest environmental hotspots in mushroom production are climate control, substrate composting or sterilization and transport of raw materials. Climate control systems alone can account for more than 40% of energy use in controlled-environment farms. Composting and substrate preparation contribute to greenhouse gas emissions, mainly due to methane and nitrous oxide. These impacts can be reduced through energy efficiency improvements, renewable energy use and better substrate management.

There are growing efforts to make mushroom farming more sustainable by integrating circular economy principles. Spent mushroom substrate can be reused as fertilizer, or even in energy and construction material production. These valorization pathways not only reduce waste but also offer additional income and resource savings. In some systems, such reuse helps reduce the total carbon footprint of mushroom production when co-product credits are included in the LCA.

However, many challenges remain. There is still limited LCA data for medicinal mushrooms and small-scale or traditional systems. Methodological issues like inconsistent system boundaries, lack of regional emission factors, and different allocation methods make comparisons difficult. Social and economic impacts are rarely considered, even though mushroom farming contributes to rural employment and food security in many parts of the world.

For the mushroom industry to fully benefit from LCA, there is a need for standardized methods, more field data, and better integration with sustainability certification and carbon reporting. Researchers, policymakers and producers can work together to build databases, develop tools and improve decision-making.

References

Aa, B., Ab, O., & Ns, Y. (2024). Mushroom cultivation in tropical Africa: Successes, challenges, and opportunities. *Journal of Agriculture Food Research, 18*, 101264. https://doi.org/10.1016/J.JAFR.2024.101264

Abed, I. A., Almarie, A. A., Yaqub, M. T., & Mahmood, E. K. (2024). Producing mushroom with high technology: Review article. *IOP Conf Ser Earth Environ Sci, 1371*, Article 062004. https://doi.org/10.1088/1755-1315/1371/6/062004

Aditya, Neeraj, Bhatia, J. N, & Yadav, A. N. (2024). Characterization and yield performance of spawn prepared from Hypsizygus ulmarius (Bull.) Redhead and some Pleurotus species (Agaricomycetes). *Biocatal Agric Biotechnol 56*, 103047. https://doi.org/10.1016/J.BCAB.2024.103047

Akter, M., Halawani, R. F., & Aloufi, F. A. (2022). Utilization of agro-industrial wastes for the production of quality oyster mushrooms. Sustainability, *14*, 994. https://doi.org/10.3390/SU14020994

Annepu, S. K., & Gupta, S. (2022). Insights into the specialty mushrooms production in China—Key takeaways to Indian farmers. *Mushroom Res 30*, 109. https://doi.org/10.36036/MR.30.2.2021.119990

Atila, F. (2021). Cultivation and utilization of shiitake mushroom. 383–413. https://doi.org/10.1007/978-3-030-74779-4_13

Bakratsas, G., Polydera, A., Katapodis, P., & Stamatis, H. (2021). Recent trends in submerged cultivation of mushrooms and their application as a source of nutraceuticals and food additives. *Future Foods, 4*, Article 100086. https://doi.org/10.1016/J.FUFO.2021.100086

Bánfi, R., Pohner, Z., & Kovács, J. (2015). Characterisation of the large-scale production process of oyster mushroom (Pleurotus ostreatus) with the analysis of succession and spatial heterogeneity of lignocellulolytic enzyme activities. *Fungal Biology, 119*, 1354–1363. https://doi.org/10.1016/J.FUNBIO.2015.10.003

Bijla, S., & Sharma, V. P. P. (2024). Status of mushroom production: Global and national scenario. *Mushroom Research, 32*(2):91–98, 2023. https://doi.org/10.36036/MR.29.1.2020.146647

Boukary, A., Olou, A., Piepenbring, M., & Yorou, N. (2024). Mushroom cultivation in tropical Africa: Successes, challenges, and opportunities. *Journal of Agriculture and Food Research, 18*, 101264. https://doi.org/10.1016/j.jafr.2024.101264

Chong, J. L., Chew, K. W., & Peter, A. P. (2023). Internet of things (IoT)-based environmental monitoring and control system for home-based mushroom cultivation. *Biosensors 13*, 98. https://doi.org/10.3390/BIOS13010098

Contato, A. G., & Conte-Junior, C. A. (2025). Lion's mane mushroom (Hericium erinaceus): A Neuroprotective fungus with antioxidant, anti-inflammatory, and antimicrobial potential-a narrative review. *Nutrients, 17*. https://doi.org/10.3390/NU17081307

Deepalakshmi, K., & Sankaran, M. (2014). Pleurotus ostreatus: An oyster mushroom with nutritional and medicinal properties. *Journal Biochemical Technology 5*, 718–726. https://doi.org/10.51847/WXXZF0N

Desisa, B., Muleta, D., & Dejene, T. (2023). Substrate optimization for Shiitake (Lentinula edodes (Berk.) Pegler) mushroom production in Ethiopia. *Journal of Fungi 9*, 811. https://doi.org/10.3390/JOF9080811

Dey, A., Patel, S., & Rashid, Md. M. (2020). Small-scale mushroom production unit for the Upliftment of rural economy and women empowerment in India: A review. *Current Journal of Applied Science and Technology, 39*, 38–46. https://doi.org/10.9734/cjast/2020/v39i230495

Dimopoulou, M., Chinou, I., & Gortzi, O. (2025). A systematic review of the seven most cultivated mushrooms: Production processes, nutritional value, bioactive properties and impact on non-communicable diseases. *Agriculture 15*, 1329. https://doi.org/10.3390/AGRICULTURE15131329

Dorr, E., Koegler, M., Gabrielle, B., & Aubry, C. (2021). Life cycle assessment of a circular, urban mushroom farm. *Journal of Cleaner Production, 288*, Article 125668. https://doi.org/10.1016/J.JCLEPRO.2020.125668

Geng, Y., Wang, Y., & Li, H. (2024). Optimization of manure-based substrate preparation to reduce nutrients losses and improve quality for growth of Agaricus bisporus. *Agriculture 14*, 1833. https://doi.org/10.3390/AGRICULTURE14101833

Ghahraei, O., Kheshtzarrina, M., & Saghafinia, A. (2023). Development of a button mushroom harvesting robot using expert system and image processing in shelf cultivation method. *Majlesi Journal of Electrical Engineering 17*, 53–61. https://doi.org/10.30486/MJEE.2023.1990853.1171

Goglio, P., Ponsioen, T., & Carrasco, J. (2024). An environmental assessment of Agaricus bisporus ((J.E.Lange) Imbach) mushroom production systems across Europe. *European Journal of Agronomy, 155*. https://doi.org/10.1016/j.eja.2024.127108

Grimm, D., & Wösten, H. A. B. (2018). Mushroom cultivation in the circular economy. *Applied Microbiology and Biotechnology, 102*, 7795–7803. https://doi.org/10.1007/S00253-018-9226-8/FIGURES/1

Gunady, M. G. A., Biswas, W., Solah, V. A., & James, A. P. (2012). Evaluating the global warming potential of the fresh produce supply chain for strawberries, romaine/cos lettuces (Lactuca sativa), and button mushrooms (Agaricus bisporus) in Western Australia using life cycle assessment (LCA). *Journal of Cleaner Production, 28*, 81–87. https://doi.org/10.1016/j.jclepro.2011.12.031

Gundoshmian, T. M., Ardabili, S., Csaba, M., & Mosavi, A. (2022). Modeling and optimization of the oyster mushroom growth using artificial neural network: Economic and environmental impacts. *Mathematical Biosciences and Engineering, 19*, 9749–9768. https://doi.org/10.3934/mbe.2022453

Jayaraman, S., Yadav, B., & Dalal, R. C. (2024). Mushroom farming: A review Focusing on soil health, nutritional security and environmental sustainability. *Farming System, 2*, Article 100098. https://doi.org/10.1016/J.FARSYS.2024.100098

Koirala, B., Zakeri, A., & Kang, J. (2024). Robotic button mushroom harvesting systems: A review of design, mechanism, and future directions. *Applied Sciences 14*, 9229. https://doi.org/10.3390/APP14209229

Kujawa, S., Wojciechowski, T., & Piekutowska, M. (2023). MushR: A smart, automated, and scalable indoor harvesting system for gourmet mushrooms. *Agriculture, 13*, 1533. https://doi.org/10.3390/AGRICULTURE13081533

Kumla, J., Suwannarach, N., & Sujarit, K. (2020). Cultivation of mushrooms and their Lignocellulolytic enzyme production through the utilization of agro-industrial waste. *Molecules, 25*, 2811. https://doi.org/10.3390/MOLECULES25122811

Leithäuser, H., Kirschner, R., & Tsai, M. J. (2025). Exploring mushroom cultivation under the 13 principles of the Agroecological transition. A review. *Journal of Sustainable Forestry*. https://doi.org/10.1080/10549811.2025.2532823

Leiva, F. J., García, J., & Martínez, E. (2017). Scenarios for the reduction of environmental impact in Agaricus bisporus production. *Journal of Cleaner Production, 143*, 200–211. https://doi.org/10.1016/j.jclepro.2016.12.129

Leiva, F. J., Saenz-Díez, J. C., & Martínez, E. (2015). Environmental impact of Agaricus bisporus cultivation process. *European Journal of Agronomy, 71*, 141–148. https://doi.org/10.1016/j.eja.2015.09.013

Leiva, F., Saenz-Díez, J. C., & Martínez, E. (2016). Environmental impact of mushroom compost production. *Journal of the Science of Food and Agriculture, 96*, 3983–3990. https://doi.org/10.1002/jsfa.7587

Lou, Z., Sun, Y., & Bian, S. (2017). Nutrient conservation during spent mushroom compost application using spent mushroom substrate derived biochar. *Chemosphere, 169*, 23–31. https://doi.org/10.1016/J.CHEMOSPHERE.2016.11.044

Lu, C. P., Liaw, J. J., Wu, T. C., & Hung, T. F. (2019). Development of a mushroom growth measurement system applying deep learning for image recognition. *Agronomy 9*, 32. https://doi.org/10.3390/AGRONOMY9010032

Luan, G., Zhao, F., & Jia, Y. (2022). Market analysis of characteristic agricultural products from the perspective of multi-source data: A case study of wild edible mushrooms. *Sustainability 14*, 14381. https://doi.org/10.3390/SU142114381

Mishurov, N. P., Selivanov, V. G., Devochkina, N. L., & Rubtsov, A. A. (2021). High-tech production of edible mushrooms on an industrial basis in the Russian federation. *IOP Conf Ser Earth Environ Sci, 723*, Article 032080. https://doi.org/10.1088/1755-1315/723/3/032080

Moxley, A., Ebel, R., Cripps, C. L., Austin, C. G., Stein, M., & Winder, M. (2022). Barriers and opportunities: Specialty cultivated mushroom production in the United States. *Sustainability, 14*(19), 12591

Mukherjee, A., Kharbikar, H., & Planning, L. U. (2024). Mushroom marvels : Empowering hill farmers of India through transformative entrepreneurship. *SATSA Mukhapatra–Annual Technical Issue, 28*, 165–181.

Muyal, A., Gayatri, & Sharma, G. (2018) Constraints faced by small, medium and large farmers in mushroom cultivation. *Agriculture Update 13*, 477–479. https://doi.org/10.15740/HAS/AU/13.4/477-479

Nabavi-Pelesaraei, A., Ghasemi-Mobtaker, H., & Salehi, M. (2023). Machine learning models of Exergoenvironmental damages and emissions social cost for mushroom production. *Agronomy, 13*. https://doi.org/10.3390/agronomy13030737

Nandeha, N. (2024). Substrates for mushroom production. Mushroom: The Fascinating Fungi, 1st ed.; Padamini, R., Rathour, SK, Dange, MM, Ali, MU, Chavda, H., Eds, 77–94

Nazir, M., Gb, H., & Gbani, M. (2014). Button mushroom cultivation. *Communication and Publication Centre, 10*, 1–27.

Nguyen, L. T., VAN Le, V., & Nguyen, B. T. T. (2023). Optimization of mycelial growth and cultivation of wild Ganoderma sinense. *Biotechnologia, 104*, 65. https://doi.org/10.5114/BTA.2023.125087

Ojha, J., & Shukla, S. K. (2023). Mushroom cultivation: A lucrative agribusiness venture. *Indian Farming, 73*(4), 33–35

Padamini, R., Rathour, S. K, & Dange, M. M. (2024). Mushroom : The Fascinating Fungi. Emerald Publishing House.

Pathak, A. P., Rathod, M. G., & Thakur, G. M. An overview on button mushroom cultivation. Bhumi Publishing, India.

Raaman, N., & Selvakumar p. (2024). Strain improvement and molecular characterization of mushrooms. https://doi.org/10.36460/Kavaka/60/sp/2024/30-53

Rehman, S. U., & Sarwar, M. S. (2025). Automated mushroom farming: An energy-efficient digital cultivation system. 0–14.

Robinson, B., Winans, K., & Kendall, A. (2019). A life cycle assessment of Agaricus bisporus mushroom production in the USA. *International Journal of Life Cycle Assessment, 24*, 456–467. https://doi.org/10.1007/s11367-018-1456-6

Rosen, M. A., Crina, Petrescu, D., & Malina, Petrescu-Mag, R. (2022). Barriers and opportunities: Specialty cultivated mushroom production in the United States. *Sustainability 14*, 12591. https://doi.org/10.3390/SU141912591

Rukhiran, M., Sutanthavibul, C., Boonsong, S., & Netinant, P. (2023). IoT-based mushroom cultivation system with solar renewable energy integration: Assessing the sustainable impact of the yield and quality. *Sustainability, 15*(18), 13968. https://doi.org/10.3390/su151813968

Rungjindamai, N., Trakunjarunkit, K., Posalee, T., & Limpanya D. (2024). Utilization of agricultural waste for the cultivation of Pleurotus mushrooms in Thailand. *Journal Pure and Applied Microbiology, 18*, 941–950. https://doi.org/10.22207/JPAM.18.2.07

Sangeeta, S. D., & Ramniwas, S. (2024). Revolutionizing mushroom processing: Innovative techniques and technologies. *Food Chem X, 23*, Article 101774. https://doi.org/10.1016/J.FOCHX.2024.101774

Sardar, H., Anjum, M. A., & Nawaz, A. (2020). Effect of different agro-wastes, casing materials and supplements on the growth, yield and nutrition of milky mushroom (Calocybe indica). *Folia Horticulturae, 32*, 115–124. https://doi.org/10.2478/FHORT-2020-0011

Sengar, R. S., Singh, A., & Singh, G. (2019) Cultivation of winter Mushroom (Flammulina velutipes). 52, 1–6

Sokół, S., Golak-Siwulska, I., & Sobieralski, K. (2016a). Biology, cultivation, and medicinal functions of the mushroom Hericium erinaceum. *Acta Mycol 50*. https://doi.org/10.5586/AM.1069

Sokół, S., Sokół, S., & Golak-Siwulska, I. (2016b). Biology, cultivation, and medicinal functions of the mushroom Hericium erinaceum. *Acta Mycol, 50*. https://doi.org/10.5586/am.1069

Sujatanagarjuna, A., Kia, S., Briechle, D. F., & Leiding, B. (2023). MushR: A smart, automated, and scalable indoor harvesting system for gourmet mushrooms. *Agriculture, 13*(8), 1533

Suntornmeth, P., Homjun, K., & Fankam-Ai, W. (2025). Development of a closed chamber system for cultivating lion's mane mushrooms using an internet of things system to increase yield and economic value. In *10th International Conference on Digital Arts, Media and Technology, DAMT 2025 and 8th ECTI Northern Section Conference on Electrical, Electronics, Computer and Telecommunications Engineering, NCON 2025 23–28*. https://doi.org/10.1109/ECTIDAMTNCON64748.2025.10962018

Ta, T. Y., Nguyen, K. L. P., & Nguyen, T. H. T. (2024). Integrated life cycle assessment with the ReSOLVE framework for environmental impacts mitigation in mushroom growing: The case in Lam Dong province. *Vietnam. Environ Dev, 51*, Article 101024. https://doi.org/10.1016/j.envdev.2024.101024

Thakur, M. P. (2020). Advances in mushroom production: Key to food, nutritional and employment security: A review. *Indian Phytopathol, 73*, 377–395. https://doi.org/10.1007/S42360-020-00244-9/METRICS

Ueawiwatsakul, S., Mungcharoen, T., & Tongpool, R. (2014). Life Cycle Assessment of Sajor-caju Mushroom (Pleurotus Sajor-caju) from different sizes of farms in Thailand. *International Journal of Environmental Science and Development, 5*, 435–439. https://doi.org/10.7763/ijesd.2014.v5.523

Veljović, S., & Krstić, J. (2020). Elaborating on the potential for mushroom-based product market expansion: Consumers' attitudes and purchasing intentions. *Bioactive Natural Products in Drug Discovery* 643–663. https://doi.org/10.1007/978-981-15-1394-7_23

Vinci, G., Prencipe, S. A., & Pucinischi, L. (2023). Sustainability assessment of waste and wastewater recovery for edible mushroom production through an integrated nexus. A case study in Lazio. *Science of the Total Environment 903*, 166044. https://doi.org/10.1016/j.scitotenv.2023.166044

Yaeger, W., Jawed, M., & Tauman, D. (2022). Modular methods for oyster mushroom cultivation in low-resource settings. In *2022 IEEE Global Humanitarian Technology Conference, GHTC 2022 30–37*. https://doi.org/10.1109/GHTC55712.2022.9911008

Yin, H., Yi, W., & Hu, D. (2022). Computer vision and machine learning applied in the mushroom industry: A critical review. *Computers and Electronics in Agriculture, 198*, Article 107015. https://doi.org/10.1016/J.COMPAG.2022.107015

Zhang, W. R., Liu, S. R., Kuang, Y. B., & Zheng, S. Z. (2019). Development of a novel spawn (Block Spawn) of an edible mushroom, Pleurotus ostreatus, in liquid culture and its cultivation evaluation. *Mycobiology, 47*, 97–104. https://doi.org/10.1080/12298093.2018.1552648

Zhang, Y., Geng, W., & Shen, Y. (2014). Edible mushroom cultivation for food security and rural development in China: Bio-Innovation, technological dissemination and marketing. *Sustainability 6*, 2961–2973. https://doi.org/10.3390/SU6052961

Zhu, S., Liu, K., & Sheng, B. (2024). Sustainable biorefinery: Life cycle assessment for combined production of herbal mushroom and bioethanol from regional biomass. *Industrial Crops and Products, 222*, Article 119577. https://doi.org/10.1016/j.indcrop.2024.119577

Zied, D. C, Maciel, W. P, & Marques, S. C. (2016). Selection of strains for shiitake production in axenic substrate. World Journal Microbiology *Biotechnolnology, 32*. https://doi.org/10.1007/S11274-016-2115-3

Chapter 8
Harvesting Biogas from Landfills for Renewable Energy, Processes for Biogas Extraction from Landfills, Advancements and Applications, Environmental and Economic Benefits

Murat Yılmaz, Mohamed A. Hassaan, and Ahmed El Nemr

Abstract Landfill biogas, which lowers greenhouse gas emissions and offers a scalable renewable energy source, mainly comprises methane and carbon dioxide. This chapter looks at modern methods for extracting biogas, including well field design, gas collecting systems, and purification processes (such as membrane separation and amine scrubbing). Recent advancements in landfill gas-to-energy (LFGTE) technology are highlighted in the chapter, such as Internet of Things-enabled monitoring devices and modular anaerobic digesters. Environmental benefits include reducing methane leakage, a potent greenhouse gas, and managing landfill odours, while economic benefits include generating cash through electricity and carbon credits. Case studies of successful projects, like the Puente Hills Landfill in California, demonstrate the viability of landfill biogas for grid injection and industrial purposes. With an emphasis on optimizing extraction effectiveness and integrating biogas into frameworks for the circular economy, topics like fluctuating gas yields and regulatory compliance are also covered.

Keywords Landfill gas-to-energy (LFGTE) · Landfill biogas · Grid injection · Circular economy · Carbon credits

M. Yılmaz
Bahçe Vocational School, Department of Chemistry and Chemical Processing Technologies, Osmaniye Korkut Ata University, Osmaniye, Türkiye
e-mail: muratyilmaz@osmaniye.edu.tr

M. A. Hassaan (✉) · A. E. Nemr
National Institute of Oceanography and Fisheries (NIOF), Kayet Bey, Elanfoushy, Alexandria, Egypt
e-mail: mhss95@mail.com

P. Verma (ed.), *Sustainable Practices in Biorefinery*,
https://doi.org/10.1007/978-981-95-6071-4_8

8.1 Introduction

Globally, landfills are recognized as the third most significant anthropogenic source of methane (CH_4), contributing approximately 11% to the total CH_4 emissions (IPCC, 2021). According to the United States Environmental Protection Agency (EPA) estimates, food waste deposited in municipal solid waste landfills accounts for approximately 58% of fugitive methane emissions (EPA, 2025a). Produced through the anaerobic breakdown of organic waste, this greenhouse gas exhibits a global warming potential of 28 to 34 times higher than carbon dioxide when considered over 100 years (IEA, 2025). Without gas recovery systems, methane released from unmanaged landfills significantly exacerbates global climate change and poses safety hazards due to the risk of explosions (Kurniawan et al., 2024).

A substantial body of research highlights the critical importance of reducing these emissions to meet the targets set by global climate accords, most notably the Paris Agreement (UNEP, 2022). Therefore, improving landfill practices through methane recovery functions as a climate mitigation strategy and a step toward sustainable waste valorization.

Landfill-derived biogas is considered a renewable energy resource, primarily composed of 45–65% methane and 35–55% carbon dioxide, along with minor constituents including hydrogen sulphide and volatile organic compounds (Jameel et al., 2024; Swinbourn et al., 2024). As a locally available and decentralized energy source, it holds considerable potential to complement other renewables like solar and wind energy (Calbry-Muzyka et al., 2022).

The utilization of this energy source not only serves as a substitute for fossil fuels but also promotes the development of distributed energy networks, supports rural electrification, and contributes to the advancement of sustainable urban infrastructure (Calbry-Muzyka et al., 2022; Swinbourn et al., 2024). Furthermore, upgrading landfill biogas to biomethane enables its incorporation into existing natural gas infrastructure, transforming it into a storable, dispatchable, and economically feasible fuel that aligns with the principles of a circular economy (Hoo et al., 2018).

8.2 Processes for Biogas Extraction

8.2.1 Landfill Gas Collection Systems

8.2.1.1 Wellfield Design: Horizontal versus Vertical Gas Wells

Effective biogas recovery from landfills begins with the engineering design of well fields—networks of wells constructed to collect landfill gas (LFG) generated through the anaerobic breakdown of organic waste (Oonk, 2012; Un, 2023). The two primary configurations utilized are vertical wells and horizontal wells.

- Vertical wells constitute the most common design and are typically drilled into the waste mass after the landfill cells have been capped. These wells provide deep access and enable efficient, continuous gas extraction. Constructed from perforated HDPE or PVC pipes surrounded by gravel backfill, they are connected to vacuum lines to facilitate gas collection (EPA, 2025a, 2025b, 2025c; Zheng et al., 2018).
- In contrast, horizontal wells are installed within the waste layers during active landfill operations. They enable initial gas capture, reduce surface emissions, and offer a cost-effective solution for temporary gas extraction. However, their effectiveness can decline over time as waste accumulates and obstructs the healthy pathways (Nec & Huculak, 2019).

An optimal design often integrates a hybrid system combining both vertical and horizontal wells, tailored to the landfill's age, waste composition, and operation length (Polat & Eren, 2021; Shaban et al., 2022). Proper spacing and depth of wells, along with effective leachate management, are critical to maintaining consistent gas flow and minimizing oxygen infiltration, which could otherwise hinder methanogenesis or cause fire hazards (Nec & Huculak, 2019; Zheng et al., 2018). Recent modelling research suggests that horizontal wells may improve gas collection efficiency by up to 30% during the early stages, whereas vertical wells provide more reliable gas capture following landfill closure (Shang et al., 2021).

8.2.1.2 Gas Extraction Technologies (Blowers, Vacuums)

To maintain sub-atmospheric pressure within the landfill, the collected gas must be continuously extracted using a vacuum-driven system. This approach helps minimize fugitive emissions and controls the subsurface movement of gas (Terraza and Willumsen, 2009). The extraction system typically includes:

- Blowers/compressors for the generation of negative pressure
- Condensate traps and moisture extraction devices
- Manifolds and control valves for regulating flow rates for each well
- Gas flow meters and analytical sensors for the measurement of CH_4, CO_2, O_2, and H_2S concentrations

Vacuum pressures are generally maintained within a range of -10 to -50 mbar. Over-extraction can lead to air ingress, resulting in aerobic zones that inhibit methane generation and increase the risk of landfill fires. Therefore, automated control systems are increasingly utilized to optimize extraction rates dynamically in real time (Sui, 2025).

8.2.2 *Purification and Upgrading*

8.2.2.1 *Removal of Contaminants* via *Membrane Separation and Amine Scrubbing*

Due to the presence of various impurities, raw landfill gas is unsuitable for direct combustion or injection into the gas grid. It contains numerous trace compounds that can damage combustion engines or lead to non-compliance with environmental emission standards (Cevallos-Mendoza et al., 2022; Gao et al., 2019; Pasichnyk et al., 2023; Rochelle, 2024). These include:

- Hydrogen sulfide (H_2S): corrosive and toxic
- Siloxanes: generate abrasive silica residues upon combustion
- Ammonia, halogenated compounds, and VOCs

Key purification techniques include:

- Membrane separation utilizes selective permeability to remove components such as CO_2, H_2S, and water vapour from methane. This method offers a modular design, high energy efficiency, and scalability, making it well-suited for various operational scales (Cevallos-Mendoza et al., 2022; Pasichnyk et al., 2023).
- Amine scrubbing, a chemical absorption process, employs monoethanolamine (MEA) solvents to selectively capture CO_2 and H_2S. Widely applied in large-scale biomethane upgrading systems, this technique can achieve methane purities exceeding 96% (Gao et al., 2019; Rochelle, 2024).

Depending on the intended application, additional treatment methods such as activated carbon adsorption, cryogenic separation, or pressure swing adsorption (PSA) may be employed to meet specific gas quality requirements (Atelge et al., 2021; Gaur et al., 2010).

8.2.2.2 Methane Enrichment for Grid Injection (Biomethane)

After eliminating contaminants, the methane-enriched stream is upgraded to biomethane, typically achieving CH_4 concentrations above 95%. To be suitable for injection into the national gas grid, the final product must comply with regulatory standards concerning energy content, dew point, and odorization (Chinea et al., 2023; Mergenthal et al., 2023).

Essential phases in enrichment and grid compatibility encompass:

- Compression of biomethane to pipeline pressure levels
- Odorant injection (e.g., tetrahydrothiophene) for leak detection
- Metering and quality assurance

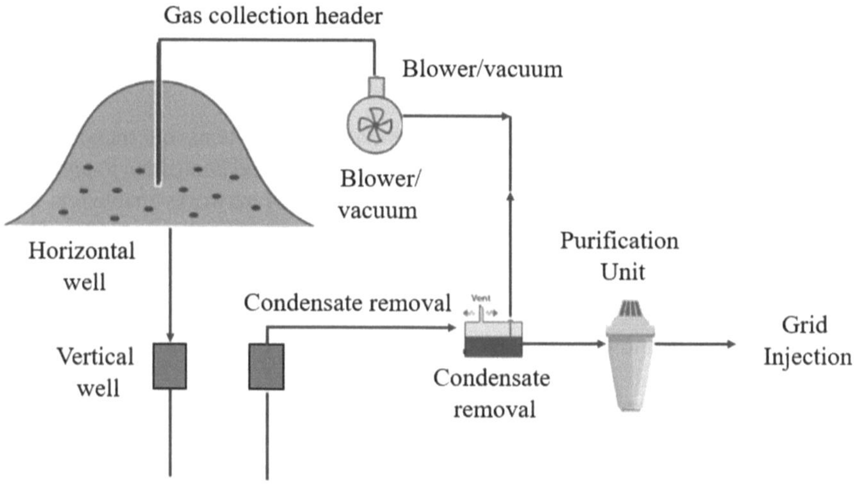

Fig. 8.1 Schematic of a typical landfill gas collection and treatment system

Studies have shown that membrane-based technologies can achieve biomethane recovery with energy efficiencies exceeding 90%, making them well-suited for decentralized production systems (Peppers et al., 2019; Rodero et al., 2024).

Biomethane can be utilized for:

- Heating for residential and industrial applications
- Electricity production with Combined Heat and Power (CHP) units
- Vehicle fuel in compressed or liquefied states (bio-CNG, bio-LNG) (Pavičić et al., 2022; Qyyum et al., 2020). Figure 8.1 illustrates a schematic of a conventional landfill gas collecting and treatment system.

8.3 Technological Advancements

Modern technological advancements have improved the efficiency of landfill gas (LFG) recovery, reduced associated environmental impacts, and increased the adaptability and sustainability of energy generation processes (Un, 2023). This section examines key technological advancements, such as Internet of Things (IoT)-enabled monitoring systems, integrated hybrid energy solutions, and modular bioreactor designs (Frontistis et al., 2023; Zhang et al., 2021).

8.3.1 IoT-Enabled Monitoring for Leak Detection and Gas Flow Optimization

By enabling remote monitoring and control of landfill gas systems, Internet of Things (IoT) technologies reduce the need for manual operation and contribute to enhanced system performance (Junus et al., 2025). Integrated sensor networks enable real-time monitoring of critical parameters such as gas flow rate, composition (including CH_4, CO_2, O_2, and H_2S), temperature, pressure, and humidity (Auelbekov et al., 2025).

These systems allow for:

- Timely identification of gas leaks thereby decreases methane emissions into the atmosphere.
- Automated regulation of vacuum levels, enhancing gas collecting efficiency, and mitigating oxygen intrusion.
- Assessment of energy production efficacy, reducing process losses (Auelbekov et al., 2025; Junus et al., 2025).

8.3.2 Hybrid Systems Integrating Biogas with Solar/Wind for Stable Energy Output

Since biogas production varies with factors like waste composition and temperature, combining it with renewable energy sources such as solar and wind in hybrid systems provides enhanced operational flexibility (Anvari et al., 2025; Nassereddine et al., 2024). These hybrid systems offer the following advantages:

- Continuous energy supply: Biogas systems are activated as supplementary energy sources when solar or wind resources are insufficient.
- Reduced need for energy storage: They ensure a reliable and continuous energy supply.
- Reduced CO_2 emissions: It is possible to establish systems entirely free of fossil fuels (Anvari et al., 2025; Nassereddine et al., 2024).

In a typical hybrid system:

- Solar panels supply energy throughout daylight hours.
- Biogas-powered generators function as backup energy sources during night-time or periods of low solar irradiance.
- Surplus energy can be stored using battery systems or thermal storage technologies (Anvari et al., 2025; Nassereddine et al., 2024).

López-Aguilar and colleagues have shown that integrating hybrid biogas-solar photovoltaic systems within landfill operations fosters innovation in the energy industry and promotes sustainability by improving waste management efficiency alongside renewable energy production. These technologies highlight their socioeconomic benefits by creating job opportunities in waste management and renewable energy sectors (López-Aguilar et al., 2025).

8.3.3 *Modular Anaerobic Digesters for Decentralized Landfill Energy*

Modular anaerobic digester systems offer decentralized, flexible, and scalable energy solutions, making them especially suitable for small to medium-sized communities (Anyaoku & Baroutian, 2018; Ellacuriaga et al., 2022). These systems are typically:

- Built within portable container units;
- Installed near landfill sites;
- Competent in processing secondary organic waste streams with landfill gas (Anyaoku & Baroutian, 2018; Ellacuriaga et al., 2022).

Advantages include:

- Short installation time (usually under 6 months);
- Operation with low capital investment;
- Eliminating energy transmission losses through local production (Anyaoku & Baroutian, 2018; Ellacuriaga et al., 2022).

Furthermore, these systems support multiple functions such as heat recovery, wastewater treatment, and the production of compost (Anyaoku & Baroutian, 2018; Ellacuriaga et al., 2022).

In the Sverdlovsk region of Russia, a wastewater treatment plant generates approximately 9.9 million cubic meters of biogas annually, which is subsequently converted into 20.8 million kWh of electricity and 24.78 million kWh of thermal energy, meeting the energy demands of the region (Huang, 2024). Figure 8.2 depicts the flow of Smart Biogas Monitoring combined with Hybrid Integration.

8.4 Environmental Benefits

The benefits of capturing and utilizing landfill gas (LFG) extend beyond energy generation. Given methane's potency as a greenhouse gas (GHG), its controlled extraction and use significantly contribute to climate change mitigation. Moreover, this process helps alleviate other environmental concerns, such as leachate production and odour emissions (Kurniawan et al., 2022, 2024). This chapter outlines the primary ecological advantages of biogas recovery from landfill sites.

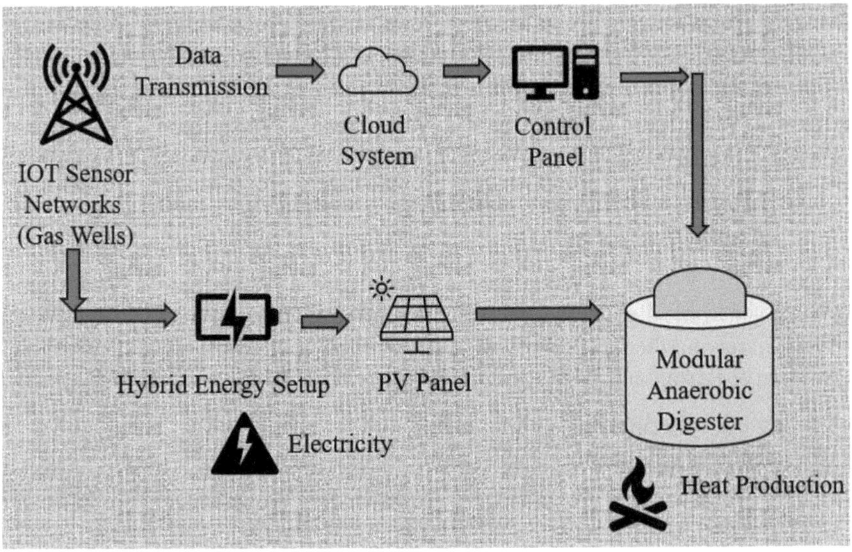

Fig. 8.2 Smart biogas monitoring and hybrid integration flow

8.4.1 Methane Emission Reduction

Methane (CH_4), the main component of landfill gas, has a global warming potential (GWP) approximately 28 to 34 times greater than that of carbon dioxide (CO_2) over a 100-year time horizon (IPCC, 2021). Approximately 11% of global anthropogenic methane emissions originate from landfills, primarily due to the anaerobic breakdown of organic waste in oxygen-limited conditions (IPCC, 2021).

Implementing gas collection systems and converting methane (CH_4) into usable energy considerably reduces direct atmospheric emissions. Additionally, the combustion of methane for energy or heat production converts it into carbon dioxide (CO_2), a greenhouse gas with substantially lower environmental impact (Alli et al., 2024; Kurniawan et al., 2024).

According to the U.S. Environmental Protection Agency (EPA), a typical landfill gas-to-energy (LFGTE) project has the potential to reduce greenhouse gas emissions by over 1 million metric tons of CO_2-equivalent each year, which corresponds to removing approximately 200,000 passenger vehicles from circulation (EPA, 2025a, 2025b, 2025c).

Moreover, methane capture supports climate change mitigation efforts aligned with international agreements such as the Paris Climate Agreement and the Global Methane Pledge (Olczak et al., 2023).

8.4.2 Landfill Leachate Management

Leachate, the liquid that percolates through landfill waste, poses a significant environmental risk because it can pollute surface water and groundwater. This liquid contains a complex mixture of organic and inorganic pollutants, including heavy metals, ammonia, and persistent organic compounds (Igwegbe et al., 2024; Wang & Qiao, 2024).

Landfill gas extraction indirectly improves leachate control through:

- Maintaining negative pressure inside the landfill reduces precipitation infiltration and limits moisture buildup.
- Regulating landfill hydraulics to confine the zones of leachate production.
- Enabling the co-treatment of leachate through the use of waste heat or digestate produced by biogas systems (Igwegbe et al., 2024; Wang & Qiao, 2024).

Improved leachate management minimizes the risk of contamination to aquatic ecosystems, thereby supporting water quality preservation and compliance with regulatory standards (Igwegbe et al., 2024; Wang & Qiao, 2024).

8.4.3 Odour Control and Public Health Improvement

Landfills are well known for their characteristic odours, which mainly result from the release of hydrogen sulphide (H_2S), mercaptans, and volatile organic compounds (VOCs) produced during the decomposition of organic material (Lim et al., 2018; Saral et al., 2009). Even at trace concentrations, these compounds have the potential to:

- Cause nuisance complaints among nearby residents.
- Trigger respiratory irritation and headaches in exposed populations
- Lower property values in areas surrounding landfill sites (Lim et al., 2018; Saral et al., 2009).

Deploying landfill gas (LFG) collection and utilization technologies reduces the release of odorous gases. Key odour control benefits include:

- Capture and combustion of sulphur-containing compounds such as hydrogen sulphide (H_2S).
- Reduction of anaerobic 'hot spots' that act as primary odour sources.
- Pressure equalization prevents uncontrolled gas emissions from landfill surfaces (Lim et al., 2018; Saral et al., 2009).

Additionally, landfill gas (LFG) recovery systems are crucial in reducing fire and explosion risks associated with methane buildup in enclosed landfill zones, where ignition from heat sources could occur (Lim et al., 2018; Saral et al., 2009).

8.4.4 *Contribution to Circular Economy and Environmental Stewardship*

The environmental benefits of landfill gas recovery align closely with the principles of the circular economy, which views waste not as a liability but as a valuable resource (Achi et al., 2024; Elroi et al., 2023). Through the transformation of landfill emissions into valuable energy and byproducts—such as compost, digestate, and CO_2 for industrial applications—biogas systems:

- Close material loops
- Reduce dependence on fossil fuels
- Promote environmental stewardship and climate resilience (Chojnacka & Moustakas, 2024; Hussain et al., 2020).

Transforming environmental liabilities into both economic and ecological assets enhances the sustainability of municipal waste management systems (Achi et al., 2024; Elroi et al., 2023; Hussain et al., 2020).

8.5 Economic Challenges

Despite offering clear environmental and energy benefits, implementing landfill gas-to-energy (LFGTE) projects is often hindered by various economic constraints (Ghosh et al., 2023; Rudd et al., 2024). These challenges include significant upfront capital costs, fluctuating gas production affecting revenue stability, and competition from low-cost fossil fuels. Understanding these economic barriers is essential for developing effective policy measures and attracting private sector investment (Ghosh et al., 2023; Rudd et al., 2024).

8.5.1 *High Upfront Costs of Gas Collection Infrastructure*

The development of a landfill biogas recovery facility entails substantial financial investment. Key cost components include:

- Wellfield construction (horizontal and/or vertical gas wells)
- Gas conveyance systems (pipelines, valves, condensate traps)
- Gas treatment and upgrading facilities (membrane separation, PSA, amine scrubbing)
- Electricity generation or grid injection infrastructure (generators, compressors, meters) (Olodu & Erameh, 2023; Zheng et al., 2018).

The total capital cost for a medium to large-scale landfill gas-to-energy (LFGTE) facility can range from \$2 million to \$15 million, depending on site size, gas composition, and system complexity (USEPA, 2022). In many cases, especially in developing countries or smaller communities, these costs exceed local budgetary resources. Furthermore, the return on investment (ROI) for such projects is typically long-term, requiring a payback period ranging from 7 to 15 years, depending on energy market prices and government incentives. As a result, many viable projects remain unrealized due to funding shortages, restricted access to credit, or insufficient investor confidence.

8.5.2 Variable Gas Yields Due to Landfill Age and Waste Composition

The economic viability of landfill gas (LFG) projects largely depends on consistent gas production, which is influenced by the following factors:

- Landfill age: Typically, gas production peaks between 5 and 7 years after waste deposition, after which it gradually declines.
- Waste composition: Biogas generation is driven by organic matter, whereas sites containing minimal biodegradable material tend to emit lower methane levels.
- Operational conditions: Temperature, humidity, compaction, and oxygen infiltration all influence microbial activity and gas production (Amini et al., 2012; EPA, 2025c).

This variability poses challenges for predicting long-term revenue, which may discourage commercial lenders and infrastructure investors. Additionally, overestimating gas production can lead to underused equipment, operational inefficiencies, and financial setbacks (WİR, 2023).

8.5.3 Market Competition with Low-Cost Natural Gas

In many regions, especially where shale gas is accessible or fossil fuels receive subsidies, natural gas remains significantly more affordable than biomethane produced from landfill sources (Hoo et al., 2018; Jameel et al., 2024). This economic disparity reduces the competitive advantage of landfill gas-to-energy (LFGTE) systems.

Factors contributing to this challenge include:

- Economies of scale in fossil fuel infrastructure
- Volatile electricity and gas market prices
- Lack of carbon pricing mechanisms or incentives for renewable gas (Hoo et al., 2018; Jameel et al., 2024).

Without financial incentives like feed-in tariffs or renewable energy credits, landfill gas projects often struggle to generate sufficient revenue to maintain profitability (Falcone, 2023). The International Energy Agency (IEA, 2021) performed a comparative analysis demonstrating that biomethane produced from landfill gas is, on average, two to three times more expensive per kilowatt-hour than pipeline natural gas, excluding subsidies. To address this cost gap, regulatory measures such as carbon taxes, renewable gas mandates, and green gas certification schemes play a vital role in levelling the competitive field and supporting the economic feasibility of landfill gas-to-energy (LFGTE) systems (Hoo et al., 2018; Jameel et al., 2024).

8.5.4 Maintenance and Operational Costs

Beyond the initial capital investment, operation and maintenance (O&M) expenses constitute a significant ongoing financial commitment, especially over the system's typical 15 to 25-year lifespan. These include:

- Routine monitoring and inspection
- Substitution of filters, membranes, and mechanical components
- Urgent repairs are necessary due to leachate infiltration, pipe obstruction, or equipment malfunction
- Skilled personnel and training requirements

In projects with limited funding, inadequate maintenance can lead to reduced efficiency, increased emissions, and eventual system failure. Therefore, securing ongoing operational financing is as crucial as the initial capital investment (Rissman et al., 2020). Table 8.1 presents the cost distribution for a typical landfill gas energy generation project.

Table 8.1 The cost distribution of a typical landfill Gas-to-Energy production project

Cost component	Approximate share (%)
Wellfield installation	25
Gas collection pipelines	15
Gas treatment/upgrading	30
Electrical/gas conversion	20
Monitoring & automation	10

8.6 Strategies for Commercialization

The commercialization of landfill gas (LFG) recovery projects is a complex process involving the navigation of financial, regulatory, and technological challenges. While the environmental and energy benefits are widely acknowledged, establishing landfill gas as a sustainable business model requires a holistic commercialization approach that aligns with government incentives, financing structures, and public–private partnerships (Casady et al., 2024; Rissman et al., 2020; UnFCCC, 2025). This chapter examines the principal instruments and institutional frameworks that facilitate implementing landfill gas-to-energy (LFGTE) systems effectively.

8.6.1 Carbon Credit Financing Under UNFCCC Protocols

Carbon credit systems, which leverage reductions in greenhouse gas emissions, represent a highly effective financing mechanism for landfill gas projects (UnFCCC, 2025). Landfill gas (LFG) projects may qualify for the following under the United Nations Framework Convention on Climate Change (UNFCCC):

- Certified Emission Reductions (CERs) according to the Clean Development Mechanism (CDM)
- Verified Emission Reductions (VERs) in voluntary carbon markets
- Article 6 carbon trading under the Paris Agreement (post-2020 mechanisms)

These credits can be traded to corporations or governments seeking to offset their carbon emissions on international markets.

Over ten years, a 5 MW landfill gas-to-energy (LFGTE) project in Brazil generated approximately 1.2 million Certified Emission Reductions (CERs), yielding an additional $9 million in carbon financing (UNEP, 2021).

To participate in these schemes, project developers are required to demonstrate measurable, reportable, and verifiable (MRV) emissions reductions, which demands rigorous documentation and independent third-party verification (Tanveer et al., 2024).

8.6.2 Public–Private Partnerships for LFGTE Projects

Public–Private Partnerships (PPPs) have emerged as a successful institutional model for developing LFGTE infrastructure, particularly in municipalities facing constraints in technical capacity or upfront capital (Ramolobe et al., 2024). In a typical PPP arrangement:

- Public entities, including local governments or waste management authorities, play a key role in providing land access, regulatory support, and oversight of waste streams.
- Private partners contribute capital for infrastructure development, manage operational activities, and bear financial risks in exchange for revenues generated from energy sales, carbon credits, or tipping fees.

PPP models can take various forms:

- Build-Operate-Transfer (BOT)
- Design-Build-Finance-Operate (DBFO)
- Concession agreements (Municipal Public–Private Partnership Framework, 2019).

By leveraging the strengths of both sectors, such partnerships ensure that initiatives are grounded in technical soundness, supported by sustainable financing, and backed by political commitment.

A notable example is the Nairobi LFG project in Kenya, which was developed through a public–private partnership framework and received support from the World Bank's Carbon Initiative for Development (Ci-Dev), covering 40% of the initial investment via carbon financing (World Bank, 2025a).

8.6.3 Policy Incentives and Regulatory Support

The success of LFGTE projects in achieving commercial viability is primarily shaped by the prevailing policy environment (Yilmaz et al., 2021). Key instruments include:

8.6.3.1 Renewable Portfolio Standards (RPS)

Many countries and regions mandate that utilities obtain some of their electricity from renewable energy sources. Including landfill gas within the eligible renewable energy mix allows LFG projects to engage in compliance markets and generate Renewable Energy Certificates (RECs) (Financing Landfill Gas Projects in Developing Countries, 2016).

8.6.3.2 Feed-In Tariffs (FiTs) and Net Metering

Feed-in Tariffs (FiTs) offer guaranteed above-market rates for electricity generated from landfill gas (LFG), ensuring a stable and predictable revenue stream over the long term. Meanwhile, net metering regulations allow on-site LFG generators to offset their energy costs by feeding excess electricity into the grid (Rezaeimozafar et al., 2022).

8.6.3.3 Tax Incentives and Grants

Some countries offer financial incentives such as tax credits, capital subsidies, or accelerated depreciation schemes, like the Modified Accelerated Cost Recovery System (MACRS) in the United States, for renewable energy investments. These measures lower the capital cost burden and improve the project's internal rate of return (IRR) (Berrydunn, 2025).

8.6.3.4 Green Gas Mandates

In developed markets, regulatory frameworks mandate the inclusion of renewable gases, such as biomethane, into existing natural gas distribution networks. This creates a niche market for refined biomethane from landfill gas and encourages private sector investment in upgrading technologies (Hoo et al., 2018).

8.6.4 Capacity Building and Institutional Support

The ability to scale LFGTE initiatives depends heavily on the readiness of institutional frameworks. To support this, national and regional authorities should:

- Develop clear permitting procedures
- Standardize protocols for environmental impact assessment (EIA)
- Train local engineers, technicians, and regulators
- Establish platforms for stakeholder engagement and knowledge exchange

8.6.5 Business Model Innovation and Risk Mitigation

Novel business models are helping to address persistent barriers to the practical commercialization of landfill gas (LFG). These include:

- **Energy-as-a-Service (EaaS):** The facility is developed and operated by private enterprises, with consumers billed based on the amount of electricity consumed, measured in kilowatt-hours.
- **Community-based biogas cooperatives:** Revenue-sharing mechanisms involve local stakeholders and help to build community support.
- **Blended finance mechanisms:** Combine public funding with concessional loans or guarantees to reduce the financial risks private sector participants face (Haessler et al., 2023; Vatankhah et al., 2023).

Additionally, tools for mitigating risk, such as political risk insurance, partial credit guarantees, and performance-based incentives, can significantly enhance the

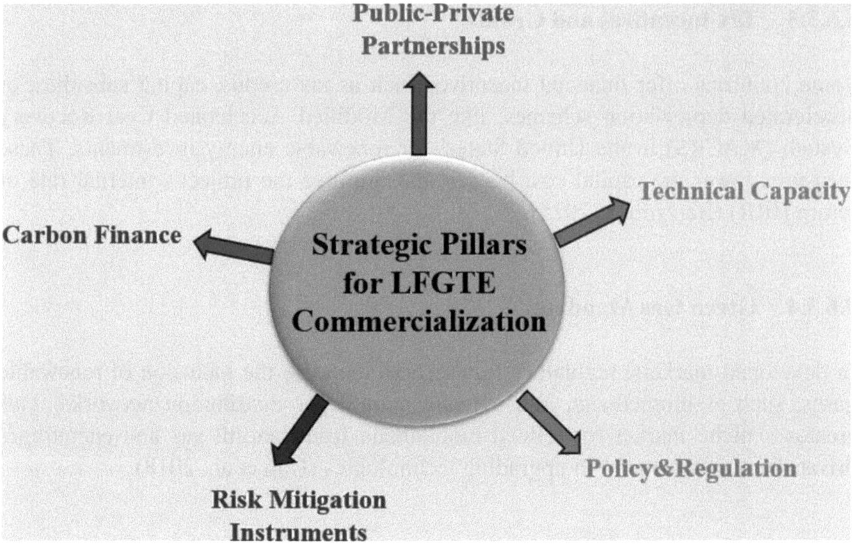

Fig. 8.3 Strategic Pillars for LFGTE Commercialization

bankability of projects. The key strategic components supporting the commercialization of LFGTE are depicted in Fig. 8.3.

8.7 Case Studies

Case studies serve as vital resources for understanding the practical challenges, outcomes, and impacts of landfill gas-to-energy (LFGTE) projects. This chapter highlights two prominent examples: the Puente Hills Landfill in the United States and the Teesside Gas-to-Grid Facility in the United Kingdom, each illustrating distinct approaches to landfill gas capture, energy conversion, and market integration.

8.7.1 Puente Hills Landfill (California, USA)

Project Overview

Located in Los Angeles County, the Puente Hills Landfill was the largest in the United States until its closure in 2013. At its peak, it received as much as 13,000 tons of municipal solid waste per day. Recognizing the site's substantial methane generation potential, the Los Angeles County Sanitation District (LACSD) developed one of the world's largest landfill gas recovery systems (LACSD, 2021).

Key Features

- **Installed capacity**: 50 MW of electricity produced by reciprocating internal combustion engines.
- **Gas collection**: More than 300 vertical and horizontal wells linked via a suction system.
- **Purification**: Fundamental filtration and desiccation for immediate application in combustion engines.
- **Energy use**: Electricity is fed directly into the Southern California Edison grid.

Environmental and Economic Impact

- Decreases by over 2.5 million metric tons of CO_2-equivalent each year.
- Supplies renewable electricity to approximately 70,000 residences.
- Produced carbon credits through the U.S. EPA Landfill Methane Outreach Program (LMOP) and aided in compliance with California's Renewable Portfolio Standard (RPS).

The Puente Hills LFGTE project received national recognition from the U.S. Department of Energy for its pioneering methods in waste-to-energy conversion.

8.7.2 *Teesside Gas-To-Grid Facility (United Kingdom)*

Project Overview

Located in northeast England, the Teesside Gas-to-Grid Facility represents a modern approach to producing biomethane from landfill gas for injection into the national gas grid. The project is operated by CoGen UK in collaboration with Northern Gas Networks (NZT, 2025).

Key Features

- **Upgraded gas volume**: Up to 3,000 Nm^3/hour of raw LFG processed.
- **Technology**: Employs membrane separation and activated carbon filtering to achieve over 97% methane purity.
- **Grid injection**: Compressed and odorized gas is introduced into the United Kingdom's low-pressure gas distribution system.
- **Real-time monitoring**: IoT-based instrumentation controls gas quality, pressure, and flow.

Environmental and Economic Impact

- Displaces ~ 25 GWh/year of fossil natural gas.
- Reduces methane emissions by over 10,000 tons CO_2-eq/year.
- Certified under the UK's Renewable Heat Incentive (RHI), offering long-term financial returns.

Innovative Aspects

- The inaugural landfill site in the UK to attain complete biomethane injection under the Green Gas Certification Scheme (GGCS).
- Connected with adjacent district heating systems, enhancing its socio-environmental advantages.

Teesside serves as a model for other EU member states seeking to decarbonize their gas networks through the adoption of renewable alternatives.

8.7.3 Lessons Learned from Global LFGTE Projects

While the cases described above represent highly successful projects, the worldwide implementation of LFGTE has revealed several recurring lessons, which are summarized in Table 8.2.

8.8 Future Directions

The advancement of landfill gas-to-energy (LFGTE) systems increasingly relies on their integration within broader frameworks encompassing climate action, energy policy, and the circular economy. As global efforts to decarbonize accelerate, landfill-derived biogas will evolve from a niche waste management solution into a critical element of renewable energy strategies and sustainable low-carbon infrastructure. This chapter explores emerging trends, innovative technologies, and strategic methodologies poised to define the next generation of LFGTE projects.

Table 8.2 Lessons emerging from the global implementation of the LFGTE

Aspect	Key insight
Policy support	Stable policy incentives, such as Renewable Portfolio Standards (RPS), Feed-in Tariffs (FiTs), and Renewable Heat Incentives (RHI), play a crucial role in reducing investment risks
Technology selection	The specific gas composition at each site should guide the selection of upgrading and energy generation technologies
Stakeholder engagement	Engaging community members and utility stakeholders at an early stage increases the chances of securing project approval
Revenue diversification	Combining revenue streams from energy sales, carbon credits, and tipping fees strengthens the overall financial resilience of the project

8.8.1 AI-Driven Predictive Modeling for Gas Yield Optimization

One major challenge in developing landfill gas-to-energy (LFGTE) systems is the fluctuation in gas production rates, which affects system design, financial forecasting, and operational management. To improve the precision of gas yield predictions, artificial intelligence (AI) and machine learning (ML) techniques are increasingly employed, leveraging both real-time and historical datasets for analysis (Praveen Kumar Kaluvakuri and Phanindra Peta, 2023).

Key AI applications include:

- **Time-series modelling** of methane output based on landfill age, waste composition, temperature, and moisture.
- **Optimization algorithms** for gas well placement and extraction pressures.
- **Anomaly detection** is used to identify equipment malfunctions or gas migration early (Behera et al., 2015; Fallah et al., 2020).

According to recent findings by Joyce et al. (2023), a deep neural network demonstrated high effectiveness in plume identification, attaining F1 scores, precision, and recall values of 0.95, 0.96, and 0.92, respectively. Additionally, the model estimated emission rates with a mean error of 24% (Joyce et al., 2023). These approaches reduce operational uncertainties and promote more effective resource allocation, thereby improving projects' financial viability.

8.8.2 Integration with Hydrogen Production via Methane Reforming

As global interest in the hydrogen economy intensifies, methane produced from landfill gas (LFG) emerges as a practical feedstock for the generation of low-carbon hydrogen via steam methane reforming (SMR) or autothermal reforming (ATR) (Alaidaros & AlZahrani, 2025; Mohd Yunus et al., 2024).

Advantages of this approach include:

- Utilizing biogenic methane contributes to a lower carbon footprint than hydrogen produced from natural gas.
- Deployment of on-site reforming technologies at large-scale landfill sites enables the development of decentralized hydrogen production hubs.

Simultaneous capture of CO_2 during the reforming process for utilization in industrial applications or for sequestration purposes (Alaidaros & AlZahrani, 2025; Mohd Yunus et al., 2024).

Landfill gas-to-hydrogen systems must incorporate carbon capture and storage (CCS) or carbon capture and utilization (CCU) technologies to ensure environmental benefits. Pilot projects in Japan and South Korea are assessing biogas-fuelled hydrogen fuel cell vchicles as part of strategies to decarbonize municipal transportation fleets (IFRI, 2018).

8.8.3 Coupling with Carbon Capture and Utilization (CCU)

Beyond energy conversion, landfill gas-to-energy (LFGTE) systems can be enhanced by integrating carbon capture and utilization technologies, allowing the conversion of CO_2 captured during biogas upgrading into (Abdelshafy & Walther, 2022; Halim, 2023):

- **Synthetic fuels** (e.g., methanol, dimethyl ether)
- **Building materials** (e.g., carbon-infused concrete)
- **Agricultural products** (e.g., algal biomass in CO_2-enriched photobioreactors) (Abdelshafy & Walther, 2022; Halim, 2023).

When combined with sustainably sourced biomass, this integration enables pathways to achieve harmful emissions, aligning with the net-zero targets set by many governments and corporations (Abdelshafy & Walther, 2022; Halim, 2023).

8.8.4 Circular Economy Synergies

Within the circular economy framework, future landfill gas-to-energy (LFGTE) projects are expected to operate as part of multi-resource recovery platforms, which include:

- **Organic waste digestion**
- **Nutrient recycling** (e.g., recovery of nitrogen and phosphorus from digestate)
- **Heat and power cogeneration**
- **Biochar production** using landfill cover material or post-digestion residues (Huang, 2024; Wang et al., 2021).

Such integrated facilities reduce environmental impacts, produce value-added products, and support regional economic development. For example, the Danish utility company operates Grøngas Vraa, an anaerobic digestion complex processing 300,000 tonnes of organic waste annually to generate biogas (Europeanbiogas, 2025).

8.8.5 Policy and Market Evolution

The transition from pilot projects to large-scale deployment will depend heavily on supportive regulatory frameworks and effective market mechanisms. Future policy trajectories encompass:

- **Renewable gas mandates** for national gas grids
- **Carbon pricing mechanisms** that internalize the environmental cost of methane leakage
- **Green gas certification systems** to ensure traceability and consumer trust
- **Cross-sectoral incentives** for coupling LFGTE with hydrogen, agriculture, or district heating (Reconciling Carbon Pricing and Energy Policies in Developing Countries, 2019; World Bank, 2025b).

Furthermore, international cooperation and climate finance will be vital in promoting the adoption of LFGTE technologies in developing countries.

8.8.6 Research and Development Priorities

Future R&D in landfill biogas recovery should focus on:

- **Advanced membrane materials** for more efficient CH_4/CO_2 separation
- **Biological upgrading** methods (e.g., using methanogenic archaea for direct conversion)
- **Sensor miniaturization** and autonomous monitoring drones for landfill management
- **Decentralized energy storage systems** to pair with intermittent gas flows (Al-Hazmi et al., 2024; Pheakdey et al., 2023).

Investment in these areas will enhance system resilience, reduce costs, and open opportunities for novel applications.

References

Abdelshafy, A., Walther, G., (2022). Coupling carbon capture and utilization with the construction industry: Opportunities in Western Germany. *Journal of CO2 Utilization 57*. https://doi.org/10.1016/j.jcou.2021.101866

Achi, C.G., Snyman, J., Ndambuki, J.M., Kupolati, W.K., (2024). Advanced waste-to-energy technologies: a review on pathway to sustainable energy recovery in a circular economy. *Nature Environment and Pollution Technology*. https://doi.org/10.46488/NEPT.2024.v23i03.002

Alaidaros, A., & AlZahrani, A. A. (2025). Integrated solar system for hydrogen production using steam reforming of methane. *International Journal of Hydrogen Energy, 140*, 1033–1048. https://doi.org/10.1016/j.ijhydene.2024.08.388

Al-Hazmi, H. E., Hassan, G. K., Kurniawan, T. A., Śniatała, B., Joseph, T. M., Majtacz, J., Piechota, G., Li, X., El-Gohary, F. A., Saeb, M. R., & Mąkinia, J. (2024). Technological solutions to landfill management: Towards recovery of biomethane and carbon neutrality. *Journal of Environmental Management, 354*,. https://doi.org/10.1016/j.jenvman.2024.120414

Alli, Y. A., Bamisaye, A., Bamidele, M. O., Etafo, N. O., Chkirida, S., Lawal, A., Hammed, V. O., Akinfenwa, A. S., Hanson, E., Nwakile, C., Kazeem, K. O., Ayanwunmi, R. J., Ige, A. S., Parga Torres, J. R., & Al Nageim, H. (2024). Transforming waste to wealth: Harnessing carbon dioxide for sustainable solutions. *Results in Surfaces and Interfaces, 17*,. https://doi.org/10.1016/j.rsurfi.2024.100321

Amini, H. R., Reinhart, D. R., & Mackie, K. R. (2012). Determination of first-order landfill gas modeling parameters and uncertainties. *Waste Management, 32*, 305–316. https://doi.org/10.1016/j.wasman.2011.09.021

Anvari, S., Medina, A., Merchán, R. P., & Hernández, A. C. (2025). Sustainable solar/biomass/energy storage hybridization for enhanced renewable energy integration in multi-generation systems: A comprehensive review. *Renewable and Sustainable Energy Reviews.* https://doi.org/10.1016/j.rser.2025.115997

Anyaoku, C. C., & Baroutian, S. (2018). Decentralized anaerobic digestion systems for increased utilization of biogas from municipal solid waste. *Renewable and Sustainable Energy Reviews.* https://doi.org/10.1016/j.rser.2018.03.009

Atelge, M. R., Senol, H., Mohammed, D., Hansu, T. A., Krisa, D., Atabani, A., Eskicioglu, C., Muratçobanoğlu, H., Unalan, S., Slimane, K., Azbar, N., & Kıvrak, H. D. (2021). A critical overview of the state-of-the-art methods for biogas purification and utilization processes. *Sustainability (Switzerland).* https://doi.org/10.3390/su132011515

Auelbekov, O., Kozbakova, A., Igibayev, K., Yessentaev, K., (2025). Development of an IoT system for monitoring the operation of a biogas plant. https://doi.org/10.20944/preprints202507.0368.v1

Behera, S. K., Meher, S. K., & Park, H. S. (2015). Artificial neural network model for predicting methane percentage in biogas recovered from a landfill upon injection of liquid organic waste. *Clean Technologies and Environmental Policy, 17*, 443–453. https://doi.org/10.1007/s10098-014-0798-4

Berrydunn, (2025). https://www.berrydunn.com/news-detail/reap-grant-key-benefits-and-tax-implications-for-businesses (Accessed 20 July 2025) [WWW Document].

Calbry-Muzyka, A., Madi, H., Rüsch-Pfund, F., Gandiglio, M., & Biollaz, S. (2022). Biogas composition from agricultural sources and organic fraction of municipal solid waste. *Renewable Energy, 181*, 1000–1007. https://doi.org/10.1016/j.renene.2021.09.100

Casady, C. B., Cepparulo, A., & Giuriato, L. (2024). Public-private partnerships for low-carbon, climate-resilient infrastructure: Insights from the literature. *Journal of Cleaner Production.* https://doi.org/10.1016/j.jclepro.2024.143338

Cevallos-Mendoza, J., Amorim, C.G., Rodríguez-Díaz, J.M., Montenegro, M. da C.B.S.M., (2022). Removal of Contaminants from Water by Membrane Filtration: A Review. Membranes (Basel). https://doi.org/10.3390/membranes12060570.

Chinea, L., Slopiecka, K., Bartocci, P., Alissa Park, A. H., Wang, S., Jiang, D., & Fantozzi, F. (2023). Methane enrichment of biogas using carbon capture materials. *Fuel, 334*,. https://doi.org/10.1016/j.fuel.2022.126428

Chojnacka, K., & Moustakas, K. (2024). Anaerobic digestate management for carbon neutrality and fertilizer use: A review of current practices and future opportunities. *Biomass and Bioenergy, 180*,. https://doi.org/10.1016/j.biombioe.2023.106991

Ellacuriaga, M., González, R., & Gómez, X. (2022). Is Decentralized Anaerobic Digestion a Solution? Analyzing Biogas Production and Residential Energy Demand. *Eng, 3*, 662–676. https://doi.org/10.3390/eng3040045

Elroi, H., Zbigniew, G., Agnieszka, W. C., & Piotr, S. (2023). Enhancing waste resource efficiency: Circular economy for sustainability and energy conversion. *Frontiers in Environmental Science, 11*,. https://doi.org/10.3389/fenvs.2023.1303792

EPA, (2025a). https://www.epa.gov/land-research/quantifying-methane-emissions-landfilled-food-waste (Accessed 20 July 2025) [WWW Document].

EPA, (2025b). www.epa.gov (Best Practices for Landfill Gas Collection System Design and Installation) (Accessed 20 July 2025) [WWW Document].

EPA, (2025c). https://www.epa.gov/lmop/basic-information-about-landfill-gas (Accessed 20 July 2025) [WWW Document].

Europeanbiogas, (2025). https://www.europeanbiogas.eu/denmark-new-300000-tpy-anaerobic-digestion-facility-opened/) (Accessed 20 July 2025) [WWW Document].

Falcone, P. M. (2023). Sustainable energy policies in developing countries: a review of challenges and opportunities. *Energies (Basel)*. https://doi.org/10.3390/en16186682

Fallah, B., Ng, K. T. W., Vu, H. L., & Torabi, F. (2020). Application of a multi-stage neural network approach for time-series landfill gas modeling with missing data imputation. *Waste Management, 116*, 66–78. https://doi.org/10.1016/j.wasman.2020.07.034

Financing Landfill Gas Projects in Developing Countries, n.d.

Frontistis, Z., Lykogiannis, G., & Sarmpanis, A. (2023). Machine learning implementation in membrane bioreactor systems: progress, challenges, and future perspectives: a review. *Environments—MDPI*. https://doi.org/10.3390/environments10070127

Gao, T., Selinger, J. L., & Rochelle, G. T. (2019). Demonstration of 99% CO2 removal from coal flue gas by amine scrubbing. *International Journal of Greenhouse Gas Control, 83*, 236–244. https://doi.org/10.1016/j.ijggc.2019.02.013

Gaur, A., Park, J. W., Maken, S., Song, H. J., & Park, J. J. (2010). Landfill gas (LFG) processing via adsorption and alkanolamine absorption. *Fuel Processing Technology, 91*, 635–640. https://doi.org/10.1016/j.fuproc.2010.01.010

Ghosh, A., Kumar, S., & Das, J. (2023). Impact of leachate and landfill gas on the ecosystem and health: Research trends and the way forward towards sustainability. *Journal of Environmental Management, 336*,. https://doi.org/10.1016/j.jenvman.2023.117708

Haessler, P., Giones, F., & Brem, A. (2023). The who and how of commercializing emerging technologies: A technology-focused review. *Technovation*. https://doi.org/10.1016/j.technovation.2022.102637

Halim, I. (2023). Coupling biogas upgrading and carbon capture and utilization for enhanced environmental performance of water reclamation plants. *Journal of Environmental Chemical Engineering, 11*,. https://doi.org/10.1016/j.jece.2023.110198

Hoo, P. Y., Hashim, H., & Ho, W. S. (2018). Opportunities and challenges: Landfill gas to biomethane injection into natural gas distribution grid through pipeline. *Journal of Cleaner Production, 175*, 409–419. https://doi.org/10.1016/j.jclepro.2017.11.193

Huang, X. (2024). The promotion of anaerobic digestion technology upgrades in waste stream treatment plants for circular economy in the context of "dual carbon": global status, development trend, and future challenges. *Water (Switzerland)*. https://doi.org/10.3390/w16243718

Hussain, Z., Mishra, J., & Vanacore, E. (2020). Waste to energy and circular economy: The case of anaerobic digestion. *Journal of Enterprise Information Management, 33*, 817–838. https://doi.org/10.1108/JEIM-02-2019-0049

IEA, 2025. https://energy.ec.europa.eu/topics/carbon-management-and-fossil-fuels/methane-emissions_en#:~:text=In%20fact%2C%20methane's%20ability%20to,on%20a%2020%2Dyear%20timescale. (Accessed 20 July 2025) [WWW Document].

IEA. (2021). International Energy Agency (IEA). (2021). Outlook for Biogas and Biomethane: Prospects for Organic Growth. (Accessed 20 July 2025) [WWW Document].

IFRI. (2018). https://www.ifri.org/sites/default/files/migrated_files/documents/atoms/files/nagashima_japan_hydrogen_2018_3.pdf (Accessed 20 July 2025) [WWW Document].

IPCC. (2021). Climate change 2021: the physical science basis. intergovernmental panel on climate change. (Access date: 15.07.2025) [WWW Document].

Igwegbe, C. A., López-Maldonado, E. A., Landázuri, A. C., Ovuoraye, P. E., Ogbu, A. I., Vela-García, N., & Białowiec, A. (2024). Sustainable municipal landfill leachate management:

Current practices, challenges, and future directions. *Desalination Water Treat*. https://doi.org/10.1016/j.dwt.2024.100709
Jameel, M.K., Mustafa, M.A., Ahmed, H.S., Mohammed, A. jassim, Ghazy, H., Shakir, M.N., Lawas, A.M., Mohammed, S. khudhur, Idan, A.H., Mahmoud, Z.H., Sayadi, H., Kianfar, E. (2024). Biogas: Production, properties, applications, economic and challenges: A review. *Results Chem*. https://doi.org/10.1016/j.rechem.2024.101549
Joyce, P., Ruiz Villena, C., Huang, Y., Webb, A., Gloor, M., Wagner, F. H., Chipperfield, M. P., Barrio Guilló, R., Wilson, C., & Boesch, H. (2023). Using a deep neural network to detect methane point sources and quantify emissions from PRISMA hyperspectral satellite images. *Atmos Meas Tech, 16*, 2627–2640. https://doi.org/10.5194/amt-16-2627-2023
Junus, M., Putradi, D.F., Soelistianto, F.A., Anshori, M.A., Ardiansyah, R., (2025). Internet of things enabled landfill pollution gas monitoring. *Indonesian Journal of Electrical Engineering and Computer Science 37*, 48–55. https://doi.org/10.11591/ijeecs.v37.i1.pp48-55.
Kurniawan, T. A., Hassan, G. K., Al-Hazmi, H. E., Othman, M. H. D., Goh, H. H., Aziz, F., Anouzla, A., Ali, I., Khan, M. I., Khan, M. M. H., & Mąkinia, J. (2024). Landfill mining: A step forward to reducing CH4 emissions and enhancing CO2 sequestration from landfill. *Journal of Hazardous Materials Advances, 100512*,. https://doi.org/10.1016/j.hazadv.2024.100512
Kurniawan, T. A., Liang, X., Singh, D., Othman, M. H. D., Goh, H. H., Gikas, P., Kern, A. O., Kusworo, T. D., & Shoqeir, J. A. (2022). Harnessing landfill gas (LFG) for electricity: A strategy to mitigate greenhouse gas (GHG) emissions in Jakarta (Indonesia). *Journal of Environmental Management, 301*,. https://doi.org/10.1016/j.jenvman.2021.113882
LACSD. (2021). Puente hills landfill gas-to-energy project report. *Los Angeles County Sanitation Districts*. (Accessed 20 July 2025) [WWW Document].
Lim, J. H., Cha, J. S., Kong, B. J., & Baek, S. H. (2018). Characterization of odorous gases at landfill site and in surrounding areas. *Journal of Environmental Management, 206*, 291–303. https://doi.org/10.1016/j.jenvman.2017.10.045
López-Aguilar, H. A., Kennedy Puentes, G., Lozoya Márquez, L. A., Chávez Acosta, O., Monreal Romero, H. A., López Meléndez, C., & Pérez-Hernández, A. (2025). Evaluation of energy potential in a landfill through the integration of a biogas-solar photovoltaic system. *Urban Science, 9*,. https://doi.org/10.3390/urbansci9010017
Mergenthal, M., Tawai, A., Amornraksa, S., Roddecha, S., Chuetor, S., 2023. Methane enrichment for biogas purification using pressure swing adsorption techniques, in: Materials Today: Proceedings. Elsevier Ltd, pp. 2915–2920. https://doi.org/10.1016/j.matpr.2022.08.003
Mohd Yunus, S., Yusup, S., Johari, S. S., Mohd Afandi, N., Manap, A., & Mohamed, H. (2024). Comparative Hydrogen Production Routes via Steam Methane Reforming and Chemical Looping Reforming of Natural Gas as Feedstock. *Hydrogen (Switzerland), 5*, 761–775. https://doi.org/10.3390/hydrogen5040040
Municipal Public-Private Partnership Framework, 2019.
Nassereddine, M., Nassreddine, G., & El Arid, A. (2024). Hybrid photovoltaic and biogas system for stable power system. *Next Energy, 5*,. https://doi.org/10.1016/j.nxener.2024.100172
Nec, Y., & Huculak, G. (2019). Landfill gas flow: collection by horizontal wells. *Transport in Porous Media, 130*, 769–797. https://doi.org/10.1007/s11242-019-01338-3
NZT. (2025). https://www.netzeroteesside.co.uk/project/ (Accessed 20 July 2025) [WWW Document].
Olczak, M., Piebalgs, A., & Balcombe, P. (2023). A global review of methane policies reveals that only 13% of emissions are covered with unclear effectiveness. *One Earth*. https://doi.org/10.1016/j.oneear.2023.04.009
Olodu, D.D., Erameh, A. (2023). Waste to energy: review on the development of land fill gas for power generation in Sub-Saharan Africa. *Black Sea Journal of Engineering and Science 6*, 296–307. https://doi.org/10.34248/bsengineering.1195247.
Oonk, H. (2012). Efficiency of landfill gas collection for methane emission reduction. *Greenhouse Gas Measurement and Management, 2*, 129–145. https://doi.org/10.1080/20430779.2012.730798

Pasichnyk, M., Stanovsky, P., Polezhaev, P., Zach, B., Šyc, M., Bobák, M., Jansen, J. C., Přibyl, M., Bara, J. E., Friess, K., Havlica, J., Gin, D. L., Noble, R. D., & Izák, P. (2023). Membrane technology for challenging separations: Removal of CO2, SO2 and NOx from flue and waste gases. *Separation and Purification Technology*. https://doi.org/10.1016/j.seppur.2023.124436
Pavičić, J., Mavar, K. N., Brkić, V., & Simon, K. (2022). Biogas and biomethane production and usage: technology development. *Advantages and Challenges in Europe. Energies (Basel)*. https://doi.org/10.3390/en15082940
Peppers, J., Li, Y., Xue, J., Chen, X., Alaimo, C., Wong, L., Young, T., Green, P. G., Jenkins, B., Zhang, R., & Kleeman, M. J. (2019). Performance analysis of membrane separation for upgrading biogas to biomethane at small scale production sites. *Biomass and Bioenergy, 128,*. https://doi.org/10.1016/j.biombioe.2019.105314
Pheakdey, D. V., Noudeng, V., & Xuan, T. D. (2023). Landfill biogas recovery and its contribution to greenhouse gas mitigation. *Energies (Basel), 16,*. https://doi.org/10.3390/en16124689
Polat, C., Eren, T. (2021). Dik ve Yatay Kuyuların Tight Gaz Kondensat Rezervuarında Kuru Gaz Enjeksiyonlu ve Enjeksiyonsuz Üretim Performanslarının Karşılaştırılması. *Deu Muhendislik Fakultesi Fen ve Muhendislik 23*, 339–348. https://doi.org/10.21205/deufmd.2021236730
Praveen Kumar Kaluvakuri, V., Phanindra Peta, V. (2023). The *Impact of AI and Cloud on Fleet Management and Financial Planning: A Comparative Analysis.*
Qyyum, M. A., Haider, J., Qadeer, K., Valentina, V., Khan, A., Yasin, M., Aslam, M., De Guido, G., Pellegrini, L. A., & Lee, M. (2020). Biogas to liquefied biomethane: Assessment of 3P's–Production, processing, and prospects. *Renewable and Sustainable Energy Reviews*. https://doi.org/10.1016/j.rser.2019.109561
Ramolobe, K. S., Khandanisa, U., & Ramolobe, K. (2024). *Africa's Public Service Delivery and Performance Review.* https://doi.org/10.4102/apsdpr
Reconciling carbon pricing and energy policies in developing countries, n.d.
Rezaeimozafar, M., Monaghan, R. F. D., Barrett, E., & Duffy, M. (2022). A review of behind-the-meter energy storage systems in smart grids. *Renewable and Sustainable Energy Reviews*. https://doi.org/10.1016/j.rser.2022.112573
Rissman, J., Bataille, C., Masanet, E., Aden, N., Morrow, W.R., Zhou, N., Elliott, N., Dell, R., Heeren, N., Huckestein, B., Cresko, J., Miller, S.A., Roy, J., Fennell, P., Cremmins, B., Koch Blank, T., Hone, D., Williams, E.D., de la Rue du Can, S., Sisson, B., Williams, M., Katzenberger, J., Burtraw, D., Sethi, G., Ping, H., Danielson, D., Lu, H., Lorber, T., Dinkel, J., Helseth, J. (2020). Technologies and policies to decarbonize global industry: Review and assessment of mitigation drivers through 2070. *Appl Energy*. https://doi.org/10.1016/j.apenergy.2020.114848
Rochelle, G. T. (2024). Air pollution impacts of amine scrubbing for CO2 capture. *Carbon Capture Science and Technology, 11,*. https://doi.org/10.1016/j.ccst.2024.100192
Rodero, M. del R., Muñoz, R., González-Sánchez, A., Ruiz, H.A., Quijano, G., 2024. Membrane materials for biogas purification and upgrading: Fundamentals, recent advances and challenges. *J Environ Chem Eng*. https://doi.org/10.1016/j.jece.2024.114106
Rudd, M. A., Jones, M., Sechrest, D., Batten, D., & Porter, D. (2024). An integrated landfill gas-to-energy and Bitcoin mining framework. *Journal of Cleaner Production, 472,*. https://doi.org/10.1016/j.jclepro.2024.143516
Saral, A., Demir, S., & Yildiz, Ş. (2009). Assessment of odorous VOCs released from a main MSW landfill site in Istanbul-Turkey via a modelling approach. *Journal of Hazardous Materials, 168*, 338–345. https://doi.org/10.1016/j.jhazmat.2009.02.043
Shaban, A., Zaki, F. E., Afefy, I. H., Di Gravio, G., Falegnami, A., & Patriarca, R. (2022). An optimization model for the design of a sustainable municipal solid waste management system. *Sustainability (Switzerland), 14,*. https://doi.org/10.3390/su14106345
Shang, S., Gu, L., Zhan, L., Qiu, H., & Lu, H. (2021). Application of horizontal well to gas production from a hydrate reservoir with free gas and high irreducible water. *J Nat Gas Sci Eng, 94,*. https://doi.org/10.1016/j.jngse.2021.104102
Sui, D. (2025). Real-Time drilling performance optimization using automated penetration rate algorithms with vibration control. *Fuels, 6*, 33. https://doi.org/10.3390/fuels6020033

Swinbourn, R., Li, C., & Wang, F. (2024). A comprehensive review on biomethane production from biogas separation and its techno-economic assessments. *Chemsuschem*. https://doi.org/10.1002/cssc.202400779

Tanveer, U., Ishaq, S., & Hoang, T. G. (2024). Enhancing carbon trading mechanisms through innovative collaboration: Case studies from developing nations. *Journal of Cleaner Production, 482*,. https://doi.org/10.1016/j.jclepro.2024.144122

Terraza, H., Willumsen, H., n.d. Guidance Note on Landfill Gas Capture and Utilization.

Un, C. (2023). A sustainable approach to the conversion of waste into energy: landfill gas-to-fuel technology. *Sustainability, 15*, 14782. https://doi.org/10.3390/su152014782

Unctad. (2023). World Investment Report 2023: Investment and sustainable energy.

UNEP. (2022). Emissions Gap Report 2022: The Closing Window—Climate crisis calls for rapid transformation of societies. *United Nations Environment Programme*. (Access Date:18.07.2025) [WWW Document].

UNEP. (2021). Carbon finance for landfill gas projects: lessons from CDM and voluntary markets. *United Nations Environment Programme*. (Accessed 20 July 2025) [WWW Document].

UNFCCC. (2025). https://unfccc.int/process-and-meetings/the-paris-agreement/article-64-mechanism (Accessed 20 July 2025) [WWW Document].

USEPA. (2022). U.S. Environmental Protection Agency (USEPA). (2022). Landfill methane outreach program: financial considerations for LFG projects. (Accessed 20 July 2025) [WWW Document].

Vatankhah, S., Bamshad, V., Altinay, L., & De Vita, G. (2023). Understanding business model development through the lens of complexity theory: Enablers and barriers. *Journal of Business Research, 155*,. https://doi.org/10.1016/j.jbusres.2022.113350

Wang, J., Okopi, S. I., Ma, H., Wang, M., Chen, R., Tian, W., & Xu, F. (2021). Life cycle assessment of the integration of anaerobic digestion and pyrolysis for treatment of municipal solid waste. *Bioresource Technology, 338*,. https://doi.org/10.1016/j.biortech.2021.125486

Wang, J., & Qiao, Z. (2024). A comprehensive review of landfill leachate treatment technologies. *Frontiers in Environmental Science*. https://doi.org/10.3389/fenvs.2024.1439128

Worldbank. (2025a). https://www.worldbank.org/en/topic/climatechange/publication/projects-reducing-emissions-earning-carbon-credits-africa (Accessed 20 July 2025) [WWW Document].

Worldbank. (2025b). https://documents1.worldbank.org/curated/en/433401585299859071/pdf/Reconciling-Carbon-Pricing-and-Energy-Policies-in-Developing-Countries-Integrating-Policies-for-a-Clean-Energy-Transition.pdf) (Accessed 20 July 2025) [WWW Document].

Yilmaz, M., Tinjum, J. M., Acker, C., & Marten, B. (2021). Transport mechanisms and emission of landfill gas through various cover soil configurations in an MSW landfill using a static flux chamber technique. *Journal of Environmental Management, 280*,. https://doi.org/10.1016/j.jenvman.2020.111677

Zhang, W., Ma, F., Ren, M., & Yang, F. (2021). Application with Internet of things technology in the municipal industrial wastewater treatment based on membrane bioreactor process. *Applied Water Science, 11*,. https://doi.org/10.1007/s13201-021-01375-8

Zheng, Q. T., Rowe, R. K., & Feng, S. J. (2018). Design of vertical landfill gas collection wells considering non-homogeneity with depth. *Waste Management, 82*, 26–36. https://doi.org/10.1016/j.wasman.2018.10.012

Chapter 9
Hydrothermal Liquefaction: An Overview of Hydrothermal Liquefaction (HTL) Technology, Processes and Potential Biofuel Products, Current Research and Future Directions

Tarek O. Said, Halil Şenol, Mohamed A. Hassaan, Emre Çolak, and Ahmed El Nemr

Abstract Hydrothermal liquefaction (HTL) enables the conversion of wet biomass into biocrude by applying high temperatures and pressures, effectively removing the necessity for energy-intensive drying steps. This chapter evaluates HTL's ability to produce biofuels like syngas, biocrude, and biochar from various feedstocks, including food waste, sewage sludge (SS), and algae. The impacts on yield and quality of three key process variables are examined: residence time, temperature (250–400°C), and catalysts (such as alkali metals). Recent innovations, including continuous-flow reactors and catalytic HTL, are discussed along with problems like reactor corrosion and nutrient recovery. While there are financial obstacles, such as high capital costs, there are also environmental advantages, such as lower carbon footprints than with pyrolysis. New applications in wastewater treatment and aviation fuel production demonstrate HTL's versatility. Research shows that HTL holds significant promise as an alternative method for processing high-moisture biomass within the energy sector. Besides the biocrude yield, operating conditions also influence the initial selection of both biomass feedstock and catalysts. When conditions are satisfied, co-processing biocrude alongside conventional crude oil allows for

T. O. Said · M. A. Hassaan · A. El Nemr (✉)
National Institute of Oceanography and Fisheries (NIOF), Kayet Bey, Elanfoushy, Alexandria, Egypt
e-mail: ahmedmoustafaelnemr@yahoo.com; ahmed.m.elnemr@gmail.com

M. A. Hassaan
e-mail: mhss95@mail.com

H. Şenol
Faculty of Engineering, Department of Energy Systems Engineering, Giresun University, Giresun, Türkiye

E. Çolak
Institute of Science, Department of Energy Systems Engineering, Giresun University, MSc Program, Giresun, Türkiye

P. Verma (ed.), *Sustainable Practices in Biorefinery*,
https://doi.org/10.1007/978-981-95-6071-4_9

using existing refinery infrastructure, thereby circumventing the need for significant capital investment in new biorefinery facilities. The chapter discusses future prospects, including integrating HTL with carbon capture technologies and applying AI-driven process optimization.

Keywords Hydrothermal liquefaction (HTL) · Biocrude · Syngas · Biochar · Biomass-feedstock

9.1 Introduction

The conversion of biomass into biofuels has attracted growing interest as an effective strategy to address climate change. Hydrothermal liquefaction (HTL) is particularly relevant among biomass conversion technologies because it can process feedstocks with high moisture content without requiring prior drying, unlike other methods such as pyrolysis. The process produces crude oil characterized by lower density, reduced heteroatom content, and enhanced energy density (Ocampo et al., 2023). HTL functions under relatively moderate conditions, generally at pressures of 100 to 200 bar and temperatures between 200 and 400 °C, significantly less severe than those used in alternative biomass conversion methods such as gasification and methanation. This section reviews the current state of research on HTL, employing bibliometric analysis and scientific metrics to highlight the field's development, emerging trends, and increasing global collaboration.

9.1.1 HTL versus Pyrolysis and Gasification: Advantages for Wet Feedstocks

At elevated temperatures exceeding the saturation pressure of water, HTL converts biomass into biocrude by thermochemically breaking down its solid structure through mechanisms such as depolymerization, bond cleavage, molecular rearrangement, and decarboxylation (Mahssin et al., 2021). Numerous studies have demonstrated the application of HTL to produce biocrude from a wide range of biomass sources, including microalgae (Miranda et al., 2022), terrestrial plants (Osorio, 2019), and fruit residues like grapefruit peels (Osorio, 2019; Wei et al., 2022). The transition to a low-carbon economy hinges on advancing technologies that harness biomass energy, with emerging biorefineries—utilizing thermochemical processes such as HTL—playing a pivotal role in converting biomass into valuable energy carriers. This study provides a comprehensive review of hydrothermal processing (HTP) of biomass, highlighting HTL as a sustainable method for converting moisture-rich and compositionally diverse feedstocks—including microalgae, lignocellulosic residues, and municipal solid waste—into biofuels and value-added bioproducts

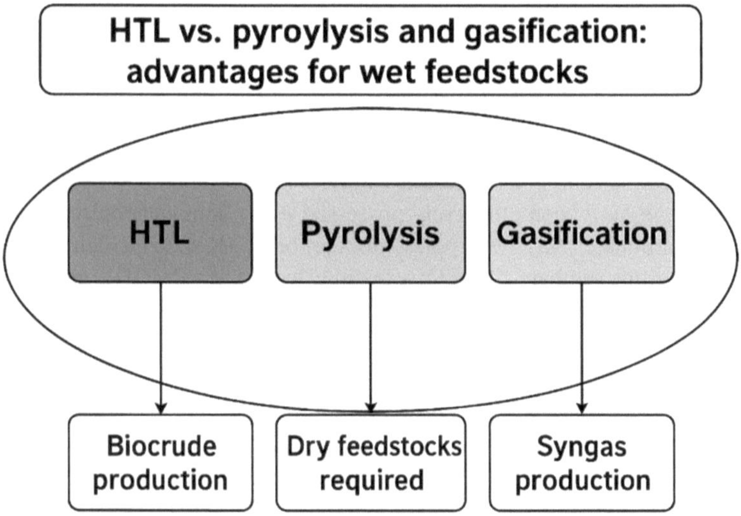

Fig. 9.1 Comparison of biomass conversion technologies: HTL, pyrolysis, and gasification in terms of feedstock moisture tolerance and processing conditions

(Rojas et al., 2025). It critically assesses recent progress in reactor design, kinetic and phenomenological modelling, and the adaptability of various feedstocks suitable for hydrothermal methods, such as sludge, food waste, and organic solid waste. Moreover, the work elucidates the structural transformations induced by the underlying chemical reactions and, to our knowledge, proposes the first models simulating transport phenomena within HTL systems. The analysis identifies key research gaps, highlights challenges in process understanding, and outlines future directions for investigation. By integrating theoretical and experimental approaches, this roadmap aims to accelerate the transition towards a circular bioeconomy and support the development of next-generation biorefineries. Among thermochemical biomass conversion technologies, HTL offers a distinct advantage in processing high-moisture feedstocks without needing energy-intensive drying steps, unlike pyrolysis and gasification. This comparative benefit is illustrated in Fig. 9.1, which contrasts the moisture tolerance and operational conditions across these methods.

9.1.2 Historical Development and Industrial Adoption

Some studies have reported that the HTL process is largely unaffected by biomass particle size, with factors such as biomass type, process conditions, and catalyst presence playing more significant roles (Zhang & Chen, 2017). The subcritical state of water enhances thermal conductivity and acts as an effective solvent, thereby reducing the necessity for extensive particle size reduction in HTL operations (Singh et al., 2015). However, recent advancements, including microwave-assisted HTL, suggest that particle size distribution can affect process efficiency by promoting improved interaction between biomass, energy input, and the reaction medium, which may accelerate conversion reactions (Zhang et al., 2023). Catalyst selection in HTL processes varies depending on the biomass feedstock to optimize performance. Both homogeneous and heterogeneous catalysts have been employed; for example, red macroalgae have been effectively processed using homogeneous catalysts such as sodium carbonate (Na_2CO_3), potassium carbonate (K_2CO_3), calcium carbonate ($CaCO_3$), sodium sulphate (Na_2SO_4), sodium hydroxide (NaOH), and potassium hydroxide (KOH) (Nallasivam et al., 2021). Magnetically recoverable catalysts have been applied in the HTL of draff (Mukundan, 2022), while heterogeneous catalysts—including zeolites, lanthanide oxides, transition metals, and alkaline metal oxides—have been utilized for the HTL of lignocellulosic biomass (Mukundan, 2022).

Although HTL has demonstrated promising results across numerous studies, it remains an emerging technology. Despite the acknowledged necessity for advancing continuous processing to facilitate industrial-scale implementation, empirical evidence supporting the practicality of continuous HTL systems is still limited. Conversely, batch processing offers a notable advantage in handling feedstocks with high dry matter content, thereby reducing challenges related to feedstock pumping and pipeline fouling commonly encountered in continuous-flow reactors (Hao et al., 2023).

Research by the Pacific Northwest National Laboratory reported biocrude yields of approximately 37 wt% in a continuous stirred-tank reactor (CSTR)-type HTL system (Fan et al., 2022a). The latest continuous HTL pilot plant, developed at Aarhus University (Denmark), has demonstrated processing capacities of up to 100 L/h for algal biomass and domestic sludge (Anastasakis et al., 2018). Findings indicate a reduction in nitrogen and oxygen content in the biocrude produced, suggesting enhanced heteroatom removal in continuous flow systems. This improvement is primarily attributed to hydrothermal reactions such as decarboxylation, dehydration, and deamination (Fan et al., 2022a).

Achieving economies of scale and fostering a high degree of integration within the shared infrastructure is critical for biorefineries to reduce operational and capital costs, representing a primary challenge in the sector. The study's findings revealed key themes influencing the knowledge and persuasion stages of the diffusion of the innovations adoption process. These insights provide valuable recommendations for technology adoption in the hotel industry and highlight the complex, dual nature of the adoption process within service sectors (Cobos et al., 2016).

9.2 HTL Processes

Hydrothermal processing is categorized into three primary methods based on the severity of operating conditions. At temperatures below 520 K, the process is called hydrothermal carbonization (HTC), which generates hydrochar—a biochar-like material exhibiting characteristics similar to low-rank coal. During HTC, lipids can often be recovered beforehand, as the lipid fraction of microalgae remains mostly intact, while the hydrochar predominantly comprises protein and carbohydrate fractions (Heilmann et al., 2010). When operated at intermediate temperatures ranging from 520 to 647 K, the process is classified as HTL, producing biocrude oil—a liquid fuel comparable to petroleum crude oil that can be further upgraded into a broad spectrum of petroleum-derived fuels. Above 647 K, hydrothermal gasification becomes dominant, yielding synthetic fuel gases. These synthetic fuels, produced via technologies such as coal-to-liquid, gas-to-liquid, and biomass-to-liquid—often utilizing Fischer–Tropsch synthesis—include products like synthetic natural gas and syngas. A significant advantage of hydrothermal gasification over liquefaction is its reduced generation of organic carbon residues. Biomass, defined as rapidly renewable organic carbon from plant and animal sources, is nature's form of solar energy storage. During gasification, biomass components remain in the aqueous phase, supporting high overall carbon efficiency (Mathimani et al., 2019; Nadarajah et al., 2024).

9.2.1 *Feedstock Preparation*

Renewable energy sources are essential to meeting greenhouse gas (GHG) emission reduction targets and mitigating the impacts of climate change. Current bioenergy production technologies are broadly categorized into two main groups: thermochemical and biological processes. Widely utilized methods include combustion/incineration, pyrolysis, gasification, anaerobic digestion (AD), fermentation, and related techniques. Each method presents distinct advantages and limitations depending on feedstock versatility, energy efficiency, operational complexity, product quality, and economic viability. Among these technologies, HTL has recently attracted significant attention from scientific and industrial communities worldwide. HTL can convert virtually any biomass type into crude bio-oil comparable to fossil crude oil, which can be refined using existing petroleum refinery infrastructure. Despite its advantages over alternative conversion methods, HTL has yet to achieve commercial-scale deployment. The literature identifies numerous operational and technological challenges that must be overcome to successfully design and scale continuous HTL systems. While extensive review and experimental studies have been conducted on process and product development at batch and pilot scales (Ghadge et al., 2022), relatively little is known about the challenges related to design, scale-up, and operation at commercial scales. This review article addresses these critical issues, outlining design considerations, scale-up obstacles, and operational challenges associated with HTL technology and proposes potential strategies to facilitate its industrial implementation.

9.2.1.1 Algae, SS, Food Waste: Moisture Content and Preprocessing

Scientific research highlights HTL as an effective and environmentally sustainable approach for valorizing sewage sludge (SS) within waste management and renewable energy sectors. Significant efforts are focused on improving conversion efficiency to enable industrial-scale deployment. This review comprehensively evaluates the current state-of-the-art HTL technology applied to SS, covering fundamental HTL principles, the impact of critical operational parameters, key industrial challenges, and integrated upgrading techniques (Fan et al., 2022b). It also discusses strategies such as pre-treatment, co-liquefaction, and post-treatment of aqueous and solid fractions (Fan et al., 2022b), along with synthesizing key results from continuous-flow HTL studies involving SS. The review concludes by offering recommendations to enhance the economic feasibility of HTL processes.

Waste SS presents significant potential as a resource and energy carrier; however, its complex composition—including high moisture and ash content, organic contaminants, and hazardous heavy metals—poses considerable challenges. These factors increase operational costs, reduce process efficiency, and negatively impact product quality. The elevated moisture content further complicates handling by generating large sludge volumes that require substantial landfill or composting capacity. Additionally, conventional conversion methods such as pyrolysis and incineration necessitate energy-intensive drying to improve process efficiency.

HTL offers a promising alternative by effectively processing high-moisture feedstocks, enabling simultaneous waste valorization and disposal. HTL has gained growing interest relative to hydrothermal carbonization (HTC) and hydrothermal gasification (HTG), primarily due to its ability to produce condensed liquid biocrude without requiring pre-drying while operating at moderate temperatures and reasonable reaction times. The application of HTL to SS has been extensively studied through batch reactor experiments and, more recently, continuous-flow systems, with ongoing efforts to optimize reaction parameters to enhance biocrude yield and quality.

In parallel, the global food waste generation—estimated at approximately 1.6 billion tonnes annually due to urbanization and industrial expansion—has driven research into alternative waste management solutions. Energy valorization of food waste represents a sustainable strategy to reduce environmental impacts associated with landfill disposal and decrease reliance on fossil-derived crude oil for liquid fuel production.

Bayat et al. (2021) investigated the HTL of food waste in a batch reactor under moderate conditions, specifically at temperatures between 240 and 295 °C, reaction times up to 60 min, and a solid loading of 15 wt%. The highest bio-crude energy content (40.2 MJ/kg) was observed at 295 °C, whereas optimal bio-crude yield (27.5 wt%) and energy recovery (49%) were achieved at 240 °C with a 30-min reaction duration. Characterization of the bio-crude involved several analytical techniques, including fatty acid methyl ester (FAME) analysis via gas chromatography with flame ionization detection, ultrahigh-resolution Fourier transform ion cyclotron resonance mass spectrometry (FT-ICR MS), CHNS elemental analysis, and thermogravimetric analysis. FT-ICR MS results indicated that the bio-crude predominantly comprised oxygenated compounds, with the O_4 class prevailing at 240 °C and the O_2 class dominant at 265 °C and 295 °C (Bayat et al., 2021).

Bench-scale experiments assessed the HTL of lipid-extracted microalgae (LEA) and the subsequent upgrading processes for liquid fuel production. Process modelling and techno-economic analysis were performed for a large-scale HTL and upgrading system based on the most reliable experimental data. The model assumed an LEA feed rate of 608 dry metric tons per day, with LEA initially converted into crude HTL bio-oil, which is then refined into liquid hydrocarbons—primarily alkanes—through hydrotreating and hydrocracking. Performance and cost evaluations demonstrated that the integrated HTL and upgrading process offers a viable and efficient pathway for producing liquid fuels from LEA (Zhu et al., 2013). The total energy efficiency, calculated using the higher heating value (HHV), was determined to be 69.5%, with an estimated annual production of 26.9 million gallons of gasoline equivalent (GGE). Sensitivity analysis indicated that the minimum fuel selling price (MFSP) ranged from $2.07 to $7.11 per GGE, depending on key process parameters. Among the most significant factors influencing production costs were the cost of the LEA feedstock, product yields, and capital expenditures associated with equipment upgrades. Furthermore, the impact of plant scale on MFSP was systematically evaluated, underscoring the economic advantages of process scale-up (Zhu et al., 2013).

Juneja et al. (2018) comprehensively analyze the fundamental structure, reaction pathways, and kinetic mechanisms underlying the decomposition of key feedstock components during the HTL process. The study also explores how critical operational parameters influence bio-oil yield. Typically, HTL produces high-heating-value biocrude or bio-oil alongside an aqueous phase, gaseous byproducts, and solid residues. HTL is particularly promising for converting high-moisture feedstocks; however, elevated solids content can impede adequate mixing within the reactor, reducing heat and mass transfer and leading to lower conversion and bio-oil yields. The chemical composition of bio-oil derived from cellulose varies depending on whether the reaction environment is acidic, neutral, or alkaline. Additionally, HTL facilitates the incorporation of nitrogen into the bio-oil. Temperature plays a crucial role in biomass depolymerization—a dominant reaction in the early stages of HTL—which requires sufficient thermal energy to overcome the activation barrier for bond cleavage (Juneja et al., 2018).

9.2.2 Reaction Mechanisms

HTL technology's capacity to convert wet biomass into petroleum-like biocrude has garnered significant scientific interest. A thorough understanding of HTL reaction mechanisms and kinetics is crucial for enhancing process insights, accurately predicting product yields, and enabling effective scale-up to industrial operations (Ahmad et al., 2025). Reaction parameters and feedstock composition strongly influence the underlying pathways and kinetic ehavior in HTL. Despite increasing attention, detailed studies on reaction mechanisms and kinetics—particularly regarding biocrude yield and product distribution in single and multi-feedstock systems—remain limited.

Ahmad et al. (2025) focused on elucidating the reaction behaviours of key biomolecular constituents, including lignocellulosic components, proteins, and lipids, under subcritical and supercritical HTL conditions. They investigated how reaction conditions affect kinetics, product distribution, and reaction pathways. Their findings reveal an inverse relationship between reaction temperature and residence time for achieving optimal biocrude yields. A high heating rate is recommended to maximize crude production and minimize secondary reactions such as cracking and recombination. Furthermore, depending on feedstock characteristics, increasing the solvent-to-feedstock ratio has improved biocrude yields. Using catalysts and reaction solvents—especially organic solvents—can raise biocrude yields by up to 70%. Among catalysts, heterogeneous types are preferred due to their ability to enhance biocrude quality and facilitate reuse. The study also explores the role of hydrothermal co-liquefaction (multi-feedstock systems) in boosting biocrude generation. Kinetic analyses suggest that HTL reactions typically follow first-order kinetics. The authors conclude by proposing future research directions to support industrial-scale HTL implementation.

Extensive research has examined reaction pathways, kinetic modelling, and predictive techniques for estimating biocrude yields and by-product formation. Prior reviews predominantly focused on feedstock characteristics, operating conditions, product yields, and general product features. However, in-depth analyses of specific chemical pathways and kinetic models remain scarce. For example, Changi et al. (2015) studied the reaction mechanisms of various biomolecular components in microalgae during HTL. Hao et al. (2021) investigated the chemical reactions of biomass during HTL and the catalytic hydrogenation process for biocrude upgrading in separate studies. Despite the growing literature, comprehensive reviews addressing reaction pathways, kinetic models, and the influence of operational parameters—especially in multi-feedstock contexts—are still limited.

To fill this gap, Ahmad et al. (2025) analyzed the reaction pathways of carbohydrate and non-carbohydrate fractions of lignocellulosic biomass at the component level, examining how changes in reaction conditions impact HTL chemistry and product distribution, with emphasis on crude yield. Building upon kinetic analyses for individual lignocellulosic components, they proposed a framework applicable to multi-feedstock systems. Finally, the study identified potential technological advancements from an industrial perspective, contributing to a deeper understanding of HTL reaction kinetics and product yields in both single and blended feedstock scenarios.

9.2.2.1 Subcritical Versus Supercritical Water Conditions

Hydrothermal treatment, which employs water as a solvent and a reactant, represents an environmentally sustainable approach for upgrading heavy oil. Nonetheless, the precise ehavior of water under subcritical and supercritical conditions remains insufficiently understood. This knowledge gap was addressed by an extensive deuterium isotope tracing study, investigating a range of temperatures (300–450 °C), pressures (8.6–42.9 Mpa), deuterium oxide to oil ratios (2 and 20), and residence times (30 and 120 min). The results demonstrated a strong dependence of water reactivity on both temperature and the ionic product of water (KW). A new theoretical model was introduced, positing that water reactivity comprises both ionic and free-radical contributions. In subcritical conditions, ionic reactions prevail where KW is elevated, while free-radical reactions become more significant as temperature increases (Chen, 2024). Approaching the phase transition point, KW initially declines gradually, followed by a steep reduction, marking the dominance of free-radical mechanisms under supercritical conditions.

Additionally, elevated pressure was found to enhance KW. Accordingly, overall water reactivity displays distinct response patterns to variations in both temperature and pressure. Chen (2024) concluded that water functions as a hydrogen donor during the hydrothermal upgrading heavy oil under both subcritical and supercritical conditions. Experimental results demonstrate that the overall reactivity of water arises from the combined effects of ionic and free-radical mechanisms. This finding offers an enhanced understanding of water's reactive ehavior during hydrothermal upgrading, highlighting the ionic product of water (KW) as a critical parameter controlling ionic reaction pathways in subcritical systems.

9.2.2.2 Role of Catalysts

To enhance biocrude yields and improve product quality tailored for specific applications, various catalytic strategies have been developed within the HTL process. Recent literature encompasses numerous studies employing homogeneous and heterogeneous catalysts across diverse catalyst types. Catalysis also plays a crucial role in upgrading HTL-derived biocrude into refined fuels, which has witnessed considerable advancements in recent years. This review aims to provide a comprehensive, up-to-date synthesis of catalytic applications in HTL by integrating the current body of knowledge (Shah et al., 2022). By comparing catalytic and non-catalytic approaches, the distinct effects of each catalyst type on HTL product yields and characteristics are quantitatively assessed, enabling the evaluation of catalyst effectiveness across various biomass feedstocks. The advantages and limitations of each catalytic strategy are critically examined, highlighting emerging challenges and potential research directions.

Catalytic HTL of SS and *Chlorella vulgaris* was performed at 325 °C with a 30-min residence time to investigate the effects of $NiMo/Al_2O_3$ and $CoMo/Al_2O_3$ catalysts on biocrude yield and quality (Prestigiacomo et al., 2019). Both catalysts exhibited significant catalytic activity, substantially enhancing biocrude quality while exerting minimal influence on overall yield. CoMo and NiMo catalysts reduced the O/C molar ratio in biocrude from 0.42 in non-catalytic runs to 0.21 and 0.19, respectively. Biocrude yield increased by 3% with CoMo but decreased by 3% with NiMo, likely due to the formation of light, water-soluble compounds diverting carbon from the biocrude phase in the NiMo-catalysed reaction. Both catalysts effectively reduced sulfur and oxygen contents in biocrude derived from *Chlorella vulgaris*, with similar reductions in O/C and S/C ratios observed for SS-derived biocrude.

The nanostructured nickel catalyst, characterized by a unique flower-like morphology, inhibited char formation attributed to nickel-promoted hydrogenation during biomass conversion, resulting in a 36.63% increase in crude yield. Both catalysts demonstrated excellent catalytic performance, enhancing the higher heating value (HHV) and hydrogen-to-carbon (H/C) ratio of the biocrude (de Caprariis et al., 2020). Furthermore, their magnetic properties facilitated facile post-reaction recovery, with average recovery efficiencies of approximately 90%.

9.2.3 *Product Separation*

Fossil fuel reserves are rapidly depleting due to excessive consumption and accelerating global industrialization, underscoring the urgent need to develop cost-effective, environmentally sustainable, and renewable energy sources for future fuel and chemical production (Demirbas, 2009; Huber et al., 2006). The HTL process produces four main output streams: biocrude, aqueous phase, gaseous by-products, and solid residues. These outputs are separated after the reaction using phase-based separation techniques, as depicted in the product flow schematic (Fig. 9.2) (Hao, 2023; Heilmann et al., 2010; Shahir et al., 2014; Yang et al., 2016).

9.2.3.1 Biocrude, Aqueous Phase, Biochar, and Syngas Recovery

When produced efficiently, biofuels generate significantly lower greenhouse gas emissions than fossil fuels (Börjesson, 1996; Nigam & Singh, 2011; Yang et al., 2015). The pyrolysis, gasification, and combustion processes necessitate energy-intensive pre-drying of high-moisture feedstocks, thereby increasing operational costs (Huber & Dumesic, 2006; Huber et al., 2006). In contrast, HTL presents a promising alternative by directly converting wet biomass into biocrude oil with substantially reduced oxygen content and enhanced calorific value without requiring

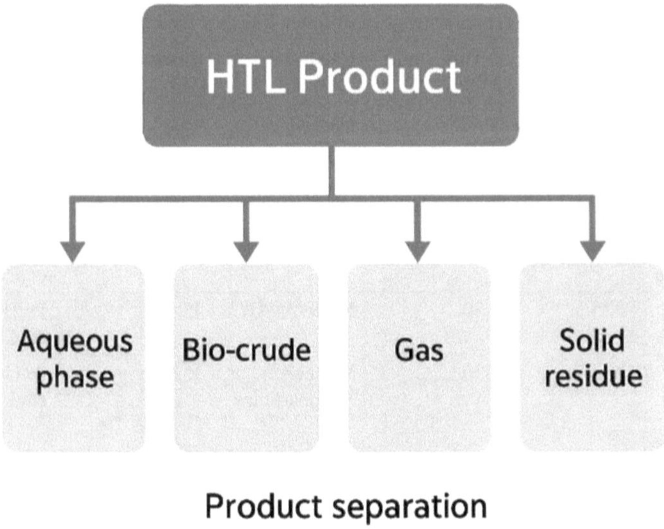

Fig. 9.2 Product separation pathways following hydrothermal liquefaction (HTL): Distribution of aqueous phase, biocrude, gas, and solid residue

drying. This process operates at elevated pressures (100–350 bar) and temperatures (250–450 °C), employing water near its critical point. Under these conditions, water's lowered viscosity and dielectric constant improve the solubility of organic compounds and boost catalytic activity for acid–base reactions via increased ionic product.

Effective upgrading of biocrude through hydrotreatment is essential for producing transportation-grade fuels that can substitute conventional petroleum-based gasoline (Castello et al., 2018; Peterson et al., 2008). Numerous comprehensive reviews in the literature examine biocrude production via HTL, emphasizing the influence of key operational parameters such as temperature, pressure, catalyst type, residence time, and feedstock properties (Akhtar & Amin, 2011; Dimitriadis et al., 2017; Gollakota et al., 2018; Huang & Yuan, 2015; Scarsella et al., 2020; Toor et al., 2011; Xue et al., 2016; Yang et al., 2019).

Current research on HTL places significant emphasis on applying homogeneous and heterogeneous catalysts to increase biocrude yield while enhancing its quality. This review evaluates how these catalytic systems influence biocrude upgrading and the broader spectrum of HTL products. Synthesizing evidence from the literature clarifies the role of various catalysts in feedstock conversion and subsequent biocrude refinement. Shah et al. (2022) examined categories of homogeneous and heterogeneous catalysts, including alkali salts, metal oxides, transition metals, organic acids, and activated carbon. Additionally, several commercial catalysts have been evaluated for biocrude upgrading. To address existing challenges and research needs, the paper also suggests possible remedies. A quantitative comparison of biocrude yields

Table 9.1 Comparative HTL performance of different biomass feedstocks

Biomass type	Temperature (°C)	Time (min)	Catalyst	Biocrude yield (%)	References number
Microalgae	320	30	Na_2CO_3	45.3	Miranda et al. (2022)
Food waste	295	30	None	27.5	Bayat et al. (2021)
Red macroalgae	300	20	K_2CO_3	41.7	Nallasivam et al. (2021)
SS	325	30	$NiMo/Al_2O_3$	33	Prestigiacomo et al. (2019)
Oak wood	330	30	Nickel Nanoparticles	36.6	de Caprariis et al. (2020)

from various feedstocks is provided in Table 9.1, which complements the following discussion on product separation.

9.2.4 *Technological Challenges*

The opportunities and challenges associated with hydrothermal carbonization (HTC) include the following: (1) As a relatively novel technology, many of HTC's underlying mechanisms remain poorly understood. Additionally, HTC must compete with other renewable energy sources and contend with existing waste disposal practices. (2) The logistics systems supporting HTC operations can be costly and time-consuming. (3) It is reasonable to expect that the capital expenditure for constructing HTC facilities will be significant. Although hydrochar's price is comparable on an energy-equivalent basis, it remains more expensive than coal in terms of equivalent energy content (Joules). (4) Due to the complexity and variability of biomass feedstocks used and the risk of feedstock contamination, uncertainty may exist regarding the final quality of the produced hydrochar.

While HTC offers numerous advantages, recognizing and addressing these limitations is essential to facilitate its broader adoption in future applications. The following sections outline several key challenges presently faced by HTC technology, alongside potential solutions that have been proposed or merit further investigation. Although HTC plants are operational worldwide, it is essential to emphasize that the technology is still in an early developmental stage and is considered relatively immature despite growing interest. For example, Scottish Water's National Sludge Strategy categorizes pyrolysis of wastewater sludge—and gasification—as 'relatively high risk' technologies, citing their commercially unproven status and noting that their planning and procurement timelines are comparable to or exceed those of conventional incineration plants. Furthermore, these technologies are frequently associated with substantial capital investment and high operational costs.

9.2.4.1 Reactor Corrosion and Material Durability

Thermochemical methods transform biomass into biofuels through heat and chemical reactions, with various terms used interchangeably in the literature depending on reactor conditions (Bevan et al., 2020). The choice of reactor conditions is determined by factors such as reactor scale, feedstock type, intended product application, and technology provider. A critical difference among these methods is their ability to process feedstocks with high moisture levels, typically 75% to 90%. Conversely, feedstocks containing approximately 50–70% moisture are generally not economically suited for dry pyrolysis, gasification, or torrefaction, as these processes require substantial energy for drying beforehand. This drying step is both energetically costly and financially inefficient, often making it more practical to exclude high-moisture biomass from such treatments (Libra et al., 2011). Consequently, HTC presents a valuable alternative, as it can effectively handle feedstocks with elevated moisture content.

9.2.5 Energy-Intensive High-Pressure Systems

HTL is a thermochemical technique used to convert biomass feedstocks into liquid fuels. The process operates in an aqueous environment under high pressure (5–20 MPa) and temperatures ranging from 250 to 370 °C. Within these subcritical conditions, hydrolysis and re-polymerization reactions break down complex biomass into smaller, energy-dense molecules, making it essential to maintain water pressure within these specified limits (Mathimani et al., 2019). Benjamin et al. (2019) aimed to develop a novel standard procedure for integrating heat and mass flows in the HTL process to co-locate the facility alongside an existing Kraft pulp mill to facilitate efficient biocrude production.

HTL is an energy-intensive process that produces biocrude oil resembling conventional crude by operating at elevated temperatures and pressures. Situating an HTL plant adjacent to a Kraft pulp mill presents strategic advantages, including optimized supply chain and logistics integration, asset reuse, and utilizing black liquor as an HTL feedstock. The study employed a systematic design methodology focused on maximizing energy efficiency through iterative mass and heat integration, optimizing material and energy flows alongside process assets. Implementing this method reduced the number of heat exchangers by half, from 14 to 7. Substituting conventional fuels with bio-crude derived from this integrated HTL process could lower transport fuel-related carbon emissions by approximately 11.3 kg CO_2-equivalent per gigajoule.

The HTL process involves reacting polymeric substances such as cellulose, lignin, and synthetic polymers with near-critical or supercritical water, producing low molecular weight liquids analogous to natural oils formed over geological timescales. With energy efficiencies reaching up to 90%, HTL significantly outperforms other biomass conversion methods like pyrolysis and AD, which typically achieve around 30%

efficiency. However, scaling classical HTL to industrial levels remains challenging due to the necessity for extremely high temperatures (250–450 °C) and pressures (100–350 bar) (Liiv et al., 2022).

9.2.6 Nutrient Recovery from Aqueous Phase Byproducts

Wet biomass undergoes thermochemical conversion via HTL, producing biocrude oil alongside a byproduct known as the hydrothermal liquefaction aqueous phase (HTL-AP). This nutrient-rich wastewater can promote crop growth and elevate inorganic nitrogen levels, particularly nitrate (NO_3^-), when appropriately treated. This study aimed to enhance the inorganic nitrogen content—specifically ammonia/ammonium (NH_3/NH_4^+) and nitrate—in HTL-AP through fungal remediation for potential application in hydroponic systems. The white-rot fungus *Trametes versicolor*, noted for its ability to degrade a wide range of organic pollutants, was applied to a 5% diluted HTL-AP and incubated for nine days (Vitoria et al., 2025). Although no visible fungal biomass was detected during incubation, laccase enzyme activity confirmed the presence of *T. versicolor*. After three days of fungal treatment, nitrate and ammonia/ammonium nitrogen concentrations increased by 17-fold and eightfold, respectively, indicating an optimal treatment window. Subsequent inoculation with nitrifying bacteria further doubled nitrate concentrations compared to fungal treatment alone, demonstrating enhanced nitrogen conversion. Chemical oxygen demand (COD) decreased by 51.33% within one day, likely reflecting fungal degradation of organic matter; however, COD levels subsequently increased, possibly due to metabolites released by the fungus. These findings suggest T. versicolor as a promising agent for augmenting inorganic nitrogen in HTL-AP. Future research should focus on mitigating HTL-AP toxicity, assessing hydroponic crop performance post-fungal treatment, and optimizing methods to reduce ammonia/ammonium concentrations while increasing nitrate availability (Vitoria et al., 2025).

Shanmugam et al. (2017) investigated the removal of nutrients—specifically phosphorus and nitrogen—as struvite from the aqueous phase generated during the HTL of algae-derived bio-oil. The study examined the effects of key process variables, including pH, temperature, and reaction time, on struvite formation. Ammonium nitrogen removal ranged from 40 to 100% under all tested conditions, while phosphorus removal consistently exceeded 99%. Biogas production assays demonstrated that methane yields from the struvite-recovered aqueous phase were approximately 3.5 times higher (182 ± 39 mL/g COD) than those from the non-struvite recovered phase. These results indicate that the aqueous phase from algal HTL can be effectively utilized for both methane production and nutrient recovery via struvite precipitation. It is estimated that around 69.5 kg of struvite can be generated per metric tonne of dried algae processed by HTL. The enhanced methane production associated with the struvite-recovered phase suggests that the removal of ammonium nitrogen (NH_4^+-N) promotes increased methanogenesis. The aqueous phase derived from algal HTL presents valuable opportunities for integrated nutrient recovery and supplementary energy generation.

9.3 Economic Viability

HTL stands out among thermochemical processes as one of the most promising methods for producing liquid biofuels. Although the production costs of HTL-derived biofuels remain relatively high, Brazil's well-established biomass supply chain and highly competitive sugarcane industry provide a strong foundation for large-scale HTL deployment. To evaluate the economic feasibility of HTL within the Brazilian context, Deuber et al. (2021) conducted a techno-economic analysis considering sugarcane bagasse as the primary feedstock under two scenarios: an HTL facility integrated within the Brazilian sugarcane industry and a standalone HTL plant. Previous studies have investigated HTL and biocrude upgrading using various feedstocks, including assessments of environmental and economic impacts (Hussain & Anastasakis, 2025). However, developing a cost-effective, integrated processing strategy for full-scale HTL implementation remains challenging, mainly due to the complex characteristics of HTL process water (HTL-PW). Recent research suggests that wet oxidation can substantially reduce the COD of HTL-PW—by up to 85% with a residence time of 15 min (Kilgore et al., 2023; Vadlamudi et al., 2024).

9.3.1 Capital Expenditure for Continuous-Flow HTL Reactors

Aierzhati et al. (2021) investigated the feasibility of HTL of food waste using a transportable pilot-scale reactor and assessed its techno-economic potential as a commercially viable renewable energy source. The biocrude yield obtained from a 35 L pilot reactor, operating at 0.15 gallons per minute, 300 °C, and a 60-min retention time, was significantly higher (29.5 wt%) than that from laboratory-scale reactors (21.9 wt%). Comparative analyses of elemental composition, oil content, and heating values revealed similar characteristics between biocrudes produced at both scales. TEA estimated the minimum selling price of the biocrude at $3.48 per gallon of gasoline-equivalent (GGE) under base-case conditions. Transportation costs for feedstock and oil products were compared between onsite and mobile HTL reactor scenarios, indicating that mobile units are economically advantageous when feedstock sources are widely dispersed over distances exceeding 106 miles. By integrating pilot-scale data with scenario-based assessments, the study provides valuable insights into the sustainability of scaling HTL technology. Additionally, findings showed that continuous reactors yield higher biocrude quantities than batch reactors, although pilot-scale biocrude contained a greater proportion of heavy oil molecules and fewer nitrogen-containing heterocycles. The techno-economic evaluation supports the conclusion that mobile HTL units may offer improved cost-effectiveness for broadly distributed biomass resources, providing a robust foundation for future food waste HTL deployment at pilot and commercial scales.

9.3.2 Biocrude Upgrading Costs (Hydrotreating, Fractionation)

Capital cost estimates for HTL and wastewater treatment were carried out using Aspen Process Economic Analyser version 11. Furthermore, cost data for upgrading units—such as hydrotreating, hydrocracking, and hydrogen production—were sourced from the literature and adjusted according to the economies of scale power law with appropriate scaling factors to improve accuracy (Knorr et al., 2013). Annual operating costs were calculated using a service factor 0.9 (Watson et al., 2019). Instead of catalytic hydrothermal gasification, this study employed a two-stage fermentation process to treat the aqueous phase, following the methodology outlined by Watson et al. (2019). The proposed biocrude upgrading process was modelled based on procedures detailed in relevant technical reports (Jones et al., 2014; Snowden-Swan et al., 2017). Further upgrading of biocrude is necessary to meet transportation fuel standards. Although in-situ applications of homogeneous and heterogeneous catalysts have been explored to improve bio-crude quality (Yang et al., 2022), these approaches have only achieved limited nitrogen and oxygen content reductions. Consequently, current research mainly focuses on catalytic hydrotreatment (CHT) for biocrude upgrading.

9.3.3 Market Competition with Fossil-Derived Crude Oil

HTL has attracted increasing attention due to its distinct advantage over alternative methods: it can process wet biomass directly, removing the requirement for energy-intensive drying and thus lowering overall operational costs (Mishra et al., 2022). Although hydrous pyrolysis and HTL are sometimes synonymous, HTL operates at comparatively lower temperatures and heating rates. Specifically, HTL is defined as converting feedstocks into liquid fuels under intermediate pressures (10–35 MPa) and temperatures (250–400 °C) using hot, pressurized water. Key benefits of HTL compared to conventional pyrolysis include enhanced energy efficiency and markedly reduced tar production.

As global crude oil trade expands with rising demand, competition among importers intensifies, increasing pressure on importing nations. This study quantifies, and maps import competition pressure by modelling importers as nodes and competitive relationships as directed edges within a crude oil import trade competition network. The direction of each edge indicates the flow of competitive pressure, while the edge's weight reflects the extent of competition imposed on each importer. Applying complex network theory, the research analyses the evolution of crude oil import competition from 2000 to 2020 (Hao et al., 2023). Key findings include: (1) competition is more intense among Asian importers than European ones; (2) Saudi Arabia and Russia are the most competitive crude oil exporters, with China showing greater dependence on Saudi Arabia than on the United States; (3) crude oil trade relationships fall into four categories—import dependence, importer-oriented, close cooperation, and loose trade links; and (4) China's influence over Angola and Saudi Arabia has declined recently, while Germany and the Netherlands have increased competitive pressure on Russia. Based on these results, the study recommends diversifying supply sources, expanding reliable global trade partnerships, and implementing risk mitigation strategies. Overall, this work assists nations in recognizing competitive pressures in the crude oil market and offers guidance to enhance their strategic positioning.

9.4 Applications and Innovations

As traditional fossil fuel reserves diminish and pollution concerns escalate, the search for sustainable and renewable fuel alternatives becomes increasingly critical. Biomass-derived biocrude represents a promising option, with HTL as a key technology in its production. HTL exhibits remarkable flexibility, enabling the transformation of a wide variety of biomass and waste materials into biocrude, with yields ranging from approximately 60% to 86%, depending on the feedstock (Usman et al., 2024). This detailed review addresses recent advancements in HTL, including the role of catalysts in enhancing process efficiency, challenges related to scale-up, and the prospects for commercializing continuous HTL systems that incorporate aqueous phase recycling. Moreover, it explores the utilization of machine learning for optimizing the HTL process, highlighting how these sophisticated computational approaches can improve product quality and process performance. Following subsequent hydrotreatment, HTL forms an essential component of biomass-to-fuel conversion technologies. The review stresses the ongoing requirement for biocrude upgrading and refining research, presenting HTL as a transformative pathway that offers a viable alternative to fossil fuels while tackling issues linked to heteroatoms and contaminants within biocrude. The paper concludes by discussing practical applications of recent developments and suggesting a strategic direction for future research and innovation.

9.4.1 Aviation Fuel Production *via* HTL Biocrude Refining

At the Pacific Northwest National Laboratory (PNNL), biocrude is produced via HTL directly from the solid content of wet wastes, circumventing the need for expensive catalysts, solvents, or energy-demanding drying steps commonly associated with alternative technologies like pyrolysis and gasification (Yang et al., 2020). HTL provides a consistent feedstock supply by utilizing wet wastes such as sewage sludge (SS), often at a negative net cost. Using SS as a feedstock has the potential to reduce fuel production costs by roughly USD 1.5 to 7 per gallon by offsetting disposal expenses, given that urban municipalities pay between USD 200 and 600 per dry tonne (or USD 40 to 120 per wet tonne assuming 50% solids) for disposal (Seiple et al., 2017, 2020; Snowden-Swan et al., 2020). The 2021 state-of-technology (SOT) evaluation from PNNL projected a minimum fuel-selling price (MFSP) slightly above USD 3 per gallon of (GGE) for fuels derived from wet-waste HTL, not accounting for disposal cost savings. With an overall carbon yield near 60–70% (Cronin et al., 2021), HTL produces a thermally stable biocrude containing approximately 70–80 wt.% carbon and a heating value of around 35–40 MJ/kg, comparable to conventional crude oil at 45 MJ/kg (Snowden-Swan et al., 2020). To function as drop-in fuels similar to petroleum, these biocrudes require hydrotreatment, significantly lowering heteroatom concentrations—mainly oxygen and nitrogen—from the typical 10–15 wt.% found in WWHTLB (Cronin et al., 2021). However, HTL biocrudes generally exhibit elevated levels of metals such as potassium, sodium, silicon, iron, and calcium (Haider et al., 2018; Vardon et al., 2011), along with oxygenated compounds like fatty acids, when compared to conventional crude oils, resulting in higher total acid numbers (TAN) (Haarlemmer et al., 2016).

9.4.2 *Wastewater Treatment Synergies*

Disposing of SS and food waste digestate residues presents considerable challenges, primarily due to difficulties in dewatering and environmental risks posed by heavy metals and pathogens. This research investigated a synergistic approach combining hydrothermal pretreatment (HP), AD, and pyrolysis to improve dewatering efficiency, recover energy, and produce biochar capable of immobilizing heavy metals. Findings revealed increased solid content of centrifuged cakes following HP of SS at 180 °C when DR was added at 25% and 50% mass proportions (Li et al., 2024). The resulting centrate, characterised by elevated COD, underwent AD treatment at 37 °C with 50% and 75% DR additions, resulting in cumulative methane productions of 193.75 and 210.39 mL/g COD input, respectively. Higher DR ratios induced a shift in methanogenic activity from hydrogenotrophic to acetoclastic pathways. Heavy metals such as copper, zinc, lead, and nickel were predominantly retained within biochar generated by pyrolysis at 700 °C after co-HP with 50% DR. Chemical fractionation demonstrated that over 85% of copper, zinc, lead, and chromium were sequestered in residual fractions, corresponding to a low ecological risk index of 15.22. Moreover, using methane produced from AD of the co-HP centre (50:50, w/w) to fuel the HP process reduced energy requirements by 89%. This integrated treatment method facilitates effective carbon recovery from solid wastes and contributes significantly to lowering carbon emissions.

9.4.3 Catalytic HTL for Nitrogen/oxygen Removal

In the context of hydroprocessing for drop-in biofuel production, HTL biocrude originating from non-lignocellulosic feedstocks often contains high levels of inorganic elements, oxygen, and notably elevated nitrogen content. Removing nitrogen is particularly challenging, requiring severe processing conditions that may jeopardize operational stability and alter the distribution of hydrocarbon fractions. Castello et al. (2024) showed that microalgae-derived biocrude can be effectively treated over extended periods using a multi-stage process with various sulphide catalysts despite its elevated metal and nitrogen levels. Although nitrogen removal remained complex, hydrodeoxygenation was accomplished under relatively mild operating conditions. Enhanced nitrogen elimination was linked to increased hydrogen consumption, necessitating higher temperatures around 400 °C and reduced space velocities. While the severity of hydrotreatment had a limited effect on middle distillate production, it caused a notable shift in boiling point profiles towards lighter gasoline-range products. Moreover, the denitrogenation process appeared to promote the breakdown of larger molecules within the heavier fractions of the biocrude.

9.5 Case Studies

This research evaluates the potential application of advanced hydrothermal HTC technologies in small-scale communities in the United Kingdom, focusing on Chirnside, a town in the Scottish Borders that produces sewage sludge and biodegradable municipal waste. The study theoretically investigates the HTC process developed for treating both types of waste. Alongside mass and energy balance analyses, it explores this technology's environmental, social, and economic implications and opportunities. The proposed HTC plant, designed to process waste at 72.5 kg per hour, shows a positive net energy balance (Bevan et al., 2020). The hydrochar generated is expected to produce 1,452 MWh annually, satisfying about 35.6% of Chirnside's projected energy needs for 2041. The paper discusses the expected advantages and potential hurdles of HTC adoption, offering essential perspectives to guide sustainable technology development in comparable settings.

9.5.1 Steeper Energy's HTL Pilot in Denmark

The European Green Deal aims to achieve carbon neutrality by promoting decarbonized fuels and enhancing waste management systems (Fetting, 2020). WWTPs are crucial for sustainable development, environmental protection, water conservation, nutrient recycling, energy generation, and economic growth (Obaideen et al., 2022). Denmark, with a population equivalent (PE) of 7.5 million, treats 680 million m^3 of wastewater annually across over 700 treatment facilities. In 2022, these plants processed and disposed of approximately 123,000 tonnes of solid waste, as reported by the Danish water sector. Disposal methods must comply with legal regulations; for instance, sludge containing specific micropollutants or heavy metals is prohibited from agricultural use. Smaller WWTPs generally employ mineralization or dewatering techniques, while larger plants commonly utilize AD to valorize sludge and produce biogas biologically. Methane, the valuable component of biogas, accounts for only about 60%, with the remainder lost as carbon dioxide. The large quantities of digestate necessitate proper disposal, often incurring substantial operational costs, particularly since treatment plants typically pay for digestate disposal and distribute it to local farmers as fertilizer. Hussain and Anastasakis (2025) conducted a TEA on decentralised HTL units integrated into medium-sized WWTPs (0.1 to 1.0 million PE). Their case study focused on a typical Danish WWTP serving 150,000 PE.

9.5.2 Pacific Northwest National Laboratory (PNNL) Algae-To-Biocrude Projects

Experimental findings indicate that HTL of wastewater-grown algae enhances biocrude yield by 34%, compared to 29% on an ash-free dry weight basis. This increase is linked to the lower ash content in freshly harvested algal biomass (Abhishek Kumar et al., 2024). To maximize biomass availability for HTL, it is recommended that algal biomass be co-processed with AD biosolids and other waste streams. Transport logistics for biomass feedstocks to centralized HTL facilities also require careful consideration. Two promising biomass sources at WRRFs for conversion into value-added products are the wet sludge from primary and secondary treatment stages and biosolids produced from AD of this sludge. A recent report evaluates the co-HTL of algae alongside wet sludge or biosolids to mitigate seasonal feedstock variability and leverage existing WRRF infrastructure for biocrude production (Abhishek Kumar et al., 2024). The produced HTL biocrude is subsequently sent to refineries to upgrade into final fuel products. Operating and capital costs for the HTL process are derived from process modelling, with the MFSP of the finished fuels estimated by factoring in upgrading expenses (Xu et al., 2024). According to industry expert inputs in the 2021 PNNL report, algae production yields from primary effluent and liquid wastewater are projected at 0.15 and 0.8 metric tons per million gallons, respectively. This study utilizes phosphorus content in each wastewater stream and assumes a phosphorus demand of 1 g per 100 g of algae to estimate optimal algae production levels (Clippinger & Davis, 2021).

9.6 Future Directions

The 2024 case study explored the potential for improving wastewater treatment processes by integrating algae cultivation with HTL. Various scenarios indicated that growing algae can effectively remove excess nutrients from primary, secondary, and digester effluents, thereby enhancing wastewater management. Co-processing wastewater-grown algae with residual solids, such as sludge and digested biosolids, through HTL presents a viable route for fuel production (Abhishek Kumar et al., 2024). Although nitrogen and phosphorus must be recovered as valuable co-products, producing algal biomass onsite at WRRFs could reduce the need for external nutrient sourcing and recycling.

Future research priorities for cost-effective algal feedstocks and HTL technology development should include reducing capital expenditure by designing smaller, economically viable HTL plants. Additionally, refining processes to target fertilizer production more precisely—rather than alternatives such as cement additives—may improve cost efficiency. HTL applied to various feedstocks, mainly biomass, has shown considerable promise in generating high biocrude yields with improved quality. Nevertheless, despite these technological advancements, HTL remains at an early commercialization stage. This review synthesizes and critically evaluates existing research on biocrude production via HTL, focusing on its technological capacity to satisfy biofuel industry requirements, ongoing advancements in feedstock thermochemical conversion, and innovative reactor design development.

9.6.1 AI-Optimized Reaction Parameters for Yield Maximization

Critical parameters, including temperature, pressure, and residence time, must thoroughly examine the feedstock composition to maximize biocrude yield and quality (Wodołażski & Smoliński, 2025). Adjusting the ratios of biomass constituents—proteins, carbohydrates, and lipids—or employing co-liquefaction with complementary materials can substantially influence the outcomes due to their significant impact on biocrude properties. Identifying key operational factors like reagent flow rates and biomass concentration is essential; however, maintaining consistent HTL conditions remains challenging because of variations in reactor designs, residence times, and feedstock characteristics across different studies (Lababpour & Patel, 2015).

Lababpour and Patel (2015) conducted a detailed analysis of fundamental operational variables such as heat input, system pressure, biomass concentration, and reaction time. To optimize product composition, Chen et al. (2014) and Ruiz et al. (2013) performed experiments in small-scale reactors to investigate how different feedstocks affect HTL performance. The design of continuous reactors necessitates a comprehensive understanding of reaction kinetics, fluid dynamics, and thermal behaviour. Ranganathan and Savithri (2015) developed a two-dimensional computational fluid dynamics (CFD) model integrating HTL kinetics to assess the effects of temperature, pressure, and slurry flow rate on biocrude yield from sewage sludge within a continuous tubular reactor. Similarly, Xiao et al. (2013) utilized CFD simulations to examine temperature distribution and its correlation with reaction rates in tubular reactors. Joshi et al. (2022) applied CFD modelling to simulate the influence of variables such as temperature, pressure, and residence time on biocrude production, emphasizing their relationship to the Prandtl number. Recent pilot-scale research has incorporated diverse process parameters into continuous HTL reactors, comparing simulation outcomes with experimental data (Elliott et al., 2015). These modelling efforts support the optimization of reactor geometry and operational conditions, thereby advancing process design. Establishing reliable HTL process models and simulations is crucial for scaling production and enabling commercialization. A summary of studies employing experimental, computational, and AI-driven methods for HTL reaction optimization is provided in Table 9.2.

Table 9.2 Summary of AI, experimental, and computational studies optimizing HTL reaction parameters for biocrude yield enhancement

Approach/ method	Feedstock	Key parameters investigated	Main outcome/yield insight	References
Experimental + sensitivity	Lignocellulosic biomass	Heat input, pressure, biomass concentration	Critical influence of biomass loading on yield	Lababpour and Patel (2015)
Bench-scale experiment	Algae + Swine manure	Feedstock interaction	Co-liquefaction improved yield and quality	Chen et al. (2014)
Experimental design	Agricultural residues	Biomass variability	Feedstock-specific optimization needed	Ruiz et al. (2013)
2D CFD simulation	Sewage sludge	Temperature, pressure, flow rate	Performance simulated for continuous reactor	Ranganathan and Savithri (2015)
CFD simulation	Lignin-rich biomass	Temperature profiles	Temperature gradients affect reaction rate	Similarly, Xiao et al. (2013)
CFD modelling	Slurry with particles	Temp., residence time, Prandtl number	Prandtl number correlated with yield	Joshi et al. (2022)
Pilot-scale integration	Mixed wet biomass	Multiple parameters	Simulation–experiment agreement for upscaling	Elliott et al. (2015)

9.6.2 Co-Locating HTL Plants with Wastewater Treatment Facilities

The rapid expansion of urban populations demands the advancement of more efficient and environmentally sustainable technologies for resource recovery and waste treatment. HTL emerges as a promising method for converting organic waste into bio-crude oil. Thomsen et al. (2024) examined HTL-derived products from feedstocks collected at four wastewater treatment facilities in Denmark, processing a variety of waste streams, including digestate, primary and secondary sludge, food waste, fats, oils, and greases (FOG). The study also assessed the impact of co-processing mixed waste streams. HTL trials were performed at a dry matter content of 16.7%, with residence times fixed at 20 min and temperatures set at 300, 325, and 350 °C. Except for FOG processed at 300 °C, all feedstocks exhibited peak bio-crude yields at 325 °C. Blending different waste streams produced synergistic effects from biochemical interactions, resulting in energy recoveries ranging from 62 to 76% and bio-crude yields exceeding predicted values. Based on feedstock composition and biochemical characteristics, two predictive models were developed to forecast bio-crude yields, demonstrating absolute errors between 4 and 5%. Furthermore, the study thoroughly reviewed sludge from wastewater treatment plants, evaluating key process water parameters, nutrient recovery capabilities, and heavy metal concentrations in solid residues.

The surging global energy demand, propelled by accelerating urbanization, highlights the critical need for enhanced urban waste management solutions. Sewage sludge (SS) production from municipal wastewater treatment plants (WWTPs) is expected to rise markedly. In 2020, annual municipal wastewater generation was estimated to be between 360 and 380 cubic kilometres, with projected increases of 24% by 2030 and 51% by 2050 (Giacomo & Romano, 2022)). Approximately half of this volume undergoes treatment across roughly 60,000 WWTPs worldwide, whereas the remaining portion is released untreated into the environment (Macedo et al., 2022; Qadir et al., 2020).

References

Abhishek Kumar, A., Watkins, J., Cronin, D., Fox, S., Schmidt, A., Valdez, P. (2024). Case study: hydrothermal liquefaction of biomass sources at a wastewater treatment facility. PNNL-37230 the U.S. Department of Energy under Contract DE-AC05–76RL01830. Pacific Northwest National Laboratory Richland, Washington 99354.

Ahmad, F., Doddapaneni, T. R. K. C., Toor, S. S., & Kikas, T. (2025). Reaction mechanism and kinetics of hydrothermal liquefaction at sub- and supercritical conditions: a review. *Biomass, 5*(1), 9. https://doi.org/10.3390/biomass5010009

Aierzhati, A., Watson, J., Si, B., Stablein, M., Wang, T., & Zhang, Y. (2021). Development of a mobile, pilot scale hydrothermal liquefaction reactor: Food waste conversion product analysis and techno-economic assessment. *Energy Conversion and Management: X, 10*, Article 100076. https://doi.org/10.1016/j.ecmx.2021.100076

Akhtar, J., & Amin, N. A. S. (2011). A review on process conditions for optimum bio-oil yield in hydrothermal liquefaction of biomass. *Renewable and Sustainable Energy Reviews, 15*, 1615–1624.

Anastasakis, K., Biller, P., Madsen, R. B., Glasius, M., & Johannsen, I. (2018). Continuous hydrothermal liquefaction of biomass in a novel pilot plant with heat recovery and hydraulic oscillation. *Energies, 11*(10), 1–23. https://doi.org/10.3390/en11102695

Bayat, H., Dehghanizadeh, M., Jarvis, J. M., Brewer, C. E., & Jena, U. (2021). Hydrothermal liquefaction of food waste: effect of process parameters on product yields and chemistry. *Frontiers in Sustainable Food Systems, 5*, Article 658592. https://doi.org/10.3389/fsufs.2021.658592

Benjamin, H., Ong, Y., Walmsley, T. G., Atkins, M. J., Varbanov, P. S., & Walmsley, M. R. W. (2019). A heat- and mass-integrated design of hydrothermal liquefaction process co-located with a Kraft pulp mill. *Energy, 189*, Article 116235. https://doi.org/10.1016/j.energy.2019.116235

Bevan, E., Fu, J., & Zheng, Y. (2020). Challenges and opportunities of hydrothermal carbonisation in the UK; case study in ChirnsideRSC. *Adv, 10*, 31586–31587.

Börjesson, P. I. I. (1996). Energy analysis of biomass production and transportation. *Biomass and Bioenergy, 11*, 305–318.

Castello, D., Haider, M. S., Chiaberge, S., & Rosendahl, L. A. (2024). Understanding catalytic hydrotreating of hydrothermal liquefaction nitrogen-rich biocrude in a two-stage continuous hydrotreater. *Chemical Engineering Journal, 481*, Article 148333. https://doi.org/10.1016/j.cej.2023.148333

Castello, D., Pedersen, T. H., & Rosendahl, L. A. (2018). Continuous hydrothermal liquefaction of biomass: a critical review. *Energies, 11*, 3165.

Changi, S. M., Faeth, J. L., Mo, N., & Savage, P. E. (2015). Hydrothermal reactions of biomolecules relevant for microalgae liquefaction. *Industrial and Engineering Chemistry Research, 54*, 11733–11758.

Chen, W. T., Zhang, Y., Zhang, J., Schideman, L., Yu, G., Zhang, P., & Minarick, M. (2014). Co-liquefaction of swine manure and mixed-culture algae: Interactions between feedstock components improve bio-crude yield and quality. *Applied Energy, 120*, 63–70.

Chen, Z. (2024). New insight into subcritical and supercritical water reactivity during non-catalytic hydrothermal upgrading of heavy oil. *Fuel, 366*, Article 131380. https://doi.org/10.1016/j.fuel.2024.131380

Clippinger, J., Davis, R. (2021). Techno-Economic assessment for opportunities to integrate algae farming with wastewater treatment. *Technical Report NREL/TP-5100–75237* https://doi.org/10.2172/1821631.

Cobos, L. M., Mejia, C., Ozturk, A. B., & Wang, Y. (2016). A technology adoption and implementation process in an independent hotel chain. *International Journal of Hospitality Management, 57*, 93–105. https://doi.org/10.1016/j.ijhm.2016.06.005

Cronin, D., Schmidt, A. J., Billing, J., Hart, T. R., Fox, S. P., Fonoll, X., Norton, J., & Thorson, M. R. (2021). Comparative study on the continuous flow hydrothermal liquefaction of various wet-waste feedstock types. *ACS Sustain Chem Eng, 10*, 1255–1256.

de Caprariis, B., Bracciale, M. P., Bavasso, I., Chen, G., Damizia, M., Genova, V., Marra, F., Paglia, L., Pulci, G., Scarsella, M., et al. (2020). Unsupported Ni metal catalyst in hydrothermal liquefaction of oak wood: Effect of catalyst surface modification. *Science of the Total Environment, 709*, Article 136215.

Demirbas, A. (2009). Biorefineries: Current activities and future developments. *Energy Convers Manag, 50*, 2782–2801.

Deuber, R. D. S., Fernandes, D. S., Bressanin, J. M., Watson, J., Chagas, M. F., Bonomi, A., Fregolente, L. V., & Watanabe, M. D. B. (2021). Techno-economic assessment of HTL integration to the Brazilian sugarcane industry: An evaluation of different scenarios. *Industrial Crops and Products, 173*, Article 114139. https://doi.org/10.1016/j.indcrop.2021.114139

Dimitriadis, A., & Bezergianni, S. (2017). Hydrothermal liquefaction of various biomass and waste feedstocks for biocrude production: A state of the art review. *Renewable and Sustainable Energy Reviews, 68*, 113–125.

Elliott, D. C., Biller, P., Ross, A. B., Schmidt, A. J., & Jones, S. B. (2015). Hydrothermal liquefaction of biomass: Developments from batch to continuous process. *Bioresource Technology, 178*, 147–156.
Fan, Y., Hornung, U., & Dahmen, N. (2022a). Hydrothermal liquefaction of sewage sludge for biofuel application: A review on fundamentals, current challenges and strategies. *Biomass and Bioenergy, 165*, Article 106570. https://doi.org/10.1016/j.biombioe.2022.106570
Fan, Y., Prestigiacomo, C., Gong, M., Tietz, T., Hornung, U., & Dahmen, N. (2022b). Comparative investigation on the value-added products obtained from continuous and batch hydrothermal liquefaction of sewage sludge Front. *Environmental Sciences, 10*, 1–13. https://doi.org/10.3389/fenvs.2022.996353
Fetting, C. (2020). The european green deal. ESDN Report, December, ESDN Office, Vienna).
Ghadge, R., Nagwani, N., Saxena, N., Dasgupta, S., & Sapre, A. (2022). Design and scale-up challenges in hydrothermal liquefaction process for biocrude production and its upgradation. *Energy Conversion and Management: X, 14*, Article 100223. https://doi.org/10.1016/j.ecmx.2022.100223
Giacomo, G.D., Romano, R. (2022). Evolution and prospects in managing sewage sludge resulting from municipal wastewater purification. *Energies 15* (15), p. 5633.
Gollakota, A. R. K., Kishore, N., & Gu, S. (2018). A review on hydrothermal liquefaction of biomass. *Renewable and Sustainable Energy Reviews, 81*, 1378–1392.
Haarlemmer, G., Guizani, C., Anouti, S., Déniel, M., Roubaud, A., & Valin, S. (2016). Analysis and comparison of bio-oils obtained by hydrothermal liquefaction and fast pyrolysis of beech wood. *Fuel, 174*, 180–188.
Haider, M. S., Castello, D., Michalski, K. M., Pedersen, T. H., & Rosendahl, L. A. (2018). Catalytic hydrotreatment of microalgae biocrude from continuous hydrothermal liquefaction: heteroatom removal and their distribution in distillation cuts. *Energies, 11*, 3360.
Hao, B., Xu, D., Wang, Y., Wang, Y., Kapusta, K., Guo, Y. (2023). Catalytic hydrothermal liquefaction of municipal sludge for biocrude production over non-noble bimetallic catalyst in ethanol solvent. *Fuel 331* (P1), Article 125812, https://doi.org/10.1016/j.fuel.2022.125812.
Hao, B., Xu, D., Jiang, G., Sabri, T. A., Jing, Z., & Guo, Y. (2021). Chemical reactions in the hydrothermal liquefaction of biomass and in the catalytic hydrogenation upgrading of biocrude. *Green Chemistry, 23*, 1562–1583.
Hao, X. (2023). Import competition and pressure in the international crude oil trade: A network analysis. *Resources Policy, 82*, Article 103468. https://doi.org/10.1016/j.resourpol.2023.103468
Heilmann, S. M., Davis, H. T., Jader, L. R., Lefebvre, P. A., Sadowsky, M. J., Schendel, F. J., von Keitz, M. G., & Valentas, K. J. (2010). Hydrothermal carbonization of microalgae. *Biomass and Bioenergy, 34*(6), 875–882. https://doi.org/10.1016/j.biombioe.2010.01.032
Huang, H., & Yuan, X. (2015). Recent progress in the direct liquefaction of typical biomass. *Progress in Energy and Combustion Science, 49*, 59–80.
Huber, G. W., & Dumesic, J. A. (2006). An overview of aqueous-phase catalytic processes for production of hydrogen and alkanes in a biorefinery. *Catalysis Today, 111*, 119–132.
Huber, G. W., Iborra, S., & Corma, A. (2006). Synthesis of Transportation Fuels from Biomass: Chemistry, Catalysts, and Engineering. *Chemical Reviews, 106*, 4044–4098.
Hussain, A., & Anastasakis, K. (2025). Technoeconomic evaluation of integrating hydrothermal liquefaction in wastewater treatment plants. *Bioresource Technology, 419*, Article 132030. https://doi.org/10.1016/j.biortech.2024.132030
Jones, S.B., Zhu, Y., Anderson, D.B., Hallen, R.T., Elliott, D.C., Schmidt, A.J., Albrecht, K.O., Hart, T.R., Butcher, M.G., Drennan. C., Snowden-Swan, L.J. (2014). Process design and economics for the conversion of algal biomass to hydrocarbons: whole algae hydrothermal liquefaction and upgrading (No. PNNL-23227). Pacific Northwest National Lab. (PNNL), Richland, WA (United States).
Joshi, T., Parkash, O., & Krishan, G. (2022). Computational fluid dynamics (CFD) simulation of slurry flow in a pipeline with suspended particles. *Particuology, 60*, 58–67.

Juneja, A., Kumar, D., Tumuluru, J.H. (2018). Hydrothermal Liquefaction a Promising Technology for High Moisture Bioma SS Conversion Bookbiomass Preprocessing and Pretreatments for Production of Biofuels. 1st Edition Imprint, CRC Press, 25p. eBook ISBN9781315153735.
Kilgore, U.J., Subramaniam, S., Fox, S.P., Cronin, D.J., Guo, M.F., Schmidt, A.J., Ramasamy, K.K., Thorson, M.R. Wet air oxidation of HTL aqueous waste. *Biomass Bioenergy 176* (2023), Article 106889.
Knorr, D., Lukas, J., Schoen, P. (2013). Production of advanced biofuels via liquefaction - hydrothermal liquefaction reactor design, NREL/SR-5100–60462. *National Renewable Energy Laboratory, Golden, CO.*
Lababpour, A., & Patel, S. (2015). Process simulation and techno-economic analysis of lignocellulosic ethanol production. *Fuel, 148*, 183–192.
Li, C., Wang, Y., Xie, S., Wang, R., Sheng, H., Yang, H., & Yuan, Z. (2024). Synergistic treatment of sewage sludge and food waste digestate residues for efficient energy recovery and biochar preparation by hydrothermal pretreatment, anaerobic digestion, and pyrolysis. *Applied Energy, 364*, Article 123203. https://doi.org/10.1016/j.apenergy.2024.123203
Libra, J. A., Ro, K. S., Kammann, C., Funke, A., Berge, N. D., Neubauer, Y., Titirici, M.-M., Fühner, C., Bens, O., & Kern, J. (2011). *Biofuels, 2*, 71–76.
Liiv, J., Mäeorg, U., Vaino, N., Rikmann, E. (2024). The role of negative emissions technologies in 2050 Decarbonation PathwaysSci. Tech. Energ. *Transition 79*(3), 8p. https://doi.org/10.2516/stet/2023043.
Macedo, H.E., et al. (2022). Distribution and characteristics of wastewater treatment plants within the global river network. *Earth Syst Sci Data 14* (2), 559–577
Mahssin, Z.Y. et al. (2021). Converting biomass into bio-asphalt - a review IOP Conf. Ser. Earth Environ Sci 682 (1), https://doi.org/10.1088/1755-1315/682/1/012066.
Mathimani, T., Baldinelli, A., Rajendran, K., Prabakar, D., Matheswaran, M., van Leeuwen, R. P., & Pugazhendhi, A. (2019). Review on cultivation and thermochemical conversion of microalgae to fuels and chemicals: Process evaluation and knowledge gaps. *Journal of Cleaner Production, 208*, 1053–1064. https://doi.org/10.1016/j.jclepro.2018.10.096
Miranda, A.M., Hernandez-Tenorio, F., Ocampo, D., Vargas, G.J., Sáez, A.A. (2022). Trends on CO2 capture with microalgae: a bibliometric analysis. *Molecules 27* (15), 1–14, https://doi.org/10.3390/molecules27154669.
Mishra, R. K., Kumar, V., Kumar, P., & Mohanty, K. (2022). Hydrothermal liquefaction of biomass for bio-crude production: A review on feedstocks, chemical compositions, operating parameters, reaction kinetics, techno-economic study, and life cycle assessment. *Fuel, 316*, Article 123377. https://doi.org/10.1016/j.fuel.2022.123377
Mukundan, S., Xuan, J., Dann, S.E., Wagner, J.L. (2022). Highly active and magnetically recoverable heterogeneous catalyst for hydrothermal liquefaction of biomass into high quality bio-oil. *Bioresour Technol 369*, Article 128479, https://doi.org/10.1016/j.biortech.2022.128479.
Nadarajah, K., Rodriguez-Narvaez, O.M., Ramirez, J., Bandala, E.R., Goonetilleke, A. (2024). Lab-scale engineered hydrochar production and techno-economic scaling-up analysis. *Waste Management 174*, 568–574, ISSN 0956–053X, https://doi.org/10.1016/j.wasman.2023.12.024.
Nallasivam, J. et al. (2021). Valorization of red macroalgae biomass via hydrothermal liquefaction using homogeneous catalysts. *Bioresour Technol 346*, Article 126515, https://doi.org/10.1016/j.biortech.2021.126515.
Nigam, P. S., & Singh, A. (2011). Production of liquid biofuels from renewable resources. *Progress in Energy and Combustion Science, 37*, 52–68.
Obaideen, K., Shehata, N., Sayed, E.T., Abdelkareem, M.A., Mahmoud, M.S., Olabi, A.G. (2022). The role of wastewater treatment in achieving sustainable development goals (SDGs) and sustainability guideline Energy. *Nexus 7,* Article 100112.
Ocampo, E., Beltrán, V. V., Gómez, E. A., Ríos, L. A., & Ocampo, D. (2023). Hydrothermal liquefaction process: Review and trends. *Current Research in Green and Sustainable Chemistry, 7*, Article 100382. https://doi.org/10.1016/j.crgsc.2023.100382

Osorio, A., Gómez, E., Ocampo, D., & Rios, L. A. (2019). Solvothermal liquefaction of acacia wood (acacia mangium). *Inf Tecnol, 30*(2), 211–222. https://doi.org/10.4067/S0718-07642019000200211

Peterson, A. A., Vogel, F., Lachance, R. P., Fröling, M., Antal, M. J., Jr., & Tester, J. W. (2008). Thermochemical biofuel production in hydrothermal media: A review of sub- and supercritical water technologies. *Energy & Environmental Science, 1*, 32.

Prestigiacomo, C., Costa, P., Pinto, F., Schiavo, B., Siragusa, A., Scialdone, O., & Galia, A. (2019). Sewage sludge as cheap alternative to microalgae as feedstock of catalytic hydrothermal liquefaction processes. *Journal of Supercritical Fluids, 143*, 251–258.

Qadir, M., et al. (2020). Global and regional potential of wastewater as a water, nutrient and energy source. In: Natural resources forum. Wiley Online Library.

Ranganathan, S. V., & Savithri, S. (2015). Two-dimensional CFD modeling of hydrothermal liquefaction of sewage sludge. *Journal of Supercritical Fluids, 97*, 22–30.

Rojas, M., Manrique, R., Hornung, U., Funke, A., Mullen, C. A., Chejne, F., & Maya, J. C. (2025). Advances and challenges on hydrothermal processes for biomass conversion: Feedstock flexibility, products, and modeling approaches. *Biomass and Bioenergy, 194*, Article 107621. https://doi.org/10.1016/j.biombioe.2025.107621

Ruiz, H. A., Rodríguez-Jasso, R. M., Fernandes, B. D., Vicente, A. A., & Teixeira, J. A. (2013). Hydrothermal processing, as an alternative for upgrading agriculture residues and marine biomass according to the biorefinery concept: A review. *Renewable and Sustainable Energy Reviews, 21*, 35–51.

Scarsella, M., de Caprariis, B., Damizia, M., & De Filippis, P. (2020). Heterogeneous catalysts for hydrothermal liquefaction of lignocellulosic biomass: A review. *Biomass and Bioenergy, 140*, Article 105662.

Seiple, T. E., Coleman, A. M., & Skaggs, R. L. (2017). Municipal wastewater sludge as a sustainable bioresource in the United States. *Journal of Environmental Management, 197*, 673–680.

Seiple, T. E., Skaggs, R. L., Fillmore, L., & Coleman, A. M. (2020). Municipal wastewater sludge as a renewable, cost-effective feedstock for transportation biofuels using hydrothermal liquefaction. *Journal of Environmental Management, 270*, Article 110852.

Shah, A. A., Sharma, K., Haider, M. S., Toor, S. S., Rosendahl, L. A., Pedersen, T. H., & Castello, D. (2022). The role of catalysts in biomass hydrothermal liquefaction and biocrude upgrading. *Processes, 10*(2), 207. https://doi.org/10.3390/pr10020207

Shahir, S. A., Masjuki, H. H., Kalam, M. A., Imran, A., Fattah, I. M. R., & Sanjid, A. (2014). Feasibility of diesel–biodiesel–ethanol/bioethanol blend as existing CI engine fuel: An assessment of properties, material compatibility, safety and combustion. *Renewable and Sustainable Energy Reviews, 32*, 379–395.

Shanmugam, S. R., Adhikari, S., & Shakya, R. (2017). Nutrient removal and energy production from aqueous phase of bio-oil generated via hydrothermal liquefaction of algae. *Bioresource Technology, 230*, 43–48. https://doi.org/10.1016/j.biortech.2017.01.031

Singh, R., Prakash, A., Balagurumurthy, B., Bhaskar, T. (2015). Hydrothermal liquefaction of biomass. *Recent Adv. Thermochem Convers Biomass*, 269-291, https://doi.org/10.1016/B978-0-444-63289-0.00010-7

Snowden-Swan, L.J., Zhu, Y., Bearden, M.D., Seiple, T.E., Jones, S.B., Schmidt, A.J., Billing, J.M., Hallen, R.T., Hart, T.R., Liu, J., Albrecht, K.O., Fox, S.P., Maupin, G.D., Elliott, D.C. (2017). Conceptual Biorefinery Design and Research Targeted for 2022: Hydrothermal Liquefaction Processing of Wet Waste to Fuels (No. PNNL-27186). Pacific Northwest National Lab. (PNNL), Richland, WA (United States).

Snowden-Swan, L.J., Billing, J.M., Thorson, M.R., Schmidt, A.J., Jiang, Y., Santosa, D.M., Seiple, T.E., Daniel, R.C., Burns, C.A.M., Li, S. (2020). Wet Waste Hydrothermal Liquefaction and Biocrude Upgrading to Hydrocarbon Fuels: 2020 State of Technology; Pacific Northwest National Lab. (PNNL): Richland, WA, USA, 2021.

Thomsen, L. B. S., Anastasakis, K., & Biller, P. (2024). Hydrothermal liquefaction potential of wastewater treatment sludges: Effect of w astewater treatment plant and sludge nature on products distribution. *Fuel, 355*, Article 129525. https://doi.org/10.1016/j.fuel.2023.129525
Toor, S. S., Rosendahl, L., & Rudolf, A. (2011). Hydrothermal liquefaction of biomass: A review of subcritical water technologies. *Energy, 36*, 2328–2342.
Usman, M., Cheng, S., Boonyubol, S., & Cross, J. S. (2024). From biomass to biocrude: Innovations in hydrothermal liquefaction and upgrading. *Energy Conversion and Management, 302*, Article 118093. https://doi.org/10.1016/j.enconman.2024.118093
Vadlamudi, D.P., Lei, X.G., Goldfarb, J.L., Tester, J.W. (2024). Wet oxidation of aqueous phase byproducts from uncatalyzed and acid-catalyzed hydrothermal liquefaction of manure. *Chemical Engineering Journal 498*, Article 155524.
Vardon, D. R., Sharma, B., Scott, J., Yu, G., Wang, Z., Schideman, L., Zhang, Y., & Strathmann, T. J. (2011). Chemical properties of biocrude oil from the hydrothermal liquefaction of Spirulina algae, swine manure, and digested anaerobic sludge. *Bioresource Technology, 102*, 8295–8303.
Vitoria, F.C., Leme, V.F.C., Lopez, K., Costa, T., Conerty, B., Leonelli, L.B., Zhang, Y., Davidson, P.C. (2025). Hydrothermal liquefaction aqueous phase my core mediation to increase inorganic nitrogen availability. *Heliyon 10*(11), 2024, e31992, ISSN 2405–8440, https://doi.org/10.1016/j.heliyon.2024.e31992.
Watson, S.B., J., Aierzhati, A., Yang, L., Liu, Z., Zhang, Y. (2019). Biohythane production of post-hydrothermal liquefaction wastewater: a comparison of two-stage fermentation and catalytic hydrothermal gasification. *Bioresour Technol 274*, 335–342.
Wei, Y. et al. (2022). Synergistic citric acid-surfactant catalyzed hydrothermal liquefaction of pomelo peel for production of hydrocarbon-rich bio-oil Sci. *Total Environ 857*, Article 159235, https://doi.org/10.1016/j.scitotenv.2022.159235.
Wodołażski, A., & Smoliński, A. (2025). Optimization study of hydrothermal liquefaction sewage sludge to biocrude oil in continuous multiphase plug flow reactor. *Processes, 13*(4), 976. https://doi.org/10.3390/pr13040976
Xiao, L. P., Sun, Z. J., Shi, Z. J., Xu, F., & Sun, R. C. (2013). Impact of hot compressed water pretreatment on the structural features and the enzymatic hydrolysis of lignin. *Industrial Crops and Products, 50*, 657–664.
Xu, Y., Edmundson, S., Zhu, Y., Hart, T., Cronin, D., Fox, S., Schmidt, A., Valdez, P. (2024). 2023 Business case study: hydrothermal liquefaction of algal bloom biomass. PNNL-35507. https://doi.org/10.2172/2482043.
Xue, Y., Chen, H., Zhao, W., Yang, C., Ma, P., & Han, S. (2016). A review on the operating conditions of producing bio-oil from hydrothermal liquefaction of biomass. *International Journal of Energy Research, 40*, 865–877.
Yang, J., He, Q. (Sophia), Yang, L. (2019). A review on hydrothermal co-liquefaction of biomass. *Appl Energy 250*, 926–945.
Yang, C., Wang, S., Jiang, Z., Li, J., He, C., Xu, T., & Xu, D. (2022). Catalytic hydrotreatment upgrading of biocrude oil derived from hydrothermal liquefaction of animal carcass. *Fuel, 317*, Article 123528. https://doi.org/10.1016/j.fuel.2022.123528
Yang, C., Wang, S., Yang, J., Xu, D., Li, Y., Li, J., & Zhang, Y. (2020). Hydrothermal liquefaction and gasification of biomass and model compounds: A review. *Green Chemistry, 22*, 8210–8232.
Yang, J., Caldwell, C., Corscadden, K., He, Q. S., & Li, J. (2016). An evaluation of biodiesel production from Camelina sativa grown in Nova. *Scotia Ind Crops Prod, 81*, 162–168.
Yang, L., He, Q. S., Corscadden, K., & Udenigwe, C. C. (2015). The prospects of Jerusalem artichoke in functional food ingredients and bioenergy production. *Biotechnol Rep, 5*, 77–88.
Zhang, Y., Chen, W.T. 2017. Hydrothermal Liquefaction of Protein-Containing Feedstocks, 2 Elsevier Ltd., https://doi.org/10.1016/B978-0-08-101029-7.00004-7.
Zhang, B., Biswal, B. K., Zhang, J., & Balasubramanian, R. (2023). Hydrothermal treatment of biomass feedstocks for sustainable production of chemicals, fuels, and materials: Progress and perspectives. *Chemical Reviews, 123*(11), 7193–7294. https://doi.org/10.1021/acs.chemrev.2c00673

Zhu, Y., Albrecht, K. O., Elliott, D. C., Hallen, R. T., & Jones, S. B. (2013). Development of hydrothermal liquefaction and upgrading technologies for lipid-extracted algae conversion to liquid fuels. *Algal Research, 2*(4), 455–464. https://doi.org/10.1016/j.algal.2013.07.003

Chapter 10
Renewable Natural Gas (RNG) from Biomethane: Production and Applications, Production Processes for RNG from Biomethane. Applications and Benefits of RNG, Market Trends and Regulatory Considerations

Mohamed A. Hassaan, Khouloud M. Barakat, and Ahmed El Nemr

Abstract Derived from improved biomethane, renewable natural gas (RNG) is a carbon–neutral energy source essential for decarbonizing industries that are difficult to electrify. The manufacturing processes described in this chapter include gasification of woody biomass and anaerobic digestion of organic waste, which are followed by purification (e.g., pressure swing adsorption and water scrubbing). Case studies like the EU's "Green Gas Initiative" demonstrate market acceptance. Applications include grid injection, industrial heat, and transportation fuel (such as CNG automobiles). The role that regulatory frameworks like the EU RED II and the U.S. Renewable Fuel Standard (RFS) play in providing incentives for RNG projects is reviewed. Emerging trends, including decentralized, modular systems and hydrogen-RNG blends, are being investigated as potential answers to the problems of high upgrading costs and feedstock unpredictability. The chapter ends with a plan for growing RNG to reach net-zero goals.

Keywords Biomethane · Renewable natural gas (RNG) · Decarbonizing · Woody biomass · Anaerobic digestion · Organic waste · Green gas initiative · Hydrogen-RNG

M. A. Hassaan (✉) · K. M. Barakat · A. El Nemr
National Institute of Oceanography and Fisheries (NIOF), Kayet Bey, Elanfoushy, Alexandria, Egypt
e-mail: mhss95@mail.com

P. Verma (ed.), *Sustainable Practices in Biorefinery*,
https://doi.org/10.1007/978-981-95-6071-4_10

10.1 Introduction

10.1.1 RNG as a Carbon-Negative Energy Carrier

Biomethane referred to as renewable natural gas (RNG), is a renewable fuel derived from biogas that has been refined to a level comparable to that of fossil natural gas and contains 90% or more methane (Al Mamun & Torii, 2017). The RNG may be distributed via the current gas pipeline infrastructure since biogas has a high enough methane concentration once carbon dioxide and other contaminants are removed. RNG can be utilized in existing appliances, including natural gas-powered cars (Usman et al., 2022). Anaerobic digestion is the most popular method of gathering biogas to produce biomethane. Anaerobic digestion facilities can be purpose-built wastewater treatment plants or facilities that break down manure or organic waste from homes. Another result of organic materials breaking down in landfills is biogas.

Additionally, RNG can be generated by mechanizing hydrogen and carbon dioxide/monoxide using the Sabatier method, bio-methanolation, or electrochemical cells that resemble fuel cell (Newswire, 2018). Methanating carbon dioxide from carbon capture facilities or synthetic gas (syngas), which is created when wood or other lignocellulosic materials are gasified, can be accomplished using these methods. These RNG-creation techniques are still in the beginning stages and account for a very tiny percentage of global production.

10.1.2 Global RNG Production Capacity and Incentive Programs

Despite being a relatively new business, renewable natural gas (RNG) is expanding quickly because of its advantages for the environment and government backing. The global RNG market is expected to expand at a compound annual growth rate (CAGR) of 25% between 2024 and 2030, reaching $12 billion (Akbari & Kumar, 2024). Demand for new renewable energy sources is raising due to governments worldwide establishing aggressive goals for renewable energy. RNG is a clean and renewable energy source that can assist in achieving these goals. Additionally, governments are offering a range of incentives, including: grants tax credits, and subsidies to promote the production and use of RNG. RNG is becoming more accessible and appealing to producers and consumers due to these incentives.

Lastly, improvements in RNG production technology are making the process more economical and efficient. As a result, RNG is becoming a more appealing substitute for fossil natural gas. Notwithstanding the market's potential for expansion, several issues must be resolved: high production costs and the cost of feedstock and equipment contribute to the continued relatively high cost of RNG manufacturing. Limited infrastructure: RNG still has a relatively small infrastructure, especially regarding storage and shipping (Usman et al., 2022).

Public awareness: many people are unaware of RNG's advantages. Because of this, it is challenging to generate demand for the fuel. Despite these obstacles, the RNG business has several development prospects: By broadening the feedstock base, RNG's feedstock base can be broadened to encompass a range of sources, including landfill gas, industrial wastewater, and food waste from homes. As a result, RNG will become more widely available and reasonably priced. Furthermore, new RNG applications are being developed. RNG can be utilized for several purposes, such as heating, power generation, and transportation. As a result, the fuel is finding new markets. Entering new markets: although the RNG market is still tiny, it could grow significantly over the next several years. New players in the market are benefiting from this. In the coming years, the worldwide RNG market will have the potential to expand considerably, making it a promising business. Growing demand for renewable energy, government assistance, and improvements in RNG manufacturing technology are driving the market (Zhang et al., 2025).

10.2 Production Processes

The fuel known as Renewable Natural Gas (RNG) is derived from a range of waste materials. Anaerobic digestion, thermal gasification, or power-to-gas technologies capture biogas as that waste decomposes. The biogas is converted into biomethane after removing carbon dioxide, hydrogen sulfide, and other gases (Kumar & Samadder, 2020). Biomethane can be pumped into natural gas distribution networks or consumed locally, and it is completely interchangeable with natural gas (Fig. 10.1).

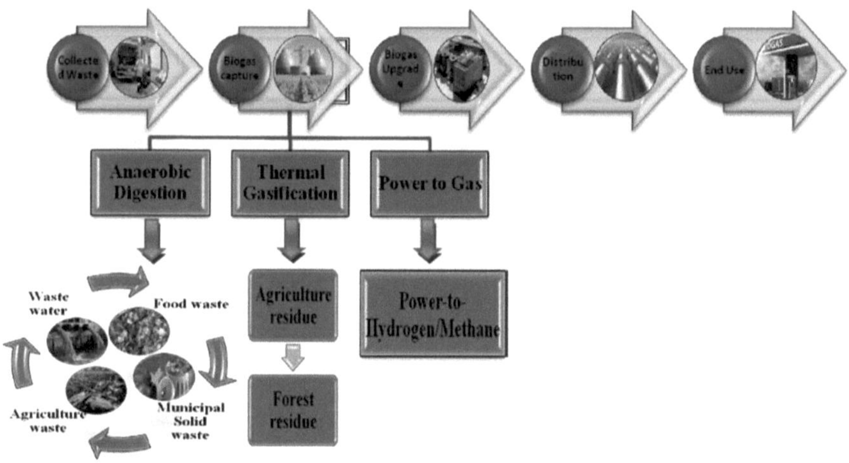

Fig. 10.1 Biomethane or RNG production process

10.2.1 Anaerobic Digestion

A biological activity called anaerobic digestion occurs when bacteria break down biodegradable materials without oxygen. Most biogas comprises methane (CH_4) and carbon dioxide (CO_2). There are two stages to the anaerobic fermentation process used to create biogas (HoSt): (1) Hydrolysis phase: Organic matter is converted to carbon dioxide, fatty acids, and hydrogen. (2) The methanogenic phase, during which methane is produced by breaking fatty acids (Archana et al., 2024). Proper mixing, a continual process of adding organic matter to the digester and removing the processed waste, and suitable conditions like temperature, pH, N balance, etc., are necessary for a stable anaerobic fermentation process.

10.2.1.1 Wet versus Dry Digestion Systems

Anaerobic digestion methods for treating biodegradable wastes can be divided into two categories: (1) Systems for wet anaerobic digestion that employ organic compounds with a dry matter content of no more than 10–20%.

(2) Systems of dry anaerobic digestion for materials including at least 20–40% dry matter. The dry matter content determines whether dry digestion or wet digestion should be used for the organic fermentation (Subbarao et al., 2023).

In full-scale applications, dry digestion can be carried out in a continuous or discontinuous system. Because of biogas production's sequential loading and unloading phases, dry digestion is considered discontinuous. Over time, several digesters will work in tandem to continuously produce biogas. Over time, several digesters will work in tandem to continuously produce biogas.

Advantages of Dry Digestion:

- Very tolerant system for impurities (sand, fibers, big particles, etc.);
- Dry matter/total solids 20–40% as opposed to the maximum of 20% for wet digestion.
- Low power and heat requirements;
- Mobile biogas plants (containers) are possible;
- Multiple digesters can be managed concurrently;
- Less critical equipment (pumps, agitation systems, feeding equipment) is needed;
- land-applied solid digestate that resembles manure is produced;
- Less water is needed;
- Less maintenance is needed;
- The system is simpler than wet AD systems;
- Different substrates are used per digester unit.

Drawbacks of Dry Digestion:

- It requires special technologies for digester loading and unloading;
- It involves the management of biogas and heat production variation;
- It is not completely mixed;

- In discontinuous systems, the microbial process must begin for each batch;
- it usually produces fewer methane production than wet AD systems;
- It usually requires a lot of structural material (much digester space is consumed for structure material).

Using a wet digester to process dry biomass has several benefits. Wet anaerobic digestion's primary benefit is its ability to produce huge amounts of biogas through ideal mixing. The investment and operational expenses are cheaper than a dry anaerobic digestion system. The lightest particles that stay on the surface and the inert particles that flow will separate during dry matter fermentation in a wet digester.

Wet digesters have the following benefits:

- More versatility in terms of the materials to be handled;
- Minimal startup and running costs;
- Integrated biological desulphurization

Wet digesters have the following drawbacks:

- Must add liquid to lower the mixture's dry matter;
- Needs expensive and sturdy mixing equipment;
- Requires a large amount of energy from the facility to run pumps and agitators;
- Produces wet digestate that can alter land application procedures and result in additional investments.

A dry anaerobic digestion system is recommended when the introduced biomass comprises many non-biodegradable elements, such as synthetic materials or more than 10% sand. This is true for green waste (more than 20% sand and some household waste).

10.2.1.2 RIN and Co-Digestion of Agricultural and Food Waste

The long-awaited Set Rule final text for the U.S. Environmental Protection Agency's Renewable Fuel Standard (RFS) went on scale in late June 2023. Other significant changes affecting the biogas and renewable natural gas (RNG) industries were kept in place, even if the pathway for the creation of Renewable Identification Number (RIN) credits linked to renewable power and car charging (eRINs) was eliminated. The allocation of RINs between D3 and D5 RINs is one of those significant changes. This means that digesters can now continue to produce D3 RINs using biogas or RNG from wastewater or manure, and they can also produce D5 RINs using any extra biogas or RNG that is created from accepting and co-digesting food waste. As a result, digesters can collect D3 RIN revenue, which was previously impossible (Rowan et al., 2022).

10.2.2 Thermochemical Conversion

Agricultural biomass, kitchen trash, cattle dung, and microalgae—which are made up of soluble saccharide, lignocellulose, protein, and fats—are the four primary groups into which biomass resources can be divided (Brosowski et al., 2019). Among the resources listed above, agricultural biomass is used the most since it has the simplest elements (Mao et al., 2019). Thermochemical conversion is a practical and often investigated method of turning biomass into biofuels. It can eliminate undesirable byproducts and produce a high selectivity of desired products by optimizing process parameters and adding additives (Jha et al., 2022; Seo et al., 2022). However, the carbon loss from changing land use should be considered when accounting for net carbon gains properly. The carbon sequestration lost directly and indirectly due to land-use change must be surpassed by the carbon produced by replacing fossil fuels to make a carbon benefit (IPCC, 2022; Mishra et al., 2022). A segmentation of the thermochemical processes by which biomass could contribute to the energy mix of the future is shown schematically in Fig. 10.2.

Thermochemical conversion involves obtaining biomass-producing solid fuel and burning it to power a steam cycle, generating electricity (National Grid Live, 2022). Torrefaction, liquefaction, pyrolysis, and gasification are the thermochemical conversion processes of biomass that can yield syngas, charcoal, and bio-oil.

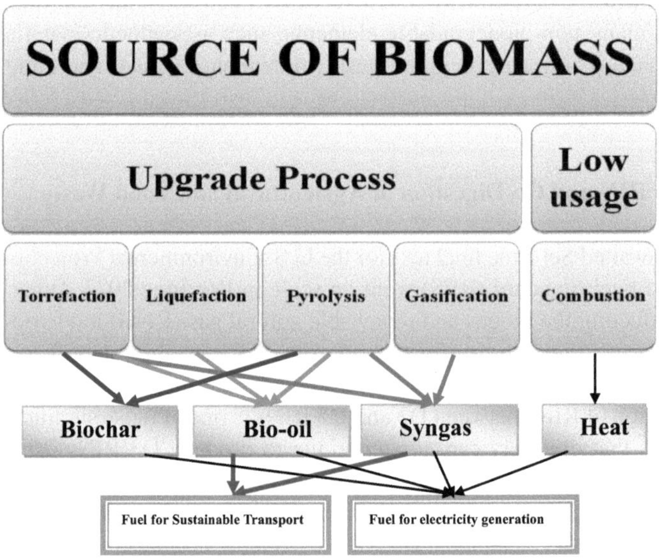

Fig. 10.2 Diagram showing the potential routes for integrating biomass into the future energy mix is called "Biomass Thermochemical Conversion."

10.2.2.1 Gasification of Woody Biomass and Syngas Cleaning

One of the best processes for turning biomass into various energy forms is biomass gasification. Gasification is the process by which biomass is partially oxidized at high temperatures to produce syngas. To transform biomass's biological makeup—which includes proteins, fats, and carbohydrates—into syngas that contains alkane hydrocarbons like: CO, H_2, CH_4, C_mH_n, and others, gasification technology relies on a series of basic reactions, including dehydration, pyrolysis/devolatilization, and gasification (Ai et al., 2022). Depending on the reactor and parametric conditions, gasification has 70% to 90% conversion efficiency (Pinto et al., 2017). Because syngas from biomass gasification are easier to transport and store than solids, their uses are more efficient and cleaner than those of direct burning (Razmi et al., 2021). Figure 10.3 illustrates the use of syngas from biomass gasification. Due to its about 30% lower energy density than natural gas, syngas is not suitable for distribution. But it can also make other chemicals like petroleum, methanol, synthetic natural gas, and fuel for cars and fuel cells (Rauch et al., 2014).

In recent years, biogasification technology has advanced quickly as a new energy development technology, and several investigations in this field have been carried out by numerous international and national researchers (Gao et al., 2023). Most of these researches concentrated on how the performance of gasification reaction was affected by the biomass feedstock and gasification parameters (Couto et al., 2013). Few studies summarize the effects of feedstock properties, gasification parameters, and gasifier

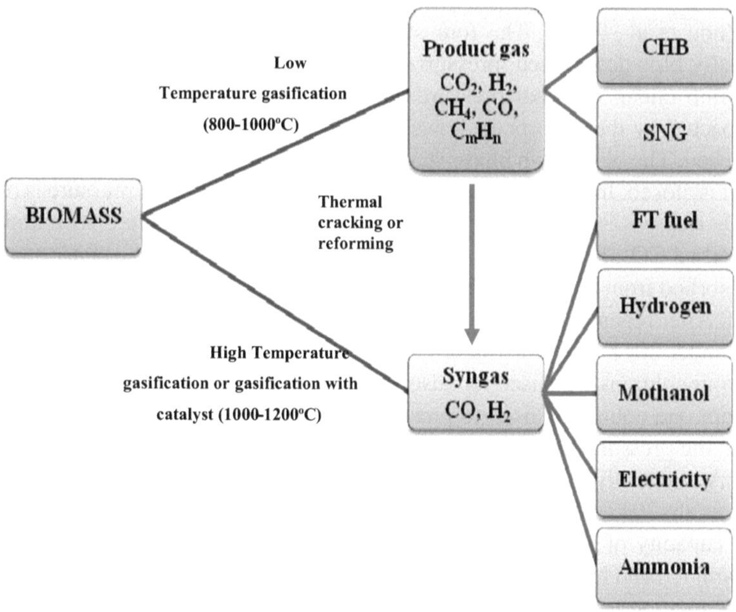

Fig. 10.3 Applications of biomass gasification to syngas

use although it is well recognized that the concentration, yield, quality, and features of each syngas component in the biomass gasification process are significant for downstream applications (Gu et al., 2019).

10.2.3 Upgrading Technologies

Nowadays, pressure swing adsorption, amine absorption, water scrubbing absorption, physical absorption, cryogenic, and membrane are the most widely used technologies to improve biogas. According to Angelidaki et al. (2018), approximately 35% of the current facilities use water-scrubbing to create biogas, followed by pressure swing adsorption (30%) and amine absorption (23%).

10.2.3.1 Pressure Swing Adsorption (PSA) vs. Water Scrubbing

Contact between the gas molecules and the adsorbent is used in a dry process known as pressure swing adsorption to separate the gases. To maximise gas-adsorbent interaction, porous materials with high specific areas are used as adsorbents. The most often used adsorbents are either kinetic type, which adsorbs CO_2 more quickly than CH_4 because of managed diffusion rates, or equilibrium form, which adsorbs a much bigger load of CO_2. Activated carbons, carbon molecular sieves (CMS), titanosilicates, silica gels, and natural and manufactured zeolites are frequently utilized materials (Zhou et al., 2011). The four stages of a pressure swing adsorption system are usually blowdown, feed, pressurization and purge. The raw gas is injected into the column under 5–10 bar pressure during the feed phase. While CH_4, which is not impacted by the adsorbent, flows through the column, CO_2 is adsorbed in the column bed. The blowdown phase starts when the column bed is filled with CO_2 and the inlet is closed. In order to desorb CO_2 from the adsorbent, the pressure is reduced and CO_2-rich gas is discharged from the column. Some methane is lost along with the desorbed CO_2. Lastly, at the lowest column pressure, the purge phase starts. The CO_2 desorbed from the column bed is extracted by blowing upgraded gas through the column. After regeneration, the column is repressurised with either raw or improved gas (Grande, 2011). As illustrated in Fig. 10.4, a PSA system typically comprises two to four columns, one used for adsorption and the others for regeneration. The gas flow from one column is used to pressurize another column during the blow-down phase in the pressure equalization phase. To lessen methane loss, these columns are joined. Additionally, this phenomenon lowers energy usage throughout the process (Imtiaz et al., 2022).

The capacity of the methods above to convert biogas into fuel-grade methane was examined and highlighted in numerous research published in the literature. One practical method for upgrading biogas to high-purity biomethane is pressure swing adsorption (PSA). Using a special plate design, Ali et al. (2022) investigated the efficiency of the pressure swing adsorption process to upgrade a biogas mixture

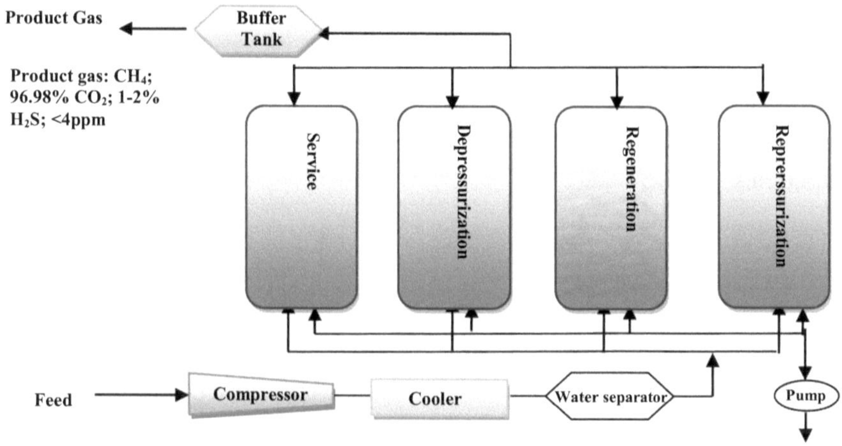

Fig. 10.4 Upgrade pressure swing adsorption system to improve biogas Product

consisting of 30% CO_2 and 70% CH_4 to promote the traditional PSA system's operation under non-adiabatic/non-isothermal circumstances. The concept could achieve 97 percent biomethane quality with a specific energy demand of 0.1052 kW/mole CH_4 at ambient temperature and system pressure of 2 bar. Ferella et al. (2017) used pressure swing adsorption over zeolite and activated carbon to improve biogas at low bed pressure. They found that 98% of the biomethane was pure and less than 5% leaked into the waste stream. Liu et al. (2011) upgraded biogas that included 50% CO_2 and 50% CH_4 using a simulation of a vacuum-pressure swing adsorption system. Their process used 0.22 kWh/kg of specific energy to produce 96.9% recovered and 99.4% pure biomethane.

Water scrubbing, one of the most well-known and widely used procedures, removes H_2S and CO_2 from raw gas since these gases dissolve more easily in water than CH_4. Water is supplied to the counter once the gas comes up from the bottom of the column, and the working pressure for water scrubbing is 10 bar (Wantz et al., 2022). As seen in Fig. 10.5, the raw gas is delivered to the bottom of the absorption column at a temperature of 35 to 40 °C and an operating pressure of 10 bar. Water is typically added at the top of the column to enhance the gas–liquid contact area, and the bottom is generally packed randomly. To ensure maximum efficiency, liquid and gas must flow counter currently. Water absorbs CO_2 and a negligible amount of CH_4. Compared to CH_4, CO_2 is more soluble in water, which significantly impacts process selectivity (Imtiaz et al., 2022). The pressure in a flash column is lowered to 3 bar to minimize the methane that escapes into the off-gas stream from the water scrubber. Wastewater thoroughly saturated with H_2S, CO_2, and a small amount of CH_4 upon exiting the scrubber's bottom is returned to the absorption column after being restored (Abatzoglou & Boivin, 2009). Regeneration is accomplished through desorption column's air stripping and lowering pressure. If the H_2S content is significant, stripping air is not advised since the water rapidly becomes sulphur-impacted,

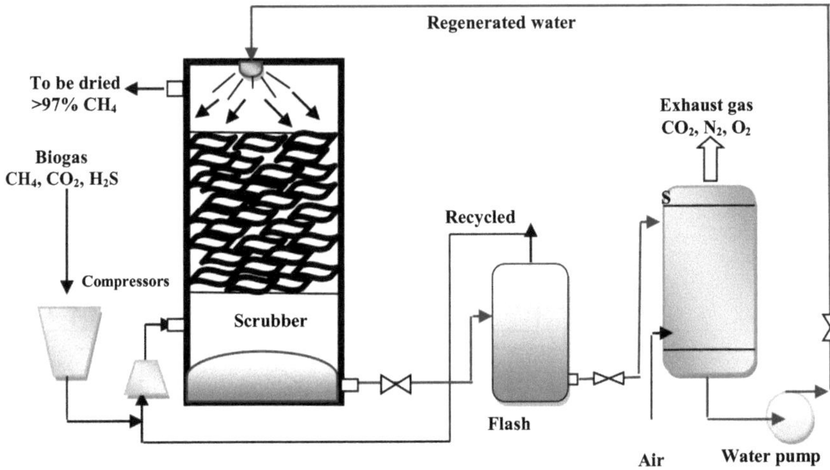

Fig. 10.5 Upgrade Water scrubbing system to improve biogas product

leading to corrosion and operational problems. If an inexpensive water source is available, using fresh water is advised. When there is a significant concentration of H_2S, pre-removal of H_2S is required during the water scrubbing process (Sun et al., 2015). Rotunno et al. (2017) assessed the technology's ability to upgrade biogas mixtures with 40% CO_2 and 60% CH_4 to the fuel of vehicle. They verified that water-scrubbing absorption is a viable method for producing biomethane from raw biogas with an energy efficiency of 89.8% and a purity of 98.1%.

10.2.3.2 Membrane Separation for CO_2 Removal

At a specific pressure, high permeability gases—such as those with small molecular sizes and low affinity—can pass through the membrane, whereas low permeability gases are retained. This is how membrane permeation is designed (Imtiaz et al., 2022). Low permeability CH_4 is retained and recovered at the hollow column's end, but high permeable pollutants, including O_2, CO_2,and H_2O, flow as penetrate through the membrane, as seen in Fig. 10.6. Haider et al. (2016) investigated different membrane types for raise a biogas mixture with 70% CH_4 and 30% CO_2 under varying system pressures. They achieved a 97% purity rate for biomethane with an accurate energy consumption of 0.22 kWh/Nm3 of the untreated biogas.

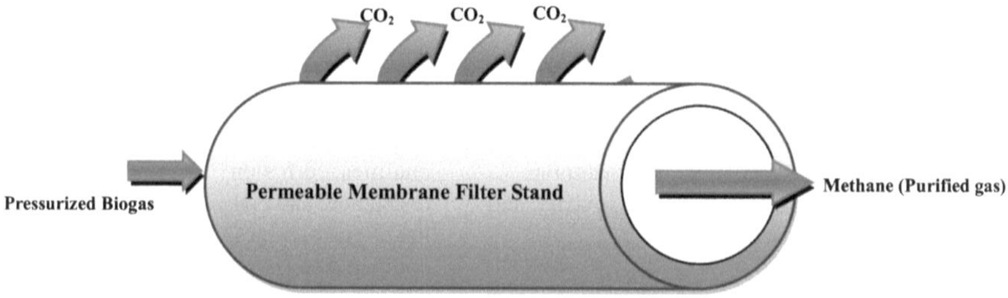

Fig. 10.6 Membrane separation diagram for CO_2 removal and purified methane obtained

10.3 Technological Challenges

10.3.1 Impurity Removal (H_2O, CO2, H_2S, VOCs)

Biogas, which is mostly composed of carbon dioxide and methane with a number of contaminants such water vapor (H_2O), siloxanes, NH_3, and volatile organic compounds (VOC), It is generated by anaerobic digestion of wastewater or biodegradable waste (Wasajja et al., 2020). The kind of biomass supplied to the digester that generates biogas and the source of its feedstock have an impact on the biogas composition (Papurello et al., 2016; Saadabadi et al., 2019). These pollutants have an adverse effect on biogas conversion devices and have negatively impact on the environment and human health as emissions when they are present in excess of their threshold values (Table 10.1) (Werkneh et al., 2022).

After methane, which is created in certain stages of the production of biogas process, biogas main constituent is carbon dioxide (CO_2). Because its composition in raw biogas depends on several operating variables, including temperature, pressure, and digester liquid content, CO_2 can be used by methanogenic microbes to operate as an electron acceptor (Atelge et al., 2021). When water and CO_2 are combined, carbonic acid is created, and harms processed apparatus (Deng et al., 2020). Carbon dioxide from biogas was extracted from raw biogas inflow using removal technologies to concentrate methane. While the maturity of carbon dioxide separation technologies varies greatly, they are categorized based on the physical–chemical processes that were employed to separate them (Hoyer et al., 2016). Some techniques have the advantage of concurrently eliminating carbon dioxide and other contaminants, while others necessitate a pretreatment unit to eliminate biogas contaminants.

PSA and water scrubbing (primarily at higher pH) remove both hydrogen sulfide and carbon dioxide simultaneously, whereas chemical scrubbing and membrane separation methods require a pre-treatment step to remove hydrogen sulfide using amines before carbon dioxide separation and are crucial to preventing membrane poisoning (Nguyen et al., 2021). The pre-treated biogas can be further processed to remove carbon dioxide in order to increase the biogas to the level of biomethane. These technologies include the following applications in a multi-phase process: To achieve the

Table 10.1 Impacts of some biogas impurities on the environment, human health, and process machinery

Impurities	Human health and environment	Effects on equipment	References
NH_3	NOx production and release following combustion, Toxic to Anaerobic bacteria, Health issues, toxicity, and unpleasant odor	Engine anti-knock qualities, corrosion resistance, and NH_3's lower corrosiveness compared to H_2S	Atelge et al. (2021)
H_2S	Harmful to the environment, producing acid rain (H_2SO_4) and SO_2 and SO_3 production with unpleasant odor, irritating to the eyes, strong nerve toxin	Extremely caustic, toxic to PSA adsorbents, and poisonous to catalytic converters	Atelge et al. (2021),
N_3	Negative environmental impact. Lowering the calorific content	corrosion and anti-knock properties	Wasajja et al. (2020)
Siloxanes	In charge of the post-combustion emissions control catalytic system's fouling	Producing "glassy microcrystalline silica," which shortens equipment lifespan	Soreanu et al. (2011)
Water vapor	CO_2 and H_2S combine with water vapor to produce acids	Corrosion brought on by NH_3 reactions	Awe et al. (2017)

Wobbe index requirements, i) In order to concentrate methane, an upgrading process uses inert gases, mostly CO_2; ii) trace elements detrimental to natural gas grid end users are eliminated throughout the cleaning process (Allegue & Hinge, 2012).

Several methods, including chilling, compression, adsorption, absorption, and refrigerating through heat exchangers—typically by raising pressure and decreasing temperature—can extract *water* from biogas (Biernat and Samson-Bręk, 2012). According to current environmental regulations, the condensed water droplets are either returned to the digester or evacuated as effluent (Ryckebosch et al., 2011). Even though adsorbent renewal can be accomplished by heating, the moisture in biogas can be eliminated by employing adsorption dryers with high-water dryer adsorbents, such as activated carbon, aluminum oxide, magnesium oxide, silica gel, and molecular sieves (Nguyen et al., 2021). Among them, the most popular chemical drying technique is alumina or adsorption using zeolites or molecular sieves (Allegue & Hinge, 2012). Another popular method is water absorption, which can be used with hygroscopic salts and water-binding substances like triethylene glycol or glycol. Once these salts have been dissolved by absorbing moisture from the biogas, the saturated salt solution is subsequently released from the bottom side of the jar (Allegue & Hinge, 2012). Water is removed from biogas at the same time as gaseous pollutants and water-soluble aerosols (Lopez et al., 2012).

The most common component of biogas, *hydrogen sulfide*, is an odorous gas that damages the environment and human health (Paglini et al., 2022). Its corrosive properties can harm end users and biogas conversion equipment (Lanzini et al., 2017). According to Van Loosdrecht et al. (2016), organically bound sulfur compounds, which are present in proteins and SO_4^{2-} through sulfate-reducing bacteria (SRB), considering the main source of H_2S.

However, the concentration of H_2S can increase to several thousand parts per million depending on the type of biomass (Lanzini et al., 2017). Through oxidation in boilers and combustion engines, hydrogen sulfide may contribute to the creation of NOx ($SO_3$and SO_2), or sulfur oxides, which are discharged as exhausted gas emissions into the atmosphere (Munawer, 2018). The human respiratory system is impacted by these irritative gas and harmful properties toward mucous membranes (Khan et al., 2019). The elimination of hydrogen sulfide is accomplished by a series of treatment processes, ranging from primary to tertiary (Hoyer et al., 2016). By adding iron salts in the form of $FeSO_4$, $FeCl_2$ or $FeCl_3$, into the digester, the first step is the hydrogen sulfide precipitation. As a result, an insoluble iron sulfide precipitate (FeS) is produced, which is eliminated along with the digester and prevents further downstream transportation (Petersson & Wellinger, 2009). The secondary and tertiary processes are the biological and activated carbon adsorption methods, which have been used to extract hydrogen sulphide from biogas. A strain of bacteria (*Thiobacillus* and *Sulfolobus*) that feeds sulphur on a carrier material is inoculated to carry out the biological processes. The most often used technique is tertiary removal, which is predicated on the interaction of hydrogen sulfide with the pore surface of activated carbon when oxygen is present (Hoyer et al., 2016). This process is carried out in the gas phase at lower pressures and temperatures, whereas heating prior to the adsorption process controls water condensation (in the biogas and activated carbon). On the other hand, the activated carbon filters have experienced both chemical and physical adsorption (Hoyer et al., 2016).

Other components of biogas include *volatile organic compounds (VOC)*, which include alcohols, halogens, aromatic compounds, and alkanes. The concentration of these compounds varies according to the kind of biomass and the anaerobic digestion conditions (Paglini et al., 2022). Halogens also have an impact on downstream machinery and pipelines, primarily because of the corrosive products that are created when halogens, such as chlorine, react with anode-side Ni-based catalysts "followed by the sublimation of the reaction product" (Bona et al., 2020). However, no further treatment is required to eliminate the chlorine because it is present in very small amounts in the raw biogas (Rout et al., 2021).

10.3.2 Energy Losses During Biogas Upgrading

Between 0.4% and 8.6% of the CH_4 produced is emitted throughout the biogas generation process, according to ground-based remote sensing observations at agricultural and biowaste treatment plants (Bakkaloglu et al., 2021; Bühler et al., 2022; Hrad et al., 2021). Many researches revealed that the total CH_4 losses in wastewater treatment facilities (WWTP) varied from 2.2% to 14.9% (Delre et al., 2017; Samuelsson et al., 2018; Scheutz & Fredenslund, 2019). Measurements conducted on-site revealed various emission sources and leaks, based on the operating systems and technology. Typical hotspots were digestate storage tanks that were open and not gastightly enclosed (Reinelt et al., 2017) and the off-gas from biogas utilization units (Kvist & Aryal, 2019). While some of the input CH_4 is emitted by combined heat and power (CHP) facilities due to incomplete combustion, the efficiency of the upgrading technology's carbon dioxide (CO_2) removal determines how much CH_4 slips from biomethane production (Kapoor et al., 2019). Furthermore, during the receipt and storage of substrates, CH_4 can be emitted through the air ventilation of biowaste reception and processing halls (Fredenslund et al., 2018) and from non-gastight storage, mixing, and hydrolysis tanks (Schories et al., 2018). Additionally, anaerobic digesters can serve as CH4 sources since CH4 can pass through the membranes of single membrane and air-inflated double-membrane roofs (Liebetrau et al., 2017). Lastly, CH_4 emissions may result from leaks and other process disruptions (Reinelt & Liebetrau, 2019).

10.4 Economic and Regulatory Considerations of RNG

10.4.1 Cost Comparison: RNG versus Fossil Natural Gas

RNG has both economic and environmental advantages. In the first half of 2023, natural gas prices averaged $2.41 per MMBtu, according to the Henry Hub Natural Gas Spot Price. However, because of its climate-offsetting benefits, RNG sells at a premium to market prices. As mentioned, state and federal incentive schemes allow RNG to be priced at more than $100 per MMBtu. Because RNG is a renewable natural gas, specific buyers will also pay more for it (Ridley-Kaye et al., 2024). Currently, producing RNG is more expensive than extracting fossil natural gas. Commercial viability is hampered by the high infrastructure cost of processing and upgrading biogas into RNG, such as anaerobic digesters. In addition to the initial capital requirements, RNG production costs can range from $3 to over $30 per MMBtu, according to the World Resources Institute. The expenses related to fossil natural gas, such as testing and verification for pipeline standards and pipeline interconnection fees, are also borne by RNG. Some states have also introduced targeted subsidies to help with RNG's initial expenses. Lastly, several variables, such as the initial infrastructure expenses, the operations scale, the carbon intensity of the RNG produced, and any relevant financial credits, will determine whether or not a RNG producer realizes net economic advantages (Jaffee et al., 2016).

10.4.1.1 Renewable Fuel Standard (RFS) Credits and Low Carbon Fuel Standard (LCFS)

The Energy Independence and Security Act of 2007 (EISA) considerably enlarged the Clean Air Act's, the Energy Policy Act (EPA) of 2005 created the *Renewable Fuel*

Standard program (Renzi, 2019). According to Broder (2009), the RFS program is a national policy that mandates a specific amount of renewable fuel to replace or decrease the amount of fossil fuel in jet fuel, home heating oil, and transportation fuel. Under the RFS program, there are four types of renewable fuels:

- Diesel powered by biomass
- Cellulosic biofuel
- Total renewable fuel
- Advanced biofuel

The RFS program was greatly expanded by the 2007 enactment of EISA, which also brought about several significant improvements, such as:

- Increasing and prolonging the annual volume requirements until 2022.
- Including clear criteria for renewable fuels to be eligible, such as lifecycle greenhouse gas (GHG) emissions and renewable biomass.
- Establishing grandfathering provisions for quantities from specific current facilities.
- Adding particular kinds of waiver powers.

Fuel must meet the requirements of both the Act and the implementing RFS rules for the EPA to classify it as a renewable fuel under the RFS program (EPA, 2009). Among other things, fuels must reduce GHG emissions by a specific amount compared to a petroleum baseline from 2005. Under the RFS program, the Environmental Protection Agency (EPA) has authorized fuel routes for the four renewable fuel categories (Mufson & Eilperin, 2009). Renewable compressed natural gas from dumps, cellulosic ethanol made from crop waste, jet fuel made from soybean oil, and ethanol made from sugarcane and numerous other advanced biofuel paths have already received approval (RFS2, 2010).

- Biomass-based diesel needs to meet a 50% lifecycle GHG reduction and be made from eligible renewable biomass.
- Cellulosic biofuel must have a 60% lifespan GHG reduction and be made from cellulose, hemicellulose, or lignin.
- Advanced biofuel must have a 50% lifespan GHG reduction and be made from eligible renewable biomass, except corn starch.
- Ethanol made from maize starch is commonly referred to as renewable fuel (or conventional biofuel), and it must achieve a 20% lifespan GHG reduction.

A *low-carbon fuel standard* (LCFS), an emission trading rule, aims to lower the average carbon intensity of transportation fuels in a particular jurisdiction relative to traditional petroleum fuels like gasoline and diesel. Providing power to electric vehicles, delivering hydrogen fuel to fuel cell vehicles, and incorporating biofuels like ethanol, biodiesel, renewable natural gas, and renewable diesel into fossil fuels are the most popular ways to lower transportation carbon emissions (Kahn, 2009). The main objective of a low-carbon fuel standard is to lower the CO_2 emissions from cars with various internal combustion engine types while taking into account the vehicle's whole life cycle in order to reduce the carbon footprint of transportation.

In 2007, California enacted the first low-carbon fuel standard law in history; the California Air Resources Board (CARB) established the eligibility requirements in April 2009, but the law didn't go into effect until 2011 (Buchanan, 2009). British Columbia approved similar laws in April 2008 (Penner, 2008), while the European Union introduced and accepted identical legislation in January 2007 (EP, 2008).

Similar nationwide regulations for low-carbon fuels, albeit with less strict requirements than California, have been proposed in several US laws (Daniel & Gordon, 2009). None had been authorized as of the beginning of 2010. In 2010, the U.S. Environmental Protection Agency (EPA) published the final rule for the expanded Renewable Fuel Standard (RFS2) for 2010 and beyond (RSF2, 2010). Direct emissions and considerable indirect emissions from land use changes were considered in this ruling, which was required under the Energy Independence and Security Act of 2007 (EISA) (GhGRT, 2010).

10.4.2 EU RED II Mandates for Biomethane Blending

Another issue with biofuels is that blending requirements may result in consumers paying more for fuel (Lundberg et al., 2023). As the price of oil climbed globally in 2022, fuel prices in many EU nations skyrocketed. To mitigate the impact on consumers, some governments chose to suspend or halt their blending regulations (ePURE, 2022). Countries must simultaneously prepare to fulfill RED III's new, more aggressive goals for reducing transportation and biofuel emissions. Recognizing the extent to which national blending regulations reduce emissions, investments in the manufacturing of conventional and advanced biofuels, and their effects on consumer fuel prices is crucial because they have been and continue to be the most effective policy tool for reaching emission reduction targets for the transportation sector. However, mandates vary depending on whether they are based on energy, volume, or emission reduction and whether they target gasoline and diesel fuels independently or in tandem. Because of this, it is impossible to compare mandates across nations directly and to evaluate their effects statistically at the EU level.

Prior research on biofuel regulations has typically concentrated on specific nations, including the Netherlands (Hoppe & Bueren, 2017), Sweden and Finland (Hedeler et al., 2020), Germany (Kaup & Selbmann, 2013), or on offering a more comprehensive, qualitative summary of biofuel policies worldwide (Su et al., 2015). While Ebadian et al. (2020) provide quantitative data for combining obligation and insights into the role of policies in the development of biofuel markets, Brynge-mark and Söderholm (2022) provide an econometric analysis of the relationship between biofuel policy and biofuel output. However, the blending regulations are not converted to a single unit, and the applicability is limited to ethanol (Ebadian et al., 2020).

10.5 Applications

10.5.1 Transportation: CNG/LNG Vehicles and Marine Fuel

Several applications exist for the transportation industry's liquefied natural gas (LNG). As we work to cut carbon and greenhouse gas emissions in order to create cleaner air, the United States and nations worldwide increasingly use LNG to fuel trucks, buses, and ships (Anderson et al., 2015). According to experts, LNG has a promising future as a fuel for transportation. The opportunities and problems associated with LNG's use as a fuel are listed below (GIIGNL, 2018). On January 1, 2020, the International Maritime Organization ordered that ulphur emissions from marine vessels be capped (IMO, 2020). CLNG is in ulphu of IMO, 2020's implementation. Many shipping companies, builders, and operators around the world are using LNG as a cleaner alternative fuel to meet the new emissions standards because: (1) it reduces traditional pollutants like Nox; (2) it's safe, affordable, and abundant; (3) only emits trace amounts of ulphur oxide, which the IMO has capped; (4) lowers carbon emissions, potentially enabling shipping operators to adhere to future carbon restrictions.

According to DNV GL, the number of ships fuelled by LNG will reach around 1,800 by 2020 (DNV, 2018). While compressed natural gas (CNG) and liquefied natural gas (LNG) are utilized as car fuels, heavy-duty vehicles travelling long distances are better suited for LNG. Whether in the form of CNG or LNG, the increased usage of natural gas as a transportation fuel can aid in lowering carbon emissions and air pollution from the transportation industry. The natural gas vehicle industry's voice, NGV America, claims (REE, 2017): Throughout their well-to-wheel lifecycle, natural gas-powered automobiles emit 13–21% lower greenhouse gas emissions than their gasoline and diesel counterparts. Because natural gas-powered cars generate roughly 80% fewer non-methane hydrocarbons and 50% fewer Nox gas, they can also help to enhance the quality of the surrounding air.

10.5.2 Industrial Decarbonization: Cement and Steel Industries

By developing technologies for high-performance energy storage and renewable energy generation, materials science has significantly reduced CO_2 emissions from the electrical industry (Daehn et al., 2022). Cement and steel emissions are very high, making up 7–8% of worldwide CO_2-eq emissions apiece (GCCA, 2021; IEA, 2020). Global steel output increased by a factor of 17 or 4.1% between 1950 and 2021(Wang et al., 2021; Worldsteel, 2022), and the average yearly growth in cement production was a factor of 30, or 4.9% (U.S. Geological Survey, 2023). Cement CO_2 emissions rose 3.7% yearly on average between 1990 and 2019, according to Chen et al. (2022); steel CO_2 emissions increased 2.9% annually on average between 1990 and 2015, according to Wang et al. (2021); and Future emissions for both industries are predicted by Van Ruijven et al. (2016) using different levels of carbon pricing. The direct emissions from the production of cement and steel could be further reduced by implementing five different decarbonization strategies: (1) increasing process/system efficiencies; (2) electrifying processes to use electricity; (3) switching to alternative fuels; (4) carbon capture and storage (CCS/CCU); and (5) transferring to different raw materials. The technological maturity, the timing of the various choices' commercial availability, and their significance in future decarbonization remain unclear despite study on all five options in the manufacturing of cement and steel (Tautorat et al., 2023).

10.5.3 Grid Injection for Residential Heating

It was compelled to affect household heating decisions and how natural gas appliances can provide affordable decarbonization options. The focus is shifting to the future, where cutting-edge technologies like gas heat pumps and renewable natural gas (RNG) are expected to revolutionize residential heating and significantly reduce emissions. Pumps are first heated by natural gas. As was evident in earlier installments of this series, installing a natural gas heat pump is almost as expensive as installing a state-of-the-art electric heat pump. On the other hand, electric heat pumps transfer heat rather than produce it. Heat is also transferred by a natural gas heat pump. It can generate its own heat using natural gas, but when temperatures drop too far, there isn't enough heat to move effectively (Kay, 2024). Compared to electric-only heat pumps, natural gas heat pumps are less expensive to operate because they run on natural gas, which is now a third of the price of electricity and is expected to stay that way for decades. Compared to an electric cold-climate heat pump, a residence with a natural gas heat pump would save $651 annually or nearly $10,000 over the equipment's fifteen-year lifespan. Apart from their low operating costs, natural gas heat pumps also offer the advantage of having far lower emissions than all-electric heat pumps (O'Brien, 2023).

10.6 Case Studies

10.6.1 Ameresco's Sacramento Bio-Digester (U.S.)

California has long been at the forefront of implementing sustainable transportation methods, and now it can claim ownership of another first-of-its-kind land project in the US. Two companies in the Sacramento area, by gathering and reusing food waste from a nearby landfill, (disposal Industries) Clean; World and Atlashave launched the Sacramento Biodigester, the first closed-loop organic waste operation in the country. The garbage that Atlas Disposal delivers powers a portion of its garbage fleet. Atlas Disposal delivers food and organic garbage to the South Area Transfer Station in Sacramento from surrounding restaurants, supermarkets, food processing plants, and residences. There, Clean World has built a commercial facility to use anaerobic digestion to convert the waste into energy and car fuel which produces a mixture of carbon dioxide and methane. Renewable natural gas (RNG), the close chemical equivalent of pipeline natural gas, describes this biogas after it has been "refined" by the use of a biogas upgrading system that BioCNG, LLC designed and built. Clean Energy Fuels constructed the adjacent compressed natural gas filling station, which is also California's first sustainable natural gas refueling station dispenses the RNG stored in tanks. The refueling station is powered by electricity from a modest amount of biogas. The Sacramento Biodigester is already operational and converting 25 tons of food waste daily into RNG; however, it is now being scaled up to a 100-ton capacity. When fully expanded, the facility will produce over 700,000 diesel gallon equivalents (DGEs) of RNG per year, which will be provided to Atlas' CNG vans as well as other public and private fleets, such as some of the city cars in Sacramento through the public access refueling station. The following are some of the project's financial and environmental advantages: (1) every year, about 40,000 tons of food waste is kept out of landfills; (2) 5,800 tons of greenhouse gas is reduced annually; (3) 700,000 diesel gallon equivalents are replaced annually; (4) Sixteen long-term green jobs were created; (5) over $1.1 million in combined municipal tax revenue was received annually; (6) co-products of high-value organic soil amendments were offered for sale.

10.6.2 Nature Energy's RNG Plants in Denmark

Denmark's biggest biogas producer is Nature Energy. It now owns and runs ten biogas facilities and is working on expanding existing plants, like Månsson and Midtfyn, and developing new ones. The company has begun capturing CO_2 for use in the food and beverage industries at the Korskro biogas facility. This further lowers the biogas plant's CO_2 emissions, enhancing sustainability and demonstrating how biogas is a practical example of the circular economy that extends beyond energy, transportation fuel, and agriculture. Denmark is in a perfect position to benefit from biogas (Table 10.2). A third of its yearly consumption can be stored in the enormous caverns that make up its gas grid. "Denmark's grid has 85,000 times the storage capacity of Elon Musk's battery." The Danish grid is entirely different; it is an excellent method of backup solar and wind power, which must naturally be environmentally friendly. This is a fantastic chance for the gas grid. The goal is to be able to accept all organic waste that is locally sourced within a 25-km radius. The industry's short-term objective in Denmark is to have 50% of the grid run on biomethane by 2025 and 100% by 2040. "The tipping point is fifty percent." At that point, biogas will be discussed in the same way as wind and solar energy,

Table 10.2 Nature Energy project's feedstock, financial and environmental advantages in South of Odense, Denmark

Factors	Nature energy
Feedstock	350,000 tons per year tpa. (This will bc 500,000 tonnes after expansion.): To promote biology and maintain maximum output, glycerol and beet molasses, 25% industrial waste, and 75% manures and slurries are given irregularly
Output	• 1,500 m^3/hr of biomethane to the grid without the need for propane. 2.750 m^3/h following expansion • A natural fertilizer of 325,000 tpa is put back into the soil • Three operators, eight full-time drivers, and one on-site manager • Delivers and picks up from 47 nearby farms
Financials	• The estimated plant cost is DKK 165,000,000, or £19,500,000 • To make it economically viable, all feedstock is gathered from within a 25-km radius • The estimated cost of facility enlargement is £17,241,000, or DKK 145,000,000 • The best feedstocks cost money
Interesting factors	• To save OPEX and improve road safety—a crucial PR factor—Nature Energy owns, operates, and employs local truck drivers • Work is now being done to expand the capacity to 550,000 tpa • The expansion will only handle organic manures and is independent of the existing plant • It was Denmark's third Nature Energy plant to be constructed

acknowledging waste as the primary source of gas rather than fossil fuels. The circular economy will then be solidified as a reality.

10.7 Future Prospects

10.7.1 Hydrogen-RNG Blends for Energy Storage

It describes the risks of expanding investments in fossil gas infrastructure that uses hydrogen and RNG instead of electricity and sustainable energy to meet electrical needs. Renewable Natural Gas Systems May Be Climate-Intensive at Scale, this states that "RNG is not inherently climate-friendly. Considering both the source of methane used to produce RNG and the likely alternative fate of that methane, and using reasonable assumptions about likely system methane leakage, it is unlikely that a RNG system could deliver GHG-negative, or even zero GHG, energy at scale."

Researchers at the National Renewable Energy Laboratory (NREL), a national U.S. Department of Energy laboratory, integrated hydrogen into the gas network. NREL's report highlights the knowledge gaps surrounding hydrogen blending, despite the fact that a number of gas utilities are conducting pilot programs and claiming that hydrogen can help achieve net zero emission targets. NREL discovered that "the presence of hydrogen significantly affects both fatigue crack growth and fracture resistance for pipeline steel utilized in the transportation and distribution system." Furthermore, "hydrogen can impact the physical properties, such as density and degree of crystallinity, of polyethylene materials," the researchers discovered. Stated differently, the physical characteristics of plastic pipes positioned across the gas distribution system may be impacted by hydrogen blending. According to this peer-reviewed study, which was written by scientists and engineers from the Hydrogen Science Coalition, Environmental Defense Fund, and Environmental Defense Fund Europe and published in Energy Science & Engineering, every component on the gas infrastructure value chain is "challenged by reuse" because of the substantial, fundamental physical and chemical differences between hydrogen and methane. Without de-rating to lower pressures, hydrogen in the current gas system is useless, resulting in significant investments, retrofits, replacements, or decreased energy flow rates. Furthermore, there has been a minimal decrease in greenhouse gas emissions: "While repurposing the natural gas system for use with hydrogen may, at first, seem appealing, the limited practicality, risks, and data gaps strongly suggest that like-for-like gas substitution proved limited benefits for increased risks."

10.7.2 Decentralized Modular Upgrading Units for Rural Areas

Decentralized renewable energy (DRE) has emerged as a viable alternative to responsibly fulfill our growing power demands in the wake of the recent incredible shift in the global energy environment. Instead of conventional centralized power systems, decentralized renewable energy concentrates on producing electricity using regional renewable resources. In contrast to centralized power facilities, decentralized renewable energy generation generates electricity locally and at lower scales using renewable resources. It entails using distributed energy systems to capture the power of renewable resources, including solar, wind, hydro, and biomass. By generating power closer to the point of use, these decentralized systems lessen reliance on long-distance transmission and help communities achieve self-sufficiency. The traditional concept of centralized power networks, which mostly rely on fossil fuels and transmit power over great distances, is broken by decentralized renewable energy. Instead, it uses smaller-scale facilities to capture the plentiful energy from renewable sources. This change releases communities from the fragility of centralized grid networks and enables them to become self-sufficient. The capacity of DRE to produce dependable and robust energy sources is one of its main benefits. Decentralized renewable energy offers a localized option in isolated and rural locations where grid connectivity is either unstable or prohibitively expensive. Communities can benefit from a continuous power supply by producing electricity closer to the point of use, which lessens reliance on outside sources and lessens the effects of system outages and natural disasters. In addition, energy poverty is a serious issue in many parts of the world, particularly in rural and isolated places. By providing accessible and sustainable power solutions to those who need them most, DRE can play a significant role in closing this gap. Communities may take charge of their energy supply by supporting local energy generation, which opens up possibilities for better healthcare, education, economic development, and quality of life. In addition to providing social and financial advantages, the shift to localized renewable energy also helps create a cleaner and greener future. By utilizing renewable resources, we can lessen our dependency on fossil fuels, restrict carbon dioxide emissions, and fight climate change.

Furthermore, localized renewable energy projects can guarantee sustainable cohabitation with the natural world by minimizing environmental effects and adapting to particular local ecosystems. DRE initiatives have a great deal of potential to boost regional economies. Communities can stimulate entrepreneurship, draw in investment, and create jobs by investing in renewable infrastructure. In addition to creating economic opportunities, local procurement of materials, installation, and maintenance services supports the general development of rural and isolated communities.

References

Abatzoglou, N., & Boivin, S. (2009). A review of biogas purification processes. *Biofuels, Bioproducts & Biorefining, 3*, 42–71. https://doi.org/10.1002/bbb.117

Ai, N., Chen, L., & Fu, Y. (2022). A novel analysis on pyrolysis and gasification process of rice straw feedstock. *Sustain Energy Technolo Assess, 51*, Article 101866. https://doi.org/10.1016/j.seta.2021.101866

Akbari, M., & Kumar, A. (2024). The development of data-intensive techno-economic models for the comparison of renewable natural gas production from six different biomass feedstocks for the decarbonization of energy demand sectors. *Fuel, 358*, Article 130107. https://doi.org/10.1016/j.fuel.2023.130107

Al Mamun, M. R., & Torii, S. (2017). Enhancement of methane concentration by removing contaminants from biogas mixtures using combined method of absorption and adsorption. *International Journal of Chemical Engineering, 2017*, 1–9. https://doi.org/10.1155/2017/7906859.ISSN1687806X.S2CID55761019

Ali Abd A., Shabbani H.J.K., Helwani Z., Othman M.R. (2022). Novel design of pressure swing adsorption using compact plates for adsorption heat recuperation of CO_2 capture in biomethane upgrading process. *Energy Convers Manag*, 15: 115999. https://doi.org/10.1016/j.enconman.2022.115999 Get rights and content

Allegue L.B., Hinge J. (2012). Biogas and Bio-Syngas Upgrading Report, 1. *Danish Technol Instit*, p. 97. www.teknologisk.dk › _root › media

Anderson, M., Salo, K., & Fridell, E. (2015). Particle—and gaseous emissions from an LNG powered ship. *Environ Sc Technol, 49*(20), 12568–12575. https://doi.org/10.1021/acs.est.5b02678

Angelidaki, I., Treu, L., Tsapekos, P., Luo, G., Campanaro, S., Wenzel, H., & Kougias, P. G. (2018). Biogas upgrading and utilization: Current status and perspectives. *Biotechnology Advances, 36*(2), 452–466. https://doi.org/doi.org/10.1016/j.biotechadv.2018.01.011

Archana, K., Visckram, A. S., Kumar, P. S., Manikandan, S., Saravanan, A., & Natrayan, L. (2024). A review on recent technological breakthroughs in anaerobic digestion of organic biowaste for biogas generation: Challenges towards sustainable development goals. *Fuel, 358*, Article 130298. https://doi.org/10.1016/j.fuel.2023.130298

Atelge, M. R., Senol, H., Djaafri, M., Hansu, T. A., Krisa, D., Atabani, A., Eskicioglu, C., Muratçobanoglu, H., Unalan, S., Kalloum, S., Azbar, N., & Kıvrak, H. D. (2021). A Critical overview of the state-of-the-art methods for biogas purification and utilization processes. *Sustain, 13*, 11515. https://doi.org/10.3390/su132011515

Awe O.W., Zhao Y., Nzihou A., Minh D.P., Lyczko N. (2017). A review of biogas utilization, purification and upgrading technologies: Review. *Waste Biomass Valor, 8*(2):267–283. https://link.springer.com/article/https://doi.org/10.1007/s12649-016-9826-4

Bakkaloglu, S., Lowry, D., Fisher, R. E., France, J. L., Brunner, D., Chen, H., & Nisbet, E. G. (2021). Quantification of methane emissions from UK biogas plants. *Waste Managem, 124*, 93. https://doi.org/10.1016/j.wasman.2021.1001.1011

Biernat K., Gis W., Samson-Bręk I. (2012). Review of technology for cleaning biogas to natural gas quality. Environ Sc, Engin Corpus ID: 115139099. https://www.semanticscholar.org/632995b880f624e967b9d203c3afa171cca06a21

Bona, D., Beggio, G., Weil, T., Scholz, M., Bertolini, S., Grandi, L., Baratieri, M., Schievano, A., Silvestri, S., & Pivato, A. (2020). Effects of woody biochar on dry thermophilic anaerobic digestion of organic fraction of municipal solid waste. *Journal of Environmental Management, 267*, Article 110633. https://doi.org/10.1016/j.jenvman.2020.110633

Broder J.M. (2009). With something for everyone, climate bill passed. *New York Times*. https://www.nytimes.com/2009/07/01/us/politics/01climate.html

Brosowski, A., Krause, T., Mantau, U., Mahro, B., Noke, A., Richter, F., Raussen, T., Bischof, R., Hering, T., Blanke, C., Müller, P., Thrän, D. (2019). How to measure the impact of biogenic residues, wastes and byproducts: development of a national resource monitoring based on the example of Germany. *Biomass Bioenergy, 127*: Article 105275. doi. https://doi.org/10.1016/j.biombioe.2019.105275

Bryngemark E., Söderholm P. (2022). Green industrial policies and domestic production of biofuels: an econometric analysis of OECD countries Environ Econ Pol Stud, 24: 225–261. https://link.springer.com/article/https://doi.org/10.1007/s10018-021-00320-y

Buchanan W. (2009) Air Resources Board moves to cut carbon use. *San Francisco Chronicle*. https://www.sfgate.com/green/article/air-resources-board-moves-to-cut-carbon-use-3243880.php

Bühler M., H¨ani C., Ammann C., Br¨onnimann S., Kupper T. (2022). Using the inverse dispersion method to determine methane emissions from biogas plants and wastewater treatment plants with complex source configurations. *Atmosph Environ*, X 13: 100161. 100110.101016/j.

Chen C., Xu R., Tong D., Qin X., Cheng J., Liu J., Zheng B., Yan L., Zhang Q. (2022). A striking growth of CO_2 emissions from the global cement industry driven by new facilities in emerging countries. *Environ Res Lett, 17*: Article 044007, https://doi.org/10.1088/1748-9326/AC48B5

Couto, N., Rouboa, A., & Silva, V. (2013). Influence of the biomass gasification processes on the final composition of syngas. *Energy Procedia, 36*, 596–606. https://doi.org/10.1016/j.egypro.2013.07.068

Daehn K., Basuhi R., Gregory J., Berlinger M., Somjit V., Olivetti E.A. (2022). Innovations to decarbonize materials industries. *Nature Rev Mater, 7*: 275–294 https://www.nature.com/articles/s41578-021-00376-y

Daniel S., Gordon D. (2009) Two billion cars: driving toward sustainability. Oxford University Press, New York. Pp. 194–196. ISBN 978–0–19–537664–7.

Delre A., Monster J., Scheutz C. (2017). Greenhouse gas emission quantification from wastewater treatment plants, using a tracer gas dispersion method. Sci Total Environ, 605–606: 258–268. 210.1016/j.scitotenv.2017.1006.1177.

Deng L., Liu Y., Wang W. (2020). Biogas cleaning and upgrading. *Chapter: Biogas Technology. Springer, Singapore*, pp. 201–243. https://link.springer.com/chapter/https://doi.org/10.1007/978-981-15-4940-3_6

DNV (2018). LNG status update, https://www.dnvgl.com/maritime/mydnvgl-service-overview/lng-intelligence-lngi/

Ebadian, M., van Dyk, S., McMillan, J.D., Saddler, J. (2020) Biofuels policies that have encouraged their production and use: an international perspective Energy Pol, 147: Article 111906. https://doi.org/10.1016/j.enpol.2020.111906
EPA (2009). Proposes new regulations for renewable fuel standard to implement requirements of EISA; GHG reduction and indirect land use change effects included. Green Car Congress. https://www.greencarcongress.com/2009/05/epa-nprm-20090505.html
ePURE (2022). Updated for 2022: Overview of Biofuels Policies and Markets across the EU. https://www.epure.org/news/updated-for-2022-overview-of-biofuels-policies-and-markets-across-the-eu/
Ferella, F., Puca, A., Taglieri, G., Rossi, L., Gallucci, K. (2017). Separation of carbon dioxide for biogas upgrading to biomethane. J Clean Prod, 164: 1205–1218 https://doi.org/10.1016/j.jclepro.2017.07.037 Get rights and content
Fredenslund, A.M., Hinge, J., Holmgren, M. A., Rasmussen, S.G., & Scheutz, C. (2018). Onsite and ground-based remote sensing measurements of methane emissions from four biogas plants: A comparison study. *Bioresource Technol, 27*, 88–95. https://doi.org/10.1016/j.biortech.2018.1008.1080
Gao, Y., Wang, M., Raheem, A., Wang, F., Wei, J., Xu D., Song, X., Bao, W., Huang, A., Zhang, S., Zhang, H. (2023). Syngas production from biomass gasification: influences of feedstock properties, reactor type, and reaction parameters. *ACS Omega 8*(35): 31620−31631. http://pubs.acs.org/journal/acsodf
GCCA. (2021). Getting the numbers right project: emissions report 2019 London. https://gccassociation.org/2050-net-zero-roadmap-one-year-on/
U.S. Geological Survey, (2023). Mineral commodity summaries 2023. https://doi.org/10.3133/mcs2023.
GIIGNL. (2018). The LNG industry, annual report 2018 https://giignl.org/sites/default/files/PUBLIC_AREA/Publications/rapportannuel-2018pdf.pdf
Grande C.A. (2011). Biogas upgrading by pressure swing adsorption. In Biofuel's Engineering Process Technology; IntechOpen: London, UK, pp. 65–84. https://doi.org/10.5772/18428
Gu, H., Tang, Y., & Yao, J. (2019). Study on biomass gasification under various operating conditions. *Journal of the Energy Institute, 92*(5), 1329–1336. https://doi.org/10.1016/j.joei.2018.10.002
Haider, S., Lindbråthen, A., & Hägg, M.-B. (2016). Techno-economical evaluation of membrane based biogas upgrading system: A comparison between polymeric membrane and carbon membrane technology. *Green Energy Environ., 1*(3), 222–234. https://doi.org/10.1016/j.gee.2016.10.003
Hedeler, B., Hellsmark, H., Söderholm, P., Donner-Amnell, J. (2020). The dynamic between policy mixes and the emergence of sustainable value chains: comparative perspectives from biofuel development in Finland and Sweden. *Presented at the 11th International Sustainability Transition Conference (IST 2020), IST 2020* 283–283 https://www.researchgate.net/publication/344041670
Hoppe T., van Bueren E. (2017). From frontrunner to laggard: The netherlands and europeanization in the cases of RES-E and biofuel stimulation. *Guide EU Renew Energy* Pol, Pp. 65–84. https://research.tudelft.nl/en/publications/
Hoyer, K., Hulteberg, C., Svensson, M., Jernberg, J., Nørregård, Ø. (2016). Biogas upgrading—technical review. Energiforsk, 1–71. https://www.hivos.org/sites/default/files/biogas_and_household_air_quality_30–10–15_0.pdf.
Hrad, M., Vesenmaier, A., Flandorfer, C., Piringer, M., Stenzel, S., & Huber-Humer, M. (2021). Comparison of forward and backward Lagrangian transport modelling to determine methane emissions from anaerobic digestion facilities. *Atmospheric Environment X, 12*, 10013. https://doi.org/10.1016/j.aeaoa.2021.100131
IEA (2020). Energy technology perspectives 2020. https://www.iea.org/reports/energy-technology-perspectives-2020.

IMO (2020). Fourth greenhouse gas study 2020, Key findings from the Fourth IMO GHG Study 2020: https://www.imo.org/en/OurWork/Environment/Pages/Fourth-IMO-Greenhouse-Gas-Study-2020.aspx.

Imtiaz, A., Othman, M. H. D., Jilani, A., Khan, I. U., Kamaludin, R., Iqbal, J., & Al-Sehemi, A. G. (2022). Challenges, opportunities and future directions of membrane technology for natural gas purification: a critical review. *Membranes, 12*, 646. https://doi.org/10.3390/membranes12070646

IPCC Intergovernmental Panel on Climate Change. (2022) IPCC special report on climate change, desertification, land degradation, sustainable land management, food security, and greenhouse gas fluxes in terrestrial ecosystems https://www.ipcc.ch/site/assets/uploads/2019/08/4.pdf.

Jaffee A.M., Dominguez-Faus R. (2016). Final draft report on the feasibility of renewable natural gas as a large-scale, low carbon substitute, Uc Davis Inst Transp Stud Program, 2 https://ww2.arb.ca.gov/sites/default/files/classic/research/apr/past/13-307.pdf.

Jha, S., Okolie, J.A., Nanda, S., Dalai, A.K. (2022). A review of biomass resources and thermochemical conversion technologies. Chem Eng Technol, 45: 791–799. https://doi.org/10.1002/ceat.202100503

Kahn, D. (2009). California Adopts Low-Carbon Fuel Standard. *Scientific American*. https://www.scientificamerican.com/article/california-adopts-low-car/.

Kapoor, R., Ghosh, P., Kumar, M., Vijay, V.K. (2019). Evaluation of biogas upgrading technologies and future perspectives: a review. *Environ Sc Poll Res, 26*: 11631–11661. https://link.springer.com/article/https://doi.org/10.1007/s11356-019-04767-1

Kaup, F., & Selbmann, K. (2013). The seesaw of Germany's biofuel policy—tracing the evolvement to its current state. *Energy Pol, 62*, 513–521. https://doi.org/10.1016/j.enpol.2013.08.024

Kay A. (2024) Building for efficiency: The RNG revolution, American gas association (AGA). https://www.aga.org/building-for-efficiency-the-rng-revolution/

Khan, M. A. H., Rao, M. V., & Li, Q. (2019). Recent advances in electrochemical sensors for detecting toxic gases: NO_2, SO_2 and H_2S. *Sensors, 19*, 905. https://doi.org/10.3390/s19040905

Kumar, A., & Samadder, S. R. (2020). Performance evaluation of anaerobic digestion technology for energy recovery from organic fraction of municipal solid waste: A review. *Energy, 197*, Article 117253. https://doi.org/10.1016/j.energy.2020.117253

Kvist, T., Aryal, N. (2019). Methane loss from commercially operating biogas upgrading plants. *Waste Manage, 87*: 295–300. 210.1016/j.

Lanzini, A., Madi, H., Chiodo, V., Papurello, D., Maisano, S., Santarelli, M., & Van Herle, J. (2017). Dealing with fuel contaminants in biogas-fed solid oxide fuel cell (SOFC) and molten carbonate fuel cell (MCFC) plants: Degradation of catalytic and electrocatalytic active surfaces and related gas purification methods. *Progress in Energy and Combustion Science, 61*, 150–188. https://doi.org/10.1016/j.pecs.2017.04.002

Liebetrau J., Reinelt T., Agostini A., Linke B. (2017). Methane emissions from biogas plants. Methods for measurement, results and effect on greenhouse gas balance of electricity produced, IEA Bioenergy: Task 37: 2017: 12. URL: https://www.ieabioenergy.com/wp-content/uploads/2018/01

Liu, Z., Grande, C. A., Li, P., Yu, J., & Rodrigues, A. E. (2011). Multi-bed vacuum pressure swing adsorption for carbon dioxide capture from flue gas. *Separation and Purification Technology, 81*(3), 307–317. https://doi.org/10.1016/j.seppur.2011.07.037

National Grid Live, National grid: Live. (2022). https://grid.iamkate.com/.

Van Loosdrecht, M.C.M., Brdjanovic, D., Lopez-Vazquez, C.M., Nielsen, P.H. (2016). Biological sulphate-reduction, experimental methods in wastewater treatment. *Intern Water Assoc, 362*: 54–72. https://doi.org/10.2166/9781780404752.

Lopez, M.E., Rene E.R., Veiga M.C., Kennes C. (2012). Biogas Technologies and cleaning techniques. In: Lichtfouse, E., et al. (Eds.), Environmental Chemistry for a Sustainable World: Volume 2: Remed Air Water Poll, Springer, pp. 347–377. https://link.springer.com/chapter/https://doi.org/10.1007/978-94-007-2439-6_9.

Lundberg, L., Sanchez, O. C., & Zetterholm, J. (2023). The impact of blending mandates on biofuel consumption, production, emission reductions and fuel prices. *Energy Pol, 147*(2020), Article 113835. https://doi.org/10.1016/j.enpol.2023.113835

Mao, G., Huang, N., Chen, L., Wang, H.M. (2018). Research on biomass energy and environment from the past to the future: a bibliometric analysis. *Sci Total Environ, 635*:1081–1090, https://doi.org/10.1016/j.scitotenv.2018.04.173.

Mishra, A., Humpenöder, F., Churkina, G., Reyer, C.P.O., Beier, F., Bodirsky, B.L., Schellnhuber, H.J., Lotze-Campen, H., Popp, A. (2022). Land use change and carbon emissions of a transformation to timber cities. *Nat Commun, 13*: 4889, https://doi.org/10.1038/s41467-022-32244-w.

Mufson, S., Eilperin, J. (2009). EPA proposes changes to biofuel regulations. The Washington Post. https://www.washingtonpost.com/wp-dyn/content/article/2009/05/05/AR2009050503731.html

Munawer, M. E. (2018). Human health and environmental impacts of coal combustion and post-combustion wastes. *J Sustain Min, 17*, 87–96. https://doi.org/10.1016/j.jsm.2017.12.007

SoCalGas and Opus 12 Successfully Demonstrate Technology That Simplifies Conversion of Carbon Dioxide into Storable Renewable Energy". prnewswire.com (Press release). (2018). PR Newswire. https://www.sempra.com/socalgas-and-opus-12-successfully-demonstrate-technology-simplifies-conversion-carbon-dioxide.

Nguyen, L. N., Kumar, J., Vu, M. T., Mohammed, J. A. H., Pathak, N., Commault, A. S., Sutherland, D., Zdarta, J., Tyagi, V. K., & Nghiem, L. D. (2021). Bio-methane production from anaerobic co-digestion at wastewater treatment plants: A critical review on development and innovations in biogas upgrading techniques. *Science of the Total Environment, 765*, Article 142753. https://doi.org/10.1016/j.scitotenv.2020.142753

O'Brien, B. (2023). Natural gas homes are lowest-cost and lowest-emissions, even compared to homes with electric cold-climate heat pumps. High-efficiency natural gas appliances in homes can lower utility bills and emissions. https://www.aga.org/report-finds-gas-heating-beats-cold-climate-heat-pumps-on-cost-and-emissions/

Paglini, R., Gandiglio, M., & Andrea, L. A. (2022). Technologies for deep biogas purification and use in zero-emission fuel cells systems—a review. *Energies, 15*(3551), 1–30. https://doi.org/10.3390/en15103551

Papurello, D., Silvestri, S., Tomasi, L., Belcari, I., Biasioli, F., & Santarelli, M. (2016). *Biowaste for SOFCs. Energy Proc, 101*, 424–431. https://doi.org/10.1016/j.egypro.2016.11.054

European Parliament. (2008). "Texts adopted Wednesday,: Monitoring and reduction of greenhouse gas emissions from fuels". https://eur-lex.europa.eu/legal-content/EN/TXT/PDF/?uri=CELEX:52024AP0145

Penner, D. (2008). Government brings in low-carbon fuel bill. The Vancouver Sun. https://web.archive.org/web/20120314153812, http://www2.canada.com/vancouversun/news/business/story.html.

Petersson, A., Wellinger, A. (2009). Biogas upgrading technologies–developments and innovations. *IEA Bioenergy, 20*: 1–19. https://www.ieabioenergy.com/.

Pinto, F., Costa, P., Miranda, M. (2017). Thermochemical treatment. In: Algal Biofuels; CRC Press: Pp.140–188. eBook ISBN:9781315152547 https://www.taylorfrancis.com/chapters/edit/https://doi.org/10.1201/9781315152547-5

Rauch, R., Hrbek, J., Hofbauer, H. (2014). Biomass gasification for synthesis gas production and applications of the syngas. *Wiley Interdiscip. Rev.: Energy Environ, 3* (4): 343– 362. https://doi.org/10.1002/wene.97

Razmi, A. R., Afshar, H. H., & Pourahmadiyan, A. (2021). Investigation of a combined heat and power (CHP) system based on biomass and compressed air energy storage (CAES). *Sustainable Energy Technologies and Assessments, 46*, Article 101253. https://doi.org/10.1016/j.seta.2021.101253

Reinelt, T., Delre, A., Westerkamp, T., Holmgren, M.A., Liebetrau J., Scheutz, C. (2017). Comparative use of different emission measurement approaches to determine methane emissions from a biogas plant. *Waste Manage, 68*: 173–185. 110.1016/j.wasman.2017.1005.1053.

Reinelt, T., & Liebetrau, J. (2019). Monitoring and mitigation of methane emissions from pressure relief valves of a biogas plant. *Chemical Engineering and Technology, 43*, 18. https://doi.org/10.1002/ceat.201900180

Renzi, D. (2019). Recent developments in environmental law. *Tulane Environ Law J, 32* (2): 277–286. https://journals.tulane.edu/elj/article/view/2521.

RFS2. (2010). Renewable Fuel Standard Program Regulatory Impact Analysis. Environ Prot Agency, https://www.eesi.org/files/420r10006.pdf

Ricardo Energy & Environment (REE). (2017). A review of the NAEI shipping emissions: Methodology—Final report. Report for the *Department for Business, Energy & Industrial Strategy PO number 1109088*, https://ukair.defra.gov.uk/assets/documents/reports/cat07/1712140936_ED61406_NAEI_shipping_report_12Dec2017.pdf

Ridley-Kaye, M., Roberts, N., Warnberg, C., Nicholas, C. (2024). Renewable natural gas: legal landscape, private sector interest, and future opportunities for investment texas journal of oil, gas, and energy Law19 Tex. *J. Oil Gas & Energy L.* 67 pp 1–39. https://www.hoganlovells.com/

Rotunno, P., Lanzini, A., Leone, P. (2017). Energy and economic analysis of water scrubbing based biogas upgrading process for biomethane injection into the gas grid or use as transportation fuel. *Renewable Energy, 102*: Part B, 417–432 https://doi.org/10.1016/j.renene.2016.10.062

Rout, P. R., Zhang, T. C., Bhunia, P., & Surampalli, R. Y. (2021). Treatment technologies for emerging contaminants in wastewater treatment plants: A Review. *Science of the Total Environment, 753*, Article 141990. https://doi.org/10.1016/j.scitotenv.2020.141990

Rowan, M., Umenweke, G. C., Epelle, E. I., Afolabi, I. C., Okoye, P. U., Gunes, B., & Okolie, J. A. (2022). Anaerobic co-digestion of food waste and agricultural residues: An overview of feedstock properties and the impact of biochar addition. *Digital Chem Eng, 4*, Article 100046. https://doi.org/10.1016/j.dche.2022.100046

Ryckebosch, E., Drouillon, M., Vervaeren, H. (2011). Techniques for transformation of biogas to biomethane. *Biomass Bioenergy, 35* (5): 1633–1645. https://doi.org/10.1016/j.biombioe.2011.02.033 Get rights and content

Saadabadi, S. A., Thattai, A. T., Fan, L., Lindeboom, R. E. F., Spanjers, H., & Aravind, P. V. (2019). Solid oxide fuel cells fuelled with biogas: Potential and constraints. *Renewable Energy, 134*, 194–214. https://doi.org/10.1016/j.renene.2018.11.028

Samuelsson J., Delre A., Tumlin S., Hadi S., Offerle B., Scheutz C. (2018). Optical technologies applied alongside on-site and remote approaches for climate gas emission quantification at a wastewater treatment plant. *Water Res. 131*: 299- 309. https://doi.org/210.1016/j.watres.2017.1012.1018.

Scheutz, C., & Fredenslund, A. M. (2019). Total methane emission rates and losses from 23 biogas plants. *Waste Management, 97*, 38–46. https://doi.org/10.1016/j

Schories, G., Cordes, C., Winterberg, R. (2018). AcEta: Bioprozesstechnische Optimierung zweistufiger landwirtschaftlicher Biogasanlagen. Abschlussbericht zu F¨orderkennzeichen 22015412 und 22011413. Fachagentur für Nachwachsende Rohstoffe e.V., Bremerhaven. URL: https://www.fnr-server.de/ftp/pdf/berichte/22011413.pdf

Seo, M.W., Lee, S.H., Nam, H., Lee, D., Tokmurzin, D., Wang, S., Park, Y-K. (2022). Recent advances of thermochemical conversion processes for biorefinery. *Bioresour Technol, 343*: Article 126109, https://doi.org/10.1016/j.biortech.2021.126109.

Soreanu, G., Beland, M., Falletta, P., Edmonson, K., Svoboda, L., Al-Jamal, M., Seto, P. (2011). Approaches concerning siloxane removal from biogas – a review. *Canad Biosys Eng, 53*: 1–18.https://library.csbe-scgab.ca/docs/journal/53/C0815.pdf.

Su, Y., Zhang, P., Su, Y. (2015). An overview of biofuels policies and industrialization in the major biofuel producing countries. *Renew Sustain Energy Rev, 50*: 991–1003. https://doi.org/10.1016/j.rser.2015.04.032 Get rights and content

Subbarao P.M.V., D'Silva T.C., Adlak K., Kumar S., Chandra R., Vijay V.K. (2023). Anaerobic digestion as a sustainable technology for efficiently utilizing biomass in the context of carbon neutrality and circular economy. *Environ Res, 234*:116286. https://doi.org/10.1016/j.envres.2023.116286.

Sun, Q., Li, H., Yan, J., Liu, L., Yu, Z., & Yu, X. (2015). Selection of appropriate biogas upgrading technology—A review of biogas cleaning, upgrading and utilisation. *Renewable and Sustainable Energy Reviews, 51*, 521–532. https://doi.org/10.1016/j.rser.2015.06.029

Tautorat, P., Lalin, B., Schmidt, T. S., & Steffen, B. (2023). Directions of innovation for the decarbonization of cement and steel production – A topic modeling-based analysis. *J Cleaner Prod, 407*(25), Article 137055. https://doi.org/10.1016/j.jclepro.2023.137055

Greenhouse Gas Reduction Thresholds (GhGRT). (2010). U.S. environmental protection agency. https://www.epa.gov/system/files/documents/2023-08/ghgrp-overview-fact-sheet.pdf

Usman, I. M. T., Ho, Y. C., Baloo, L., Lam, M. K., & Sujarwo, W. (2022). A comprehensive review on the advances of bioproducts from biomass towards meeting net zero carbon emissions (NZCE). *Bioresource Technology, 366*, Article 128167. https://doi.org/10.1016/j.biortech.2022.128167

Van Ruijven, B. J., Van Vuuren, D. P., Boskaljon, W., Neelis, M. L., Saygin, D., & Patel, M. K. (2016). Long-term model-based projections of energy use and CO_2 emissions from the global steel and cement industries Resour. *Conservation & Recycling, 112*, 15–36. https://doi.org/10.1016/j.resconrec.2016.04.016

Wang, P., Ryberg, M., Yang, Y., Feng, K., Kara, S., Hauschild, M., Chen, W.Q. (2021). Efficiency stagnation in global steel production urges joint supply- and demand-side mitigation efforts. *Nat. Commun, 12*: Article number: 2066. https://doi.org/10.1038/S41467-021-22245-6.

Wantz, E., Benizri, D., Dietrich, N., & Hébrard, G. (2022). Rate-based modeling approach for High Pressure Water Scrubbing with unsteady gas flow rate and multicomponent absorption applied to biogas upgrading. *Applied Energy, 312*, Article 118754. https://doi.org/10.1016/j.apenergy.2022.118754

Wasajja, H., Lindeboom, R. E. F., van Lier, J. B., & Aravind, P. V. (2020). Techno-economic review of biogas cleaning technologies for small scale off-grid solid oxide fuel cell applications. *Fuel Processing Technology, 197*, Article 106215. https://doi.org/10.1016/j.fuproc.2019.106215

Werkneh, A.A. (2022). Biogas impurities: environmental and health implications, removal technologies and future perspectives *Heliyon, 8*: e10929. https://doi.org/10.2139/ssrn.4152685.

Worldsteel (2022) World steel in figures 2022 Brussels. https://worldsteel.org/data/world-steel-in-figures/world-steel-in-figures-2022/.

Zhang, Y., Fan, M., Wang, H., Wang, H., & Lu, Y. (2025). A comprehensive comparison of three renewable natural gas production technologies: Energy, exergy, economic, and environmental assessments. *Energy Conver Manag, 328*, Article 119615. https://doi.org/10.1016/j.enconman.2025.119615

Zhou, W.H., Guo, J.P., Tan, H.Y. (2011). Upgrading of methane from biogas by pressure swing adsorption. *In Advanced Materials Research; Trans Tech Publications Ltd.*: Zurich, Switzerland, https://doi.org/10.4028/www.scientific.

Chapter 11
Sustainable Aviation Fuels (SAFs): Future Prospects and Challenges, Development and Production of Sustainable Aviation Fuels. Technological and Regulatory Challenges, Future Prospects for SAFs in Reducing Aviation Emissions

Tarek O. Said, Mohamed A. Hassaan, and Ahmed El Nemr

Abstract Sustainable Aviation Fuels (SAFs), biofuels, are used instead of traditional jet fuel because they reduce aviation emissions and have footprint of a lower carbon. Compared to kerosene, they can cut CO_2 emissions by up to 65% because they are made from non-fossil resources. SAFs are essential to reaching the aviation sector's 2050 net-zero goals. With a focus on feedstock flexibility and ASTM certification, this chapter examines manufacturing paths such as fatty acids (HEFA) and hydro-processed esters, power-to-liquid (PtL), and alcohol-to-jet (ATJ) technologies. Regulatory obstacles like disjointed international policies juxtapose technological difficulties like poor energy density and expensive manufacturing costs. Synthetic biology, algae-derived SAFs, and catalytic process innovations are cited as game-changing innovations. Case studies, including Neste's MY Sustainable Aviation Fuel, demonstrate scalability, while future prospects explore hydrogen-SAF hybrids and carbon pricing mechanisms. The chapter also underscores the need for cross-sector collaboration to overcome adoption barriers and align SAF production with global climate goals.

Keywords Sustainable aviation fuels (SAFs) · Emissions · Footprint · Power-to-Liquid (PtL) · Alcohol-to-Jet (ATJ)

T. O. Said · M. A. Hassaan · A. El Nemr (✉)
National Institute of Oceanography and Fisheries (NIOF), Alexandria, Egypt
e-mail: ahmedmoustafaelnemr@yahoo.com; ahmed.m.elnemr@gmail.com

P. Verma (ed.), *Sustainable Practices in Biorefinery*,
https://doi.org/10.1007/978-981-95-6071-4_11

11.1 Introduction

11.1.1 Aviation's Carbon Footprint and ICAO's CORSIA Framework

With a large carbon footprint, the aviation sector contributes considerably to global CO_2 emissions. The International Civil Aviation Organization (ICAO) devised the Carbon Offsetting and Reduction Scheme (CORSIA) to solve this problem. CORSIA mandates that airlines offset emissions beyond a certain baseline in an effort to stabilise net CO_2 emissions from international travel. International aviation emissions have not been incorporated into the global climate system governed by the United Nations Framework Convention on Climate Change (UNFCCC) since they are not addressed by nationally determined climate action. Instead, the ICAO handles these pollutants (ICAO, 2023). As the world grapples with the urgent need to address climate change and cut carbon emissions, the aviation sector is not immune to criticism. The industry is at a turning point and contributes 2% of global anthropogenic greenhouse gas emissions. The demand for environmentally friendly travel is rising to unprecedented levels, and global climate rules are gaining traction. There is increasing pressure on the aviation sector to lower emissions. To do so, businesses in this industry must first identify the sources of their greenhouse gas emissions (Ritchie, 2024). Despite being one of the most carbon-intensive activities, flying only contributes 2.5% of world carbon emissions. How does this add up? As it happens, almost nobody in the world is a pilot. According to research, only 10% of people worldwide fly in most years. A single but when profits rise, this will change. The leading causes of increased aviation emissions during the last 50 years have been rising demand and technological advances. The "Kaya identity"—population, income, economic energy efficiency, and energy's carbon intensity—is frequently invoked to explain total CO_2 emissions. We might gain a better understanding of the origins of airplane emissions by adopting a similar strategy.

11.1.2 ASTM Certification Pathways for SAF (Annex 7)

Specific production routes must be evaluated and approved in order for ASTM to certify SAF, leading to the creation of annexes to the ASTM D7566 standard. For instance, Annex 7 allows up to 10% blending with conventional fuel and concentrates on a particular kind of SAF made from hydroprocessed hydrocarbons, esters, and fatty acids (ASTM, 2020). With assistance from the Commercial Aviation Alternative Fuels Initiative (CAAFI), ASTM International has authorized and released a seventh annex to D7566, the SAF specification. The 6th annex to D7566 establishes standards for the manufacture and application of catalytic hydrothermolysis jet fuel (CHJ), a form of synthetic kerosene, which was authorized and published by ASTM International in February 2020. Criteria for the manufacture and application of a particular kind of synthetic paraffinic kerosene from hydrocarbon-hydroprocessed esters and fatty acids (HC-HEFA-SPK) are outlined in Annex A7. The standard states that up to 10% by volume of HC-HEFA-SPK fuel, whose development was led by IHI Corporation, can be combined with ordinary jet fuel. The D1655 standard for conventional jet fuel and the ASTM D7566 specify the fuel quality requirements for each authorized SAF manufacturing process. The fuel must undergo a rigorous testing process to determine the maximum blend ratio with traditional jet fuel and show that the blend is suitable for its intended use before a new SAF production pathway can be added in D7566. ASTM D4054 describes this process. Since D7566 is the only internationally recognized fuel standard for SAF qualification in the aviation industry, certification is essential to the commercialization of any SAF technology.

11.2 Production Pathways

11.2.1 HEFA: Hydroprocessing of Fats/Oils

Hydrotreated Vegetable Oil (HEFA), often known as HVO, is a renewable diesel fuel that is produced by using hydrogen to convert oils and lipids into hydrocarbons. By breaking down the feedstock's oxygen and carbon double bonds, a process known as hydroprocessing produces a fuel that is chemically identical to petroleum diesel and can be utilized in diesel engines that are already in place without any changes (HEFA/HVO, 2016). A wide range of vegetable oils and fats can be used to make HVO. Triglycerides and fatty acids from vegetable oils (including rapeseed, soybean, and corn oil) and tall oil, a byproduct of the pulp and paper industries, are also included in this, in addition to animal fats. Triglycerides and H2 react under high pressure to remove oxygen from oils, a process known as hydrotreatment, which produces HVO. The hydrocarbon chains that are produced are chemically identical to those found in petroleum-based diesel fuel. Propane is typically produced as a byproduct. HVO has far higher investment costs than biodiesel manufacture, which requires large-scale production facilities to make the process commercially viable. Production can occur in integrated plants that also produce fossil fuels or in standalone units that produce HVO. The bulk of the raw materials used in the manufacturing of HVO in Sweden are of Swedish and European origin, although coming from non-European countries. Each HVO (RED) is required to comply with the sustainability standards of the Renewable Energy Directive. Similar to the Fuel Quality Directive, RED sets sustainability guidelines for biofuels and bioliquids. The availability of sustainable feedstock may be a limiting factor in the production of HVO since many raw resources are limited and may have conflicting applications. The main components of the HVO marketed in Sweden are 35% slaughterhouse wastes, 23% vegetable or animal waste oils, 22% crude tall oil, 15% palm oil, and 5% animal fat. Globally, the usage of vegetable and palm oils is growing (HEFA/HVO, 2016).

11.2.2 Alcohol to Jet (ATJ): Conversion of Ethanol to Isobutanol

Alcohols can be converted to an alternative jet fuel blendstock using the alcohol-to-jet (ATJ) process, which is based on catalytic procedures used in the petrochemical and petroleum refining industries for a long time. This route provides a temporary chance for the aviation industry to meet the rising demand for SAJF and for alcohol manufacturers to join the SAJF market. It also allows for sustainable alternative jet fuel (SAJF) utilizing various resources. Here, the technical foundation is reviewed, and certain variations of the ATJ technique are evaluated. Some ATJ conversion strategies were evaluated using modelling and simulation, emphasizing contrasting the usage of an ethanol or isobutanol intermediate (Geleynse et al., 2018).

11.2.3 Power-To-Liquid (PtL): CO_2Hydrogenation with Green H_2

Green hydrogen (H_2) and collected CO_2 are used in PtL technology to transform renewable electricity into liquid fuels. This procedure creates synthetic fuels that can replace fossil fuels in existing infrastructure, frequently using hydrogenation reactions such as Fischer–Tropsch synthesis (FTS). Since PtL and power-to-gas (PtG) technologies may effectively convert CO_2 into high-value products like liquid hydrocarbons and synthetic natural gas (SNG), as well as being a viable method of storing intermittent renewable energy, there has been a lot of focus on CO_2 mitigation using these processes lately. Based on earlier studies on the PtL and PtL/PtG processes made of Fe-based FTS, Gao et al. (2021) proposed a PtL process and a PtL/PtG process in conjunction with the reverse-water–gas-shift (RWGS) and Co-based FTS, which, respectively, produce liquid hydrocarbons only and the combination of liquid hydrocarbons and high-calorie SNG. They used process modelling and comparative techno-economic analysis to identify the key performance indicators of the proposed PtL and PtL/PtG processes, including the rate of CO_2 reduction, energy efficiency, total product cost, and CO_2 mitigation cost. Using the suggested PtL and PtL/PtG technologies to produce SNG and high-value liquid hydrocarbons might reduce waste CO_2. Furthermore, the PtL/PtG and indirect PtL methods helped to enhance the output of liquid hydrocarbons. Conversely, indirect PtL and direct PtL/PtG processes encourage CO_2 reduction and energy efficiency.

11.3 Technological Challenges

The adoption of SAF is hampered by both market and technological issues. The main obstacles are regulatory barriers, high production costs, and restricted feedstock availability. The implementation of SAF is further made more difficult by the requirement for substantial infrastructure development and the necessity to balance supply and demand in the market. Airlines operating in competitive markets find it challenging to use SAF due to its higher cost than regular jet fuel (Lau and Wang, 2024). Shorter-term, more restricted tax credits are typically not as desirable for SAF producers as long-term, stable incentive schemes like the RFS or Canada's Clean Fuel Regulation, which is modelled after state-level low-carbon fuel standard programs in the US (Lau and Wang, 2024). These initiatives, which were first created for on-road fuels, should develop to completely incorporate aviation fuel. The Inflation Reduction Act's SAF blenders tax credit is a good step that acknowledges SAF's contribution to aviation's ecarbonisation.

11.3.1 Catalyst Deactivation in Hydro-Processing

Coke formation, metal deposition, and sintering are the main processes that cause hydro-processing deactivation because they obstruct catalytic sites and lower activity. These deposits can impede the hydro-processing reactions, resulting in a lower product yield and higher costs. This is especially true of coke from asphaltenes and metal compounds (such as vanadium and nickel) from the feedstock. In heavy oil hydro-processing, catalyst regeneration and deactivation are essential steps. In heavy oil hydro processing, catalyst regeneration and deactivation are essential steps. Pham et al. (2025) thoroughly summarize the elements that lead to catalyst deactivation, such as active metal sintering, coke production, and poisoning from metals and other hetero-elements. They explored the mechanisms behind these deactivation processes and discussed how they affect reactor operations and catalyst performance. The review also examines different methods of catalyst renewal, including gasification and combustion. They assessed how well these techniques remove coke and revive catalytic activity. They also go over strategies for reducing coke production, such as creating catalysts that are more resistant to coke and adding solvents and surfactants. Understanding the reasons behind catalyst deactivation and the efficacy of various regeneration strategies can help refineries streamline operations, increase product yields, and reduce their environmental impact.

Deactivation and regeneration of catalysts are essential to heavy oil hydro processing's sustainability and efficiency. The main factors influencing catalyst deactivation, such as coke production, metal poisoning, and sulphur poisoning, are thoroughly examined in this paper. It explores the fundamental mechanisms and how they negatively impact reactor operations and catalyst performance. Several regeneration methods are included (Pham et al., 2025), including gasification and combustion using steam, hydrogen, and carbon dioxide. It assesses how well these techniques work to remove coke and restart catalytic activity. Pham et al. (2025) also look at ways to reduce coke production, such as the pretreatment of feedstock, using coke-delayed agents, and creating stronger catalysts. Refineries can improve product yields, streamline operations, and reduce environmental effects by comprehending these crucial factors. This review provides insightful information for engineers and researchers looking to further the topic of heavy oil hydro-processing.

11.3.2 Scalability of PtL Systems and Electrolyzer Costs

In producing green hydrogen, scalability, PtL, systems, electrolyzer, and costs are all intimately related. The cost and scalability of these systems directly impact the total cost of green hydrogen. Electrolyzer technology, particularly PEM electrolyzers, is essential for effectively converting power into hydrogen (Capuano, 2022). An important factor in raising electrolyzer efficiency and cutting expenses is the porous transport layer (PTL). To enable rapid and broad decarbonisation in the electric power and industrial sectors, high levels of renewable energy deployment are expected to be required, facilitated by technologies that store and transform renewable electricity into other appropriate forms like hydrogen. Low-carbon-intensity hydrogen as a fuel and chemical building block is becoming a viable short-term option to lessen the reliance on fossil fuels in hard-to-decarbonize industries like heavy-duty transportation and organic chemicals. Conventional steam methane reforming H_2 generation uses natural gas; in contrast, water-splitting electrolysis uses only energy and water as inputs. Electrolysis is a significant step toward cross-sectoral decarbonisation when fuelled by low-carbon electricity (Badgett et al., 2024). However, to enable rapid computational characterisation of SAF molecules, an integrated method is required due to the limitations of both DFT and ML alone.

11.3.3 Cold Flow Properties of SAF Blends

For dependable operation in various temperatures and climates, SAFs, particularly blends, are made to preserve strong cold flow characteristics. An important characteristic is a low cloud point and a freezing point below –40 °C. These characteristics are essential for avoiding gasoline gelling or crystallizing in cold weather, which could cause problems with operation. To meet performance requirements in cold environments, SAF blends carefully evaluate specific cold flow features, including freezing and cloud points. The aviation industry must use sustainable fuels (SAFs) to lessen its environmental impact. According to ASTM D7566 fuel standards, High-energy–density hydrocarbons with ideal characteristics are required for SAFs. These include a maximum net heat of combustion of 42.8 MJ kg^{-1}, a freezing point below

–40 °C, and a density of 775 to 840 kg m^{-3} at 15 °C. If it were feasible to anticipate these qualities for a molecule with a specific structure, SAF implementation and optimization would go more quickly. Conventional experimental techniques are precise yet expensive and time-consuming. Machine learning (ML) and density functional theory (DFT) are two computational methods that can be more rapid and less expensive (Rijal et al., 2025).

11.4 Economic and Regulatory Barriers

11.4.1 High Production Costs (3–6/Gallonvs.3–6/Gallonvs.1.5/Gallon Fossil Jet Fuel)

Depending on the price of fossil jet fuel, renewable feedstocks, associated processing expenses, and other factors, Because of its small production volume, SAF often costs three to five times as much as regular jet fuel. Meanwhile, price levels are naturally impacted by supply and demand dynamics (Kjelgaard, 2024). There are negative environmental effects associated with the aviation sector's usage of fossil fuels. Hence a global switch to sustainable renewable fuels is required. As a possible replacement for non-renewable fossil fuels, SAF, which is derived from renewable bio-based resources, has attracted much attention lately. The footprint of CO_2 emissions from the SAF is substantially smaller than that of fossil fuels. Despite the environmental benefits, SAF costs a lot and is not commercially viable. Therefore, to encourage the aviation industry's broad adoption of SAF, several organizational activities, financial incentives from the government, and sensible legislation are needed (Shahriar & Khanal, 2022). By lowering the risks and uncertainties involved in launching commercial-scale biorefinery operations, investigating supply chain requirements, and enhancing technical understanding of the production processes, the incentives are also required to make SAF competitive with fossil fuels. The global techno-economic state of SAF technology is examined in this review.

Additionally, it examines current and historical organizational activities and policies to promote SAF's wider adoption in the aviation sector. This study also critically examines the environmental effects of SAF use, including water use and carbon offset. A thorough comparison of multiple bio-conversion techniques employing different feedstocks is also investigated (Shahriar & Khanal, 2022). The assessment also outlines several obstacles and areas that require more investigation to successfully transition from conventional fuels to SAF. The SAF has the potential to drastically lower aviation's CO_2 emissions and make a substantial contribution to the fight against climate change, despite the fact that there are still legal, financial, and technological obstacles to be addressed.

11.4.2 Fragmented Global Policies and Subsidy Disparities

A combination of policies is required to get beyond the various obstacles impeding sustainability transitions. Coherence in policy is thus needed. The breadth of their applicability is limited since most policy coherence studies in the literature on sustainability transitions are focused on European experiences. This article examines how policy combinations about biogas systems and the coherence problems they raise affect the production and consumption of biogas in Brazil. We found policy coherence over time and within and between biogas-related sectors, demonstrating how Brazilian states' prerequisites for production, distribution, and usage vary significantly (Kanda et al., 2022). This suggests that decentralized governance mechanisms are required to facilitate policy differentiation in addition to policy consistency. The essay concludes that in hierarchical market economies like Brazil, where resource mobilization, allocation, and governance are highly centralized, the locally rooted character of biogas systems poses a challenge.

The vertical aspect of the governance of biogas systems is described at the administrative level. Policies about biogas can be found at the national, regional/local, continental, and international levels (Gustafsson & Anderberg, 2021). Policies are linked together from the local to the global level, creating a hierarchy of complexities. Climate change and other global social challenges set the stage for administration-level policy goals and agreements. It is necessary to operationalize and adapt global goals at the local, regional, and national levels. While policies at the state and regional levels can be more ambitious, those at the international and continental levels can be established at a basic level of ambition that many member nations can implement. The production, distribution, and use of biogas differ significantly at the local level according to local socioeconomic factors (such as industrial structure, raw resources, climate objectives, and legislation). Last, policy synergies, conflicts, contradictions, and unforeseen repercussions may arise on several vertical and horizontal administrative levels.

11.5 Innovations

11.5.1 Algae-Derived SAFs with High Lipid Productivity

Microalgae have drawn much interest as a substitute feedstock for biofuel synthesis, especially when combined with genetic modification techniques to increase lipid output. Reducing the use of fossil fuels is viewed as a top priority to address climate change challenges, and biofuel made from microalgae is one possible sustainable energy source for a range of uses. These photosynthetic microalgae use carbon dioxide and solar energy to create energy-rich substances (lipids and starch), which can then be transformed into various biofuels. The most environmentally friendly alternative to fossil fuel-based petroleum diesel for transportation is biodiesel made from transesterifying triacylglycerol (Khoo et al., 2023). However, there is a significant gap in the path to commercialized microalgae-based biofuel due to obstacles like low productivity, high production costs, and difficulties scaling up the algal technology. This review article initially provides a thorough summary of essential information on microalgae, including classification of the algae, factors influencing microalgae growth during culture, and various upstream processing procedures. Recent developments in the downstream processing of microalgal biorefineries are also covered in this review (Table 11.1) (Mata et al., 2020).

Furthermore, Khoo et al. (2023) examined several recent genetic modification strategies and their viability for increased lipid yield in microalgae. Last but not least, they highlight the present difficulties and prospects for microalgae-based biofuels by going over several topics, such as the sustainability of producing biofuel from microalgae, the state of the algae-based industry at the moment, and the dangers and legal implications of genetically modifying microalgae. Microalgae are categorized as third-generation biofuel feedstock because of their capacity to use solar energy to create lipids. Because lipids like Triacylglycerol (TAG) and diacylglycerol (DAG) are easily converted into biodiesel through transesterification, they are preferred as feedstock for biofuel over starch. The use of microalgae to produce biofuel is not currently commercially and economically viable due to poor productivity and technology, despite benefits including ease of culture and assistance in mitigating CO_2.

Table 11.1 The importance of microalgae compared to alternative feedstocks in biodiesel production

Plant source	Oil*	Oil**	Land use*#	Biodiesel#
Soybean (*Glycine max*)	18	636	18	562
Jatropha	28	741	15	656
Microalgae (low oil content)	30	58,700	0.2	51.927
Palm oil (*Elaeis gunieenis*)	36	5366	2	4747
Suflower (*Helianthus annuus*)	40	1070	11	946
Canola/Rapeseed	41	974	12	862
Corn/Maize (*Zea mays*)	44	172	66	152
Cstor (*Ricinus communis*)	48	1307	9	1156
Microalgae (medium oil content)	50	97,800	0.1	86,515
Microalgae (high oil content)	70	136,900	0.1	121,104

* = Composition by wt. in biomass (%); ** = Productivity (L oil/ha/year); * # = (m^2 year/kg biodiesel); # = Productivity (kg biodiesel/ha/year)

11.5.2 Electrofuels (E-Fuel) from Direct Air Capture (DAC)

Electrofuels, sometimes known as e-fuels, are artificial fuels made by mixing hydrogen, which is frequently obtained by electrolysis, with collected CO_2. A key component of this process is Direct Air Capture (DAC), which removes CO_2 from the atmosphere to make carbon–neutral fuels possible (Fig. 11.1) (D'Adamo et al., 2024). European regulation will require new cars to have zero emissions starting in 2035, and the ecological shift in the transportation industry is a significant issue in combating environmental pollution. Much attention is being paid to using synthetic fuels, such as electrofuels (e-fuels), to lessen the impact of gasoline and diesel cars. This study aims to investigate a levelized cost (LCO) analysis of e-fuel production utilizing a renewable energy source. A photovoltaic plant plus the additional processes needed to create e-fuel—direct air capture, electrolysis, and the Fischer–Tropsch process—are anticipated to provide the process's energy (D'Adamo et al., 2024). According to their data, the baseline scenario's LCOe-fuel is approximately 3.1 €/l, with the energy generation component having the most impact, followed by the hydrogen component. Sensitivity, scenario, and risk assessments are also conducted to assess alternative scenarios. The results show that, in 84% of the situations, LCOe-fuel falls between 2.8 and 3.4 €/l. The findings show that developing e-fuels encourages environmental preservation even though the price is not competitive with fossil fuels. The concepts of pragmatic sustainability, incentive programs, technical innovation, industrial symbiosis, economies of scale, and learning economies can all help to reduce this cost by encouraging the decarbonisation of the transportation industry.

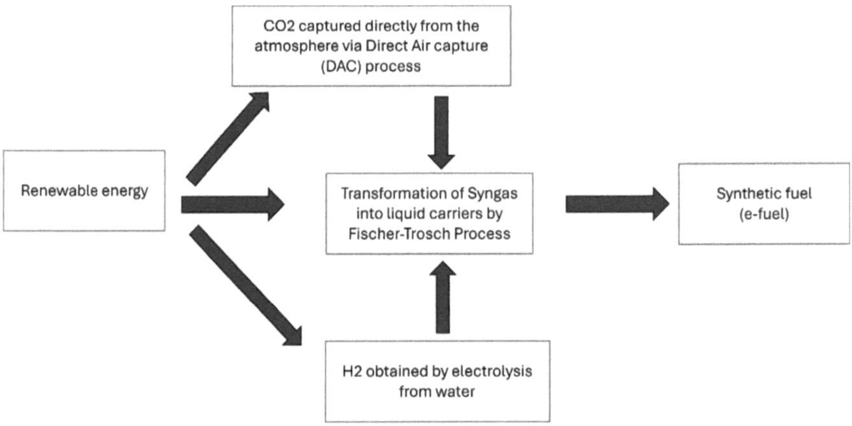

Fig. 11.1 CO_2 captured from atmosphere via DAC process

11.5.3 Blockchain for SAF Supply Chain Transparency

Digital technologies, especially those related to Industry 4.0, are causing significant advancements in supply chains. One example of such a technology is blockchain. The consensus mechanism, ecarbonisation, anonymity and identification, overall performance and expectations, data and system dependability, and transparency of information are some of the characteristics that set blockchain apart as a revolutionary technology. Supply chains may increase transparency by using blockchain to provide end-to-end visibility and traceability. An increasing number of supply chains are looking at transparency and blockchain technology, with many ecarbon on system development. To comprehend the guiding principles of its design, Sunmola and Burgess (2023) investigated transparency in blockchain-based supply chains. Alongside data-driven analysis, a systematic assessment of the literature is employed. Their findings outline the tenets of a framework for supply chains based on blockchain that prioritizes transparency by design. Their study evaluates the findings and contributions of previous publications to apply a data-driven approach to a systematic evaluation of the literature. The findings revealed 120 principles in three main areas: blockchain design, applications, enablers, and technical features. The research's framework for transparency by design for blockchain-based supply chains lays out the concepts in the literature review. There are seven findings drawn. (1) The principles include 11 system design considerations, 78 enablers and applications, and 31 technological features. The suggested framework incorporates the ideas that appeared more frequently in the results: seven enablers and applications, five system design considerations, and ten technical features. (2) When designing for transparency in blockchain-based supply chains, privacy and security are crucial technical features that must be managed appropriately. (3) Smart contracts could aid in resolving privacy and security issues. (4) Two essential elements of transparency that must be considered in the design are traceability and visibility. (5) System architecture development and testing are essential when designing for transparency since they will aid the system's beneficial development and implementation. (6) By enhancing monitoring and forecasting, system integration can increase supply chains based on blockchain technology's openness. (7) Context-awareness can boost the applicability of the suggested framework and facilitate the necessary adjustments between system architecture, technological features, enablers, and applications. One of the research's limitations is its theoretical approach. Future research should concentrate on using the design by transparency concept in an empirical investigation. Supply chain stakeholders and experts should validate the ideas, dimensions, and general framework (Sunmola & Burgess, 2023).

11.6 Case Studies

11.6.1 Neste's SAF Production in Singapore and Rotterdam

Neste, the world's largest manufacturer of SAF, has begun manufacturing SAF at its refinery for renewable goods in Rotterdam, the Netherlands. Neste can now generate up to 500,000 tonnes of SAF annually thanks to modifications made to the refinery. Nestle is now able to produce 1.5 million tons of SAF annually, or about 1.875 billion litters, globally as a result. We must keep moving forward with reducing the effects of aviation on the climate. This milestone demonstrates Neste's unwavering commitment to helping its aviation industry clients lower their greenhouse gas emissions. The Refuel EU Aviation Regulation and other SAF mandates may be implemented with a major contribution thanks to the Rotterdam-based SAF production capabilities. They must continue to press us to high standards since regulations such as these are essential to increasing SAF production and consumption. At the same time, to speed up the energy transition and associated emission reductions, the entire aviation ecosystem must support and work closely together," stated Heikki Malinen, Neste's president and CEO (Maula, 2025).

With a yearly production capacity of one million tons, Neste's refinery in Singapore is the biggest SAF production plant in the world. The largest renewable diesel refinery in the world was built in 2010 and enlarged in 2023. It is situated in Tuas, southwest of Singapore. It uses Nestle's NEXBTLTM technology to turn waste fats, oils and greases into SAF. Singapore can produce 2.6 million tons of renewable products annually, including SAF, renewable diesel, and renewable raw ingredients for chemicals and polymers (Sieppi, 2024). This partnership with Neste is a significant step toward the Singapore Airlines (SIA) Group's goal of using at least 5% sustainable aviation fuel in our overall fuel mix by 2030. Our strong collaboration with our partners and stakeholders in Singapore and globally is essential to achieving their long-term ecarbonisation goals. If the aviation industry is more sustainable, future generations will continue to benefit from the global connectivity, economic expansion, and interpersonal relationships that air travel fosters (Sieppi, 2024).

11.6.2 Lanza Jet's ATJ Facility in Georgia, U.S

The first commercial ethanol-based ATJ SAF production unit in the world is located at Lanza Jet's Freedom Pines Fuels facility in Soperton, Georgia. Leading renewable fuels technology business Lanza Jet is committed to embracing the recycling economy to accelerate the energy revolution. As a manufacturer of proprietary ATJ technology and a supplier of SAF technology, Lanza Jet is opening doors for future generations by speeding up the adoption of SAF and other clean technologies essential to solving the climate issue and revolutionizing the world economy. This Lanza Jet, Inc. network facility is scheduled to start up in 2025 and will generate 10 million gallons of renewable diesel and SAF each year. The facility uses Lanza Jet's ATJ technology to produce renewable diesel and SAF from low-carbon ethanol (US Department of Energy, 2024).

11.7 Future Directions

11.7.1 Hydrogen-Powered Aircraft and SAF Compatibility

Although they tackle separate aspects of the issue, hydrogen-powered aircraft and SAF are essential steps in the aviation industry's decarbonisation process. Since SAF is a "drop-in" fuel, it can be used in aircraft that are already in operation by mixing it with conventional jet fuel without requiring major modifications. Although promising, hydrogen necessitates major engine design and infrastructure upgrades for power generation and fuel storage. Civil aviation provides a vital transportation network that links people worldwide and promotes economic expansion. Next-generation aircraft must have far lower climatic impacts to preserve these advantages while fulfilling environmental goals. In addition to reducing or eliminating other emissions, hydrogen-powered aircraft can operate on current routes without carbon emissions (Table 11.2)(Adler & Martins, 2023). Adler and Martins (2023) analysed existing technology and thoroughly explained the basic physics of hydrogen-powered aircraft. Adler and Martins (2023) talked about how these technologies affect the environment, certification, cost, and design of airplanes. The most attractive long-term substitute for the current generation of kerosene-fueled aircraft is a hydrogen-powered aircraft. New technologies like fuel cells and superconducting electronics can be developed using hydrogen, perhaps leading to aircraft ideas that are not possible with kerosene fuel. Although they need a lot of study and development, hydrogen-powered aircraft are technically possible. One of the key innovations is the use of lightweight liquid hydrogen tanks into the aircraft. If big, fuel cell-powered freight aircraft are to become a reality, fuel cells must get stronger, lighter, and more resilient. Pollutants can be eliminated in flight using fuel cells. Even though hydrogen turbofans are much less dangerous than kerosene turbofans, they have these desirable characteristics. The viability of hydrogen aircraft is contingent upon the efficient generation of green hydrogen, which requires substantial investments in energy infrastructure and airframe and motor technologies. Their proposed approach to sustain the civil aviation industry in an eco-friendly way is using hydrogen-powered aircraft. Many academics and engineers consider them the most viable long-term alternative to kerosene-fuelled aircraft. Aircraft powered by hydrogen can accomplish more than just long-term objectives. H_2FLY and Deutsche Aircraft, Universal Hydrogen, and Zero Avia want to transport people on regional propeller aircraft fuelled by hydrogen before the end of this decade. Hydrogen aeroplanes are theoretically possible even though much more study and development are required (Adler & Martins, 2023).

Table 11.2 Characteristics of gaseous (GH_2) and liquid hydrogen (LH_2) as well as approximate tank gravimetric efficiency (a lighter tank is indicated by a greater value). The lower heating value (LHV) is used to specify certain energies. In certain situations, condensation of water vapor in the exhaust may extract more energy than the LHV recommends

Property	Unit	Jet A-1	LH_2	GH_2 (350 bar)	GH_2 (700 bar)
Storage temperature	(K)	RT	20	RT	RT
Storage pressure	(bar)	RT	~ 2	350	700
Energy density	(MJ/L)	34.9	8.5	2.9	4.8
Specific energy	(MJ/kg)	43.2	120	120	120
Tank gravimetric efficiency	(%)	100	~ 30–90	1–15	1–15

RT: Room temperature

11.7.2 Carbon Pricing Mechanisms to Bridge Cost Gaps

Pricing mechanisms such as taxes and cap-and-trade schemes seek to close the cost difference between conventional and low-carbon choices by giving carbon emissions a monetary value. This ultimately aids in addressing the climate catastrophe by motivating companies and individuals to cut emissions, invest in greener technologies, and embrace sustainable habits. Carbon pricing is seen as a crucial policy tool to unlock the building sector's potential, which provides a significant lever for lowering carbon emissions. However, there are problems with carbon pricing in residential structures, particularly in rental housing, where landlords and renters may share the costs and, as a result, the incentives to reduce carbon emissions. This leads to a principal-agent dilemma that may be unpopular and produce conflict. Kaestner et al. (2025) examine the support for various ideas to divide the financial burden of carbon pricing between landlords and tenants using broad survey data from over 12,000 households. With special emphasis on the function of perceived cost, efficacy, and fairness, they experimentally examined how public preferences are impacted by revenue utilization and the carbon price level. According to their findings, price level and revenue consumption have minimal bearing on support, but tenancy and self-interest, as well as the perceived fairness of the sharing notion, strongly connect with preferences. Overall, a sharing mechanism based on the building's energy efficiency is the cost allocation strategy that their members prefer (Kaestner et al., 2025). In the building industry as well, carbon pricing is regarded as a crucial measure to lower greenhouse gas emissions. However, it raises the expense of heating, which aggravates renters the most because they cannot choose whether to install energy retrofits for their homes. There is a glaring motivation issue because landlords make this decision and do not benefit from decreasing energy costs. Thus, the issue of who would foot the bill for rising energy costs brought on by increasing carbon pricing is a significant concern. Contrary to the literature on support for carbon pricing generally, there is no proof that the carbon price level that Kaestner et al. (2025) randomly selected in their experiment had any impact on general preferences for cost-sharing notions or income redistribution (Kotchen et al., 2017; Saeen & Kallbekken, 2011).

11.8 Future Prospective

The drive in the global aviation sector to lower carbon emissions is driving up demand for SAF. SAF has much fewer carbon emissions than traditional kerosene-based aviation fuel. Many methods are used to achieve this reduction, including carbon capture devices and biogenic-carbon fuels like biomass, which collectively reduce emissions. However, the lack of awareness among nations and the lack of pertinent rules limits the use of SAF as a new alternative fuel. Using global regulatory expertise and shared manufacturing pathways, this article highlights the benefits of sustainable aviation fuel, analyzes the market and development prospects for sustainable aviation fuel, and explains the current status of kerosene-based sustainable aviation fuel (Wang et al., 2024). In addition to establishing certification procedures and criteria for the system, participants also discussed the technical and economic feasibility, technological maturity, and environmental benefits of SAF, particularly in reducing carbon emissions. Finally, recommendations were made for future expansion of SAF to guide the green transformation in the aviation industry and its widespread adoption (Fig. 11.2) (Strategy, 2023).

In recent years, the aviation sector has had to adjust to the global emphasis on carbon emissions. According to statistics, the aviation sector is responsible for almost 2% of global greenhouse gas emissions, substantially contributing to global warming (Abrantes et al., 2021). The aviation sector has a significant impact on global warming. According to estimates, the aviation sector will raise world temperatures by 0.1 °C by 2050 if adequate countermeasures are not implemented (Klöwer

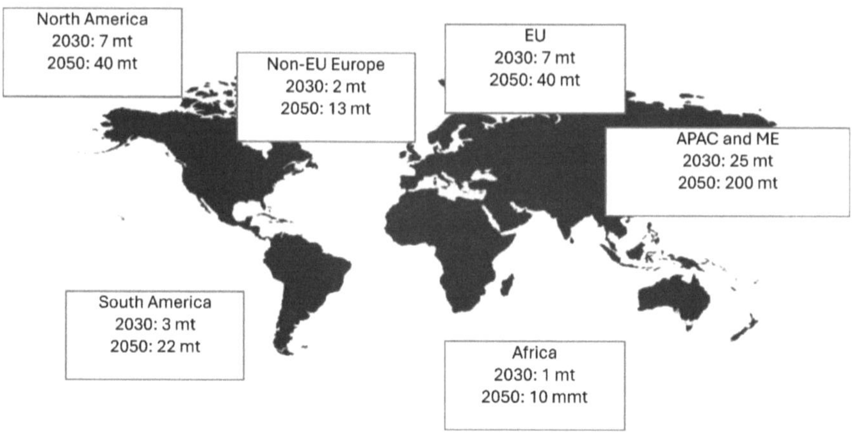

Fig. 11.2 Potential production capacity of SAF worldwide by region

et al., 2021). In response, ICAO (2016) has advocated for several actions, including enhancing the emission compliance criteria for aircraft engines and increasing the aviation industry's carbon emission compliance standards. Nevertheless, these actions have not mitigated the underlying cause of the aviation sector's carbon emission issue (ICAO, 2019). The aviation sector is being forced to adapt due to the growing global oil prices and the problems with carbon emissions from fossil fuels. Low-carbon or carbon–neutral aviation fuels must be developed, along with more stringent emission regulations and aircraft that use less fuel. A variety of organic solid wastes (OSWs) may be utilised to create SAF (US Department of Energy, 2024). These include energy crops, maize grain, oilseeds, algae, oily wastes, agricultural and forestry wastes, lumber mill wastes, municipal rubbish, livestock manure and municipal sludge (Energy, 2023). Additionally, the International Air Transport Association (IATA) data and observations show notable geographical variations in the kinds of OSWs utilized for SAF manufacture worldwide. According to the World Bank, the Food and Agriculture Organisation of the United Nations (FAO), and the International Food Policy Research Institute (IFPRI), approximately 7.34 billion tonnes of OSWs (comprising of food wastes, agricultural wastes, and municipal solid wastes) were produced globally in 2020. By 2050, the annual output of OSWs is anticipated to reach 12.71 billion tonnes due to increased urbanization and population growth (FAO, 2022).

Converting these OSWs into SAF could replace conventional petroleum fuels and significantly reduce carbon emissions throughout the aviation fuel lifecycle, in addition to lowering greenhouse gas emissions, groundwater contamination, and deteriorating air quality through traditional waste management techniques (such as landfilling and incineration). US Department of Energy (2024) predicts that 50–60 billion gallons (or 151.6–181.9 million tons) of SAF might be produced from one billion tons of dry OSWs (Energy, 2023). Theoretically, 110.1–132.12 billion gallons (or 333.8–400.6 million tonnes) of SAF could be generated using the worldwide OSW production numbers for 2020 (with a 70% moisture content); by 2050, this could reach 190.65–228.78 billion gallons (or 578.1–693.7 million tonnes) of SAF.

In summary, SAF's quick growth can help with the global OSW treatment problem while enhancing resource efficiency, promoting a circular economy, and slowing climate change. Furthermore, this technique reduces dependency on external energy sources and improves energy security, both critical for resource-constrained countries. Due to cost and technological advances, SAF from OSWs is expected to play a bigger role in the global energy market and in reducing carbon footprints in the future.

References

Abrantes, I., Ferreira, A.F., Silva, A., Costa, M. (2021). Sustainable aviation fuels and imminent technologies - CO_2 emissions evolution towards 2050. *Journal of Cleaner Production. 313*, Article 127937. https://doi.org/10.1016/j.jclepro.2021.127937.

Adler, E. J., & Martins, J. R. R. A. (2023). Hydrogen-powered aircraft: Fundamental concepts, key technologies, and environmental impacts. *Progress in Aerospace Sciences, 141*, Article 100922. https://doi.org/10.1016/j.paerosci.2023.100922
ASTM. (2020). Green Car Congress. Approves 7th annex to D7566 sustainable jet fuel specification: HC-HEFA.
Badgett, A., Brauch, J., Thatte, A., Rubin, R., Skangos, C., Wang, X., Ahluwalia, R., Pivovar, B., Ruth, M. (2024). Updated manufactured cost analysis for proton exchange membrane water electrolyzers. *Technical Report* NREL/TP-6A20–87625.
Capuano, C. (2022). Enabling Low-Cost PEM electrolysis at scale through optimization of transport components and electrode interfaces. Project ID: P198. Nel Hydrogen. Hydrogen Program 2022 Annual Merit Review and Peer Evaluation Meeting DOE Project Award #DE-EE0009238.
D'Adamo, I., Gastaldi, M., Giannini, M., & Nizami, A.-S. (2024). Environmental implications and levelized cost analysis of E-fuel production under photovoltaic energy, direct air capture, and hydrogen. *Environmental Research, 246*, Article 118163. https://doi.org/10.1016/j.envres.2024.118163
Energy, O.O.E.E.R., (2023). Sustainable aviation fuels: bioenergy technologies office. https://www.energy.gov/eere/bioenergy/sustainable-aviation-fuels.
FAO, (2022). Technical platform on the measurement and reduction of food loss and waste. https://www.fao.org/platform-food-loss-waste/flw-data/en/.
Gao, R., Zhang, C., Jun, K-W., Kim, S.K., Park, H-G., Zhao, T., Wang, L., Wan, H., Guan, G. (2021). Green liquid fuel and synthetic natural gas production via CO2 hydrogenation combined with reverse water-gas-shift and Co-based Fischer-Tropsch synthesis, *Journal of CO_2Utilization 51*, 101619. https://doi.org/10.1016/j.jcou.2021.101619.
Geleynse, S., Brandt, K., Garcia-Perez, M., Wolcott, M., & Zhang, X. (2018). The Alcohol-to-Jet conversion pathway for drop-in biofuels: techno-economic evaluation. *Chemsuschem, 11*(21), 3728–3741. https://doi.org/10.1002/cssc.201801690
Gustafsson, M., Anderberg, S. (2021). Dimensions and characteristics of biogas policies—modelling the European policy landscape Renew. Sust. Energ. Rev. **135**, Article 110200, https://doi.org/10.1016/j.rser.2020.110200.
HEFA/HVO. (2016). Hydroprocessed esters and fatty acids. F3 Fact sheets. Fuels 5. The Swedish knowledge centre for renewable transportation fuels f3, c/o Clamers industriteknik Sven Hultins plats 1 SE-412 58 Goteborg.
ICAO (International Civil Aviation Organization) (2009). Summary of conclusions and recommendations from the first meeting. https://www.icao.int/Meetings/caaf2009/Documents/CAAF-09_SD001_en.pdf#search=CAAF%2F09%2DSD%2F1.
ICAO (International Civil Aviation Organization) (2016). Civil aviation and the environment. https://www.icao.int/Meetings/a39/Documents/WP/wp_051_zh.pdf.
ICAO (International Civil Aviation Organization). (2023). Annex 16—Environmental Protection—Volume IV. Carbon offsetting and reduction scheme for international aviation (CORSIA). 2nd Edition of Annex 16, Volume IV became effective on 31 July 2023 and became applicable on 1 January 2024. p. 124
Kaestner, K., Sommer, S., Berneiser, J., Henger, R., & Oberst, C. (2025). Cost sharing mechanisms for carbon pricing: What drives support in the housing sector? *Energy Economics, 142*, Article 108134. https://doi.org/10.1016/j.eneco.2024.108134
Kanda, W., Zanatta, H., Magnusson, T., Hjelm, O., & Larsson, M. (2022). Policy coherence in a fragmented context: The case of biogas systems in Brazil. *Energy Research & Social Science, 87*, Article 102454. https://doi.org/10.1016/j.erss.2021.102454
Khoo, K. S., Ahmad, I., Chew, K. W., Iwamoto, K., Bhatnagar, A., & Show, P. L. (2023). Enhanced microalgal lipid production for biofuel using different strategies including genetic modification of microalgae: A review. *Progress in Energy and Combustion Science, 96*, Article 101071. https://doi.org/10.1016/j.pecs.2023.101071
Kjelgaard, C. (2024). The sustainable aviation fuel pricing challenge. AvBuyer Magazine. Aircraft Ownership.

Klöwer, M., Allen, M., Lee, D., Proud, S., Gallagher, L., Skowron, A. (2021). Quantifying aviation's contribution to global warming. Environ. Res. Lett. *16*, Article 104027, https://doi.org/10.1088/1748-9326/ac286e.

Kotchen, M.J., Turk, Z.M., Leiserowitz, A.A. (2017). Public willingness to pay for a US carbon tax and preferences for spending the revenue Environ. *Res. Lett. 12* (9) (2017), Article 094012.

Lau, J.I.C., Wang, Y.S. (2024). Tiffany Ang, James Chai Fah Seo, Sabeeha N.B.A. Khadaroo, Jiuan Jing Chew, Andrew Ng Kay Lup, Jaka Sunarso, Emerging technologies, policies and challenges toward implementing sustainable aviation fuel (SAF), *Biomass and Bioenergy 186*, 107277. https://doi.org/10.1016/j.biombioe.2024.107277.

Mata, T. M., Martins, A. A., & Caetano, N. S. (2010). Microalgae for biodiesel production and other applications: A review. *Renewable and Sustainable Energy Reviews, 14*, 217–232.

Maula, H. (2025). Neste started producing sustainable aviation fuel (SAF) at its renewable's refinery in Rotterdam, the Netherlands. *Neste Corporation, Press Release.* https://www.neste.com/media/subscribe.

Pham, P. T. H., Pham, C. Q., Dam, T.-T., Nguyen, Q.-A., & Nguyen, T. M. (2025). A comprehensive review of catalyst deactivation and regeneration in heavy oil hydroprocessing. *Fuel Processing Technology, 267*, Article 108170. https://doi.org/10.1016/j.fuproc.2024.108170

Rijal, D. (2025). Predicting the properties of sustainable aviation fuels. *Nature Reviews Clean Technology., 1*, 312. https://doi.org/10.1038/s44359-025-00056-y

Ritchie, H. (2024). What share of global CO_2 emissions come from aviation?" Published online at Our World in Data. Org. Retrieved from: 'https://ourworldindata.org/global-aviation-emissions' [Online Resource].

Saeen, H., & Kallbekken, S. (2011). A choice experiment on fuel taxation and earmarking in Norway. *Ecol. Econom., 70*(11), 2181–2190.

Shahriar, M. F., & Khanal, A. (2022). The current techno-economic, environmental, policy status and perspectives of sustainable aviation fuel (SAF). *Fuel, 325*, Article 124905. https://doi.org/10.1016/j.fuel.2022.124905

Sieppi, S. (2024). Singapore Airlines Group orders sustainable aviation fuel from Neste. *Neste Corporation, Press Release.* https://www.neste.com/for-media/releases-and-news/subscribe.

Strategy (2023). The potential of sustainable aviation fuels. https://www.strategyand.pwc.com/de/en/industries/aerospace-defense/sustainable-aviation-fuel.html.

Sunmola, F., & Burgess, P. (2023). Transparency by Design for Blockchain-Based Supply Chains. *Procedia Computer Science, 217*, 1256–1265. https://doi.org/10.1016/j.procs.2022.12.324

US Department of Energy. (2024). First ethanol alcohol-to-jet sustainable aviation fuel production facility unveiled. *Bioenergy Technologies Office.*

Wang, B., Ting, Z. J., & Zhao, M. (2024). Sustainable aviation fuels: Key opportunities and challenges in lowering carbon emissions for aviation industry. *Carbon Capture Science & Technology, 13*, Article 100263. https://doi.org/10.1016/j.ccst.2024.100263

Chapter 12
Nanotechnology's Role in Revolutionizing Biofuel Production, Applications of Nanotechnology in Biofuel Production, Innovations and Potential Benefits: Challenges and Future Research Directions

Tarek O. Said, Mohamed A. Hassaan, and Ahmed El Nemr

Abstract Through advancements in process optimization, feedstock pretreatment, and catalytic efficiency, nanotechnology can completely transform biofuel manufacturing. This chapter examines how nanomaterials, such as conductive materials like graphene and carbon nanotubes, can increase biofuel's sustainability and output. Particular attention is paid to biochar, a carbon-rich by-product of biomass pyrolysis, and its dual function as a soil supplement and nanocatalyst support to increase agricultural production, which indirectly affects food security and nutritional effects. The potential of innovations like conductive materials for microbial fuel cells, enzymatic hydrolysis facilitated by nanoparticles, and the nutrient retention properties of biochar to decarbonize energy systems and promote circular economies are examined. Nanomaterials' toxicity, scalability, and economic feasibility are among the challenges evaluated seriously. To meet the demands for food and energy simultaneously, the chapter ends with recommendations for future research areas and integrated systems that combine biofuel production with agro-environmental advantages.

Keywords Catalytic efficiency · Nanotechnology · Transform · Biofuel manufacturing · Pyrolysis · Decarbonize

---

T. O. Said · M. A. Hassaan · A. El Nemr (✉)
National Institute of Oceanography and Fisheries (NIOF), Cairo, Egypt

P. Verma (ed.), *Sustainable Practices in Biorefinery*,
https://doi.org/10.1007/978-981-95-6071-4_12

12.1 Introduction

12.1.1 Overview of Nanotechnology's Transformative Potential in Biofuels

Biofuels have been considered as a potential substitute for fossil fuels due to their rapid depletion. In addition to being limited, burning fossil fuels releases greenhouse gases that pose a serious risk to human health and the environment. However, the industrial synthesis of biofuels is expensive and time-consuming because of technological limitations. Nanoparticles (NPs) present a viable way to improve feedstock usage regarding energy efficiency, specificity, and time management at a reduced cost to address this problem (Anekwe et al., 2024). Recently, a number of these methods have been used, and other NPs—such as metal, magnetic, and metal oxide particles—are currently being used to improve the production of biofuel. Because of their remarkable properties, which include structure, stability, a larger surface area in relation to volume, catalytic activity, and reusability, NPs are advantageous additions to biofuels. In order to encapsulate enzymes and enhance the production of biofuel, nanomaterials have evolved into stable and reasonably priced catalysts. This chapter gives a summary of the problems and opportunities facing nanotechnology, how it helps achieve the Sustainable Development Goals (SDGs), and how new nanomaterials provide biofuel.

Due to the urgent need to develop alternative energy sources and replace fossil fuels, bioenergy production (using biotechnology) has attracted a lot of attention worldwide as a viable substitute. Anaerobic processes, microbial fermentation, algae biotechnology, and nanotechnology are biotechnological methods for producing biofuel. A technology that uses NPs with sizes ranging from 1 to 100 nm is referred to as "nanotechnology". By enabling the intelligent regulation of farming inputs including fertilizer applications, herbicides, and irrigation systems, it can increase the amount and quality of agricultural products. NPs mitigate most environmental problems caused by traditional contemporary agriculture's continued reliance on chemical fertilizers and pesticides (Sirelkhatim et al., 2015). Nanotechnology can transform the food and agriculture sectors by offering new ways to improve plants' nutritional absorption, resistance to molecular disease, and quick disease detection. Numerous studies have examined the part nanotechnology plays in preventing disease as a direct result. However, thorough knowledge regarding the function of NPs in disease prevention, particularly as it relates to fruits and vegetables, is lacking.

12.1.2 Intersection of Bioenergy and Food Systems: Role of Biochar in Bridging Energy Production and Agriculture

In recent decades, biochar—a carbon-rich solid made from biomass through thermal decomposition—has attracted a lot of attention as an appealing adsorbent (Demiral & Gündüzoħlu, 2010). Its many advantages include price, accessibility, well-developed pore structures, and a high specific area with functional groups that contain oxygen (Zhang et al., 2020a). Numerous processes, such as ligand exchange, surface precipitation, ion exchange, electrostatic contact, interaction with surface functional groups, and hydrogen bonding performance, aid in the adsorption of nutrients (NH_4^+, NO_3^-, and PO_4^{3-}) (Almanassra et al., 2021; Zhang et al., 2020b). Although unmodified biochar (BC) has a limited capacity for adsorption, phosphate adsorption can be improved by doping BC with elements such as lanthanum, aluminium, calcium, iron, and magnesium. In compared to unmodified BC, it has been demonstrated that the addition of a cationic polymer, specifically polydiallyldimethylammonium chloride (pDADMAC), greatly increases anionic exchange capacity and amplifies phosphorous adsorption by a factor of 1000 (Wang et al., 2020). Iron-based modifications can provide the added benefit of magnetic recovery. The temperature, pH, pyrolysis temperature, feedstock, and doping agent all significantly affect the BC's effectiveness and characteristics. Cui et al. (2016) examined the physicochemical characteristics and adsorption capability for nitrate and phosphate of BC made from two distinct plants. It has been demonstrated that ions like Cl^- and HCO_3^- hurt the elimination of NO_3^- and/or PO_4^{3-}, whereas cations like Mg^{2+}, Ca^{2+}, K^+, and Na^+ compete with NH_4^+.

BC is one of the most well-known carbon drawdown methods that has emerged recently and has undergone extensive testing and study. "BC is a porous, carbonaceous material that is produced by pyrolysis of biomass and is applied in such a way that the contained carbon remains stored as a long-term C (carbon) sink", according to the European BC Certification (EBC, 2022). Not at all a novel. Moreover, BC has a long history of use in agriculture worldwide as a soil improvement. However, the interest it generates due to its capacity to sequester carbon has grown. Any organic substance may often be used as the feedstock for manufacturing BC using the proper technique. Generally speaking, BC has been used in agriculture for a long time as a raw soil additive that can hold onto water and nutrients, therefore resulting in lower fertilizer consumption and higher crop yields. Research indicates that when fertilizer and BC were applied together, the average yield increased by 15% compared to the same fertilization method without the BC (Schmidt et al., 2021). This perspective states that BC addresses many SDG targets, particularly SDG 2 (Zero hunger).

As the world's population and level of living rise, there is rising concern about the future of food, energy, and water supplies. Based on earlier studies and advancements in food-energy-water systems, Hersh et al. (2019) provide prospects for sustainable growth through biomass-based products (bioproducts), such as BC, a newly discovered by-product of biofuel manufacturing. Although still in their infancy, bioproducts are expanding gradually thanks to advancements in production methods and other cost-cutting measures. Through narrative and methodical literature studies, viewpoints on possibilities and solutions that can support the ecological integrity and socioeconomic resilience of local food, energy, and water resources are found. The economic and environmental factors that affect stakeholders' choices regarding adopting and applying technology solutions are considered while analysing these solutions. It has been demonstrated that BC is one of these products that can increase productivity, especially in organic farming, by increasing carbon sequestration, organic matter efficiency, and water-nutrient holding capacity.

Additionally, BC's textural qualities and sorption capabilities have shown that it is a special remedy for removing a wide range of contaminants from water, such as metals and toluene. However, the creation of market-responsive bioproducts was severely hindered by the costs associated with biomass conversion, transportation, and collection. According to the results, the current focus on food-energy-water systems has created opportunities for bioproduct research, which might close the gaps and offer creative concepts for further study and advancement. Initiatives that focus on addressing problems in the food-energy-water nexus are also much needed both domestically and internationally, it has been discovered.

12.2 Applications of Nanotechnology in Biofuel Production

Global warming and greenhouse effects are two detrimental environmental repercussions of fossil fuels. As a result, prosperous and industrialized nations are looking for alternate resources rather than fossil fuels. Biofuels like bioethanol and biodiesel can replace fossil fuels like gasoline and petro-diesel (Esmaeili et al., 2021). These clean and renewable fuels have garnered a lot of interest. According to reports, the synthesis of bioethanol and biodiesel is significantly impacted by various kinds of NPs. Several feedstocks can be used as an oil source to produce biodiesel when a catalyst or nanocatalyst is present. Nanocatalysts' high activity, specific surface area, and high conversion yield have led to their widespread application in the production of biodiesel in recent years. Bioethanol is one useful fuel that has shown a great deal of sustainable and eco-friendly promise.

Fermentation technology can also produce bioethanol and convert carbohydrates into biofuel. Numerous nanomaterials and nanocatalysts for the synthesis of biodiesel from various oil sources are examined in this chapter. The yield of biodiesel conversion for each type of oil is examined and compared. The effect of the nanocatalyst's specific surface area on the production of biodiesel is also discussed. Research on the reusability of nanocatalysts for biodiesel production has also shown that they can be used for several cycles of biodiesel synthesis without noticeably losing their effectiveness. Furthermore, the impact of nanomaterials on the production of bioethanol and the immobilization of biocatalysts (enzymes) is highlighted (Esmaeili et al., 2021).

12.2.1 Conductive Materials

12.2.1.1 Graphene, Carbon Nanotubes (CNTs), and MXenes

MXene is a special material with a layered structure like graphene, composed mostly of relatively light components including C and N as well as early transition metals. Numerous fields, including electronics, sensors, energy, and catalysis, have extensively studied it. High conductivity, optical qualities, and high dispersibility in polar solvents are just a few of MXene's numerous distinctive attributes. MXene's strong conductivity is anticipated to enhance electrode materials' capabilities (Takeda et al., 2025). The primary subjects are MXene's electrical properties and suitability for fuel cell electrode materials, especially biofuel cells (Takeda et al., 2025). Research on fuel cells and the materials used for their electrodes is first presented as background information. The following section discusses MXene's preparation and its physical characteristics, including its shape, particle size, thermal stability, and electrical characteristics. The electrical characteristics of MXene as an electrode material are covered in this chapter, and comparisons to other electrode materials like carbon nanotubes and examples from practical applications are provided. The application of MXene as an anode and cathode material for biofuel cells is also covered in this section.

Fibres that are electrically conducting and physically robust, particularly those with high specific capacitances, are promising fibre-shaped electrodes for fibre- and textile-based energy storage devices like fibre-shaped supercapacitors (FSCs). However, in order to construct fibre electrodes with adequate mechanical strength, a substantial loading of fillers or bridging agents is typically needed, which reduces electrical conductivity and energy storage capacity. Zhao et al., (2022) described a straightforward, scalable wet-spinning technique that uses a balanced mixture of MXene and CNT in water and acetic acid as a coagulation bath to produce multifunctional Ti_3C_2Tx MXene/carbon nanotubes (MXene/CNT) hybrid fibres. The hybrid fibre exhibited exceptional energy storage ability ($\sim$295 F g^{-1} at 5 mV s^{-1}), high strength (61 $\pm$ 7 MPa), and excellent conductivity (1142.08 $\pm$ 40.04 S cm^{-1}) at a comparatively low CNT concentration of almost 1 weight per cent. When the CNT loading was increased to roughly 9 weight per cent, the conductivity increased to 1715 $\pm$ 22 S cm^{-1}, and the greatest strain at breakage was 161 $\pm$ 19 MPa. Hybrid fibres can be sewn into energy-storing textiles due to their improved mechanical qualities. The built-in FSCs have energy and power densities of about 6.08 mW h cm^{-3} and 6440 mW cm^{-3}, respectively. Shortly, wearable and textile-based device development will have new prospects thanks to MXene/CNT fibre's outstanding performance and good viability for scalable production. The advantages of employing MXene as electrode material in biofuel cells, an overview of electrode uses, and projected future trends are discussed.

12.2.1.2 Enhancing Electron Transfer in Microbial Fuel Cells

Over millions of years, plant and animal remains were heated and compressed by sedimentary and igneous strata, producing these fossils (Ma et al., 2023). This fossil fuel is widely used daily and can produce electricity effectively enough to run automobile engines, industrial machinery, and electronic devices. However, fossil fuels are unsustainable due to their limited supply. Because of this, there is a growing need to transition from fossil fuels to sustainable and renewable energy sources, and modern strategies to advance industrial civilization are also being developed (Obileke et al., 2021). To overcome the drawbacks of expensive and ineffective electrode materials, Christwardana et al. (2025) examined the effect of calcination temperature on eggshell-derived anodes for microbial fuel cells (MFCs). Eggshells were calcined at 550, 700, and 850°Cafter being activated with NaOH. The eggshells at 700 °C showed the highest electron transfer rate constant (ks = 1.64 s^{-1}) due to their enhanced structural integrity and crystallinity. With a steady voltage output of 185 mV and a maximum power density of 70 mW m^{-2}, the 700 °C calcined anode performed better than other configurations, according to electrochemical characterization. The optimized calcined eggshell anode offers better electron transfer, biofilm development, and cost-effectiveness than traditional carbon-based anodes. This work improves MFC technology and overcomes earlier problems like low electron transfer rates and expensive material costs by converting waste into sustainable anodes. These results demonstrate the promise of materials obtained from trash for environmentally acceptable, scalable energy solutions.

12.2.1.3 Catalysing Transesterification for Biodiesel Production

Glycerol and an ester are produced by the catalytic reaction of alcohol, oil, or fat, a process known as transesterification. Transesterification is a quick and inexpensive method of creating biodiesel that results in fuel with a higher cetane number and improved performance. A common process for creating biodiesel from vegetable oils, such as Eriobotrya japonica seed oil, is transesterification (Akhtar et al., 2017) and non-vegetable oils like *Tamarindus indica* (*T. indica*) seed oil as dicotyledonous plants. They can withstand extended drought and thrive in poor soils, they are perfect for low input (Manaf et al., 2019). Sajjad et al., (2022) sought to manufacture biodiesel by transesterifying *T. indica* seed oil with an alkali catalyst while optimizing the reaction conditions.

To determine the quantity of fatty acids in oil and biodiesel, gas chromatographic analysis was employed. Under the optimal conditions of an alcohol-to-oil molar ratio (6:1), catalyst (1.5% w/w), and reaction time of one hour, a 93.5% biodiesel yield was generated. The catalyst amount (20.7%) and the alcohol molar ratio to oil (74.9%) made the most contributions. In another instance, an 82.5% biodiesel yield was obtained using a catalyst (1.5% w/w), an alcohol-to-oil molar ratio (9:1), and a reaction duration of 1.5 h. Under optimal circumstances, *T. indica* methyl esters' fuel qualities fell within the bounds of ASTM D6751 biodiesel. According to the study's findings, *T. indica* may be chosen as a viable and feasible option for large-scale biodiesel production, which would replace Petro-diesel. Biodiesel can be produced using a variety of methods, including as transesterification, direct usage and mixing, thermal cracking, and micro-emulsion. Fuel produced using a micro-emulsion technique has a lower cetane number and viscosity. Although it costs more, biodiesel made by thermal cracking is comparable to gasoline made from petroleum. Although gasoline has a higher viscosity, a direct usage and mixing strategy offers the advantage of creating more portable fuel because it is liquid (Qi et al., 2010).

12.2.2 Biochar as a Nanomaterial

For the electrochemical detection of 17β-estradiol, Dong et al. (2018) created a sensitive and reasonably priced sensor based on highly conductive and adsorptive BC NPs. As long as the conductivities are ensured, BC, which is widely available and has the benefits of a large specific surface area, affordability, and good stability, may be used to make electrodes. After obtaining nano-sized BC particles (BCNPs), they examined their electrochemical characteristics under various pyrolysis conditions. High conductivity BCNPs (BCNP800) were acquired to build reliable and repeatable electrochemical sensors. The more conductive BCNP800 sensor showed better amperometric responses, such as decreased impedance, decreased anodic potential, and increased current signal towards 17β-estradiol, as compared to the pure glassy carbon electrode.

Additionally, a significant amplification of the sensing signal was produced by the adsorption-accumulation of 17β-estradiol by BCNP800. The BCNP800 sensor's excellent adsorption and conductivity qualities produced a detection limit of 11.30 nM. Global and regional climate change is being caused by greenhouse gas emissions and changes in land use. The amount of carbon compounds and gases emitted into the environment increases along with the population and industrial and agricultural activity levels. As a result, the ecosystem is polluted, and energy is squandered. With the correct tools and supervision, such gas emissions can be reduced to carbon solids. Agriculture is one of the many industries that use these "BC"-like carbon solids. Therefore, such procedures may change BC into nano-BC (Hussein et al., 2022).

12.2.2.1 *Production* via *Pyrolysis and Functionalization for Catalytic Activity*

Chaos-Hernández et al. (2022) provided a detailed explanation of how to maximize the pyrolysis, functionalization, and activation of heterogeneous catalysts derived from coconut endocarp and employ them in transesterification to generate fatty acid methyl esters (FAME). The use of KOH and Ca $(NO_3)_2$ for catalyst functionalization was investigated in detail. The best conditions for making coconut-based catalysts to maximize FAME synthesis were found using signal-to-noise ratio analysis. The findings shown that in order to enhance the characteristics of catalysts functionalized with calcium nitrate and potassium hydroxide, heat activation is required. Coconut endocarp was pyrolyzed for an hour at 600 °C to form the ideal catalyst, which was subsequently functionalized using KOH and Ca $(NO_3)_2$ and activated at 500 °C. A FAME formation of 90.8% was the outcome of this. When it came to producing biodiesel by transesterification, this catalyst's performance was on par with other catalysts. The findings indicate that using the novel catalyst to produce biodiesel might be cost-effective. The heterogeneous catalyst fabrication using the endocarp of coconuts to make biodiesel has been examined in their study. To optimize the preparation conditions and increase the generation of FAME, a thorough examination of the catalyst functionalization with KOH and Ca $(NO_3)_2$ as well as heat activation has been conducted. According to their research, transesterification of biodiesel may benefit from KOH functionalization of the support derived from coconut endocarp pyrolysis.

12.2.2.2 Use in Anaerobic Digestion and Syngas Purification

The digestate produced by an anaerobic digester is fed a feedstock, such as sludge, from a municipal wastewater treatment plant. A cake is created by dewatering the digestate. A thermal drier, for instance, might be used to dry the cake further. A pyrolysis apparatus processes the cake, yielding charcoal and a synthesis gas. The gas is routed to either the same digester or another to boost its methane output. It is possible to employ the char as a soil enhancer. A viable alternative for the shift to a circular economy powered by sustainable and renewable energy is methane from biogas. Many different technologies available today may effectively remove the contaminants found in biogas to create biomethane. A prototype plant's genuine biogas from anaerobic digestion was cleaned and upgraded in the current investigation using the chemical absorption technique. Anaerobic digestion biogas at a WWTP was to be upgraded and purified in order to provide a high methane concentration for biofuel in automobiles (Sánchez et al., 2022). Mono-ethanolamine (MEA) and N-methyl diethanolamine (MDEA) in aqueous solutions at 20% and 40% concentrations were employed as absorbents. The most successful solution at a 20% concentration was MEA because it had the highest CO_2 removal efficacy (94%) and, consequently, the highest CH_4 richness (96%). Finally, the chemical absorption process produced 62 Nm^3 biofuel for every 100 m^3 of biomethane.

12.2.3 Nanocatalysts

The synthesis of conducting polymers, nanocarbons, noble metal NPs, and nanocomposites is covered (Kant et al., 2022). By means of direct writing, inkjet printing, screen printing, and three-dimensional printing, these nanomaterials may be integrated into a flexible matrix (carbon paper, cloth, paper, and polyethylene terephthalate) and a non-flexible substrate (glass and glassy carbon electrodes). Additionally discussed are the fluidic properties of printing nano-ink on different surfaces for proper electrode preparation in electrochemical sensing applications. In order to investigate pharmaceutical, biological, food, and environmental contaminants such medications, toxicants, metal ions, insecticides, and biomolecules, the printed electrodes are ultimately compiled. The electrochemical sensors development is one facet of the growth of electrochemical devices, which will continue to produce novel, approachable sensors for all upcoming applications.

It has been noted that adding different catalysts enhances the production of hydrogen. The primary enzymes in dark fermentation that produce hydrogen are hydrogenases. There have been reports of including several nanocatalysts, including titanium oxide, gold, nickel, copper, iron, and silver. Rapid electron transport from the donor to the acceptor is made possible by nanocatalysts, which also serve as oxygen scavengers and cofactors for the enzymes nitrogenase and hydrogenase. Nanocatalysts can also act as micronutrients, which promotes the growth of microorganisms. Bhatia et al. (2023) investigated the impact of Fe_3O_4 NPs during dark fermentation of algal biomass feedstock to boost hydrogen production.

12.2.4 Metal Oxide NPs for Lipid Extraction from Algae

High-throughput, novel materials called NPs have transformed almost every aspect of human existence. A very advantageous environmentally friendly option in the quest for biofuel generation is microalgae. Microalgal biomass may be used to create biofuels including syngas, biodiesel, bioethanol, bio-hydrogen, and biomethane feed. Microalgae cannot be utilized to produce biofuels on a large scale since they are not yet commercially feasible. NPs can improve light conversion in the microalgae photobioreactor and raise the yield of CO_2 absorption when added to microalgal cultures. The most recent developments and possible uses of NPs in microalgae are comprehensively covered in this article. It looks into possible morphological toxicity and how NPs could affect microalgae's metabolic processes (Pahariya et al., 2024). To examine their effects on the pace of growth, biomass production, and intracellular chemical accumulation, different concentrations of NPs have been introduced into microalgae cells. These compounds are supplements that have been introduced to the diet to promote the growth and lipid synthesis of photosynthetic microalgae cells. A detailed assessment is conducted of the effects of various NPs on light conversion, toxicity, cellular damage, intracellular chemical accumulation, and microalgal metabolic pathways. By encouraging research on the optimal use of NPs in microalgae culture and harvesting, Pahariya et al. (2024) aimed to improve the energy-efficient commercialization of microalgae for a variety of application channels. The life cycle of metal oxide NPs (MONPs) invariably results in their release into the environment. In the environment, transformation processes such as aggregation, deposition, and dissolution will predominate in the forms of MONP occurrence. The toxicity, mobility, and bioavailability of MONPs will be influenced by their prevailing forms. Data on how MONPs change in response to pH, ionic strength (IS), and natural organic matter (NOM) are gathered in order to completely comprehend how they interact in the environment. The effects of MONPs on the physiological and biochemical traits of microalgae as well as their toxicity mechanisms were investigated in freshwater environments (Yu et al., 2025). They highlighted how altered MONP occurrence forms and their ecotoxicity brought on by changes in water quality parameters are related. Notably, it is challenging to forecast the forms of MONPs that will emerge in surface waters due to the uncertainty surrounding their transformation pathway under the impact of environmental conditions. The combined effect of these factors on MONP behaviour in their natural watery habitat must therefore be taken into account. The primary goals of this review are to increase understanding of the environmental risks associated with nanotechnology in aquatic environments and to establish a scientific basis for its sustainable development. Under the impact of aquatic environmental conditions, MONPs undergo various modifications that change their original shapes and their incidence, distribution, and destiny in aquatic environments. This incident emphasizes how crucial it is to consider the complex interactions between MONPs and aquatic environmental elements when evaluating their potential effects on the ecosystem.

The creation of NPs with antibacterial properties, like iron oxide NPs (IONPs), is made possible by nanotechnology (Fig. 12.1) (Zúñiga-Miranda et al., 2023). Because IONPs can interact with multiple biological components and impede microbial growth, they are a viable solution to antimicrobial resistance or pathogenicity. This study summarizes the key discoveries made in the last ten years on green IONP synthesis techniques utilizing plants, fungi, bacteria, and organic waste (Zúñiga-Miranda et al., 2023). They discussed the main issues that arise when using a variety of organisms and organic materials for green synthesis. Additionally, they include the most widely used techniques for characterizing these IONPs. They highlighted the potential uses of these IONPs as antiviral, antifungal, antibacterial, and antiparasitic drugs.

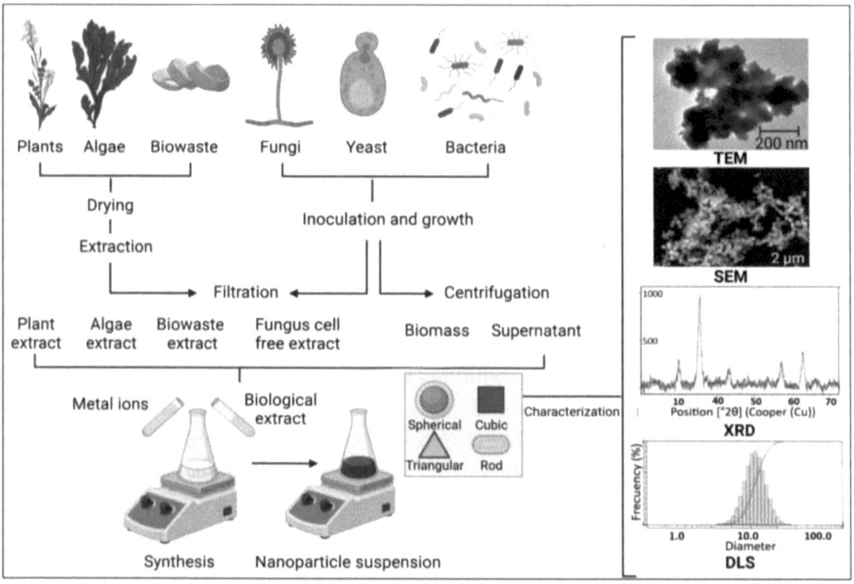

Fig. 12.1 Diagrammatic illustration of the environmentally friendly production of iron oxide NPs

12.2.5 Magnetic NPs for Enzyme Immobilization in Lignocellulosic Ethanol Production

The production of biofuels and other renewable energy sources is one of the many industrial processes that nanotechnology has revolutionized. Raw materials' complicated and resistant structure poses serious obstacles to biofuel manufacturing, particularly regarding lignocellulosic biomass. To make more fermentable sugars available, the lignocellulosic biomass—which is mostly made up of cellulose, hemicellulose, and lignin—must be properly digested. New efficient and sustainable pretreatment methods must be created because conventional pretreatment methods are usually costly, energy-intensive, and detrimental to the environment. Nanotechnology provides innovative approaches to enhance biofuel production, from biomass pretreatment to conversion into useable fuels (Esmaeili et al., 2021). The need for energy, which fossil fuels supply, has increased due to the world's continuously growing population. But it also increases the greenhouse gas influence on the environment. Concerns regarding environmental safety have been raised by the depletion of fossil fuels brought on by their rapid consumption in recent years. Using lignocellulosic biomass is one possible way to deal with these issues. Earth's plentiful lignocellulosic biomass may be converted into bioethanol and/or biochemical products by the use of appropriate pretreatment techniques, such as physical, chemical, and biological processes. However, because these techniques are expensive and time-consuming, they have a number of disadvantages (Arora et al., 2020). By creating a new, innovative, economical, practical, and environmentally friendly approach—nanotechnology—these constraints have been addressed, and a possible replacement for the current pretreatment techniques has been found.

Arora et al. (2020) critically examined several traditional pretreatment techniques and develop nanobiotechnological approaches in lignocellulosic pretreatment techniques. With a focus on lignocellulosic biomass pretreatment, Rathi (2009) examined the vital role that NPs play in enhancing the production of biofuel. Because of their notable benefits in catalysis and enzyme immobilization, nanomaterials including metallic NPs, carbon-based nanostructures (such graphene and carbon nanotubes, or CNTs), and magnetic NPs (MNPs) are suitable for biofuel applications. Cobalt (Co), nickel (Ni), and platinum (Pt)-based metallic NPs are efficient nanocatalysts in processes like transesterification, which is essential for the production of biodiesel. Furthermore, magnetic NPs make collecting and reusing enzymes easy, which significantly lowers operating costs and enhances process sustainability. With a focus on using nanomaterials in the pretreatment of lignocellulosic biomass, they looked at the most current developments in nanotechnology applications in biofuel manufacture. A thorough investigation is conducted into the function of nanocatalysts, nanoenzymes, and nanostructured materials, emphasizing improving biofuel production processes' scalability, sustainability, and efficiency. By increasing process efficiency and reducing environmental impact, nanotechnology holds great promise for the future of biofuel production and will aid in the global transition to more sustainable energy sources. The characterization techniques for NP are presented in Table 12.1 (Buarki et al., 2022).

It is well known that BC, which is made by pyrolyzing biomass like wood, trash, animal dung, and agricultural waste, is stable and beneficial to plant development and soil health (Fig. 12.2 & Table 12.2) (Gabhane et al., 2020). Its potential to improve soil physicochemical characteristics, such as structure, water retention, and nutrient availability, is attracting increasing attention from studies on its application in forestry. This will increase plant growth, drought tolerance, and disease and pest resistance.

Table 12.1 Methods for characterizing NPs

Property	Characterization techniques
Surface charge	Zeta potential, EPM
Crystal structure	HRTEM, XRD, STEM, EXAFS, electron diffraction
Shape	AFM, HRTEM, TEM, SEM, FMR, EPLS, STEM, 3D tomography
Size	AFM, MALDI, TEM, NTA, HRTEM, XRD, DLS, EXAFS, SAXS, SEM, DCS, FMR, UV–Vis, ICP-MS, NMR, EPLS, TRPS, magnetic susceptibility
Chemical composition	ICP-OES, XRD, NMR, XPS, LEIS, SEM–EDX, MFM, EELS
Magnetic properties	Mossbauer, MFM, SQUID, FMR, XMCD, VSM, magnetic susceptibility

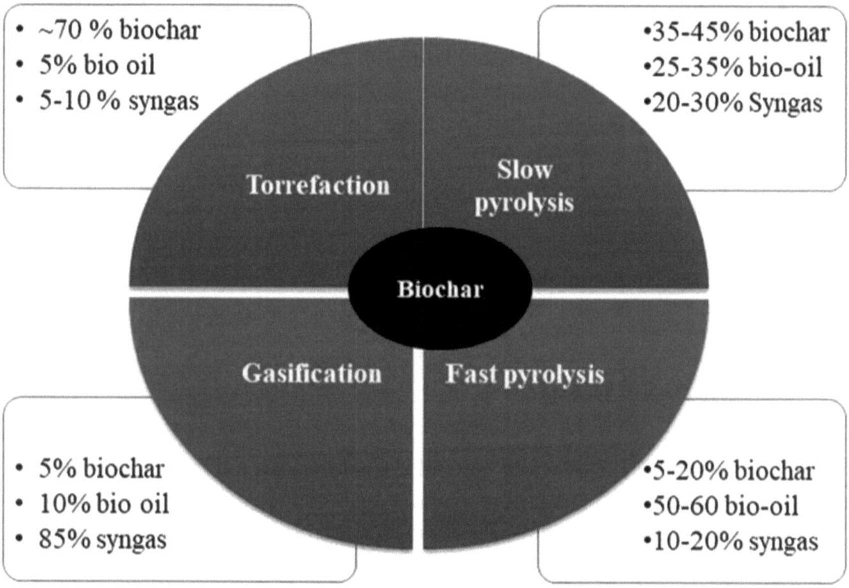

Fig. 12.2 Effects of different pyrolysis methods on biochar yields

Table 12.2 Typical ranges for the primary product yields for each of the most popular biochar production procedures now in use, such as slow and fast pyrolysis, gasification, and torrefaction

Biochar production procedures	Unit	Pyrolysis		Gasification	Torrefaction
		Slow	Fast		
Feedstock particle size	mm	5–50	2	0.2–10	0.2
Heating rate	°C/s	0.1–10	10–200	5–100	–
Temperature	°C	300–800	350–1000	700–100	200–300
Solid residence time		Hours to days	0.5–10 s	>1 h	> 1 h
Biochar yield	(%)	35–45	5–20	5	60–80
Bio-oil yield	(%)	25–35	50–60	10	5
Syngas yield	(%)	20–30	10–20	85	5–10

12.3 Biochar's Effect on Soil Health and Dietary Outcomes

However, the soil kind, the tree species, the rate of application, and the BC's composition all affect how effective the product is. Increased pH in alkaline soils, decreased leaching of hazardous components, and nutrient immobilization are possible hazards to using BC (Antonangelo et al., 2025). The broad use of BC in forestry is hampered by issues like information gaps, a dearth of site-specific research, and doubts about its economic feasibility despite its potential. Over 150 publications on using BC in forestry from the last 20 years have been compiled in this qualitative assessment.

It evaluates how BC affects tree crops and soil health, emphasizing how it might increase soil fertility and encourage tree development. The study highlights important discoveries, like the beneficial effects of BC on plant and soil health, and lists current knowledge gaps that require filling. The study summarizes existing research and suggests future paths to maximize the use of BC in sustainable forestry management, highlighting the necessity of customized strategies and financial analyses to enable wider adoption. While urging more research to clarify doubts and enhance its usefulness, the findings highlight the potential contribution of BC to improving forestry practices (Antonangelo et al., 2025).

12.3.1 Soil Amendment

According to the evidence, the BC amendment shows definite advantages for trees that thrive in nutrient-deficient soils and under challenging environmental conditions, even though it might not be a method that can generally promote forest health (Johanis et al., 2022). As previously stated, adding BC to the soil results in improved soil structure, increased plant-accessible water, and nutrient addition, all contributing to tree crop development and productivity Zhang et al. (2020a). Together, Zhang et al. (2020b) developed a mutually beneficial connection and concluded that BC produced by pyrolyzing agriculture and forest wastes was an effective supplement for restoring China's deteriorated forest soils. The authors briefly outlined the benefits of applying BC, which include (1) improving the physicochemical characteristics of the soil, (2) reducing greenhouse gas emissions, and (3) increasing the nutrient efficiency usage, which in turn promotes tree development. These positive outcomes were caused by a number of factors, including the type of raw material, the temperature at which pyrolysis took place, the rate of application, the post-application aging process, and the specifics of the soil and plantation in question.

12.3.2 Biochar's Role in Improving Soil Fertility, Water Retention, and Crop Yields

Globally, forest plantations must maintain soil fertility, ensure tree health, and advance sustainability (Liao et al., 2012). By enhancing soil properties and encouraging tree development, BC as a soil supplement provides a possible solution for these issues. Much support and attention has been given to BC's many potential benefits in forestry and agricultural systems, ranging from enhanced soil health and plant development to reduced greenhouse gas emissions and carbon absorption. It is important to keep in mind that, despite the numerous excellent results that have been published, certain research in the literature have produced inconsistent or conflicting results (Wang et al., 2020). This variety highlights how crucial it is to take specific parameters into account, since they can have a big influence on how successfully BC is administered. These factors include crop species, soil characteristics, application rates, and the kind of BC. As a result, the scientific community agrees that systematic research is essential to determining the complex links between BC production technologies, BC characteristics, and BC's performance in forestry and agricultural systems (Wang et al., 2020). This variation emphasizes how crucial it is to consider particular factors, such as the kind of BC, application rates, soil properties, and crop species, as these can significantly impact how well BC is applied. The scientific community has concluded that systematic investigations are necessary to understand the complex links between BC production technologies, BC characteristics, and their performance in agricultural and forestry systems (Wang et al., 2020). Depending on the species, age, and particular growing conditions, tree crops react differently to the application of BC.

Regarding growth, productivity, and fruit quality, several tree crops—like fruit trees—have responded favourably to BC. The response of BC to the soil's nutritional condition and citrus fruit quality has been evaluated by Zhang et al. (2021). They demonstrated that the application of BC had a good impact on the soil's physicochemical properties, including pH, organic matter, and nutrient levels. Peel, edibility, soluble solids, and the ratio of soluble solids to titratable acidity—all favourable indicators of citrus fruit—reflected this. Sarauer et al. (2019) discovered no effect on tree growth after adding BC to forest soil northwest of the U.S. at a rate of 25.0 mg ha^{-1}. However, BC had no adverse effects on plants or soil and successfully sequestered carbon from the soil (Sarauer et al., 2019). When making decisions, the kind and the soil texture must also be considered. BC amendments are more likely to increase agricultural production in sandy, coarse-textured soils than in rich, fine-textured soils, claim (Alkharabsheh et al., 2021). This is probably because heavy-textured (clayey) soils do not have limiting characteristics such as poor CEC, water, or nutrient retention. Therefore, BC is anticipated to have a more noticeable beneficial impact on soils with a coarse texture.

12.3.3 Reduction of Heavy Metal Toxicity in Agricultural Soils

Under low or no oxygen supply, biomass undergoes gradual or rapid pyrolysis to create carbonaceous (BC) material. In order to reduce metal toxicity, BC supplementation of soil is usually used to decrease the metals mobility and bioavailability. By increasing the soil's sorption capacity, BC can improve metal immobilization and thus slow down plants' uptake of metals. Its applications range from mitigating the effects of climate change to cleaning up environmental contaminants. However, BC's ability to bring about these changes depends on its physicochemical characteristics, indicating that function-specific BC should be used to accomplish a specific goal. The fundamental attributes of BC and how various modification techniques impact them are summed up by Nkoh et al. (2022). It also examines how BC may be used to remediate heavy metal pollution, how to reduce heavy metal toxicity to plants, how it affects physiological traits, and how to mitigate the consequences on human health. The physicochemical characteristics of BC are known to be influenced by the feedstock and manufacturing circumstances. For example, the ash content of BC rises as the pyrolysis temperature increases, and the pH of BC and the pyrolysis temperature have a substantial linear connection ($R^2 = 0.53$, n = 112).

Furthermore, BC's cation exchange capacity falls as the pyrolysis temperature rises. When applied, BC interacts with contaminants and soil, and depending on how it functions, it can treat poisons. While BC with negative surfaces, like acid-modified BC, mainly fix cationic pollutants, BC with positive surfaces, such mineral-doped BC, has a significant ability to repair anionic contaminants. According to the meta-analysis, adding BC to polluted soils typically lowers the amount of contaminants that plants absorb, with a few outliers for Fe and Mn. The anticipated declines were as follows: 3.03% (Pb), 18.3% (Zn), 22.8% (Mn), 25.8% (Cu), 26.2% (Cd), 33.0% (Ni), 41.5% (As), and 56.0% (Cr). Ion exchange, physical trapping of charged metals on BC surfaces, and changes in soil chemistry are some of the fundamental causes of this decline in the bioavailability of heavy metals in soils. Adding BC to heavy metal-polluted soils decreased the risk of cancer (30.6%), hazard quotient (30.0%), and heavy metals total daily intake (12.5%). These effects, however, might differ significantly according to the qualities of the BC, the chemistry of the heavy metals in issue, and the soil features. Our research offers a basic comprehension of how BC influences the heavy metals bioavailability in polluted soils and how these changes impact plants and animals (Nkoh et al., 2022).

BC has developed into a unique and affordable adsorbent based on research discoveries over the past 20 years. To lessen the harmful effects of heavy metals (HMs) on plants and animals, it has been proposed that BC be used to immobilize HMs. BCs play various roles in pollution remediation because they are heterogeneous materials with different functional groups. When choosing which type of BC to utilize for the remediation of a particular contamination or group of contaminants, it is crucial to consider the feedstock type, manufacturing conditions, and modification procedures that impact the BC's functioning. How pollutants, soil, and BC interact when applied to soil affects plant uptake, bioavailability, and speciation (Nkoh et al., 2022).

Furthermore, the properties of BC in soil change over time, which has important implications for the movement and speciation of pollutants. Therefore, optimizing BC's potential as an adsorbent and soil amendment material requires a full understanding of how it interacts with pollutants and soil. This can be accomplished through (i) understanding BC's surface chemistry and how it changes under different conditions, (ii) critically analysing BC-soil particle interactions to identify patterns and how these interactions impact the soil's physicochemical properties, and (iii) balancing the observed changes in the soil and BC's physicochemical properties with the outcomes of pollutant retention and bioavailability (Nkoh et al., 2022).

12.4 Food Security Implications

Food insecurity has several significant effects. One substantial effect is on health, particularly in children, where it may raise the risk of chronic illnesses and cause malnutrition. Food insecurity can also have social and economic effects, such as making people more susceptible to starvation and famine and possibly encouraging dangerous business practices. Lastly, food price increases and heightened resource competition are two ways food insecurity can fuel sociopolitical instability (Darnton-Hill et al., 2005; Han et al., 2015; Ricachenevsky et al., 2019; Yang et al., 2025).

12.4.1 Enhanced Nutrient Availability for Staple Crops

Nutrition is a basic requirement for all living things to carry out vital tasks, including growth, development, and production (Ricachenevsky et al., 2019). Despite being the main source of calories, these staple crops lack essential nutrients, which is why poor and emerging countries have focused more on increasing agricultural accessibility and productivity. Thus, nutrient deficits cause health problems in many nations, including growth retardation, anaemia (iron deficiency), night blindness (vitamin A deficiency), and poor mental health (Darnton-Hill et al., 2005). Much of the study on staple crops is on different approaches and strategies to improve agricultural nutrition, including micro- and macronutrients. With eight necessary amino acids in appropriate amounts, rice is a notable source of protein that supports healthy skin, hair, heart, and lungs and a healthy neurological system (Han et al., 2015). Global food security depends on staple crops like rice, wheat, and maize, yet it is still very difficult to improve their quality. Additionally emphasized are ten unanswered concerns about the regional distribution of proteins and starch, epigenetic control, and the impact of environmental factors on qualitative traits. There is an opportunity to develop high-yield "super-crop" varieties with enhanced nutritional content, processing capabilities, and consumer-preferred features by fusing multi-omics techniques with rational design tactics (Yang et al., 2025). These issues must be resolved to advance sustainable agriculture and accomplish the twin goals of environmental preservation and food security.

Rice's nutritional value is a significant issue, as is the requirement to increase productivity to feed the world's expanding population. The development of high-yielding rice varieties with improved nutritional content is required to address malnutrition, a worldwide health issue. Unquestionably, breeding methods have made a substantial contribution to increasing rice output and enhancing its nutritious content. To address the nutritional demands of the contemporary population, novel technologies including genetic engineering, gene editing, omics techniques, and agronomic practices are required in addition to conventional breeding methods. Comprehensive information on how rice varieties can be made more nutrient-dense through the use of genetic engineering techniques to increase their protein content, micro-

and macronutrients, vitamins, and oil quality was supplied by Zafar and Jianlong (2023). Additionally, they discovered QTLs linked to rice's proteins, amino acids, and micronutrients. Additionally, omics approaches offer a variety of instruments and methods for efficiently examining resources and comprehending the biological processes behind the development of traits. To improve rice nutrition, omics branches such as transcriptomics, proteomics, genomics, and metabolomics are effectively used. Therefore, they might be able to successfully alter the rice genome and directly improve the nutritional content of rice types by utilizing the knowledge gained from these procedures and combining all of these innovative ways. In the years to come, this will aid in addressing the problems associated with malnutrition.

12.4.2 Mitigating the Food Versus Fuel Debate by Boosting Agricultural Productivity

Palm oil is a vital part of the worldwide biofuel economy because of its high oil output and affordability, making it an ideal feedstock for biodiesel manufacturing. However, serious socioeconomic and environmental concerns are now due to the oil palm plantations growth. The detrimental impacts of palm oil biodiesel on the environment, including greenhouse gas emissions, deforestation, biodiversity loss, and soil and water resources deterioration, are carefully considered (Purnama et al., 2025). They also examined the "food versus fuel" controversy, highlighting how rivalry for resources and land between food production and biodiesel production impacts global food security, especially in underdeveloped countries. This research stands noteworthy because it focuses on Southeast Asian producers, especially Indonesia and Malaysia, where land-use changes and biodiesel policies have specific intersections with food and environmental systems.

In contrast to other research, they explored the frequently disregarded effects of peatland conversion, emphasizing how it exacerbates carbon emissions and biodiversity loss. Through thoroughly examining the sustainability issues and socioeconomic trade-offs associated with palm oil biodiesel, the paper sheds light on the intricate relationship between environmental stewardship, food security, and renewable energy. Additionally, they assessed best practices and technology advancements that can lessen adverse effects. Additionally, their study critically analyses the degree to which certification schemes such as the Indonesian Sustainable Palm Oil (ISPO) and the Roundtable on Sustainable Palm Oil (RSPO) promote sustainable practices. Their paper uses case studies to show how these ideas are used in actual circumstances and offers useful recommendations to scholars, industry stakeholders, and policymakers (Purnama et al., 2025).

There has been a notable shift towards sustainable and renewable energy sources as the need to mitigate climate change and cut greenhouse gas (GHG) emissions becomes more pressing globally. Biodiesel is a well-liked alternative to fossil fuels that can lessen the environmental impact of conventional fuels made from petroleum as well as carbon emissions. Among the several feedstocks available for the manufacturing of biodiesel, palm oil stands out due to its high oil output, efficiency, and affordability, particularly in tropical locations like West Africa and Southeast Asia (Purnama et al., 2024).

The "food versus fuel" controversy makes matters more difficult. Lowering the land available for food crops and converting agricultural resources and land to biodiesel production threaten global food security. Given the expanding world population and increased need for food, this issue is especially pressing and calls for a careful balance between food production and energy production (Naylor & Higgins, 2018). This discussion has been influenced by several viewpoints, including institutional, ethical, and policy aspects. Kuchler and Linnér (2012) provided a genealogical analysis, demonstrating how international organizations have reframed the issue as a larger food-versus-food dilemma that reshapes rural production priorities. Thompson (2012) discussed the moral ramifications of prioritizing fuel over food within agricultural systems.

12.5 Innovations and Potential Benefits

Nanotechnology offers significant potential to revolutionize biofuel production by improving efficiency, yield, and sustainability. NPs, with their unique properties, can be used as catalysts, pretreatment agents, and in other processes to enhance biofuel production. This involves promoting greater microalgal development, raising biofuel output, and improving biomass digestion. NPs have garnered a lot of interest for application in the production of biofuel due to their exceptional qualities, which include a high surface-area-to-volume ratio, enhanced dispersibility, and higher reactivity. Sher et al. (2024) examined the groundbreaking role that nanomaterials—particularly carbon nanotubes, metal–organic frameworks, biomass waste materials, and graphene-based catalysts—play in improving a variety of biofuel synthesis processes. The use of metal-modified graphene oxide composite catalysts, such as aluminium and ferric, is one well-known example. These catalysts show a remarkable 25% decrease in the content of free fatty acids and a 15% increase in the production of methyl hexadecenoic. Additionally, the stable and cost-effective manufacturing of TiO_2 NPs under environmental conditions consistently produced high biodiesel yields, reaching 95% over 10 cycles. However, it is important to recognize the potential drawbacks of employing nanomaterials in the production of biofuel. Careful thought must be given to environmental issues such nanoparticle emission during production processes, their effects on ecosystems, and safety risks associated with nanoparticle exposure. Green synthesis, hydrothermal-assisted carbonization, biomass hydrolysis with gold nanoparticles, and the impact of nanofuel technology on engine characteristics were all covered by Sher et al. (2024). The sustainability of novel catalysts and processes, such as magnetic MOF-derived materials and metal–organic frameworks functionalized with sulfonic acid, is closely examined. The assessment concludes with a detailed examination of the economic and environmental effects, highlighting the possible advantages and difficulties involved in integrating nanotechnology into manufacturing biofuels.

12.5.1 Hybrid Systems: BC-Conductive Material Composites for Simultaneous Energy Production and Soil Enrichment

Every city has to deal with the global issue of managing municipal solid waste (MSW), which is mainly made up of plastic and biomass. The waste-to-energy concept is presented as a means of fully utilizing MSW as an energy source in order to meet the increasing need for energy. Here, a thermal energy recovery technique from biomass and spent coloured plastic bottles was investigated using a low-temperature char-optimized reactor. Using SEM–EDS, BET, TGA/DTA, and FTIR analysis, BC—which was produced by co-carbonizing Daniella Oliver leaves with PET—was investigated. Biomass and hybrid BC produced 32.87 and 38.6 weight per cent at high temperatures of 279 and 259 °C, respectively (Adeniyi et al., 2023). Several polar groups in the BC samples suggest they could be applied as adsorbents and soil additives to remove pollutants. According to EDS analysis, the hybrid BC included a lot of inorganic components, whereas the biomass BC had more carbon. The BET surface areas of the biomass and hybrid BCs were 342.1 and 114 m^2/g, respectively. Unlike other feedstocks, the method has generated new products for a variety of uses while recycling the two most difficult MSW components for environmentally acceptable and sustainable energy.

Because they can combine unique properties from two or more components to increase performance for a variety of applications, composite materials have attracted a lot of attention. Two promising materials, graphene oxide (GO) and BC, are incorporated into composite designs (Kalderis et al., 2025). While GO has a 2D structure with improved porosity and adjustable electrical characteristics, BC, which is made from biomass, has special physicochemical qualities. Nonetheless, there is a substantial study gap in methodically comprehending the combined impacts of GO and BC in composite materials, especially their performance in various applications, environmental impact, and synthesis methods. By thoroughly examining the most recent techniques for creating BC-GO composites, their multifunctional qualities, and their possible uses, Kalderis et al. (2025) fill this knowledge gap. Because of their increased surface area and functional groups, BC-GO composites show remarkable efficacy in adsorbing organic pollutants and heavy metal ions. Various physical and chemical interactions in the adsorption mechanisms achieve superior affinities over individual materials. Additionally, BC-GO composites show great promise for use as electrodes for microbial fuel cells and supercapacitors in electrochemical applications. These multipurpose materials have enormous potential for addressing the problem of water contamination and advancing sustainable practices. They highlight the remarkable adaptability of BC-GO composites as sustainable materials by offering in-depth insights into their synthesis methods, characteristics, and applications (Kalderis et al., 2025).

12.5.2 Waste Valorization: Converting Agricultural Residues into BC for Circular Bioeconomy

An estimated 350 million tonnes of agricultural leftovers are produced annually in Asia. In addition to being utilized as green manure, the Ministry of Power estimates that many tonnes of this trash are thrown away annually (Nguyen et al., 2022). It outlined the process for turning agricultural waste into the most valuable BC and some of its essential physical and chemical characteristics. The positive impacts of bio and phytoremediation on soil contaminated with metal(lloid) are also examined in this review. BC derived from agricultural biomass is an interesting organic residual material that may be utilized as a responsible remedy for soil improvement and remediation of metal(lloid)-polluted soil. Massive cleanup demands can be met by plants with higher biomass and faster growth. Recent years have seen notable progress in converting agricultural biomass into BC and in our knowledge of the processes behind the accumulation and movement of metal(lloid) in plants used to restore soil contaminated by metal(lloid). In soil contaminated with metal(lloid)s, BC derived from various agricultural biomass can enhance phytoremediation effectiveness and encourage the growth of native plants. This carbon-enriched BC encourages natural microbial activity because it neutralizes pH and provides sufficient nutrients. The possibility of turning biomass from agricultural waste into BC is thus critically examined in this analysis, together with the effects on the potential for plant and microbial remediation in soil contaminated by metal(lloid).

In the pursuit of a sustainable future, the bioeconomy and biorefineries have become important change agents. A review paper provides a thorough and comprehensible examination of the complex bioeconomy environment (Wagh et al., 2024). The primary factors driving this sustainable paradigm are customer demand for bio-based and renewable products, resource scarcity, and environmental concerns. The primary suppliers of the feedstock required by biorefineries are the agricultural sector and the agro-industry. They support rural development and sustainable farming methods and boost the bioeconomy, creating a win–win situation. The backbone of the bioeconomy, biorefineries maximize resource use, reduce waste, and provide various bio-based goods. At the forefront are cutting-edge biorefinery processes that are increasing the variety of feedstocks and revolutionizing efficiency to produce derivatives with better value. The market is moving towards a more environmentally friendly and circular economy thanks to these value-added goods, which include biofuels, bio-plastics, and more. Waste minimization and advancing circular economy concepts demonstrate the bioeconomy's dedication to sustainability. By encouraging bio-based enterprises and preferring eco-friendly alternatives, policy, legislation, and market developments form the bio-economy and foster a competitive and healthy environment (Wagh et al., 2024).

12.5.3 *Carbon Sequestration: BC's Long-Term Carbon Storage Potential*

The return of BC from biomass to the soil is one method of sequestering carbon (CS). To evaluate the long-term biochar CS potential, it is essential to incorporate the complex physical interferences and biological interactions of the soil. Yin et al. (2022) developed a daily-resolution simulator and integrated BC into a biogeochemical field model to evaluate the 5-, 50-, and 500-year CS potential upon soil-BC-plant interaction. BC may maintain 483–557 kg C/t BC-C after 500 years of natural decomposition by simulating the situation of burying 7.5–75 t/ha BC-C in a 50 cm-depth rainfed agricultural soil with maize growing.

Additionally, BC changed the long-term soil climate and supplied labile-C to offset microbial decomposition, reducing soil organic carbon degradation by 44–265 kg C/t BC-C. Additionally, by providing exogenous nutrients—the equivalent of collecting 66–1039 kg C/t BC-C over 50 years—BC enhanced plant photosynthetic capacity. However, after reaching an upper limit (1030–1722 kg C/t BC-C), total CS declines annually because BC restricts endogenous nutrient release and impedes plant development when foreign resources are depleted. After 500 years, 651–725 kg C/t BC-C might be sequestered. Additionally, BC has greater potential in arid and infertile soils. Our analysis shows that BC-soil implantation is a potential carbon-negative technique and that biogeochemical reactions must be considered when evaluating BC's long-term CS. In order to examine BC's carbon sequestration while taking into account its carbon persistence, impacts on soil organic carbon, and plant development, the "Biogeochemical Field" hypothesis and the BC database were combined. Through the identification of interacting biochemical interactions in the BC-soil–plant system, the complex parameters impacting BC's capacity to sequester carbon over five, fifty, and five hundred years were quantified.

12.6 Challenges

12.6.1 *Technical: Nanoparticle Aggregation, BC's Variable Porosity*

Various thermochemical processes produce BC, a carbonaceous by-product of lignocellulosic biomass. BC may be reduced in size to the nanometre level to become "nano-BC". In contrast to macro-BC, nano-BC exhibits exceptional physicochemical properties, such as increased stability, a distinct nanostructure, enhanced catalytic activity, a greater specific surface area, increased porosity, enhanced surface functionality, and surface-active sites. In addition to hazardous pollutants (heavy metals, pesticides, and antibiotics), nano-BC effectively controls the transit and absorption of essential micro- and macronutrients. However, a thorough grasp of the most current nano-BC investigations is necessary for large-scale implementations, including development, physicochemical characteristics, and targeted application (Bhandari et al., 2023).

12.6.2 Environmental: Toxicity Risks of Nanomaterials in Ecosystems

Due to widespread industrialization, urbanization, and modern agricultural practices, a wide range of toxic substances have accumulated in the various environmental matrices, including pesticides, pharmaceutical and personal care products, antibiotics, hormones, organic compounds, nano-compounds, endocrine disruptors, steroids, surfactants and their metabolites, industrial additives, and heavy metals (Bhatt et al., 2022). Anthropogenic activities can cause pollutants to accumulate in many settings at levels ranging from 1 $\mu g\ kg^{-1}$ to 10 $mg\ kg^{-1}$. Hospitals, factories, power plants, oil refineries, mining, improper waste treatment, agriculture, and domestic tasks are some of these activities (Zhou et al., 2021). A thorough evaluation of nano-BC's toxicity to various creatures and its indirect impact on humans is necessary for large-scale applications. This review provides a comprehensive understanding of nano-BC research concerning (1) compositions and qualities, (2) development methodology, (3) potentiality as an emerging sorbent, photocatalyst, or enzyme carrier for environmental application, (4) and characterization methods, (5) environmental issues (Bhandari et al., 2023).

12.6.3 Economic: High Costs of Conductive Materials and BC Functionalization

Many toxic compounds have collected in many environmental matrices as a result of modern farming methods, urbanization, and extensive industrialization. Examples include steroids, surfactants and their metabolites, heavy metals, organic chemicals, pesticides, hormones, endocrine disruptors, steroids, organic chemicals, nano-compounds, and industrial additives (Bhatt et al., 2022). Hospitals, factories, power plants, oil refineries, mining, poor waste treatment, agriculture, and domestic activities are examples of anthropogenic activities that can cause pollutants to build up in different ecosystems at concentrations between 1.0 $\mu g\ kg^{-1}$ to 10.0 $mg\ kg^{-1}$ (Zhou et al., 2021).

12.7 Future Research Directions

Because of urbanization and population increase, the usage of fossil fuels is increasing at an accelerated rate, eventually leading to the depletion of fuels produced from petroleum. The world's limited supply of fossil fuels is one of the most pressing problems we are now confronting (Rai et al., 2016). Furthermore, the excessive dependence on fuels derived from petroleum has sparked debate on its detrimental effects on the economy, the environment, and energy conservation. Consequently, a great deal of effort has been made to identify an alternative source that can reduce the amount of fuels that are obtained from fossil fuels. In the current situation, when fossil fuels are progressively running out, biofuel is one of the finest substitutes for fuels made from petroleum. Greenhouse gases are emitted into the atmosphere as fossil fuels burn, endangering both the ecology and human health. Due to various limitations in the technologies currently in use and increased expenses, the generation of industrial biofuel takes a long time.

Additionally, a variety of processes are employed to transform different feedstocks into the desired outcome due to the wide range of materials and techniques (Arya et al., 2021). NPs are among the best and most economical ways to address the present problems with biomass consumption in terms of selectivity, energy efficiency, and time management. Many of these techniques have gained popularity recently, and some NPs—such as metal, magnetic, and metal oxide—are being employed to boost the production of biofuel. NPs are advantageous additions to biofuel due to their special qualities, which include their design, stability, enhanced surface area to volume ratio, catalytic activity, and reusability. Furthermore, nanomaterials such carbon nanotubes, carbon nanofibers, and carbon nanosheets have been shown to include stable catalysts for enzyme immobilization at reasonable prices, which enhance the production of biofuel. Arya et al. (2021) thoroughly analysed the main obstacles and potential future developments in utilizing different nanomaterials in biofuel production. Because of their unique qualities, biofuels are regarded as a substitute for fossil fuels and have attracted international interest recently (Bhattarai et al., 2011). Almost every continent uses a variety of plant sources as feedstock for the manufacture of biofuel, such as vegetables, maize, soybeans, sugarcane, palm oil, and jatropha (used in Africa) (Shalaby, 2013). In countries like the USA and Brazil, bioethanol works well as biodiesel for otto-cycle engines when combined with gasoline (Rai et al., 2016). But one important kind of biofuel that might either complement or replace diesel made from fossil fuels is biodiesel. Transesterification of renewable lipids is used to create biodiesel.

12.7.1 Developing Low-Cost, Scalable Synthesis of Conductive BC

Mittal et al. (2023) illustrate two sustainable methods for producing electroactive BCs and their use in electroactive built wetlands (CWs) to provide a cyclical pathway for biomass consumption and technological advancement for wastewater treatment and power generation. Based on the production method, the current study developed two different BCs with different physico-(electro)chemical properties using Canna indica biomass generated during CW operations. Compared to the amorphous BC material made by the drum kiln-processed BC (KB) method, this study's ultrafast biochar (PB) created by plasma-based processing in minutes produced more crystalline BC with excellent electrical conductivity. These BCs were employed in the electroactive built wetlands coupled with microbial fuel cells (CW-MFC) development process. They were operated in batch mode alongside a control CW-MFC based on a commercial granular graphite (GG) substrate. While KB was created in large quantities using a semi-controlled combustion process in a kiln approach and required three to four days prior to the final BC preparation, PB was produced using high-temperature plasma processing in 6.0 min. The sequence KB < GG < PB was found for the electrical conductivity (EC) of the BC and GG materials, suggesting that PB was a highly conductive substance that promoted electron transit between microbes. Therefore, PB generated the greatest densities with current and power densities of 628 mA m^{-3} and 126 mW m^{-3}, respectively. The COD elimination in CW-MFC-KB, CW-MFC-GG, and CW-MFC-PB was $72.32 \pm 2.98\%$, $72.42 \pm 2.61\%$, and $59.91 \pm 3.21\%$, respectively (Forde et al., 2014).

12.7.2 AI-Driven Design of Nanomaterials for Targeted Biofuel Pathways

Artificial intelligence (AI) is increasingly used in biofuel research, especially in nanomaterials, optimizing metabolic pathways, and choosing feedstocks. In biofuel production, AI-driven models can increase CO_2 fixation, biomass productivity, and yields of high-value compounds. AI is also being utilized to design and synthesize nanomaterials, such as those used in biodiesel manufacturing, to improve conversion yields and reaction rates. By investigating new nanomaterials to develop highly effective treatments, AI is revolutionizing the field of nanomedicine. AI analyses bigger datasets to identify desired nanoproperties for various therapeutic goals, ultimately improving the efficacy and safety of nanomaterials. AI uses genetic and clinical data from patients to guide therapies, anticipate results, and optimize drug forms and dosages to maximize benefits and reduce adverse effects. Data fusion, ethics, and regulation are some of the issues facing AI-supported nanomedicine, necessitating improved instruments and interdisciplinary cooperation. Mazumdar et al. (2024)

emphasize the value of AI in patient care and call on researchers, practitioners, and policymakers to embrace AI for improved results.

12.7.3 Field Studies on BC's Long-Term Agricultural and Dietary Impacts

According to extensive field research, BC in agriculture can affect soil, crops, and human health in beneficial and perhaps detrimental ways. Although BC, a substance that resembles charcoal and is made from biomass, can increase soil fertility and carbon sequestration, it may also change the availability of micronutrients in the soil and perhaps have an effect on the micronutrient content of crops, which may have an impact on human dietary intakes. In addition to their many agricultural and environmental advantages, BCs have enormous potential to help mitigate climate change. The long-term effects of increased BCs, particularly in boreal regions, are poorly understood. The impact of a single application of softwood BCs over eight years on two distinct boreal agricultural soils with high starting soil organic carbon contents—rich, fine-textured Stagnosol and nutrient-poor, coarse-textured Umbrisol—was investigated by Kalu et al. (2021). The physical properties of the soil, greenhouse gas emissions during seven to nine growing seasons, and the plant nutrient levels and nutrient absorption patterns of several field crops were also investigated. Additionally, they found that adding BCs had minimal long-term effects on crop biomass output, plant nutrient levels, and plant nutrient absorption in both soil types. Notable BC × fertilization interactions were seen regarding crop biomass yields in barley (2013) and peas (2016) three and six years after BC was applied in Stagnosol, respectively. In both situations, the BC significantly increased crop biomass yield when combined with the regular fertilization rate (100% of the recommended value) compared to a fertilization treatment devoid of charcoal. However, when the fertilization rate was reduced to 30% of the required amount, the BC had no effect. The levels of several plant nutrients for peas in 2016 and the absorption of both barley in 2013 and peas in 2016 showed similar noteworthy interactions with BC and fertilization. As a result, BC may enhance plant nutrient uptake in boreal environments, perhaps leading to an increase in agricultural biomass production. These effects, nevertheless, have been minor and erratic over time. The K/Mg ratio in plant biomass and the K content of plants were both markedly increased by BC, which may suggest that K and Mg in Umbrisol have an antagonistic interaction. In Stagnosol, a similar K hostility towards Na was noted. In Stagnosol, the applied BC similarly decreased the plant content and uptake of Al and Na over several years.

Additionally, they discovered that Umbrisol's higher plant Mn content with BC in the first few years decreased during the next several years. However, the relative plant concentrations of P, K, Mg, S, Al, Cu, Fe, and Ni in Stagnosol and Cd and Ni in Umbrisol rose with time. Over time, there was no discernible increase in crop biomass yield due to adding BC, even with these higher plant contents. The increased plant water availability and decreased bulk density that was first documented in the early years eventually diminished, most likely due to the topsoil's BC concentration being diluted. Even seven years after the application, BC's ability to influence N_2O emissions remained (Kalu et al., 2021).

12.8 Case Studies

12.8.1 Biochar in Brazil: Integration with Sugarcane Ethanol Production to Enhance Soil Fertility

Bioenergy is an essential short- and medium-term alternative as we move towards more sustainable and renewable energy sources. The growth of the global bioindustry depends on the creation of integrated multi-product systems that can effectively and sustainably convert specific organic resources into biofuels, bioelectricity, and other reasonably priced bioproducts. Using life cycle analysis, fixed capital investment, and the first and second laws of thermodynamics, a research was conducted to evaluate and compare a number of integrated bioenergetic complexes that process lignocellulosic material from sugarcane and oil palm crops concurrently (Batlle et al., 2022). These systems were created with Brazil in mind, a country that contributes significantly to bioenergy conversion because of its recognized soil and climate potential, large land area, and bioenergy expertise. Consequently, this study looks at three different scenarios: the first (CI), which is a conventional palm oil biodiesel and sugarcane ethanol system; the second (CII), which is an oil palm-sugarcane biorefinery connected to a lignocellulosic bio methanol plant; and the third (CIII), which is an extension of the second but brings in the concepts of advanced gas turbine integrated biomass gasification (BIG-GTCC) (Batlle et al., 2022). A systematic analytical technique that allows for the characterization and measurement of energy, exergy, and environmental issues connected to the energy conversion of lignocellulosic materials is developed and put into practice to achieve this. This technique makes it easier to evaluate and choose technologies that support the worldwide decarbonization of energy by offering indications. In terms of Global Plant Efficiency (53.4%), Surplus Electricity Index (86.6 kWh $tonMP^{-1}$), and Global Plant Exergy Efficiency (62.7%), CIII outperformed the other scenarios linked to BIG-GTCC integrating. The findings of the thermodynamic evaluation confirm its appeal to agribusinesses by highlighting the benefit of acquiring a more extensive energy portfolio from a variety of raw materials. Economically, integration is not possible, but fiscal incentives based on advancements in conversion technology, increased conversion yields, and reduced fossil fuel usage might greatly speed up integration. In sugarcane and palm cultivation, the LCA findings showed the possible environmental advantages of partially replacing fossil fuel with biodiesel (while accounting for methanol produced from lignocellulosic material). Consequently, the methyl technique reduced the fossil energy use for sugarcane by 79.6% and palm by 69.2%. Thus, the oil palm–sugarcane biorefinery achieves a fossil energy ratio (FER) of 9 energy units and a 52.6% life cycle energy efficiency (LCEE).

12.8.2 *Graphene-Oxide Catalysts: Biodiesel Production from Leftover Cooked Oil*

Waste cooking oil (WCO) has been used extensively as a low-cost and promising source for the generation of biodiesel. In work by Jume et al. (2020), bimetal zirconium/strontium oxide NPs and possible graphene oxide were combined to create a novel nanocatalyst (GO@ZrO_2–SrO) using the co-precipitation method. As a heterogeneous catalyst for the transesterification of WCO to provide FAMEs as biodiesel, the suggested nano composite has demonstrated encouraging potential. FTIR, SEM/EDX, and XRD were utilized to assess the surface functional groups, nanostructure/elements, and crystallinity of the nanocatalyst, respectively. They also examined the effects of the oil-to-alcohol ratio, reaction temperature, and reaction time on the yield of transesterification FAMEs. A material ratio of 1:0.5 (w/w) of GO:ZrO_2–SrO, an oil-to-methanol ratio of 1:4, a reaction period of 90 min, and a temperature of 120 °C were determined to be the conditions that produced the highest FAMEs yield of 91%. GO@ZrO_2-SrO may be an alternate heterogeneous catalyst to convert WCO into biodiesel, as this work showed.

12.9 Ethical and Regulatory Considerations

Nanotechnology has advantages and disadvantages; thus, ethical and legal issues must be carefully balanced. Potential hazards, equitable access, and public trust are moral concerns, whereas regulatory systems must handle risks and guarantee responsible development. Since nanotechnology has already started to permeate many various areas of research, it would be challenging to ignore its potential advantages and halt the advancement of related studies. Guidelines might be used in its development to ensure that the technology does not become overly potentially hazardous. As with any new technology, it is difficult to stop every well-funded organization from attempting to utilize the technology maliciously. But if the scientists working in this field establish and follow a set of ethical guidelines (like the Molecular Nanotechnology guidelines), we should be able to develop nanotechnology safely and still get the advantages that have been promised (Schulte & Salamanca-Buentello, 2007). Given nanotechnology's enormous potential risks, we must carefully consider its possible effects. Although nanotechnology may never reach the kind of power and widespread use that its proponents had hoped for, we should nevertheless work to address any potential ethical concerns before society irrevocably adopts the technology, just like we would with any other promising, near-horizon technology. We must think about the ethics of nanotechnology's development and create regulations that will encourage its advancement if we hope to eliminate or at least mitigate its detrimental effects on society as mentioned by Schulte and Salamanca-Buentello (2007).

12.9.1 Balancing Biochar Use for Energy vs. Agriculture in Resource-Limited Regions

Optimizing a slow pyrolysis-based bioenergy system to produce both energy and biochar instead of only energy was evaluated for its effect on greenhouse gas emissions. Using a life cycle approach, feedstock production simulations were investigated (Gaunt & Lehmann, 2008). They took into account the use of purpose-grown bioenergy crops (BEC) and crop wastes (CW) as feedstocks. Corn, switchgrass, and miscanthus were purposefully grown as bioenergy crops in place of winter wheat in the BEC scenarios. In the CW scenarios, winter wheat straw and maize stover are both regarded as feedstocks. In contrast to utilizing it just for fossil energy offsets, their research shows that applying biochar to agricultural land (2–19 Mg CO_2 ha^{-1} y^{-1}) decreases emissions by 2–5. The carbon retention in biochar accounts for 41–64 per cent of these emission reductions; the remaining amount is due to fertilizer savings, prevented soil emissions other than CO_2, and balancing the use of fossil fuels for energy. The energy generated per unit energy input at 2–7 MJ/MJ is higher than that of related technologies like ethanol from maize, even if the slow pyrolysis technique is adjusted to create biochar for land application, reducing the energy production by around 30% (Gaunt & Lehmann, 2008). Even before taking into consideration the carbon offset from using biochar, the lifetime emissions linked to burning fossil fuels to create electricity (600–900 kg CO_2 MWh^{-1}) are significantly greater than the C emissions per MWh of 91–360 kg CO_2 MWh^{-1} as a net production of energy. An energetically effective method of producing bioenergy is low-temperature slow pyrolysis, and applying biochar to the land lowers greenhouse gas emissions more than using it to offset emissions from fossil fuels.

12.9.2 EPA/FDA Guidelines for NPs Safety in Food-Chain Systems

Foods, cosmetics, and medical items are just a few of the FDA-regulated products that potentially benefit from the emerging technology known as nanotechnology. Compared to their larger-scale counterparts, objects in the nanoscale range, having at least one dimension in the size range of around 1 nm (nm) to 100 nm, may display distinct chemical, physical, or biological effects (Kaittanis et al., 2010). A drug product's enhanced bioavailability, lower dosage, or increased potency, reduced toxicity, improved pathogen detection, more protective food packaging materials, or better delivery of a functional ingredient or nutrient in food are just a few uses for dimension-dependent properties or phenomena.

Fertilizers, aquaculture, irrigation, water filtration, animal feed, animal immunizations, food processing, and packaging are just a few of the many agricultural applications of nanotechnology. Pheromones, nutrient delivery, fertilizers, agrochemicals, biofertilizers, biostimulants, post-harvest storage, insect and disease prevention, and genetic modification of plants for crop improvement through the use of nanomaterials as a carrier system are some of the agribusiness innovations made possible by nanotechnology in recent decades. To fulfil the rising need for food brought on by the world's population expansion, markets have already started incorporating nano-based items, such as food packaging, antimicrobials, and nano-encapsulated nutrients and agrochemicals. Applications for marketing permission for items based on nanotechnology must show that they may be used safely without endangering consumers or the environment (Kumari et al., 2023). Numerous nations have been diligently examining whether their legal systems are appropriate for managing nanotechnologies. Numerous methods have been employed to control nano-based products in agriculture, food, and feed. Here, Kumari et al. (2023) have placed international safety assessment norms and laws in context, together with a number of national restrictions pertaining to nano-based agricultural products, from food to feed.

As the science of nanomaterials advances quickly, nations and regions have started to create, enhance, and/or specify food and medical product regulations. To promote the moral advancement of nanomaterials across a range of industries, they provide funding for regulatory science and other research projects. In 2010, a project was initiated by the Working Group on Nanomaterials (WPN) of the Organization for Economic Co-operation and Development (OECD). Government-sponsored regulatory science research, regulatory strategies, legislative frameworks, and other research programmes, institutions, and infrastructure in foods and medications that employ NPs were all to be listed, summarized, and reviewed as part of the project (Subhan and Subhan, 2023), 2011–2012 saw the completion of their project. The 12 WPN delegations include representatives from the United States, the Russian Federation, Canada, France, Germany, Japan, Korea, the Netherlands, Norway, Poland, and the European Union. The publication of this study was approved by the Committee for Scientific and Technological Policy (CSTP) in January 2013. This chapter of the book covers the need for advancements in nanomaterial safety rules in the food and pharmaceutical industries.

References

Adeniyi, A. G., Amusa, V. T., Emenike, E. C., & Iwuozor, K. O. (2023). Hybrid biochar production from biomass and pigmented plastic for sustainable waste-to-energy. *Emergent Materials, 6*, 1481–1490. https://doi.org/10.1007/s42247-023-00538-4

Akhtar, T., Tariq, M. I., Iqbal, S., Sultana, N., & Wei, C. K. (2017). Production and characterization of biodiesel from Eriobotrya Japonica seed oil: An optimization study. *International Journal of Green Energy, 13*, 574–746. https://doi.org/10.1080/15435075.2017.1310107

Alkharabsheh, H. M., Seleiman, M. F., Battaglia, M. L., Shami, A., Jala, R. S., Alhammaad, B. A., Almutairi, K. F., & Al-Saif, A. M. (2021). Biochar and its broad impacts in soil quality and fertility, nutrient leaching and crop productivity: A review. *Agronomy, 11*, 993. https://doi.org/10.3390/agronomy11050993

Almanassra, I. W., Mckay, G., Kochkodan, V., Ali Atieh, M., & Al-Ansari, T. (2021). A state-of-the-art review on phosphate removal from water by biochars. *Chemical Engineering Journal, 409*, Article 128211. https://doi.org/10.1016/J.CEJ.2020.128211

Anekwe, I. M. S., Tetteh, E. K., Akpasi, S. O., & Isa, Y. M. (2024). Current advances and potentials of nanotechnology for biofuel production. In I. S. Dunmade, M. O. & Daramola, S. A. Iwarere (Eds.) *Sustainable engineering. Green energy and technology*. Springer, Cham. https://doi.org/10.1007/978-3-031-47215-2_22.

Antonangelo, J. A., Sun, X., & Eufrade-Junior, H. J. (2025). Biochar impact on soil health and tree-based crops: A review. *Biochar, 7*, 51. https://doi.org/10.1007/s42773-025-00450-6

Arora, A., Nandal, P., Singh, J., & Verma, M. L. (2020). Nanobiotechnological advancements in lignocellulosic biomass pretreatment. *Materials Science for Energy Technologies, 3*, 308–318. https://doi.org/10.1016/j.mset.2019.12.003

Arya, I., Poona, A., Dikshit, P. K., Pandit, S., Kumar, J., Singh, H. N., Jha, N. K., Rudayni, H. A., Chaudhary, A. A., & Kumar, S. (2021). Current trends and future prospects of nanotechnology in biofuel production. *Catalysts, 11*(11), 1308. https://doi.org/10.3390/catal11111308

Batlle, E. A. O., Julio, A. A. V., Santiago, Y. C., Palácio, J. C. E., Bortoni, E. D. C., Nogueira, L. A. H., Dias, M. V. X., & González, A. M. (2022). Brazilian integrated oilpalm-sugarcane biorefinery: An energetic, exergetic, economic, and environmental (4E) assessment. *Energy Conversion and Management, 268*(2022), Article 116066. https://doi.org/10.1016/j.enconman.2022.116066

Bhandari, G., Gangola, S., Dhasmana, A., Rajput, V., Gupta, S., Malik, S., & Slama, P. (2023). Nano-biochar: Recent progress, challenges, and opportunities for sustainable environmental remediation. *Frontiers in Microbiology, 19*(14), 1214870. https://doi.org/10.3389/fmicb.2023.1214870

Bhatia, S. K., Banu, J. R., Singh, V., Kumar, G., & Yang, Y.-H. (2023). Algal biomass to biohydrogen: Pretreatment, influencing factors, and conversion strategies. *Bioresource Technology, 368*, Article 128332. https://doi.org/10.1016/j.biortech.2022.128332

Bhatt, P., Bhandari, G., & Bilal, M. (2022). Occurrence, toxicity impacts and mitigation of emerging micropollutants in the aquatic environments: Recent tendencies and perspectives. *Journal of Environmental Chemical Engineering, 10*, Article 107598. https://doi.org/10.1016/j.jece.2022.107598

Bhattarai, K., Stalick, W. M., Mckay, S., Geme, G., & Bhattarai, N. (2011). Biofuel: An alternative to fossil fuel for alleviating world energy and economic crises. *Journal of Environmental Science and Health Part A Toxic, 46*, 1424–1442.

Buarki, F., AbuHassan, H., Al Hannan, F., & Henari, F. Z. (2022). Green synthesis of iron oxide nanoparticles using *Hibiscus rosa sinensis* flowers and their antibacterial activity. *Journal of Nanotechnology, 2022*, 5474645.

Chaos-Hernández, D., Reynel-Avila, H. E., Mendoza-Castillo, D. I., Bonilla-Petriciolet, A., & Aguayo-Villarreal, I. A. (2022). Functionalization and activation of carbon-based catalysts with KOH and calcium and their application in transesterification to produce biodiesel: Optimization of catalytic properties and kinetic study. *Fuel, 310*(Part B), 122066. https://doi.org/10.1016/j.fuel.2021.122066.

Christwardana, M., Prayoga, B. A., Kuntolaksono, S., Joelianingsih, J., & Maulana, A. Y. (2025). Enhanced electron transfer in microbial fuel cells using calcined eggshell anode with optimized performance. *Bioresource Technology Reports, 29*, Article 102088. https://doi.org/10.1016/j.biteb.2025.102088

Cui, X., Hao, H., He, Z., Stoffella, P. J., & Yang, X. (2016). Pyrolysis of wetland biomass waste: Potential for carbon sequestration and water remediation. *Journal of Environmental Management, 173*, 95–104. https://doi.org/10.1016/J.JENVMAN.2016.02.049
Darnton-Hill, I., Webb, P., Harvey, P. W., Hunt, J. M., Dalmiya, N., Chopra, M., Ball, M. J., Bloem, M. W., & de Benoist, B. (2005). Micronutrient deficiencies and gender: Social and economic costs. *American Journal of Clinical Nutrition, 81*(5), 1198S-1205S.
Demiral, H., & Gündüzoğlu, G. (2010). Removal of nitrate from aqueous solutions by activated carbon prepared from sugar beet bagasse. *Bioresource Technology, 101(*6), 1675–1680. https://doi.org/10.1016/J.BIORTECH.2009.09.087.
Dong, X., He, L., Liu, Y., & Piao, Y. (2018). Preparation of highly conductive biochar nanoparticles for rapid and sensitive detection of 17β-estradiol in water. *Electrochimica Acta, 292*, 55–62. https://doi.org/10.1016/j.electacta.2018.09.129
EBC (European Biochar Certificate). (2022). Guidelines for a Sustainable Production of Biochar. Arbaz, Switzerland: European Biochar Foundation.
Esmaeili, H., Nourafkan, E., Nakisa, M., & Ahmed, W. (2021). Chapter 7—Application of nanotechnology for biofuel production. In W. Ahmed, M. Booth, & E. Nourafkan, *Micro and nano technologies, emerging nanotechnologies for renewable energy*. Elsevier, pp. 149–172. https://doi.org/10.1016/B978-0-12-821346-9.00005-5.
Forde, C. J., Meaney, M., Carrigan, J. B., Mills, C., Boland, S., & Hernon, A. (2014). Chapter 12: Biobased fats (lipids) and oils from biomass as a source of bioenergy. In *Bioenergy research: Advances and applications*, pp. 185–201.
Gabhane, J. W., Bhange, V. P., Patil, P. D., Bankar, S. T., & Kumar, S. (2020). Recent trends in biochar production methods and its application as a soil health conditioner: A review. *SN Applied Sciences, 2*, 1–21.
Gaunt, J.L., & Lehmann, J. (2008). Energy balance and emissions associated with biochar sequestration and pyrolysis bioenergy production. *Environmental Science & Technology, 42*(Issue 11), 4152–4158.
Han, S. W., Chee, K. M., & Cho, S. J. (2015). Nutritional quality of rice bran protein in comparison to animal and vegetable protein. *Food Chemistry, 172*, 766–769.
Hersh, B., Mirkouei, A., Sessions, J., Rezaiel, B., & You, Y. (2019). A review and future directions on enhancing sustainability benefits across food-energy-water systems: the potential role of biochar-derived products. *AIMS Environmental Science, 6*(5), 379–416. https://doi.org/10.3934/environsci.2019.5.379.
Hussein, B. A., Mahdi, A. B., Izzat, S. E., Dwijendra, N. K. A., Parra, R. M. R., Arenas, L. A. B., Mustafa, Y. F., Yasin, G. Hammid, A. T., & Kianfar, E. (2022). Production, structural properties nano biochar and effects nano biochar in soil: A review. *Egyptian Journal of Chemistry, 65*(12), 607–618.
Johanis, H., Lehejček, J., & Tejnecký, V. (2022). An insight into long-term effects of biochar application on forest soils. *European Journal of Forest Research, 141*, 213–224. https://doi.org/10.1007/s10342-022-01440-0
Jume, B. H., Gabris, M. A., Nodeh, H. R., Rezania, S., & Cho, J. (2020). Biodiesel production from waste cooking oil using a novel heterogeneous catalyst based on graphene oxide doped metal oxide nanoparticles. *Renewable Energy, 162*, 2182–2189. https://doi.org/10.1016/j.renene.2020.10.046
Kaittanis, C., Santra, S., & Manuel, P. J. (2010). Emerging nanotechnology-based strategies for the identification of microbial pathogenesis. *Advanced Drug Delivery Reviews, 62*, 408–423.
Kalderis, D., Gholami, P., Pashalidis, I., & Khataee, A. (2025). Synergistic integration of biochar and graphene oxide in multi-functional composites: From sustainable synthesis to environmental remediation and energy storage. *Journal of Industrial and Engineering Chemistry, 144*, 210–227. https://doi.org/10.1016/j.jiec.2024.10.015
Kalu, S., Simojoki, A., Karhu, K., & Tammeorg, P. (2021). Long-term effects of softwood biochar on soil physical properties, greenhouse gas emissions and crop nutrient uptake in two contrasting

boreal soils. *Agriculture Ecosystems & Environment, 316*, Article 107454. https://doi.org/10.1016/j.agee.2021.107454

Kant, T., Shrivas, K., Dewangan, K., Kumar, A., Jaiswal, N. K., Deb, M. K., & Pervez, S. (2022). Design and development of conductive nanomaterials for electrochemical sensors: A modern approach. *Materials Today Chemistry, 24*, Article 100769. https://doi.org/10.1016/j.mtchem.2021.100769

Kuchler, M., & Linnér, B. O. (2012). Challenging the food vs. fuel dilemma: Genealogical analysis of the biofuel discourse pursued by international organizations. *Food Policy, 37*(5), 581–588. https://doi.org/10.1016/j.foodpol.2012.06.005.

Kumari, R., Suman, K., Karmakar, S., Mishra, V., Lakra, S. G., Saurav, G. K., & Mahto, B. K. (2023). Regulation and safety measures for nanotechnology-based agri-products. *Frontiers in Genome Editing, 5*, 1200987. https://doi.org/10.3389/fgeed.2023.1200987

Liao, C., Luo, Y., Fang, C., Chen, J., & Li, B. (2012). The effects of plantation practice on soil properties based on the comparison between natural and planted forests: A meta-analysis. *Global Ecology and Biogeography, 21*, 318–327. https://doi.org/10.1111/j.1466-8238.2011.00690.x

Ma, J., Zhang, J., Zhang, Y., Guo, Q., Hu, T., Xiao, H., & Jia, J. (2023). Progress on anodic modification materials and future development directions in microbial fuel cells. *Journal of Power Sources,* 556, Article 232486.

Manaf, I. S. A., Embong, N. H., Khazaai, S. N. M., Rahim, M. H. A., Yusoff, M. M., Lee, K. T., & Maniam, G. P. (2019). A review for key challenges of the development of biodiesel industry. *Energy Convers Manag, 185*, 508–517. https://doi.org/10.1016/j.enconman.2019.02.019

Mazumdar, H., Khondakar, K. R., Das, S., Halder, A., & Kaushik, A. (2024). Artificial intelligence for personalized nanomedicine; from material selection to patient outcomes. *Expert Opinion on Drug Delivery, 22*(1), 85–108. https://doi.org/10.1080/17425247.2024.2440618

Mittal, Y., Srivastava, P., Kumar, N., Kumar, M., Singh, S. K., Martinez, F., & Yadav, A. K. (2023). Ultra-fast and low-cost electroactive biochar production for electroactive-constructed wetland applications: A circular concept for plant biomass utilization. *Chemical Engineering Journal, 452*(Part 1), 138587. https://doi.org/10.1016/j.cej.2022.138587.

Naylor, R. L., & Higgins, M. M. (2018). The rise in global biodiesel production: Implications for food security. *Global Food Security, 16*, 75–84. https://doi.org/10.1016/j.gfs.2017.10.004

Nguyen, T. T. V., Phan, A. N., Nguyen, T.-A., Nguyen, T. K., Nguyen, S. T., Pugazhendhi, A., & Phuong, H. H. K. (2022). Valorization of agriculture waste biomass as biochar: As first-rate biosorbent for remediation of contaminated soil. *Chemosphere, 307*(3), Article 135834. https://doi.org/10.1016/j.chemosphere.2022.135834

Nkoh, J. N., Ajibade, F. O., Atakpa, E. O., Abdulaha-Al Baquy, M., Mia, S., Odii, E. C., & Xu, R. (2022). Reduction of heavy metal uptake from polluted soils and associated health risks through biochar amendment: A critical synthesis. *Journal of Hazardous Materials Advances, 6*, Article 100086. https://doi.org/10.1016/j.hazadv.2022.100086

Obileke, K., Onyeaka, H., Meyer, E. L., & Nwokolo, N. (2021). Microbial fuel cells, a renewable energy technology for bio-electricity generation: a mini-review. *Electrochemistry Communications, 125*, Article 107003.

Pahariya, R., Chauhan, A., Ranjan, A., Thakur, S. K., Tuli, H. S., Ramniwas, S., Shahwan, M., & Jindal, T. (2024). Impact of nanoparticles on microalgae and the prospects for biofuel production: Current advancements and future outlook. *Journal of Applied Biology & Biotechnology, 12*(3), 17–25.

Purnama, I., Trisunaryanti, W., Wijaya, K., Mutamima, A., Oh, W.-C., Boukherroub, R., & Aziz, M. (2024). Multi-pathways for sustainable fuel production from biomass using zirconium-based catalysts: A comprehensive review. *Energy Technology, 12*(2), 2300901. https://doi.org/10.1002/ente.202300901

Purnama, I., Mutamima, A., Aziz, M., Wijaya, K., Maulida, I. D., Junaidi, J., Sari, K., Effendi, I., & Dini, I. R. (2025). Environmental impacts and the food vs. fuel debate: A critical review of palm oil as biodiesel. *Global Change Biology Bioenergy, 17*(6), e700043. https://doi.org/10.1111/gcbb.70043.

Qi, D. H., Chen, H., Matthews, R. D., & Bian, Y. Z. (2010). Combustion and emission characteristics of ethanol–biodiesel–water mi-cro-emulsions used in a direct injection compression ignition engine. *Fuel, 89*, 958–964. https://doi.org/10.1016/j.fuel.2009.06.029

Rai, M., Dos Santos, J. C., Soler, M. F., Franco Marcelino, P. R., Brumano, L. P., Ingle, A. P., Gaikwad, S., Gade, A., & Da Silva, S. S. (2016). Strategic role of nanotechnology for production of bioethanol and biodiesel. *Nanotechnology Reviews, 5*, 231–250.

Rathi, E. R. (2009). Nanotechnology: Technology revolution of 21st century. 1st Edn. Vikas Publishing House Private Limited, Plot 2014.

Ricachenevsky, F. K., Vasconcelos, M. W., Shou, H. X., Johnson, A. A. T., & Sperotto, R. A. (2019). Editorial: Improving the nutritional content and quality of crops: Promises, achievements, and future challenges. *Frontiers in Plant Science, 10*, 738.

Sajjad, N., Orfali, R., Perveen, S., Rehman, S., Sultan, A., Akhtar, T., Nazir, A., Muhammad, G., Mehmood, T., Ghaffar, S., Al-Taweel, A., Jilani, M. I., & Iqbal, M. (2022). Biodiesel production from alkali-catalyzed transesterification of tamarindus indica seed oil and optimization of process conditions. *Molecules, 27*(10), 3230. https://doi.org/10.3390/molecules27103230

Sánchez, B. M., Aragón, A. J., Torres, J. C., & Osorio, F. (2022). Purification and upgrading biogas from anaerobic digestion using chemical asborption of CO2 with amines in order to produce biomethane as biofuel for vehicles: A pilot-scale study. *Energy Sources, Part a: Recovery, Utilization, and Environmental Effects, 44*(4), 10201–10213. https://doi.org/10.1080/15567036.2022.2143957

Sarauer, J. L., Page-Dumroese, D. S., & Coleman, M. D. (2019). Soil greenhouse gas, carbon content, and tree growth response to biochar amendment in western United States forests. *GCB Bioenergy, 11*, 660–671. https://doi.org/10.1111/gcbb.12595

Schmidt, H.-P., Kammann, C., Hagemann, N., Leifeld, J., Bucheli, T. D., & Monedero, M. A. S. (2021). Biochar in agriculture–a systematic review of 26 global meta-analyses. *GCB–Bioenergy, 13*(11), 1708–1730. https://doi.org/10.1111/gcbb.12889.

Schulte, P. A., & Salamanca-Buentello, F. (2007). Ethical and scientific issues of nanotechnology in the workplace. *Environmental Health Perspectives, 115*(1), 5–12. https://doi.org/10.1289/ehp.9456. PMID: 17366812.

Shalaby, E.A. (2013). Biofuel: Sources, extraction and determination. In *Liquid, gaseous and solid biofuels—conversion techniques*. InTech. https://doi.org/10.5772/51943.

Sher, F., Ziani, I., Hameed, M., Ali, S., & Sulejmanović, J. (2024). Advanced nanomaterials design and synthesis for accelerating sustainable biofuels production—a review. *Current Opinion in Green and Sustainable Chemistry, 47*, Article 100925. https://doi.org/10.1016/j.cogsc.2024.100925

Sirelkhatim, A., Mahmud, S., Seeni, A., Kaus, N. H. M., Ann, L. C., Bakhori, S. K. M., Hasan, H., & Mohamad, D. (2015). Review on zinc oxide. Nanoparticles: Antibacterial activity and toxicity mechanism. *Nano-Micro Letters, 7*, 219–242. https://doi.org/10.1007/s40820-015-0040-x

Subhan, M. A., & Subhan, T. (2023). Nanomaterial's safety regulations in food and drug industry. In U. Shanker, C. M. Hussain, & M. Rani (Eds.) *Handbook of green and sustainable nanotechnology*. Springer, Cham. https://doi.org/10.1007/978-3-031-16101-8_94.

Takeda, C., Hussain, W., Nakane, D., Ooi, H., & Akitsu, T. (2025). Role of MXenes toward enzymatic biofuel and biofuel cell design. In J. Singh, K. R. Singh, R. Verma, R. P. Singh (Eds.) *MXenes: Expanding the frontiers of energy applications. Clean energy production technologies*. Springer, Singapore. https://doi.org/10.1007/978-981-96-0491-3_4.

Thompson, P. B. (2012). The agricultural ethics of biofuels: The food vs fuel debate. *Agriculture, 2*(4), 339–358. https://doi.org/10.3390/agriculture2040339

Wagh, M. S., Sowjanya, S., Nath, P. C., Chakraborty, A., Amrit, R., Mishra, B., Mishra, A. M., & Mohanta, Y. K. (2024). Valorisation of agro-industrial wastes: Circular bioeconomy and biorefinery process—a sustainable symphony. *Process Safety and Environmental Protection, 183*, 708–725. https://doi.org/10.1016/j.psep.2024.01.055

Wang, Z., Bakshi, S., Li, C., Parikh, S. J., Hsieh, H.-S., & Pignatello, J. J. (2020). Modifcation of pyrogenic carbons for phosphate sorption through binding of a cationic polymer. *Journal of Colloid and Interface Science, 579*, 258–268. https://doi.org/10.1016/j.jcis.2020.06.054

Yang, C., Huang, L., Wang, B-C., Zhong, Y., Ma, X., Zhang, C., Sun, Q., Wu, Y., Yao, Y., & Liu, Q. (2025). Enhancing quality traits in staple crops: current advances and future perspectives. *Journal of Genetics and Genomics*. In press. https://doi.org/10.1016/j.jgg.2025.05.001.

Yin, J., Zhao, L., Xu, X., Li, D., Qiu, H., & Cao, X. (2022). Evaluation of long-term carbon sequestration of biochar in soil with biogeochemical field model. *Science of the Total Environment, 822*, Article 153576. https://doi.org/10.1016/j.scitotenv.2022.153576

Yu, F., Gao, J., Zhang, P., Tang, S., Liu, H., & Li, W. (2025). Distribution, environmental behavior, and ecotoxicity of different metal oxide nanoparticles in the aquatic environment. *Process Safety and Environmental Protection, 196*, Article 106856. https://doi.org/10.1016/j.psep.2025.106856

Zafar, S., & Jianlong, X. (2023). Recent advances to enhance nutritional quality of rice. *Rice Science, 30*(6), 523–536. https://doi.org/10.1016/j.rsci.2023.05.004

Zhang, X., Qu, J., Li, H., La, S., Tian, Y., & Gao, L. (2020a). Biochar addition combined with daily fertigation improves overall soil quality and enhances water-fertilizer productivity of cucumber in alkaline soils of a semi-arid region. *Geoderma, 363*, Article 114170. https://doi.org/10.1016/j.geoderma.2019.114170

Zhang, M., Song, G., Gelardi, D. L., Huang, L., Khan, E., Mašek, O., Parikh, S. J., & Ok, Y. S. (2020b). Evaluating biochar and its modifications for the removal of ammonium, nitrate, and phosphate in water. *Water Research, 186*, Article 116303. https://doi.org/10.1016/J.WATRES.2020.116303

Zhang, M., Zhang, L., Riaz, M., Xia, H., & Jiang, C. (2021). Biochar amendment improved fruit quality and soil properties and microbial communities at different depths in citrus production. *Journal of Cleaner Production, 292*, Article 126062. https://doi.org/10.1016/j.jclepro.2021.126062

Zhao, X., Zhang, J., Lv, K., Kong, N., Shao, Y., & Tao, J. (2022). Carbon nanotubes boosts the toughness and conductivity of wet-spun MXene fibers for fiber-shaped super capacitors. *Carbon, 200*, 38–46. https://doi.org/10.1016/j.carbon.2022.08.045

Zhou, Y., Qin, S., Verma, S., Sar, T., Sarsaiya, S., Ravindran, B., et al. (2021). Production and beneficial impact of biochar for environmental application: A comprehensive review. *Bioresource Technology, 337*, Article 125451. https://doi.org/10.1016/j.biortech.2021.125451

Zúñiga-Miranda, J., Guerra, J., Mueller, A., Mayorga-Ramos, A., Carrera-Pacheco, S. E., Barba-Ostria, C., Heredia-Moya, J., & Guamán, L. P. (2023). Iron oxide nanoparticles: Green synthesis and their antimicrobial activity. *Nanomaterials (Basel), 13*(22), 2919. https://doi.org/10.3390/nano13222919

Chapter 13
Production of Enzymes and Citric Acid by Fungi Using Cereal and Fruit Wastes: A Circular Bioeconomy Concept

Kodandoor Sharathchandra, Edayilam Anjana, and Kandikere Ramaiah Sridhar

Abstract Solid-substrate fermentation (SSF) was followed to produce extracellular enzymes and citric acid from cereal and fruit wastes using two filamentous fungi (*Aspergillus niger* and *Neurospora crassa*). The SSF was followed by two nutrient compositions of substrates. The first composition consists of two cereal flours (barley flour and wheat bran) and two fruit wastes (seed powder of clustered apple, *Annona reticulata*, and shell powder of groundnut, *Arachis hypogaea*) with sucrose and mineral solutions. The second composition consists of two cereal flours (semolina and ragi powder, *Eleusine coracana*) and two fruit wastes (seed powder of sapota, *Manilkara zapota*, and shell powder of pista, *Pistacia vera*) with sucrose and mineral solutions. Both compositions were assessed for production of enzymes (amylase, cellulase, maltase, pectinase, and xylanase) and citric acid by SSF up to 7 days. In both compositions, *A. niger* exhibited significantly high production of cellulase, pectinase, and xylanase, whereas *N. crassa* demonstrated significantly high production of maltase. Overall, in composition 2, production of all enzymes by both fungi was significantly higher than in composition 1. In the first composition, *N. crassa* produced a significantly higher quantity of citric acid than *A. niger*, while it was the opposite in the second composition. In composition 2, *A. niger* formed the highest amount of citric acid, while *N. crassa* produced almost equal quantities of citric acid in both compositions. Previous studies have discussed the application of agricultural wastes in the production of enzymes and citric acid by SSF.

Keywords Agricultural residues · *Aspergillus niger* · Cereal flours · *Neurospora crassa* · Seeds · Solid-substrate fermentation

---

K. Sharathchandra · E. Anjana · K. R. Sridhar (✉)
Department of Biosciences, Mangalore University, Mangalagangotri, Mangalore, Karnataka, India
e-mail: kandikeremanasa@gmail.com

K. R. Sridhar
Central Research Laboratory, NITTE (Deemed to be University), KS Hegde Medical Academy (KSHEMA), Mangalore, Karnataka, India

P. Verma (ed.), *Sustainable Practices in Biorefinery*,
https://doi.org/10.1007/978-981-95-6071-4_13

13.1 Introduction

Solid-substrate fermentation (SSF) is a method in which microbes grow with meagre or very low availability of water. The significance of SSF for mankind dates back several centuries, especially for food processing in the Western region (e.g., bread and cheese) and Eastern region (e.g., koji). Based on the progress in the last century and in recent times, it has become a powerful technology to produce versatile biomolecules and value-added products necessary for many industries (e.g., biochemical, bioenergy, food, pharmaceutical, and textile) (Martins et al., 2011; Pandey, 2003; Soccol & Vandenberghe, 2003; Thomas et al., 2013). As the SSF mimics the natural habitat (mainly fungi and molds), it has become eco-friendly as it demands less energy for sterilization, has a low risk of microbial contamination, has an increased yield, has increased recovery, and has low waste production compared to submerged fermentation (SmF) (De Castro & Sato, 2015). Other advantages include the production of higher-quality products, lesser use of organic solvents, lower operating costs, and reduced downstream processing (Martins et al., 2011; Singhania et al., 2009).

Agricultural residues as useful resources with large surface area, more porosity, and size of particle serve as important feedstock for SSF (Bringezu & Bleischwitz, 2009; Farinas, 2015; Ravindran et al., 2016; Savino et al., 2021). Currently, SSF is attracting new interest because agricultural residues have a wide range of applications in valorizing unexploited biomass (Thomas et al., 2013; Sadh et al., 2018). Enzyme production by SSF using agricultural wastes is lucrative, as it supports fungal growth and production of enzymes (Kumar & Kanwar, 2012; Thomas et al., 2013). In recent times, SSF is extensively employed in the fermentation industries, especially for the production of enzymes (Pandey et al., 1999). Thus, the SSF is of specific interest for countries producing abundant biomass of agro-industrial wastes, as these serve as inexpensive feedstock (Gombert et al., 1999; De la Cruz Quiroz et al., 2015). Besides, the SSF has several advantages over submerged fermentation (SmF) concerning biomolecule production, especially enzymes and others (Panda et al., 2016).

Agricultural residues commonly employed for SSF include straws of different origins, corn cobs, husks, cereal brans (oat, rice, soybean, and wheat), peels (coffee and fruits), pulps (coffee and fruits), and bagasse (cassava and sugarcane). These substrates consist of lignin, cellulose, hemicellulose, starch, pectin, and fibers (Farinas, 2015; Ray et al., 2024; Singhania et al., 2009; Soccol & Vandenberghe, 2003; Suminto et al., 2024). There are several studies concerning the use of sawdust for enzyme production (Devi & Kumar, 2012; Victor et al., 2003). In this context, cereal husk (finger millet) appears as an ideal substrate for microbial fermentation due to its low cost, easy availability, and richness in organic content (Ishchi & Sibi, 2019). Application of filamentous fungi and yeasts in developing SSF is advantageous since this method is comparable to natural habitats. They are capable to producing substantial quantities of enzymes and other value-added metabolites (Farinas, 2015). White-rot fungi are known to selectively degrade lignin, while brown-rot fungi degrade cellulose and hemicellulose (Yoon et al., 2014). Macro- and micronutrients are supplied with the medium to support the fungal growth (Farinas, 2015; Pandey, 2003; Soccol & Vandenberghe, 2003).

Show et al., (2015) and Varriale et al., (2025) reported that citric acid has economic potential due to its several applications (e.g., beverages, pharmaceuticals, and cosmetics). Its waste utilization aligns with principles of the circular economy, as it reduces the impact on the environment and produces useful bioproducts for industries like biofuel, food, pharmaceuticals, and textiles (Lima et al., 2025). It is produced by fermentation by *A. niger* (Varriale et al., 2025). West (2023) reported that the level of citric acid production by *A. niger* depends on the sugar content of fruit waste. Adeoye et al. (2015), in their study, used UV radiation for mutation and optimization of medium to improve citric acid production through the screening of five indigenous strains of *A. niger* using the feedstock of hydrolyzed cassava peel medium. Citric acid production by the mutant strains of *A. niger* optimized the physicochemical parameters by the Central Composite Design (CCD) of the Response Surface Methodology (RSM).

Currently, one of the key themes in sustainable development is the need for suitable waste utilization and management (UNEP, 2011; UNHSP, 2010). The amount of waste production was estimated to be up to 25–30% of the total raw resources produced per year from the industries using fruits, roots, tubers, and vegetables (Wadhwa & Bakshi, 2013). Such wastes, mainly composed of pomace, rinds, seeds, and skins, are often rejected as byproducts. Application of SSF for the production of industrially valued enzymes using different combinations of some agrowastes of some cereals and fruit wastes is limited. Thus, the present study was undertaken to produce enzymes and citric acid using selected cereals, cereal brans, and fruit wastes by *Aspergillus niger* and *Neurospora crassa* through SSF.

13.2 Substrates and Fungal Strains

To follow SSF, two compositions of nutrients were used along with a control to assess enzymes (Table 13.1). Schematic experimental design is presented in Fig. 13.1. Chemicals used were of analytical grade purchased from SRL, India, while PDA (potato dextrose agar) was from Hi-Media, India. Composition 1 consists of wheat bran, barley flour, and fruit waste (custard apple seed and groundnut shell powders) with sucrose and mineral solution in 250 ml Erlenmeyer flasks to inoculate fungal strains. Composition 2 consists of semolina, ragi flour, and fruit waste (sapota seed powder and pista shell powder) with sucrose and mineral solution in 250 ml Erlenmeyer flasks to inoculate fungal strains. The same compositions were used for citric acid estimation except for sucrose solution to inoculate fungal strains. Control also has the same nutrient composition in 250 ml Erlenmeyer flasks without inoculation of fungal strains. Triplicates were maintained for control to assay enzymes and citric acid. Flasks with nutrients were autoclaved and cooled to inoculate fungi. Wheat bran, barley flour, ragi flour, semolina, and fruit wastes were dried at 60 °C until attaining constant dry mass. They were mixed in desired quantities and mixed.

Table 13.1 Nutrient composition for production of enzymes and citric acid (*mineral solution: $CuSO_4.5H_2O$, 7 mg; $FeSO_4.7H_2O$, 7 mg; $ZnSO_4.7H_2O$, 7 mg; 0.2 N HCl, 100 ml; pH 5)

Media compositions	Enzymes	Citric acid
Composition 1		
Wheat bran (g)	2	2
Barley flour (g)	2	2
Custard apple seed powder (g)	1	1
Groundnut shell powder (g)	1	1
Sucrose solution 25% (ml)	0	2
Mineral solution (ml)*	2	2
Composition 2		
Shredded wheat (semolina) (g)	2	2
Ragi flour (g)	1	1
Sapota seed powder (g)	1	1
Pista shell powder (g)	2	2
Sucrose solution 25% (ml)	0	2
Mineral solution (ml)*	2	2

Alternate mixed replicate samples without sucrose or mineral solution were dried at 60 °C to find out the dry mass to express enzymes and citric acid.

Aspergillus niger (MTCC-281) and *Neurospora crassa* (MTCC-260) were procured from the Institute of Microbial Technology, Chandigarh, India. They were cultivated on the PDA (Potato Dextrose Agar) medium, which was used for SSF. From a one-week-old culture, spore suspension was prepared by transferring it into the sterile distilled water with a sterilized loop. Culture suspension (0.5 ml; ~ 400–500 spores/ml) in sterile phosphate buffered saline (PBS) was inoculated into autoclaved flasks with nutrients, which were used for enzyme and citric acid production. The control set has been maintained without fungal inoculation. Inoculated flasks with nutrients and control flasks were incubated at laboratory temperature (27 ± 2 °C) under stationary conditions in the dark for up to 7 days.

13.3 Enzyme and Citric Acid Assays

Enzymes from the fermented materials were extracted by addition of distilled water (50 ml) to each flask, kept under agitation (150 rpm, 1 h), filtered (Whatman # 1), and centrifuged (3000 g, 10 min, 25 °C). The supernatant was used for the enzyme assay. The amount of enzyme necessary to release 1 μM of the respective reducing sugars per minute has been considered as one unit of enzyme activity.

Enzymes were harvested by sodium citrate buffer (20 ml, 50 mM, pH 5.3). The slurry was centrifuged (5000 × g, 10 min, 4 °C). To assess the quantitative difference

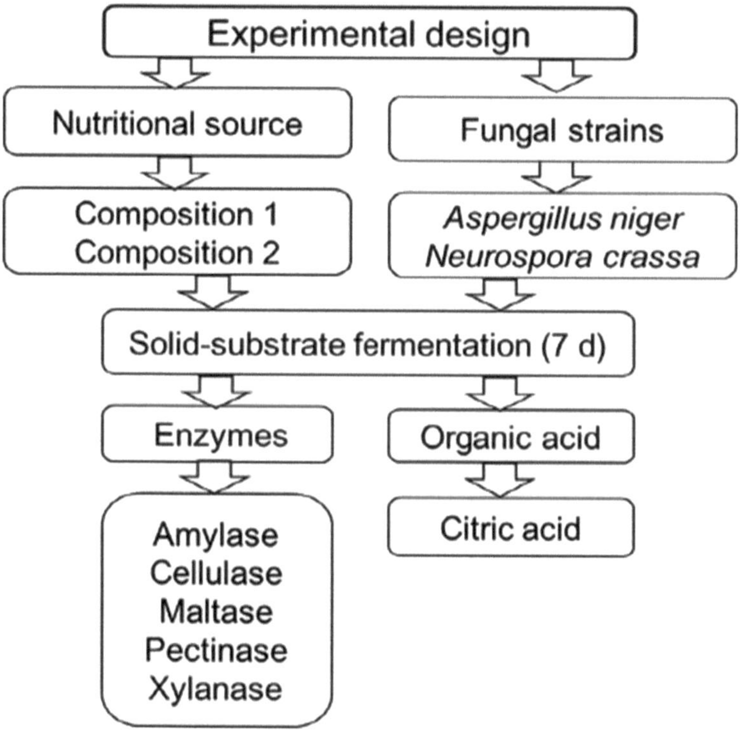

Fig. 13.1 Overview of the production of extracellular enzymes and citric acid by solid-substrate fermentation

in production of enzymes by *A. niger* and *N. crassa*, a paired *t*-test was followed (StatSoft Inc., 2008).

13.3.1 Amylase

The assay of α-amylase (EC 3.2.1.1) was by addition of enzyme extract (0.1 ml) to sodium acetate buffer (0.1 M, 0.9 ml, pH 5.0, along with 1% cornstarch). After the reaction (10 min, 50 °C), the released reducing sugar was assessed by the DNS (3,5-dinitrosalicilic acid) technique (Miller, 1959). The quantity of reducing sugar released was quantified by a glucose standard curve.

13.3.2 Cellulase

The cellulase (EC 3.2.1.4) was measured by mixing CMC (0.9 ml, 1% w/v) in Na-citrate buffer (50 mM, pH 5.3) with dilute enzyme extract (0.1 ml) and incubation (50 °C for 15 min) (Ghose, 1987). The enzyme action was terminated by the addition of DNS (1.5 ml), followed by boiling the mixture (5 min). The color was read at 540 nm, and the quantity of reducing sugar was estimated by a glucose standard curve.

13.3.3 Maltase

The activity of maltase (α-glucosidase) (EC 3.2.1.20) was determined by measurement of the production of reducing sugars using 3,5-dinitrosalicylic acid (DNSA) (Miller, 1959), after the enzymatic action of maltase on maltose by the glucose oxidase method (Trinder, 1969). The enzyme action was determined by the addition of enzyme extract (0.2 ml) to maltose solution (5.0 mM, 0.8 ml) in buffer (potassium phosphate 100 mM, pH 6.5). After the reaction (10 min, 50 °C), the reducing sugar was assessed by the DNS method and boiled (5 min) in a water bath. The color was read at 540 nm, and the quantity of reducing sugar was measured by a glucose standard curve.

13.3.4 Pectinase

The pectinase (endo-polygalacturonase) (EC 3.2.1.15) was assessed by pectin as a substrate. The enzyme extract (0.2 ml) with pectin solution (1% citric pectin, 0.8 ml in 0.1 M citric buffer, pH 5) was incubated (50 °C, 20 min); the reaction was stopped by addition of DNS reagent (1.5 ml) (Wang et al., 1997). The absorbance was measured at 540 nm. The color was read at 540 nm, and the quantity of reducing sugar was estimated by a galacturonic acid standard curve.

13.3.5 Xylanase

Xylanase or hemicellulase (endo-1,4-β-xylanase) (EC 3.2.1.8) was assessed by mixing birch wood xylan [0.9 ml, 1% (w/v) in 50 mM Na-citrate buffer, pH 5.3] along with diluted enzyme (0.1 ml) and incubating (50 °C, 5 min) (Bailey et al., 1992). The reaction was stopped by the addition of DNS (1.5 ml), followed by boiling (5 min) (Miller, 1959). After cooling, the color formed was read at 540 nm. The extent of released reducing sugar was estimated using a xylose standard curve.

13.3.6 Citric Acid

Fermented stuff was oven-dried (45 ± 2 °C), cooled, and citric acid was extracted on addition of distilled water (100 ml). On agitating the mixture on a rotary shaker for 2 h, it was filtered through Whatman # 1 filter paper. Citric acid was estimated in the supernatant.

To estimate by the titration method, the supernatant (10 ml) was transferred into a conical flask. Indicator (phenolphthalein, 2 – 3 drops) was added and titrated (against 0.1 N NaOH) till attaining a pink color (Chetan et al., 2018). The change from colorless to pink showed the presence of citric acid, and its quantity was estimated.

$$\text{Citric acid (\%)} = \frac{\text{Normality} \times \text{Volume of NaOH} \times \text{Equivalent weight of citric acid}}{\text{Volume of extract} \times 10}$$

For the confirmatory test, 2 ml of extract, 1 drop of dilute NH_4OH, and silver nitrate solution were mixed and boiled up to 15 min. A blackish silver mirror denotes the presence of citric acid. To assess the quantitative difference in production of citric acid by *A. niger* and *N. crassa*, a paired *t*-test was followed (StatSoft Inc., 2008).

13.4 Observations and Discussion

13.4.1 Enzymes

Fungi produce large quantities of extracellular enzymes, which are involved in digesting insoluble polymers such as cellulose, proteins, and starch. Several enzymes could be produced by the SSF at pilot and industrial scales (Rodríguez Couto, 2018; He & Chen, 2013).

In our study, production of fungal enzymes by SSF in composition 1 reveals a significantly higher quantity of pectinase produced by both fungi, followed by production of cellulase (Fig. 13.2). Production of amylase ($p < 0.05$), cellulase ($p < 0.001$), and xylanase ($p < 0.01$) was significantly higher in *A. niger* than in *N. crassa*, while it was the reverse for maltase ($p < 0.01$). In composition 2, *A. niger* produced the highest amount of pectinase, followed by cellulase (Fig. 13.2). Production of pectinase ($p < 0.001$), cellulase ($p < 0.01$), and xylanase ($p < 0.01$) was higher in *A. niger* than *N. crassa*, while it was the reverse for amylase ($p < 0.001$) and maltase ($p < 0.05$). Overall, in composition 2, production of all enzymes by both fungi was significantly higher than in composition 1. In both compositions, *A. niger* served as a good producer of cellulase, pectinase, and xylanase, while *N. crassa* served as a good producer of maltase.

Amylase production by *A. niger* under SSF using potato peels was studied by Mukherjee et al. (2019), and they found enhanced enzyme at initial pH 3. According

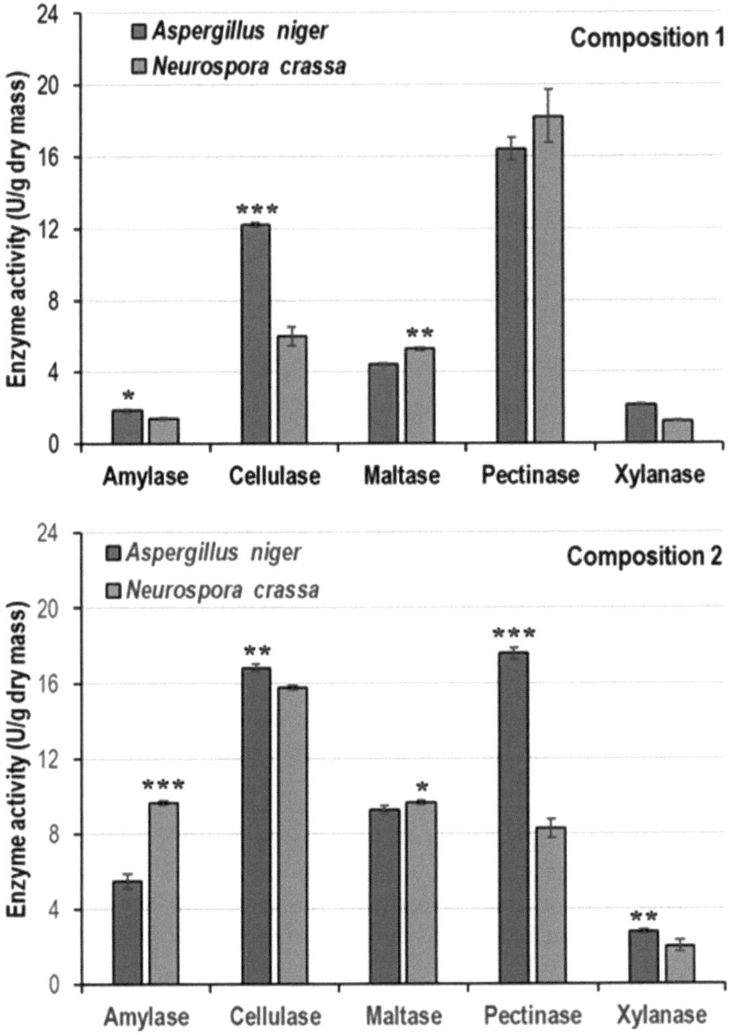

Fig. 13.2 Impact of different compositions of substrates on production of extracellular enzymes by *A. niger* and *N. crassa* by solid-substrate fermentation (n = 3, mean ± SD; *, $p < 0.05$; **, $p < 0.01$; ***, $p < 0.001$)

to Chakraborty et al. (2022), the optimum parameters necessary for maximum amylase enzyme by *A. niger* are a pH of 6.5 at 40 °C and a duration of incubation of 96 h in molasses medium. Our study revealed significantly higher production of amylase in composition 2 by *A. niger* as well as *N. crassa.*

Studies of cellulase production are of critical importance owing to the significance of the economics of biomass bioconversion into biofuels and other chemicals (Klein-Marcuschamer et al., 2012). Most commercial cellulases are produced by *Aspergillus* and *Trichoderma* (Agrawal et al., 2023; Bhat, 2000; Gusakov, 2011). Among them, *A. niger*, along with *A. oryzae*, is widely used for biotechnological applications (Hu et al., 2011). Our study revealed consistently higher production of cellulase in both compositions, with the highest in composition 2.

Performance of *A. niger* showed optimum conditions of pH 4.3 and a temperature of 80 °C (stable at 40 °C) for maltase production (del Moral et al., 2018). In our study, maltase production was higher in composition 2 by *A. niger* and *N. crassa*; however, in both compositions, *N. crassa* showed significantly higher production.

Pectin methyl esterase and endo-polygalacturonase have important roles in fruit industries, especially in clarifying juices, preparing gels, retting textile fibers, extracting olive oil, and also isolating protoplasts (Kashyap et al., 2001; Jayani et al., 2005; Kohli & Gupta, 2015). *A. niger* is a major producer of acidic pectinase, and it will be used by the fruit and wine industries (Kashyap et al., 2001). Our study showed production of pectinase was the highest in both compositions by A. niger, while N. crassa showed the highest production in composition 1.

Fungal xylanases are useful in animal feeds, for food processing, and in textile industries and the production of value-added products (e.g., xylitol and ethanol) (Salles et al., 2005; Bhardwaj et al., 2019). Use of xylanase in the pulp and paper industry is ecofriendly, as it reduces the usage of chlorine and chlorine dioxide. In our study, xylanase production was higher by A. niger in both compositions.

13.4.2 Citric Acid

Citric acid production varied between composition 1 and 2 with fungal inoculation (Fig. 13.3). Composition 1 was favorable for *N. crassa* to produce significantly higher production ($p < 0.05$) of citric acid, while composition 2 was favorable for *A. niger* ($p < 0.001$). Overall composition 2 favored the highest citric acid production by *A. niger*, while *N. crassa* produced almost equal quantities of citric acid in both compositions.

There is huge demand for citric acid owing to its production by low-cost substrates by fermentation (Verma, 2012; Chetan et al., 2018; West, 2023). In addition, extraction of citric acid is not an expensive process, as it is water soluble and pretreatment is not required (Chetan et al., 2018). As the most common organism is *A. niger*, our study revealed the highest citric acid production in composition 2.

13.5 Conclusion

Solid-substrate fermentation is an alternative technique beneficial for utilizing agroindustrial wastes without major processing for the production of value-added products (e.g., antibiotics, enzymes, and organic acids). The current pilot study showed production of extracellular enzymes by fungal strains *Aspergillus niger* and

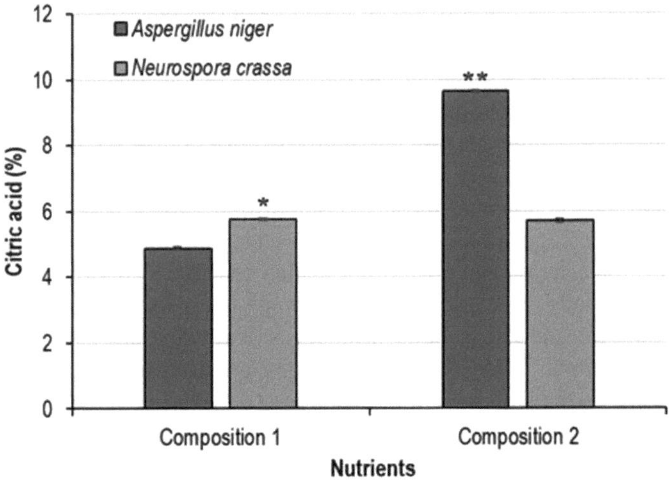

Fig. 13.3 Impact of different compositions of substrates on production of citric acid by *A. niger* and *N. crassa* by solid-substrate fermentation (n = 3, mean ± SD; *, $p < 0.05$; **, $p < 0.01$)

Neurospora crassa using cereal products and fruit wastes is useful. Among the two nutrient compositions that were offered, both compositions resulted in the highest production of pectinase by *A. niger*, followed by cellulase. *N. crassa* produced pectinase and cellulase in compositions 1 and 2, respectively. Overall, composition 2 was better than composition 1 in the production of amylase, cellulase, maltase, pectinase, and xylanase. Similar to enzyme production, composition 2 favored citric acid production by *A. niger*. This study showed that cereal and fruit wastes could be used to generate enzymes and citric acid. Further investigation is necessary for improved production of extracellular enzymes and citric acid with different pH, temperature, incubation duration, and nutrient composition. It may be advantageous to study dual inoculation or co-cultivation of *A. niger* and *N. crassa*, especially for composition 2, for enhanced production of enzymes and organic acids.

Acknowledgements The authors are indebted to the Department of Biosciences and Mangalore University for logistic support to carry out this study. We are grateful to Dr. S. Mahadevakumar, Scientist, Botanical Survey of India, Port Blair, Andamans, for constructive comments and technical support.

References

Adeoye, A. O., Lateef, A., & Gueguim-Kana, E. B. (2015). Optimization of citric acid production using a mutant strain of *Aspergillus niger* on cassava peel substrate. *Biocat Agric Biotechnol, 4*, 568–574. https://doi.org/10.1016/j.bcab.2015.08.004

Agrawal, K., Nair, L. G., Chaturvedi, V., & Verma, P. (2023). Designing microbial cellulases using genetic engineering approach: A promising strategy towards zero-waste cellulosic biorefinery. *Biocat Agric Biotechnol, 52*, Article 102830. https://doi.org/10.1016/j.bcab.2023.102830

Bhardwaj, N., Kumar, B., & Verma, P. (2019). A detailed overview of xylanases: an emerging biomolecule for current and future prospective. *Bioresour Bioprocess, 6*(1). https://doi.org/10.1186/s40643-019-0276-2

Bhat, M. K. (2000). Research review paper: Cellulases and related enzymes in biotechnology. *Biotechnology Advances, 18*, 355–383. https://doi.org/10.1016/S0734-9750(00)00041-0

Bringezu, S., & Bleischwitz, R. (2009). Sustainable resource management: Global trends, visions and policies. *Taylor & Francis, New York, USA*. https://doi.org/10.4324/9781351279284

Chakraborty, M. B., Patgiri, S. R., Sarma, M., & Upadhyaya, H. (2022). Optimizing physical parameters for amylase production using *Aspergillus niger* and ammonium molasses medium. In A. C. Shukla (Ed.), *Applied mycology*, pp 259−269. Springer Cham. https://doi.org/10.1007/978-3-030-90649-8_12

Chetan, D. M., Sarang, S. F., Nithin, N., Priyanka, N., & Bhat, R. S. (2018). Comparison of citric acid production from *Aspergillus niger* in solid and suspension state fermentation. *International Journal of Green Pharmacy, 12*, 502–509.

De Castro, R. J. S., & Sato, H. H. (2015). Enzyme production by solid state fermentation: General aspects and an analysis of the physicochemical characteristics of substrates for agro-industrial wastes valorization. *Waste Biomass Valor, 6*, 1085–1093. https://doi.org/10.1007/s12649-015-9396-x

De la Cruz, Q. R., Roussos, S., Hernández, D., Rodríguez, R., Castillo, F., & Aguilar, C. N. (2015). Challenges and opportunities of the bio-pesticides production by solid-state fermentation: Filamentous fungi as a model. *Critical Reviews in Biotechnology, 35*, 326–333. https://doi.org/10.3109/07388551.2013.857292

del Moral, S., Barradas-Dermitz, D. M., & Aguilar-Uscanga, M. G. (2018). Production and biochemical characterization of α-glucosidase from *Aspergillus niger* ITV-01 isolated from sugar cane bagasse. 3 *Biotech, 8*(7). https://doi.org/10.1007/s13205-017-1029-6

Devi, M. C., & Kumar, M. S. (2012). Isolation and screening of lignocellulose hydrolytic saprophytic fungi from dairy manure soil. *Annals of Biological Research, 3*, 1145–1152.

Farinas, C. S. (2015). Developments in solid-state fermentation for the production of biomass-degrading enzymes for the bioenergy sector.*Renewable and Sustainable Energy Reviews, 52*, 179–188. https://doi.org/10.1016/j.rser.2015.07.092

Ghose, T. K. (1987). Measurement of cellulase activities. *Pure and Applied Chemistry, 59*, 257–268. https://doi.org/10.1351/pac198759020257

Gombert, A. K., Pinto, A. L., Castilho, L. R., & Freire, D. M. (1999). Lipase production by *Penicillium restrictum* in solid-state fermentation using babassu oil cake as substrate. *Process Biochemistry, 35*, 85–90. https://doi.org/10.1016/s0032-9592(99)00036-9

Gusakov, A. V. (2011). Alternatives to *Trichoderma reesei* in biofuel production. *Tr Biotechnol, 29*(9), 419–425. https://doi.org/10.1016/j.tibtech.2011.04.004

He, F.-J., & Chen, J.-Q. (2013). Consumption of soybean, soy foods, soy isoflavones and breast cancer incidence: Differences between Chinese women and women in Western countries and possible mechanisms. *Food Science and Human Wellness, 2*(3–4), 146–161. https://doi.org/10.1016/j.fshw.2013.08.002

Hu, J., van den Brink, J., Gruben, B. S., Wösten, H. A. B., Gu, J.-D., & de Vries, R. P. (2011). Improved enzyme production by co-cultivation of *Aspergillus niger* and *Aspergillus oryzae* and with other fungi. *International Biodeterioration & Biodegradation, 65*(1), 248–252. https://doi.org/10.1016/j.ibiod.2010.11.008

Ishchi, T., & Sibi, G. (2019). Husk as substrate for cellulase production under temperature mediated solid state fermentation by *Streptomyces* sp. *American Journal of BioScience, 7*:77−81. https://doi.org/10.11648/j.ajbio.20190704.11

Jayani, R. S., Saxena, S., & Gupta, R. (2005). Microbial pectinolytic enzymes: A review. *Proc Biochem, 40*, 2931–2944. https://doi.org/10.1016/j.procbio.2005.03.026

Kashyap, D. R., Vohra, P. K., Chopra, S. M., & Tewari, R. (2001). Applications of pectinases in the commercial sector: A review. *Bioresource Technology, 77*, 215–227. https://doi.org/10.1016/S0960-8524(00)00118-8

Klein-Marcuschamer, D., Oleskowicz-Popiel, P., Simmons, B. A., & Blanch, H. W. (2012). The challenge of enzyme cost in the production of lignocellulosic biofuels. *Biotechnology and Bioengineering, 109*(4), 1083–1087. https://doi.org/10.1002/bit.24370

Kohli, P., Kalia, M., & Gupta, R. (2015). Pectin methylesterases: A review. *I Bioprocess Biotech, 5*(5), 1000227. https://doi.org/10.4172/2155-9821.100022

Kumar, A., & Kanwar, S. S. (2012). Lipase production in solid-state fermentation (SSF): recent developments and biotechnological applications. *Proceedings in Biotechnology & Molecular Biology 6*, 13–27

Lima, C. A., Contato, A. G., de Oliveira, F., da Silva, S. S., Hidalgo, V. B., et al. (2025). Trends in enzyme production from citrus by-products. *Processes, 13*, 766. https://doi.org/10.3390/pr13030766

Martins, S., Mussatto, S. I., Martínez-Avila, G., Montañez-Saenz, J., Aguilar, C. N., & Teixeira, J. A. (2011). Bioactive phenolic compounds: Production and extraction by solid-state fermentation. *A Review. Biotechnol Adv, 29*(3), 365–373. https://doi.org/10.1016/j.biotechadv.2011.01.008

Miller, G. L. (1959). Use of dinitrosalicylic acid reagent for determination of reducing sugar. *Analytical Chemistry, 31*(3), 420–428. https://doi.org/10.1021/ac60147a030

Mukherjee, R., Paul, T., Soren, J. P., Haldar, S. K., Mondal, K. C. et al. (2019). Acidophilic α-amylase production from *Aspergillus niger* rbp7 using potato peel as substrate: A waste to value added approach. *Waste and Biomass Valorization, 10*, 851–863. https://doi.org/10.1007/s12649-017-0114-8

Panda, S. K., Mishra, S. S., Kayitesi, E., & Ray, R. C. (2016). Microbial-processing of fruit and vegetable wastes for production of vital enzymes and organic acids: Biotechnology and scopes. *Environmental Research, 146*, 161–172. https://doi.org/10.1016/j.envres.2015.12.035

Pandey, A. (2003). Solid-state fermentation. *Biochemical Engineering Journal, 13*, 81–84. https://doi.org/10.1016/S1369-703X(02)00121-3

Pandey, A., Selvakumar, P., Soccol, C. R., & Poonam, N. (1999). Solid state fermentation for the production of industrial enzymes. *Current Science, 77*, 149–162.

Ravindran, R., & Jaiswal, A. K. (2016). Exploitation of food industry waste for high-value products. *Trends in Biotechnology, 34*, 58–69. https://doi.org/10.1016/j.tibtech.2015.10.008

Ray, R. C., Behera, S. S., Awogbemi, O., Sooch, B. S., Thatoi, H., et al. (2024). Beyond enzymes and organic acids, solid-state fermentation as an alternative for valorizing fruits and vegetable wastes into novel bio-products in a circular economy: A critical review. *AIMS Microbiology, 11*(2), 462–500. https://doi.org/10.3934/microbiol.2025021

Rodríguez-Couto, S. (2008). Exploitation of biological wastes for the production of value-added products under solid-state fermentation conditions. *Biotechnology Journal, 3*, 859–870. https://doi.org/10.1002/biot.200800031

Sadh, P. K., Duhan, S., & Duhan, J. S. (2018). Agro-industrial wastes and their utilization using solid state fermentation: A review. *Bioresources and Bioprocessing, 5*, 1. https://doi.org/10.1186/s40643-017-0187-z

Salles, B. C., Medeiros, R. G., Bao, S. N., Silva Jr. F. G., & Filho, E. X. F. (2005). Effect of cellulase-free xylanases from Acrophialophora nainiana and Humicola grisea var. thermoidea on eucalyptus kraft pulp. *Process Biochemistry, 40*(1), 343–349. https://doi.org/10.1016/j.procbio.2004.01.008

Savino, S., Bulgari, D., Monti, E., & Gobbi, E. (2021). Agro-industrial wastes: A substrate for multi-enzymes production by *Cryphonectria parasitica. Fermentation, 7*, 279. https://doi.org/10.3390/fermentation7040279

Show, P. L., Oladele, K. O., Siew, Q. Y., Zakry, F. A. A., Lan, J.C.-W., & Ling, T. C. (2015). Overview of citric acid production from *Aspergillus niger*. *Frontiers in Life Science, 8*(3), 271–283. https://doi.org/10.1080/21553769.2015.1033653

Singhania, R. R., Sukumaran, R. K., Patel, A. K., Larroche, C., & Pandey, A. (2009). Advancement and comparative profiles in the production technologies using solid-state and submerged fermentation for microbial cellulases. *Enzyme and Microbial Technology, 46*, 541–549. https://doi.org/10.1016/j.enzmictec.2010.03.010

Soccol, C. R., & Vandenberghe, L. P. S. (2003). Overview of solid-state fermentation in Brazil. *Biochemical Engineering Journal, 13*, 205–218. https://doi.org/10.1016/S1369-703X(02)00133-X

StatSoft Inc. (2008). Statistica Version # 8. Tulsa, Oklahoma, USA

Suminto, S., Huang, A. A., Hasanth, U., & Murcholis, W. (2024). Optimizing solid-state fermentation for metabolite enrichment by *Aspergillus tamarii* on rice bran and wheat. *Journal of Applied Biology and Biotechnology, 12*(4), 195−202. https://doi.org/10.7324/JABB.2024.179836

Thomas, L., Larroche, C., & Pandey, A. (2013). Current developments in solid-state fermentation. *Biochemical Engineering Journal, 81*, 146–161. https://doi.org/10.1016/j.bej.2013.10.013

Trinder, P. (1969). Determination of blood glucose using an oxidase-peroxidase system with a non-carcinogenic chromogen. *Journal of Clinical Pathology, 22*(2), 158–161. https://doi.org/10.1136/jcp.22.2.158

UNEP (United Nations Environmental Programme). (2011). Recycling rates of metals: A status report. International Resource Panel, p. 45

UNHSP. (2010). *United Nations Human Settlements Programme*. Global Report on Human Settlements. London and Starling, VA, Earthscan Publications.

Varriale, L., Kuka, K., Tippkötter, N., Olsson, L., & Ulber, R. (2025). Development of a consolidated bioprocess for the production of citric acid using *Aspergillus niger* as biocatalyst. *Biofuels, Bioproducts and Biorefining, 19*(6), 1622–1630. https://doi.org/10.1002/bbb.2758

Verma, M. (2012). Bioproduction and extraction optimization of citric acid from *Aspergillus niger* by rotating drum type solid-state bioreactor. *Industrial Crops and Products, 41*(1), 78–84. https://doi.org/10.1016/j.indcrop.2012.04.001

Victor, O. T., Solomon, B., Betiku, E., Layokun, S. K., & Amigun, B. (2003). Cellulase production by *Aspergillus flavus* Linn isolate NSPR 101 fermented in saw dust, bagasse and corn cob. *African Journal of Biotechnology, 2*, 150–152.

Wadhwa, M., & Bakshi, M. P. S. (2013). Fruit and vegetable wastes can be used as livestock feed and substrates to generate other value-added products. FAO. http://www.fao.org/docrep/018/i3273e/i3273e.pdf

Wang, G., Michailides, T. J., & Bostock, R. M. (1997). Improved detection of polygalacturonase activity due to *Mucor piriformis* with a modified dinitrosalicylic acid reagent. *Phytopathol, 87*, 161–163. https://doi.org/10.1094/PHYTO.1997.87.2.161

West, T. P. (2023). Citric acid production by *Aspergillus niger* using solid-state fermentation of agricultural processing coproducts. *Applied Biosciences, 2*, 1–13 https://doi.org/10.3390/applbiosci2010001

Yoon, L. W., Ang, T. N., Ngoh, G. C., & Chua, A. S. M. (2014). Fungal solid-state fermentation and various methods of enhancement in cellulase production. *Biomass and Bioenergy, 67*, 319–338. https://doi.org/10.1016/j.biombioe.2014.05.013

Chapter 14
Energy Efficiency in Bioenergy Production: Strategies and Innovations

Kandasamy Gajendiran, N. Mathiyazhagan, and D. Natarajan

Abstract Energy efficiency is crucial in assessing the sustainability and economic feasibility of bioenergy generating systems. With the escalation of global energy demands and the intensification of environmental concerns, the optimization of energy utilization in bioenergy processes has become imperative. This chapter examines essential strategies and recent advancements designed to improve energy efficiency throughout the several phases of bioenergy production, encompassing feedstock selection, conversion, and post-treatment. An extensive examination of bioenergy conversion routes, encompassing thermochemical and biochemical techniques, establishes the basis for comprehending energy dynamics within these systems. The chapter explores methodologies like process integration, heat and energy recovery, and co-generation, which markedly diminish energy losses and enhance overall system efficacy. Moreover, it emphasizes upcoming advances such as the utilization of artificial intelligence, intelligent sensors, and real-time monitoring technologies that provide intelligent process control and adaptive optimization. The amalgamation of renewable energy sources with bioenergy production systems is examined as a hybrid strategy to enhance energy efficiency and diminish carbon emissions. Case studies from various geographical regions offer practical insights into the implementation of energy-efficient measures in bioenergy facilities. These examples highlight the economic and environmental advantages of implementing such measures and provide templates for replication. The chapter delineates existing hurdles, encompassing technological, regulatory, and economic obstacles, while providing insights into prospective trends in energy-efficient bioenergy systems. This chapter functions as a thorough resource for researchers, policymakers, and industry stakeholders seeking to promote energy-efficient approaches in bioenergy production.

K. Gajendiran (✉)
PG and Research Department of Microbiology, M.G.R. College, Hosur, Tamil Nadu, India
e-mail: mailtogk87@gmail.com

N. Mathiyazhagan
Department of Biotechnology, Saveetha School of Engineering, Saveetha Institute of Medical and Technical Sciences, SIMATS, Thandalam, Chennai, Tamil Nadu, India

D. Natarajan
Department of Biotechnology, Periyar University, Salem, Tamil Nadu, India

P. Verma (ed.), *Sustainable Practices in Biorefinery*,
https://doi.org/10.1007/978-981-95-6071-4_14

Keywords Bioenergy · Energy efficiency · Process optimization · Sustainable energy · Renewable energy technologies

14.1 Introduction

In the context of climate catastrophe and depleting fossil fuel supplies, bioenergy has surfaced as a viable cornerstone of the global shift towards renewable energy sources. It provides the combined advantage of employing biomass waste while diminishing greenhouse gas (GHG) emissions (Nair et al., 2022a; Olabi et al., 2023). The sustainability and long-term viability of bioenergy are significantly contingent upon energy efficiency during the production lifetime. Energy efficiency in bioenergy pertains to optimizing the usable energy output while reducing the energy inputs necessary for cultivation, processing, conversion, and distribution (Saleem, 2022). The International Renewable Energy Agency states that augmenting the energy efficiency of bioenergy systems might improve the net energy balance (NEB) by 25–40%, contingent upon the feedstock and technology employed (Nahak et al., 2022). For instance, classic wood-burning stoves possess an energy efficiency of about 10–15%, whereas contemporary biogas digesters and sophisticated biomass gasifiers can attain efficiencies of up to 85% when coupled with heat recovery systems (Behera et al., 2019; Narayanan, 2024a). Moreover, the Energy Return on Investment (EROI) serves as a critical metric for evaluating energy efficiency. Research demonstrates that maize ethanol possesses an Energy Return on Investment (EROI) of approximately 1.3:1, whereas sugarcane ethanol can attain values up to 8:1. Additionally, algal biofuels (Kandasamy et al., 2023), despite being in the developmental stage, exhibit the potential for EROIs exceeding 5:1 with process optimization (Paramasivam et al., 2024). This diversity underscores the necessity of implementing optimal procedures and technology suited to particular feedstocks and local conditions. In energy-intensive sectors such as transportation and industry, where decarbonization poses considerable difficulties, efficient bioenergy systems could markedly diminish reliance on fossil fuels (Carmona-Martínez et al., 2024). Furthermore, energy-efficient bioenergy is essential for rural and off-grid areas, particularly in developing nations, where access to dependable electricity is still constrained. Energy-efficient bioenergy systems not only decrease operational energy requirements but also mitigate environmental effects. The life-cycle greenhouse gas emissions from bioenergy can vary significantly, from approximately 10 gCO_2-eq/MJ for biogas derived from waste to exceeding 100 gCO_2-eq/MJ for poorly generated biodiesel (Xu et al., 2022). Improving efficiency via intelligent feedstock management and optimized conversion pathways can significantly reduce this footprint. Besides emissions, efficient systems minimize land, water, and nutrient inputs per unit of energy generated. Advanced hydrothermal liquefaction technologies, when utilized with wet biomass, can circumvent drying—a significant energy drain—and conserve up to 30% of process energy relative to conventional approaches (Bassoli et al., 2024). Enhancing energy efficiency directly results in financial savings. The U.S. Department of Energy

(DOE) predicts that optimizing processes and recovering energy in biomass-to-biofuel facilities can decrease production costs by 15–30% (Nunes, 2024). Moreover, nations such as Germany and Sweden, which have established energy-efficient bioenergy systems, report favorable macroeconomic outcomes, including employment creation in rural regions and less dependence on imported fuels. Energy efficiency enhances the appeal of bioenergy technology to investors and politicians, particularly within carbon pricing frameworks. For example, within the European Union Emission Trading System (EU ETS), highly efficient bioenergy facilities can generate supplementary income via carbon credits and performance-based incentives (Scheelhaase et al., 2021). This chapter seeks to critically analyze the significance of energy efficiency in improving the sustainability, scalability, and cost-effectiveness of bioenergy production systems. It examines the complete production continuum, from feedstock management to energy conversion, pinpointing critical energy loss areas and proposing tactics and solutions to mitigate them. This chapter seeks to provide a thorough guide for the design, implementation, and scaling of energy-efficient bioenergy systems that are both environmentally sustainable and economically feasible over the long term, through an analysis of theoretical foundations and practical implementations.

14.2 Overview of Bioenergy Production Processes

The generation of bioenergy is a multifaceted, sequential process involving biomass collection, pre-treatment, conversion, and distribution. Each stage imposes distinct energy requirements, rendering energy efficiency a vital factor throughout the production process (Chopra et al., 2024). Inefficiencies at any stage can markedly diminish the overall sustainability and net energy output of the system. Consequently, a comprehensive understanding of energy flows, conversion efficiencies, and loss points is crucial for enhancing performance and directing technological advancement (Table 14.1).

14.2.1 Biomass Acquisition and Preprocessing

Biomass feedstock's, including agricultural leftovers, forest waste, energy crops, and algae, constitute the foundation of all bioenergy systems (Duca and Nair et al., 2022b; Toscano, 2022). The energy efficiency of a bioenergy route is significantly affected by the techniques employed for feedstock collection and preparation (Fig. 14.1). Biomass collection entails the harvesting and transportation of raw materials from their source to the processing facility. The energy necessary for these operations fluctuates considerably based on the type of feedstock, bulk density, and geographic distribution (Williams et al., 2016). For example, loose, low-density materials such as straw or bagasse need greater energy for handling and transportation compared

Table 14.1 Overview of Bioenergy Production Processes

Stage	Description	Key energy considerations	Examples/ Technologies
Biomass collection	Collection and accumulation of biomass from agricultural, forestry, marine, or waste sources	Energy consumption is contingent upon biomass density, transportation distance, and collection methodology	Combine harvesters, manual harvesting, transport vehicles
Biomass pre-treatment	Preparation of biomass for conversion, including size reduction, drying, and chemical or biological conditioning	Drying and grinding are energy-intensive processes; pre-treatment should be optimized for cost-effectiveness and energy efficiency	Mechanical shredders, dryers, and acid/alkaline pre-treatment units
Conversion (Thermochemical)	High-temperature procedures that convert biomass into fuels or energy through decomposition. Encompasses combustion, pyrolysis, gasification, and hydrothermal liquefaction	Requires thermal energy input; efficiency is contingent upon reactor design and feedstock characteristics	Fluidized bed gasifiers, pyrolysis reactors, and combustion boilers
Conversion (Biochemical)	Utilization of microorganisms and enzymes to transform biomass into biogas, ethanol, hydrogen, and other products	Demands optimized biological conditions and frequently necessitates pre-treatment; energy input encompasses mixing, heating, and similar processes	Anaerobic digesters, fermenters, and bioreactors
Energy recovery	Collection and application of energy resources (thermal energy, electrical energy, biofuels)	Co-generation (CHP) can enhance overall system efficiency to 80–85%	Gas engines, turbines, and combined heat and power (CHP) units
Product upgrading	Enhancement of bioenergy products for final use (e.g., biogas purification, bio-oil processing)	Supplementary energy necessary for purification, compression, or stabilization	Membrane separation, cleaning, and distillation units
Energy input–output analysis	Assessment of total energy use in relation to energy generation. Comprises indicators such as Net Energy Balance (NEB) and Energy Return on Investment (EROI)	Essential for assessing system viability and sustainability	Life cycle assessment tools, energy analysis software

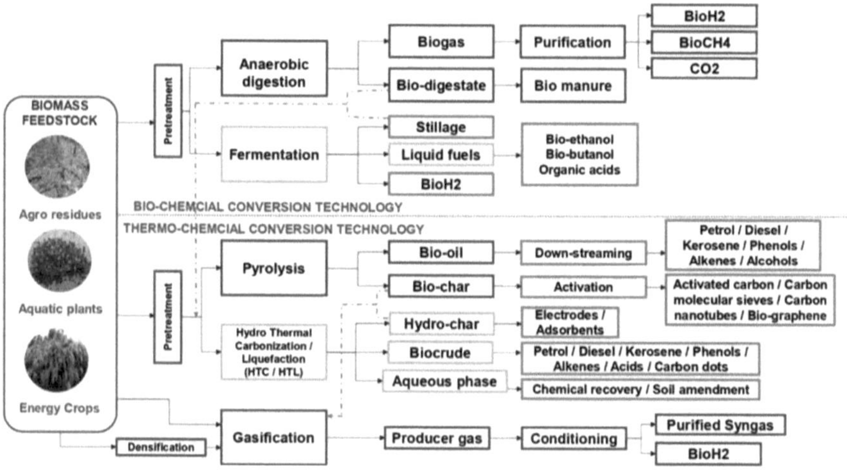

Fig. 14.1 Biorefinery methodology for biomass valorization (Thaha et al., 2025)

to compact, high-density feedstock's like wood pellets (Sarker et al., 2023; Thanh et al., 2023b). An essential inefficiency is in the elevated energy costs of transporting dispersed or bulky biomass. Densification technologies, including pelletizing and briquetting, can decrease energy consumption in transportation by 30–50% and enhance storage stability concurrently (Vaish et al., 2022).

Pre-treatment techniques are intended to optimize biomass for effective conversion. These methods may encompass size reduction, drying, and chemical or enzymatic treatments to enhance reactivity (Joshi & Manjare, 2024). Nevertheless, these processes frequently need substantial energy. For instance, dehydrating biomass to achieve ideal moisture content can need as much as 1.8 MJ per kilogramme of water extracted, signifying a substantial energy drain (John et al., 2024). This is especially vital for moist biomass varieties such as algae or food waste. In these instances, traditional drying methods are impractical; therefore, alternatives such as solar drying, dewatering membranes, or direct wet processing (e.g., hydrothermal liquefaction) should be emphasized (Arias et al., 2023). Furthermore, creating integrated pre-treatment systems that harness leftover heat or waste energy from subsequent process steps can yield significant energy savings. From a policy standpoint, subsidies or incentives for decentralized biomass processing units in proximity to farms could diminish transportation energy use and emissions.

14.2.2 *Conversion Technologies*

After pre-treatment, biomass is converted into useable energy forms, including heat, electricity, biogas, or liquid fuels (Ramos et al., 2022). These technologies are classified into two main categories: thermochemical and biochemical. Every pathway possesses distinct attributes, compromises, and efficiency metrics. Thermochemical conversion employs heat to decompose biomass into energy carriers. Combustion, the most conventional method, directly incinerates biomass to generate heat and electricity (Fig. 14.2). Although extensively utilized, its thermal efficiency is frequently constrained (20–30%) unless integrated with contemporary cogeneration systems, which can attain overall efficiencies of up to 80% (Luo et al., 2023). Pyrolysis and gasification yield superior energy products such as bio-oil and syngas, respectively. Fast pyrolysis can produce up to 70% bio-oil by weight, with energy efficiency ranging from 50 to 65% (Narayanan & Ma, 2024; Zheng et al., 2022). Nonetheless, elevated temperatures and reactor intricacies increase capital and operational energy expenditures. Hydrothermal liquefaction (HTL) offers an energy-efficient solution, particularly for moist biomass like algae, by obviating the necessity for energy-demanding drying and attaining energy recovery rates of up to 70% (Varghese et al., 2025). Biochemical conversion utilizes bacteria or enzymes to transform biomass into fuels such as bioethanol, butanol, methane, or hydrogen. Anaerobic digestion (AD) is especially advantageous for moist organic waste, achieving energy efficiency of up to 80% and facilitating nutrient recycling (Peng et al., 2020). Fermentation is typically employed to generate ethanol from sugar- or starch-laden substrates; however, lignocellulosic ethanol is more energy-intensive owing to the requirement for expensive enzymatic hydrolysis. Consolidated bioprocessing (CBP), which integrates enzyme production and hydrolysis within a single reactor, represents a viable strategy to diminish energy requirements (Olguin-Maciel et al., 2020). Furthermore, advancements in synthetic biology and metabolic engineering are crucial for improving yields and minimizing supplementary energy demands in biochemical processes. The selection of conversion technology must fit with feedstock characteristics, energy objectives, and regional limitations, underpinned by comprehensive techno-economic and life cycle evaluations (Mishra et al., 2023).

14.2.3 Energy Input–Output Assessment

Assessing energy efficiency in bioenergy systems necessitates meticulous energy input–output analysis. Two often utilized metrics are Net Energy Balance (NEB) the differential between energy output and fossil energy intake and Energy Return on Investment (EROI), which assesses the ratio of energy output to total input (Dupont et al., 2021). Elevated NEB and EROI values signify systems that are both efficient and sustainable. For instance, Brazilian sugarcane ethanol exhibits a net energy balance (NEB) of + 8.3 MJ/L and an energy return on investment (EROI) of 8:1, but U.S. maize ethanol has a marginal NEB of + 1.5 MJ/L and an EROI of merely 1.3:1. These discrepancies highlight the necessity of refining both feedstock selection and processing techniques. A thorough energy analysis must extend beyond basic accounting to include environmental and thermodynamic considerations (Rocco et al., 2014). Life Cycle Assessment (LCA) enhances the analysis by assessing greenhouse gas emissions, water consumption, and land-use alterations across the value

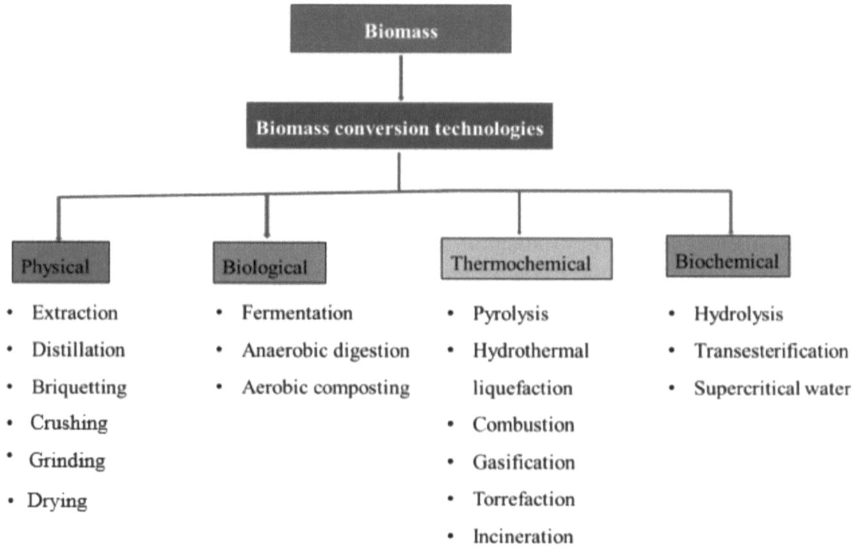

Fig. 14.2 Overview of biomass conversion technology (Tshikovhi & Motaung, 2023)

chain. For example, using heat recovery from fermentation processes or distillation columns might diminish energy use by as much as 15%, resulting in significant enhancements in carbon intensity (Kiss & Smith, 2020). Furthermore, energy analysis—a technique that assesses the quality or utility of energy—can pinpoint irreversibility's and inefficiencies at every level, facilitating focused enhancements. To improve transparency and comparability, it is essential for academics and companies to implement standardized energy accounting frameworks and verify that concealed energy costs (e.g., contained in feedstock fertilizers or water pumps) are appropriately represented. Moreover, the integration of digital technologies for real-time monitoring and predictive modelling might facilitate the ongoing optimization of energy flows (Das et al., 2024).

14.2.4 Analytical Discourse and Recommendations

Despite notable progress, the bioenergy sector still encounters obstacles in attaining comprehensive energy efficiency. A significant deficiency is the fragmentation of the supply chain, which frequently results in redundancy and energy inefficiencies (Das et al., 2024). Integrated biorefineries that concurrently produce fuels, power, and biochemicals present a possible option by optimizing value extraction from each biomass unit and attaining enhanced total energy efficiency (Narayanan et al., 2024b). An additional under examined domain is the potential for hybrid systems—integrating biological and thermochemical processes to optimize energy yield and operational flexibility. Residual solids from anaerobic digestion or fermentation might be subjected to gasification for enhanced energy recovery. Furthermore, increased implementation of co-generation and tri-generation systems, particularly in industrial bioenergy applications, might substantially enhance energy utilization rates (Lin et al., 2023). Policy initiatives are also crucial. Governments ought to prioritize financing for decentralized, modular bioenergy systems that reduce transportation energy and are customized to local biomass resources. Compulsory reporting of energy efficiency indicators and the incorporation of energy performance in subsidy eligibility criteria could enhance advancements throughout the sector. Thus, improving energy efficiency in bioenergy production is not solely a technical endeavor but a strategic necessity that demands concerted efforts in technological advancement, systems integration, and policy endorsement.

14.3 Strategies for Improving Energy Efficiency

Enhancing the energy efficiency of bioenergy production systems necessitates a holistic strategy that optimizes all phases of the production chain. Strategic interventions, including the judicious selection and management of biomass feedstock's, the implementation of integrated processing systems, and the utilization of sophisticated catalytic technologies, are crucial for minimizing energy losses and enhancing the overall energy return (Nunes, 2024) (Table 14.2).

14.3.1 Selection and Management of Feedstock

Feedstock characteristics significantly influence the energy efficiency of bioenergy production, as various biomass sources, including agricultural residues, energy crops, forest waste, and algal biomass, demonstrate considerable variability in moisture content, chemical composition, bulk density, and energy content (Duca and Toscano, 2022). These characteristics directly affect the energy input necessary for processing and the yield of final energy products. Moisture content is especially important among these elements. High-moisture biomass, such as food waste or algae, requires significant energy for drying prior to thermochemical conversion, whereas dry feedstocks like wood pellets or straw can be combusted or gasified with minimal preprocessing (Paudel et al., 2024). Choosing low-moisture or pre-dried biomass might thus decrease pre-treatment energy consumption by as much as 30%.

Lignocellulosic biomass, including wheat straw, bagasse, and corn stover, is frequently favored for its elevated carbon content and widespread availability (Paudel et al., 2024). Nonetheless, its structurally intricate composition requires energy-demanding chemical or enzymatic pre-treatment in biochemical conversion processes. In contrast, sugar-rich feedstock's such as sugarcane or sweet sorghum provide elevated bioethanol yields with less processing energy, although they present

Table 14.2 Strategies for Improving Energy Efficiency in Bioenergy Systems

Strategy	Description	Energy efficiency benefits	Examples/Applications
Feedstock selection and management	Selecting biomass with advantageous characteristics (e.g., low moisture content, high calorific value) and overseeing supply logistics	Minimises energy consumption for drying and transportation; enhances conversion efficiency	Utilizing dry feedstocks (e.g., straw, pellets); precision agriculture for energy crops
Process integration and heat recovery	Developing systems for the capture and reutilization of waste heat while integrating various unit processes	Enhances total system efficiency by 20–40%; lowers external heating and cooling requirements	Combined heat and power (CHP), steam recovery, and integrated biorefineries
Use of catalysts and enzymes	Utilizing catalysts or enzymes to enhance and optimize conversion reactions	Decreases activation energy; enhances yield; minimizes the necessity for elevated temperature or pressure conditions	Catalytic gasification and enzymatic hydrolysis of lignocellulosic materials
Advanced reactor design	Utilization of optimized configurations, including fluidized bed reactors or modular fermenters	Improves thermal transfer, reaction regulation, and product specificity	Dual fluidized bed gasifiers and plug-flow anaerobic digesters
Co-processing and Co-digestion	Integrating several biomass types to enhance reaction equilibrium and microbiological activity	Regulates the carbon-to-nitrogen ratio; enhances biogas production; mitigates fermentation inhibition	Co-digestion of manure with organic waste or energy crops
Waste minimization and valorization	Employing co-products (e.g., charcoal, glycerol, lignin) or transforming waste heat and effluents into beneficial outputs	Enhances overall energy yield and system sustainability	Utilization of lignin as boiler fuel; enhancement of glycerol for bioplastic production (Narayanan, 2023)

(continued)

Table 14.2 (continued)

Strategy	Description	Energy efficiency benefits	Examples/Applications
Automation and monitoring	Deploying intelligent sensors, artificial intelligence, and control systems for instantaneous optimization	Minimises operational inaccuracies; facilitates adaptive responses to fluctuations in feedstock and demand; enhances efficiency	Artificial intelligence-enhanced fermentation regulation; sensor-assisted anaerobic digester surveillance
Modular and scalable systems	Creating systems that are versatile and adjustable for various feedstocks and capacities	Improves deployment across many settings with no efficiency losses	Mobile biochar facilities; containerized biogas systems

issues about food-fuel competition and significant water requirements (Ameen et al., 2024). To enhance process efficiency, sophisticated feedstock management procedures, including the blending of complimentary biomass types, may be utilized. For example, combining high-lignin materials with readily degradable organic waste improves the carbon-to-nitrogen (C/N) ratio, hence increasing microbial activity in anaerobic digestion systems (Shahbaz et al., 2020). Moreover, considering seasonal and geographic availability aids in reducing energy costs linked to transit and storage (Mohanasundari et al., 2023). Innovative techniques like precision agriculture and remote sensing technologies enhance energy-efficient bioenergy production by maximizing biomass yields while minimizing fertilizer and irrigation usage. Furthermore, cultivating energy crops on marginal lands and employing waste biomass not only mitigate land-use conflicts but also improve the sustainability and energy efficiency of the entire system (Shah et al., 2023). Advancing the next generation of bioenergy systems will necessitate the creation of region-specific feedstock optimization models that incorporate energy efficiency, ecological sustainability, and economic viability (Mandley et al., 2020).

14.3.2 Process Integration and Thermal Recovery

Process integration is a highly effective strategy for improving energy efficiency in bioenergy systems. It entails the intentional and methodical design of interrelated processes to reduce redundancy, reclaim waste energy, and enhance overall resource efficiency. Techniques like pinch analysis and heat integration are frequently utilized to discern thermal synergy within and across different process units (Klemeš et al., 2018). Thermochemical bioenergy facilities release substantial thermal energy during processes such as combustion, gasification, and distillation. Instead of permitting this energy to dissipate, it can be efficiently harnessed and repurposed such as employing flue gas heat to preheat biomass feedstock or process water. Implementing heat exchangers and steam recovery systems can diminish auxiliary heating needs by 20–40%, contingent upon the facility's size and configuration (Balasamy et al., 2025). Combined Heat and Power (CHP) systems exemplify energy integration by concurrently generating electricity and useable heat from a singular fuel source. Biomass-based combined heat and power (CHP) facilities can attain total energy utilization rates of 80–85%, markedly surpassing traditional electricity-only plants, which generally achieve efficiencies of 30–40% (Mohan et al., 2006). Furthermore, tri-generation systems are being actively investigated in industrial bioenergy applications. These systems generate power and heat while also producing cooling via absorption chillers, thus fulfilling multiple energy requirements through a single integrated process. Integrated biorefineries signify a new frontier in process integration, generating a range of fuels, chemicals, energy, and value-added bio-products from a singular biomass feedstock (Pandey & Sharma, 2024). These facilities are engineered to optimize material and energy flows, hence enhancing resource utilization and economic returns. The remaining lignin from bioethanol synthesis can be utilized as boiler fuel to generate steam for upstream processes, hence diminishing fossil energy demand. This integration promotes energy efficiency and supports circular bioeconomy principles by valorizing by-products (Zabaniotou, 2018).

To maximize the potential of process integration, policymakers and engineers must prioritize the creation of modular and scalable integration frameworks. Moreover, specific incentives for the implementation of heat recovery and cogeneration systems particularly in small and medium-sized bioenergy facilities can address existing efficiency deficiencies and expedite the shift towards a more sustainable energy framework (Dobre et al., 2024).

14.3.3 Utilization of Catalysts and Enzymes

Catalysts and enzymes are essential in improving the efficiency, selectivity, and reaction rates of thermochemical and biochemical bioenergy conversion processes (Poornima et al., 2024). By decreasing activation energy barriers, they facilitate reactions at reduced temperatures and pressures, therefore minimizing overall energy consumption and enhancing product yields. In thermochemical processes like pyrolysis and gasification, the application of heterogeneous catalysts such as zeolites, nickel, and cobalt-based materials can markedly improve the quality and yield of desired products, including syngas and bio-oil (Abou Rjeily et al., 2021). Catalytic pyrolysis has demonstrated an enhancement in the output of important bio-oil fractions by 10–15%, concurrently enhancing fuel quality via the deoxygenation of heavy organic molecules (Dada et al., 2023). These advancements not only augment the energy efficiency of the conversion process but also diminish the necessity for energy-intensive downstream purification. Enzymes play a pivotal role in the biochemical conversion processes that transform lignocellulosic biomass into fermentable sugars through saccharification (Jahangeer et al., 2024). Enzymes like cellulases and hemicellulases enhance sugar recovery and diminish dependence on aggressive and energy-intensive chemical pre-treatment processes. Nonetheless, the synthesis of commercial enzymes is inherently energy-intensive, presenting a challenge to the overall energy equilibrium. Innovative methods in enzyme immobilization, thermostable enzyme formulations, and on-site enzyme manufacturing are mitigating these limits by enhancing enzyme efficiency and decreasing energy requirements in their production and administration (Narayanan et al., 2021a; Jaiswal & Jaiswal, 2024). Progress in metabolic engineering and synthetic biology is transforming this field by facilitating the creation of genetically modified microbial strains with increased tolerance to processing conditions, elevated productivity, and enhanced enzyme secretion abilities (Abdel-Mageed, 2025). These modified bacteria facilitate consolidated bioprocessing (CBP), an innovative method that integrates hydrolysis and fermentation into a singular operating phase. CBP obviates the necessity for energy-intensive intermediate separation processes and can significantly reduce overall energy requirements for the process. To guarantee that these catalytic improvements significantly aid in energy conservation, it is essential to invest in research dedicated to next-generation biocatalysts. This encompasses life cycle studies of catalyst and enzyme synthesis, utilization, and recovery to guarantee that their deployment results in a net positive energy and environmental equilibrium (Gaur et al., 2022; Kumar & Verma, 2020). Enhancing energy efficiency in bioenergy systems requires a comprehensive approach that integrates astute feedstock selection, cohesive process design, and sophisticated catalytic technology. When properly executed, these strategies can substantially augment the energy return on investment (EROI), reduce environmental consequences, and improve the economic feasibility of bioenergy (Paramasivam et al., 2024).

14.4 Advanced Methods in Process Optimization

With the increasing demand for sustainable and energy-efficient bioenergy systems, innovation in process optimization has become essential. Conventional approaches, although effective, frequently fail to optimize energy recovery, mitigate environmental impact, and decrease operational expenses (Chen et al., 2022). As a result, sophisticated technological interventions have arisen at several phases of bioenergy production, particularly in fermentation, gasification, and energy system integration.

14.4.1 Sophisticated Fermentation and Gasification Methods

Fermentation and gasification are essential processes in bioenergy production, transforming biomass into fuels such as ethanol, methane, and syngas (Kennes et al., 2016). Although conventional procedures are well-established, they frequently exhibit low substrate conversion rates, elevated energy requirements, and unsatisfactory yields. Technological advancements currently provide substantial enhancements in efficiency, production, and energy equilibrium (Armstrong et al., 2016).

14.4.1.1 Advanced Fermentation Techniques

Traditional fermentation methods frequently encounter constraints, including suboptimal sugar yields from lignocellulosic biomass, the production of undesirable by-products, and the necessity for energy-demanding downstream processing. Recent improvements in fermentation technology aim to integrate and streamline multiple process steps to improve overall energy and conversion efficiency, hence addressing these inefficiencies (Boodhoo et al., 2022). Consolidated bioprocessing (CBP) is a highly promising method that integrates enzyme production, biomass hydrolysis, and fermentation into a singular operational step (Narayanan et al., 2021b; Singhania et al., 2022). By obviating the necessity for external enzyme supplementation, CBP diminishes energy expenditure, streamlines process logistics, and decreases operational expenses. Engineered microbial strains like *Clostridium thermocellum* and *Zymomonas mobilis* have been created to directly ferment pretreated biomass, resulting in higher sugar-to-ethanol conversion efficiencies and increased resilience to fermentation inhibitors (Sar et al., 2023).

A notable advancement is simultaneous saccharification and co-fermentation (SSCF), enabling the simultaneous fermentation of hexose and pentose sugars. This method increases ethanol production by roughly 20–25% relative to conventional batch fermentation processes. Moreover, thermophilic fermentation, conducted at high temperatures, diminishes the likelihood of microbial contamination (Arora et al., 2015; Lu et al., 2023) and enhances compatibility with heat-intensive upstream processes, hence improving energy efficiency. Collectively, these sophisticated fermentation methods signify crucial advancements in enhancing bioenergy output by tackling both biochemical and thermal inefficiencies (Woźniak et al., 2025).

14.4.1.2 Advanced Gasification

Gasification is a thermochemical process that transforms biomass into a combustible synthesis gas (syngas) principally consisting of carbon monoxide (CO), hydrogen (H_2), methane (CH_4), and carbon dioxide (CO_2) (Maitlo et al., 2022). This syngas can be employed for electricity generation, synthetic fuel synthesis, or direct thermal usage. Conventional gasifiers are frequently constrained by challenges like tar production, inadequate energy efficiency, and variable gas quality (Fig. 14.3). Modern gasification systems, including dual-fluidized bed and plasma gasifiers, have been developed to address these issues. These sophisticated systems provide superior temperature regulation, increased feedstock adaptability, and improved cold gas efficiency, achieving up to 75% (Alcheikhhamdon & Hoorfar, 2016).

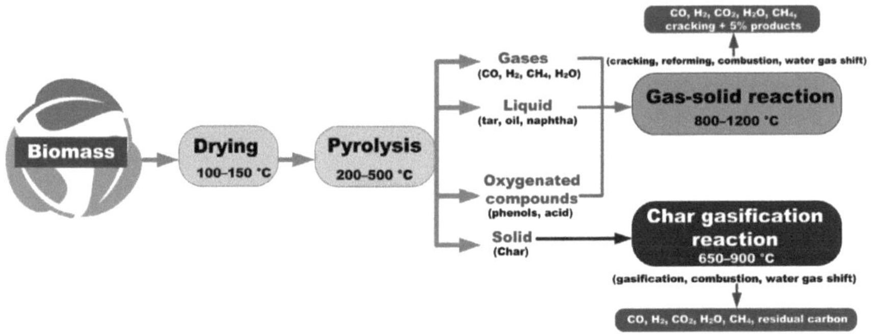

Fig. 14.3 Mechanisms and phases of pyrolysis and gasification (Glushkov et al., 2021)

Additional enhancements are attained via catalytic gasification, employing catalysts such as nickel or dolomite to decompose tars and augment hydrogen production, therefore elevating the total quality and applicability of the syngas (Ghodke et al., 2023). Moreover, integrated systems that connect gasification with subsequent processes such as Fischer–Tropsch synthesis or methanation facilitate the effective transformation of syngas into valuable products, including liquid fuels and renewable natural gas (RNG) (dos Santos & Alencar, 2020). These linkages enhance energy conversion efficiency and broaden the scope of bioenergy applications. To enhance future scalability and optimize biomass use, research should prioritize hybrid systems that integrate improved fermentation and gasification methods. Integrated techniques would provide the concurrent conversion of carbohydrate-rich and lignin-rich biomass fractions, optimizing energy recovery and system efficiency (Diment et al., 2025; Narayanan, 2024b).

14.4.2 Co-Generation and Tri-Generation Systems

One of the most efficient methods to enhance energy efficiency in bioenergy systems is to capture and utilize not just electricity but also the heat (and, in certain instances, cooling) produced during biomass conversion processes (Li et al., 2023). Co-generation (CHP) and tri-generation (CCHP) systems are vital elements of advanced energy-efficient buildings.

14.4.2.1 Co-Generation (Combined Heat and Power)

Co-generation, or combined heat and power (CHP), denotes the concurrent generation of electricity and beneficial thermal energy from a singular fuel source. In biomass-based systems, this generally entails the burning or gasification of biomass to generate electricity, while the resultant waste heat is harnessed and utilized for industrial processes, district heating, or drying operations (Li et al., 2023; Thanh et al., 2023a). This integrated method markedly enhances overall energy efficiency, with CHP systems attaining efficiencies of 75–85%, compared to the 30–40% efficiency characteristic of traditional stand-alone power plants. Biomass CHP facilities are extensively utilized in areas like Northern Europe, providing electricity and heating to residential and industrial sectors, hence enhancing energy security and diminishing reliance on fossil fuels (Cross et al., 2021). In nations such as India, sugar mills frequently employ CHP systems that harness bagasse, a by-product of sugarcane processing, for simultaneous power and steam generation. This not only guarantees optimal utilization of agricultural leftovers but also significantly diminishes the mills' dependence on external energy sources, illustrating the feasibility and economic benefits of co-generation in bioenergy applications (Thirumalaivasan et al., 2024).

14.4.2.2 Combined Cooling, Heating, and Power (CCHP)

Tri-generation systems, or combined cooling, heat, and power (CCHP) systems, enhance the advantages of traditional CHP by additionally generating cooling in conjunction with electricity and thermal energy (Dobre et al., 2024). This enhanced functionality is especially beneficial in sectors like food processing, pharmaceuticals, and data centres, where cooling is essential for operations. These systems incorporate absorption chillers fuelled by waste heat to produce chilled water or air, therefore efficiently harnessing thermal energy that would otherwise be squandered. CCHP systems can attain overall energy efficiencies of up to 90%, particularly when functioning constantly under stable base-load conditions (Akbarnataj et al., 2024). This renders them an optimal alternative for enhancing energy recovery and minimizing primary fuel usage. Governments and industries should prioritize the implementation of tri-generation technologies in hot climates and encourage the strategic co-location of bioenergy facilities with industrial operations that have consistent year-round thermal energy and cooling demands (Agonafer et al., 2022).

14.4.3 Integration with Renewable Energy Sources

Although bioenergy is fundamentally a renewable energy source, its incorporation with other intermittent renewables like solar and wind markedly improves overall system resilience, diminishes the necessity for energy storage, and facilitates the creation of more adaptable and sustainable hybrid energy systems. The integration of many sources is essential for enhancing the energy efficiency and adaptability of future energy infrastructures, especially in relation to variable energy demands and the availability of renewable resources (Ang et al., 2022; Mani et al., 2024).

A viable technique is the installation of solar-biomass hybrid systems, which utilize solar thermal energy to warm biomass or water, hence diminishing dependence on fossil fuels in processes such as steam generation, drying, or pyrolysis (Ndukwu et al., 2021). Sun-assisted biorefineries have demonstrated a reduction in overall thermal energy demand of 15–30%, contingent upon local sun irradiance levels (Singh et al., 2024). Wind-bioenergy hybrid systems are increasingly popular, particularly in off-grid or microgrid settings. In these configurations, wind turbines provide electricity for auxiliary functions such as pumps or system controls while bioenergy delivers consistent base-load power and acts as a backup during low-wind intervals, guaranteeing uninterrupted energy supply. Enhanced integration is observed in power-to-gas (P2G) technologies, which transform excess renewable electricity into hydrogen through electrolysis (Nnabuife et al., 2025). This hydrogen can then be utilized with anaerobic digestion or gasification to generate synthetic methane or to enhance biogas. These integrated procedures boost energy storage and grid stability while improving the calorific value and quality of biogas emissions. Digital platforms and intelligent energy management systems are being progressively utilized to properly handle these intricate energy flows. These technologies provide real-time monitoring, optimization, and demand-responsive control, guaranteeing that hybrid systems function at peak efficiency (Narayanan et al., 2024a; Wang et al., 2025).

To expedite the advancement and implementation of integrated bioenergy-renewable systems, financial mechanisms and supportive regulatory frameworks must prioritize research, demonstration, and deployment, particularly in areas with fluctuating renewable energy availability and ample biomass supplies (Wang et al., 2025). Thus, novel methodologies in fermentation, gasification, and energy integration are revolutionizing the efficiency paradigm of bioenergy production. These technologies enhance energy return and system reliability while augmenting the variety and value of bioenergy within a comprehensive renewable energy portfolio. As the discipline advances, attention must transition from discrete optimizations to comprehensive, intelligently interconnected systems that are adaptable, resilient, and scalable.

14.5 Technological Advancements and Automation

The bioenergy sector is experiencing a fundamental change propelled by digital transformation and automation (Pandey et al., 2023). Conventional manual and semi-automated procedures are progressively supplanted or enhanced by intelligent, adaptive technologies that streamline operations, minimize human error, and optimize energy efficiency (Zafar et al., 2024). The amalgamation of artificial intelligence (AI), machine learning (ML), Internet of Things (IoT), and data-driven decision-making platforms is facilitating a novel generation of intelligent bioenergy systems (Rajinikanth et al., 2024a; Vijayakumarr et al., 2025).

14.5.1 Artificial Intelligence and Machine Learning in Process Control

Artificial intelligence (AI) and machine learning (ML) algorithms (Basheer et al., 2025; Zaidi et al., 2025) have become crucial instruments for enhancing operational efficiency and decision-making in bioenergy systems (Mohan et al., 2024). Their ability to analyze extensive datasets, identify intricate patterns, and adjust to fluctuating conditions renders them exceptionally qualified for overseeing the variability intrinsic to biomass feedstock's and the complexities of biochemical and thermochemical conversion processes. In fermentation systems, machine learning models are utilized to forecast microbial growth rates, substrate utilization, and product synthesis by employing real-time data like temperature, pH, and substrate concentration (Vinestock et al., 2024). Methods such as random forests, support vector machines (SVM), and artificial neural networks (ANNs) (Ali et al., 2025) have exhibited significant precision in predicting ethanol yields and detecting early signs of contamination or system failure.

In thermochemical processes such as gasification and pyrolysis, artificial intelligence is employed to enhance operations by forecasting syngas composition, reducing tar production, and adjusting parameters including reactor temperature, biomass feed rate, and air-to-fuel ratios (Sakheta et al., 2023). Reinforcement learning algorithms have demonstrated the capacity to continually adjust process parameters based on real-time feedback, yielding energy savings of 10–15% in pilot-scale applications. Moreover, AI-driven control systems facilitate predictive maintenance by examining equipment utilization and identifying wear-and-tear patterns in components like pumps, turbines, and digesters (Mohamed Almazrouei et al., 2023). This predictive capability mitigates unanticipated downtime and improves overall plant dependability and availability. These intelligent systems provide adaptive control strategies that dynamically modify process parameters in reaction to variations in feedstock quality or energy demand, thus enhancing responsiveness and stability. To effectively use these potential, it is essential to promote joint research between AI developers and bioenergy engineers. These collaborations can result in the development of domain-specific AI models that are not only exceptionally accurate and resilient under varying situations but also interpretable and usable across diverse biomass conversion methods (Vassiliadis et al., 2024).

14.5.2 Intelligent Sensors and Instantaneous Monitoring

Real-time data capture constitutes the foundation of intelligent and energy-efficient bioenergy systems. The implementation of intelligent sensors across several phases of bioenergy production facilitates ongoing observation of critical process parameters, including temperature, pressure, gas composition, pH, dissolved oxygen levels, biomass concentration, and total energy consumption (Gotore et al., 2025).

These sensors furnish essential data to enhance operations, augment conversion efficiency, and avert system breakdowns. Contemporary sensors, frequently using Micro-Electro-Mechanical Systems (MEMS) and nanotechnology (Hossain et al., 2024; Narayanan, 2025), provide compact, energy-efficient, and exceptionally sensitive solutions that can be effortlessly included into pipelines, reactors, and control modules. Infrared and laser-based gas analyzers provide real-time measurements of gases such as CO, CO_2, CH_4, and H_2 in biogas or syngas streams, facilitating prompt modifications to combustion or gasification settings to ensure optimal performance (Megía et al., 2021).

In biochemical processes like fermentation and anaerobic digestion, optical and electrochemical sensors are utilized to monitor essential parameters such as biomass degradation rates, redox potential, and metabolite buildup, all of which substantially affect conversion yields (Rozina et al., 2024). Wireless sensor networks (WSNs) have augmented operational flexibility by facilitating the transmission of real-time data from decentralized or remote bioenergy facilities, including rural biogas units and open algal ponds, to centralized monitoring and control hubs. In regions with unstable or no internet connectivity, edge computing and sensor fusion technologies are being increasingly employed (Nguyen et al., 2024). These systems locally process data, enabling prompt decision-making and minimizing delay, which is particularly advantageous for off-grid or dispersed energy systems. Future sensor designs should emphasize self-calibration, self-cleaning capabilities, and non-invasive setups to boost longevity and reduce operational disturbances in the harsh and changing environments characteristic of bioenergy production. Enhancing sensor reliability and minimizing maintenance requirements would facilitate the broader implementation of real-time monitoring and control, hence promoting increased efficiency and resilience within the bioenergy sector (Nguyen et al., 2024).

14.5.3 Data-Driven Decision Support Systems

With the rising digitization of bioenergy production, the quantity of operational and environmental data created is expanding quickly. Data-driven Decision Support Systems (DSS) utilize this data to provide operators, engineers, and policymakers with prompt, informed, and strategic decision-making abilities (Elkady et al., 2024; Parveen et al., 2025). These sophisticated platforms amalgamate real-time process data, historical performance metrics, and external variables such as weather forecasts, biomass availability, and market prices to enhance various functions, including feedstock scheduling, load balancing, grid synchronization, process route selection (e.g., anaerobic digestion versus gasification), economic feasibility assessments, and life-cycle carbon intensity evaluations. In biogas facilities, DSS platforms can evaluate present operational conditions in conjunction with historical performance to suggest optimal feedstock combinations that enhance methane production while reducing the likelihood of volatile fatty acid (VFA) buildup (Beschkov & Angelov, 2025). DSS tools in biorefineries enhance the selection of downstream valorization paths for co-products such as lignin or glycerol, consequently augmenting profitability and resource efficiency. Cloud-based Decision Support System solutions, with intuitive dashboards and predictive analytics, provide real-time optimization across the whole plant, including geographically scattered locations (Talari et al., 2022). These systems can integrate with Enterprise Resource Planning (ERP) platforms to synchronize production plans with supply chain logistics, dynamic energy price, and regulatory compliance mandates.

To provide equal access to these sophisticated tools, particularly for small-scale bioenergy producers in resource-limited settings, it is imperative to create open-source, interoperable decision support system platforms that can be readily customized and implemented (Lanucara et al., 2024). Hence, the amalgamation of technical advancements such as artificial intelligence, smart sensor networks, and intelligent decision support systems is revolutionizing bioenergy production from reactive, labor-intensive methods into intelligent, self-optimizing ecosystems. These digital solutions boost energy efficiency while facilitating predictive management, adaptive control, and strategic foresight essential elements for long-term sustainability and global competitiveness in the renewable energy sector. To fully realize the potential of this transition, sustained investment in digital infrastructure, interdisciplinary collaboration, and extensive capacity-building efforts is essential.

14.6 Analyses of Energy-Efficient Practices

Practical applications of bioenergy systems offer essential insights into the conversion of theoretical and technological progress into tangible improvements in energy efficiency (Arias et al., 2024). This document presents three case studies from Europe, North America, and Asia that illustrate region-specific improvements enhancing energy efficiency in various bioenergy production systems. A mid-sized biogas facility in Bavaria, Germany, underwent extensive optimization from 2018 to 2021 (Thrän et al., 2025). The facility, initially dependent on traditional anaerobic digestion of maize silage and pig dung, implemented various efficiency enhancements. Diversifying feedstock to incorporate grass silage, food waste, and crop residues optimized the carbon-to-nitrogen ratio and increased biogas outputs by 15% (Ngabala & Emmanuel, 2024). A contemporary Combined Heat and Power (CHP) unit supplanted the obsolete system, enhancing overall energy utilization efficiency to 85% (Dobre et al., 2024). The incorporation of an AI-driven control system facilitated predictive management of digester conditions utilizing real-time data, yielding a 10% enhancement in methane production and a 12% decrease in parasitic energy use (Negi et al., 2025). This renovation enhanced the energy return on investment (EROI) from 2.5:1 to 4.1:1 and diminished carbon emissions by roughly 280 tonnes of CO_2-equivalent per year. A pioneering pilot-scale algae-based biofuel factory in California showcased the viability of energy-positive operation through the integration of solar energy with hydrothermal liquefaction (HTL) technology (Deepika et al., 2024). Microalgae were cultivated in raceway ponds powered by photovoltaic systems, utilizing CO_2 from a neighboring industrial facility to augment algal output. In contrast to traditional techniques that necessitate energy-intensive drying, the wet algal biomass was directly processed by hydrothermal liquefaction (HTL), achieving a recovery of up to 75% of the biomass's energy content and yielding high-quality bio-crude (Borazjani et al., 2025). Heat integration enhanced efficiency by utilizing thermal energy from the HTL reactor to regulate pond temperature and warm water. Nutrient-dense aqueous by-products were repurposed inside the cultivation system, reducing reliance on synthetic fertilizers (Sarker et al., 2019). This closed-loop design attained a net energy gain of + 5.4 MJ/kg of biomass and an 80% decrease in carbon intensity relative to traditional diesel fuel (Lutzu et al., 2024).

A community-scale biomass gasification initiative in rural Punjab, India, converted agricultural residues mainly rice husks and wheat straw into dependable power and thermal energy (Wakeel et al., 2023). The technology circumvented energy expenses linked to biomass drying by employing dry, locally obtained feedstocks. A downdraft gasifier generated low-tar syngas that powered a dual-fuel engine producing 1 MW of electricity. Waste heat was harnessed via heat exchangers and diverted to adjacent rice mills and residences for processing and heating, hence enhancing overall system efficiency. The project integrated intelligent load management and remote diagnostics, guaranteeing optimal performance and minimal downtime (Krishna Rao et al., 2024). This decentralized model supplied renewable energy to more than 300 families, displaced fossil fuels, and prevented over 1,500 tonnes of CO_2 emissions annually, while attaining an overall system efficiency of 68% (Tarekegne, 2021). These case studies demonstrate that site-specific solutions, stakeholder collaboration, and technological integration may significantly enhance energy efficiency throughout the bioenergy value chain. They demonstrate the significance of adaptive designs customized to feedstock availability, local infrastructure, and socio-economic situations, functioning as scalable models for future sustainable energy systems.

14.7 Obstacles and Prospective Outlooks

Although energy-efficient bioenergy technologies provide significant environmental and economic advantages, their broad adoption encounters numerous enduring obstacles. These problems encompass technological, financial, regulatory, and infrastructural areas (Falcone, 2023). A comprehensive comprehension of these obstacles is crucial for formulating effective methods to enhance energy-efficient innovations and attain long-term sustainability in bioenergy systems.

14.7.1 Technical Obstacles to Implementation

Notwithstanding considerable progress in bioenergy conversion and process optimization, numerous technological obstacles persist, impeding the scalability and extensive implementation of energy-efficient bioenergy systems (El-Araby, 2024). A significant constraint is the intrinsic variability of biomass feedstocks, which exhibit considerable differences in moisture content, ash composition, calorific value, and chemical properties based on their origin, seasonal fluctuations, and processing techniques. This inconsistency presents a considerable obstacle to sustaining stable and effective conversion processes, requiring the creation of highly flexible systems that can manage varying input characteristics without compromising energy performance (Shao et al., 2022). Pre-treatment and conversion processes, especially for intricate biomass types like lignocellulosic and algal biomass, pose significant challenges. Innovative technologies such as hydrothermal liquefaction (HTL), gasification, and consolidated bioprocessing exhibit enhanced energy efficiency; yet, they frequently entail substantial capital expenditures, intricate infrastructure demands, and necessitate meticulous operational oversight (Nunes, 2024). These limitations render implementation challenging in small- and medium-scale operations, particularly in decentralized or rural regions where technical and financial resources are scarce. Process integration and heat recovery systems can enhance total energy balance by 30–40%, contingent upon sophisticated engineering design, precise process modelling, and consistent maintenance (Beck et al., 2022). The implementation of AI-driven automation and real-time monitoring systems, while promising, relies on the presence of dependable digital infrastructure, proficient technical personnel, and strong cybersecurity measures—factors frequently absent in low-resource or developing areas. Biochemical conversion routes face problems such as the restricted thermal and operational stability of enzymes and catalysts, the elevated cost of industrial enzymes, and the complexities associated with recycling or reusing catalysts on an industrial scale (Intasian et al., 2021). These characteristics increase operational expenses and limit the long-term economic sustainability of numerous procedures. The transition from laboratory to commercial operations is further exacerbated by durability challenges, system fouling, and deterioration, resulting in frequent equipment replacement and heightened maintenance and energy costs (Osman et al., 2024). Future research and development must concentrate on devising cost-efficient, modular, and versatile bioenergy technologies that can be tailored to various operational situations. Moreover, enhanced investment in pilot-scale demonstration projects is crucial for validating and refining energy-efficient configurations in practical settings, facilitating wider uptake and commercialization.

14.7.2 Policy and Regulatory Frameworks

Robust policy and regulatory frameworks are essential for the efficient implementation and expansion of energy-efficiency bioenergy systems (Nair & Verma, 2025). Nonetheless, in several areas, current policies are fragmented, inconsistently implemented, or insufficiently enforced, creating substantial obstacles to advancement (Schipfer et al., 2022). A significant difficulty is the lack of standardized indicators and evaluation criteria specifically designed for bioenergy. In contrast to fossil fuel technologies, which adhere to established performance standards, bioenergy systems frequently lack standardized methods for evaluating energy return on investment, lifetime greenhouse gas emissions, and overall system efficiency. This inconsistency impedes performance validation and informed policy formulation. Furthermore, financial incentive mechanisms such as subsidies, feed-in tariffs, carbon credits, and renewable energy certificates typically advantage more conventional renewable sources like solar, wind, and hydroelectric power (Qadir et al., 2021). Consequently, bioenergy efforts, especially small-scale or community-based ones, are often inadequately supported and underestimated. Bureaucratic inefficiencies, such as protracted permission procedures and ambiguous long-term policy promises, further inhibit private sector investment in bioenergy infrastructure and technological innovation (Haldar et al., 2024; Narayanan & Rajinikanth, 2025).

A further concern is to the categorization of waste-to-energy technology. Notwithstanding their ecological advantages, these systems are frequently seen as waste management solutions instead of as contributors to renewable energy objectives. This misrepresentation may hinder access to renewable energy funds and hide their function in circular economy models. Furthermore, legislative ambiguities about land use, biomass categorization, and biofuel blending requirements hinder project development and sustainability evaluations. The issues are exacerbated by a pervasive absence of capacity-building programs in numerous developing nations. The lack of technical training, digital literacy programs, and sustainability education creates a skills gap that hinders the effective adoption and upkeep of contemporary, energy-efficient bioenergy systems (Mondejar et al., 2021). Governments must implement comprehensive bioenergy policies that include energy efficiency standards, lifecycle carbon accounting, and inclusive financial incentives to resolve these concerns. Clear regulations regarding land use, biomass definitions, and blending mandates are crucial, as is the optimization of approval processes to minimize delays. Promoting public–private collaborations can enhance innovation and investment. Moreover, enhancing education and training programs is essential for developing a proficient workforce that can sustain modern bioenergy infrastructure and guarantee the enduring success of these systems (Amir et al., 2023).

14.7.3 Prospective Developments in Energy-Efficient Bioenergy Systems

The future of bioenergy depends on the creation of highly efficient, intelligent, and adaptable systems that can respond to changing energy landscapes and environmental demands. Numerous new trends are set to propel the forthcoming generation of energy-efficient bioenergy production.

1. **Digital Transformation and AI-Enhanced Optimization**: As artificial intelligence and machine learning technologies advance, their incorporation into bioenergy systems will become increasingly prevalent (Shi et al., 2023). Real-time optimization algorithms, digital twins, and predictive maintenance tools will improve operational reliability and system efficiency. Cloud-based decision support systems (DSS) will allow even little producers to utilise advanced analytics, enhancing energy management and financial returns (Ryu et al., 2023).
2. **Modular and Decentralised Bioenergy Systems**: Smaller-scale, modular systems, particularly those utilizing agricultural wastes or food waste, are increasingly favored in rural and peri-urban regions (Rajendran et al., 2024). These systems can be linked with microgrids and function off-grid, rendering them suitable for distant populations and disaster-prone areas. Advancements in containerized gasification systems, plug-and-play anaerobic digesters, and portable biorefineries will facilitate this trend (Jameel et al., 2024).
3. **Hybrid Renewable Energy Systems**: Bioenergy will be progressively integrated with other renewable sources, including solar, wind, and hydropower, to develop hybrid systems that bolster grid resilience, diminish seasonal reliance, and augment energy efficiency. Solar-biomass hybrids, wind-driven digesters, and power-to-gas systems exemplify attractive domains for integrated energy solutions (Rajinikanth et al., 2024b).
4. **Integration of Circular Bioeconomy**: Future bioenergy systems will serve as pivotal elements of circular bioeconomies, characterized by waste reduction, valorization of by-products, and carbon sequestration or reutilization (Radhakrishnan & Narayanan, 2025). Technologies such as biochar production via pyrolysis, carbon capture and utilization (CCU), and nutrient recycling will provide resource-positive energy systems that transcend sustainability towards regeneration (Samoraj et al., 2024).
5. **Standardization and Certification**: International organizations are progressively anticipated to develop standardized certification frameworks for energy-efficient and sustainable bioenergy, with the objective of improving market transparency and augmenting customer confidence (Apeh & Nwulu, 2025). These certifications, based on parameters including lifetime greenhouse gas emissions, net energy balance, and biodiversity impacts, will be crucial in differentiating genuinely high-efficiency bioenergy systems from less sustainable or environmentally harmful options. The future development of energy-efficient bioenergy systems will be influenced by the integration of digital technology, circular economy principles, and progressive policy frameworks (Balsalobre-Lorente &

Shah, 2024). To achieve widespread influence, these systems must be technologically advanced, accessible, affordable, and adaptable to various geographic and socio-economic circumstances. Despite ongoing technological and regulatory obstacles, the swift progression of innovation and global energy agendas offers numerous prospects for advancement. Realizing the complete potential of bioenergy as a sustainable energy source requires a comprehensive approach that integrates advanced technologies, supportive policies, and community-focused designs [143]. An integrated strategy will be essential in establishing bioenergy as a fundamental component of a low-carbon, energy-efficient global future.

14.8 Conclusion

Energy efficiency is fundamental to sustainable and economically feasible bioenergy systems. This chapter has examined the intricate processes of bioenergy production, encompassing biomass collection, conversion, and final energy output, while identifying critical techniques to improve efficiency throughout the whole value chain. Advancements in feedstock management, process integration, catalytic improvement, and digital automation have shown considerable promise in decreasing energy consumption, enhancing energy outputs, and mitigating environmental effects. Case studies from Europe, North America, and Asia exemplify the effective implementation of these methods through modern technologies, tailored operational techniques, and collaborative stakeholder involvement. These examples underscore the significance of contextual adaptation and the amalgamation of bioenergy systems with other renewable energy sources to attain optimal outcomes. Nevertheless, numerous obstacles persist. Technical constraints, such as feedstock variability and infrastructure deficiencies, coupled with fragmented regulatory frameworks and inadequate financial backing, persist in hindering wider deployment. Confronting these difficulties necessitates synchronized endeavors in technological advancement, policy reform, educational outreach, and financial investment. The convergence of bioenergy with digitalization, artificial intelligence, the circular bioeconomy, and hybrid renewable systems is set to revolutionize its position in the global energy framework. Proactive policies that foster innovation, standardized regulations, and fair access to advanced technologies will be crucial for realizing this potential. Ultimately, energy-efficient bioenergy transcends a mere technical goal; it is a strategic necessity for attaining global objectives pertaining to sustainability, energy security, and climate resilience. Through the integration of innovation, systems thinking, and participatory governance, bioenergy may serve as a fundamental pillar of a low-carbon, resource-efficient future.

References

Abdel-Mageed, H. M. (2025). Frontiers in nanoparticles redefining enzyme immobilization: A review addressing challenges, innovations, and unlocking sustainable future potentials. *Micro and Nano Systems Letters, 13*, 1–28.

Abou Rjeily, M., Gennequin, C., Pron, H., Abi-Aad, E., & Randrianalisoa, J. H. (2021). Pyrolysis-catalytic upgrading of bio-oil and pyrolysis-catalytic steam reforming of biogas: A review. *Environmental Chemistry Letters 19*, 2825–2872.

Agonafer, T. D., Eremed, W. B., & Adem, K. D. (2022). Biogas-based trigeneration system: A review. *Results in Engineering, 15*, Article 100509.

Akbarnataj, K., Saffaripour, M., & Houshfar, E. (2024). Novel design of a CCHP system to boost nearly zero-carbon building concept. *Energy Conversion and Management, 309*, Article 118468.

Alcheikhhamdon, Y., & Hoorfar, M. (2016). Natural gas quality enhancement: A review of the conventional treatment processes, and the industrial challenges facing emerging technologies. *Journal of Natural Gas Science and Engineering, 34*, 689–701.

Ali, S. M., Vijayakumar, K., & Narayanan, M. (2025). Deep transfer learning framework for brain tumor detection in MRI slices: A study. In *2025 International Conference on Frontier Technologies and Solutions (ICFTS)*, pp. 1–6.

Ameen, M., Mahmood, A., Shehzad, A. N., Zia, M. A., & Javaid, M. M. (2024). Sorghum's potential unleashed: A comprehensive exploration of bio-energy production strategies and innovations. *Bioresource Technology Reports, 101906*.

Amir, M., Deshmukh, R. G., Khalid, H. M., Said, Z., Raza, A., Muyeen, S. M., Nizami, A.-S., Elavarasan, R. M., Saidur, R., & Sopian, K. (2023). Energy storage technologies: An integrated survey of developments, global economical/environmental effects, optimal scheduling model, and sustainable adaption policies. *Journal of Energy Storage, 72*, Article 108694.

Ang, T.-Z., Salem, M., Kamarol, M., Das, H. S., Nazari, M. A., & Prabaharan, N. (2022). A comprehensive study of renewable energy sources: Classifications, challenges and suggestions. *Energy Strategy Reviews, 43*, Article 100939.

Apeh, O. O., & Nwulu, N. I. (2025). Enhancing transparency and efficiency in green energy management through blockchain: A comprehensive bibliometric analysis. *Energy Nexus, 18*, Article 100405.

Arias, A., Nika, C.-E., Vasilaki, V., Feijoo, G., Moreira, M. T., & Katsou, E. (2024). Assessing the future prospects of emerging technologies for shipping and aviation biofuels: A critical review. *Renewable and Sustainable Energy Reviews, 197*, Article 114427.

Arias, D. M., García-Valladares, O., Besagni, G., & Markides, C. N. (2023). A vision of renewable thermal technologies for drying, biofuels production and industrial waste, gas or water recovery. *Applied Thermal Engineering, 223*, Article 120022.

Armstrong, R. C., Wolfram, C., De Jong, K. P., Gross, R., Lewis, N. S., Boardman, B., Ragauskas, A. J., Ehrhardt-Martinez, K., Crabtree, G., & Ramana, M. (2016). The frontiers of energy. *Nature Energy, 1*, 1–8.

Arora, R., Behera, S., & Kumar, S. (2015). Bioprospecting thermophilic/thermotolerant microbes for production of lignocellulosic ethanol: A future perspective. *Renewable and Sustainable Energy Reviews, 51*, 699–717.

Balasamy, S., Sakthivelan, P., Magesh, V., & Sundramoorthy, A.K. (2025). Synthesis and biocompatibility studies of 2D molybdenum carbide (MXene) nanosheets and their potential uses. *Nanomedicine* (London, England), *20*, 1537–1547.

Balsalobre-Lorente, D., & Shah, S. A. R. (2024). Stay circular economy, empowerment, and natural resource utilization factual factors for SDG 12? The principal role of digital technologies. *Journal of Environmental Management, 370*, Article 122459.

Basheer, N., Senthilnayaki, B., & Narayanan, M. (2025). Diabetic retinopathy detection in retinal OCT images with fused ResNet features. In *2025 International Conference on Frontier Technologies and Solutions (ICFTS)*, pp. 1–6.

Bassoli, S. C., da Fonseca, Y. A., Wandurraga, H. J. L., Baeta, B. E. L., & de Souza Amaral, M. (2024). Research progress, trends, and future prospects on hydrothermal liquefaction of algae for biocrude production: A bibliometric analysis. *Biomass Conversion and Biorefinery, 14*, 28781–28796.

Beck, A., Knöttner, S., Unterluggauer, J., Halmschlager, D., & Hofmann, R. (2022). An integrated optimization model for industrial energy system retrofit with process scheduling, heat recovery, and energy supply system synthesis. *Processes, 10*, 572.

Behera, B. K., Varma, A., Behera, B. K., & Varma, A. (2019). Thermal conversions of biomass. *Bioenergy for Sustainability and Security*, 301–369.

Beschkov, V. N., & Angelov, I. K. (2025). Volatile fatty acid production versus methane and hydrogen in anaerobic digestion. *Fermentation 11*, 172.

Boodhoo, K., Flickinger, M., Woodley, J., & Emanuelsson, E. (2022). Bioprocess intensification: A route to efficient and sustainable biocatalytic transformations for the future. *Chemical Engineering and Processing-Process Intensification, 172*, Article 108793.

Borazjani, Z., Azin, R., Osfouri, S., Karami, R., Kennedy, E., & Stockenhuber, M. (2025). Hydrothermal liquefaction of Caulerpa sertularioides: Optimized biocrude production and characterization with pretreatment techniques. *Biomass and Bioenergy, 194*, Article 107635.

Carmona-Martínez, A. A., Rueda, A., & Jarauta-Córdoba, C. A. (2024). Deep decarbonization of the energy intensive manufacturing industry through the bioconversion of its carbon emissions to fuels. *Fuel, 371*, Article 131922.

Chen, W., Huang, Z., & Chua, K. J. (2022). Sustainable energy recovery from thermal processes: A review. *Energy, Sustainability and Society, 12*, 46.

Chopra, J., Rangarajan, V., Rathnasamy, S., & Dey, P. (2024). Life cycle assessment as a key decision tool for emerging pretreatment technologies of Biomass-to-Biofuel: Unveiling challenges, advances, and future potential. *BioEnergy Research, 17*, 857–876.

Cross, S., Welfle, A. J., Thornley, P., Syri, S., & Mikaelsson, M. (2021). Bioenergy development in the UK & Nordic countries: A comparison of effectiveness of support policies for sustainable development of the bioenergy sector. *Biomass and Bioenergy, 144*, Article 105887.

Dada, T. K., Sheehan, M., Murugavelh, S., & Antunes, E. (2023). A review on catalytic pyrolysis for high-quality bio-oil production from biomass. *Biomass Conversion and Biorefinery, 13*, 2595–2614.

Das, O., Zafar, M. H., Sanfilippo, F., Rudra, S., & Kolhe, M. L. (2024). Advancements in digital twin technology and machine learning for energy systems: A comprehensive review of applications in smart grids, renewable energy, and electric vehicle optimisation. *Energy Conversion and Management X*, 100715.

Deepika, C., Mrinal, Pohrmen, C. B., Jaiswal, K. S., Sangmesh, B., Jaiswal, K. K., Ramasamy, A. P., & Jaiswal, A. K. (2024). Hydrothermal liquefaction of wet microalgal biomass for biofuels and platform chemicals: Advances and future prospects. *Discover Applied Sciences 6*, 245.

Diment, D., Löfgren, J., Alopaeus, M., Stosiek, M., Cho, M., Xu, C., Hummel, M., Rigo, D., Rinke, P., & Balakshin, M. (2025). Enhancing lignin-carbohydrate complexes production and properties with machine learning. *Chemsuschem, 18*, Article e202401711.

Dobre, C., Costin, M., & Constantin, M. (2024). A review of available solutions for implementation of small–medium combined heat and power (CHP) systems. *Inventions, 9*, 82.

dos Santos, R. G., & Alencar, A. C. (2020). Biomass-derived syngas production via gasification process and its catalytic conversion into fuels by Fischer Tropsch synthesis: A review. *International Journal of Hydrogen Energy, 45*, 18114–18132.

Duca, D., & Toscano, G. (2022). Biomass energy resources: Feedstock quality and bioenergy sustainability. *MDPI, 57*

Dupont, E., Germain, M., & Jeanmart, H. (2021). Estimate of the societal energy return on investment (EROI). *Biophysical Economics and Sustainability, 6*, 1–14.

El-Araby, R. (2024). Biofuel production: Exploring renewable energy solutions for a greener future. *Biotechnology for Biofuels and Bioproducts, 17*, 129.

Elkady, S., Hernantes, J., & Labaka, L. (2024). Decision-making for community resilience: A review of decision support systems and their applications. *Heliyon, 10*, Article e33116.

Falcone, P. M. (2023). Sustainable energy policies in developing countries: A review of challenges and opportunities. *Energies, 16*, 6682.

Gaur, V. K., Gautam, K., Sharma, P., Gupta, S., Pandey, A., You, S., & Varjani, S. (2022). Carbon-based catalyst for environmental bioremediation and sustainability: Updates and perspectives on techno-economics and life cycle assessment. *Environmental Research, 209*, Article 112793.

Ghodke, P. K., Sharma, A. K., Jayaseelan, A., & Gopinath, K. (2023). Hydrogen-rich syngas production from the lignocellulosic biomass by catalytic gasification: A state of art review on advance technologies, economic challenges, and future prospectus. *Fuel, 342*, Article 127800.

Glushkov, D., Nyashina, G., Shvets, A., Pereira, A., & Ramanathan, A. (2021). Current status of the pyrolysis and gasification mechanism of biomass. *Energies, 14*, 7541.

Gotore, O., Nguyen, T. T., Masere, T. P., Shumba, A., Gumbo, A., Sittisom, P., Heritier, M. A., & Itayama, T. (2025). Biochar-synergy in anaerobic digestion of animal wastes for total pollution control and bioenergy production: A sustainable integrated perspective. *Cleaner Chemical Engineering, 11*, Article 100177.

Haldar, S., Hoffman, J., Verma, M., Peddibhotla, A., & Bazaz, A. (2024). Reimagining energy infrastructure for justice: Power, politics, and institutional work in India's 2.05 GW Pavagada solar park. *Energy Research & Social Science 116*, 103645.

Hossain, N., Mahmud, M. Z. A., Hossain, A., Rahman, M. K., Islam, M. S., Tasnim, R., & Mobarak, M. H. (2024). Advances of materials science in MEMS applications: A review. *Results in Engineering, 22*, Article 102115.

Intasian, P., Prakinee, K., Phintha, A., Trisrivirat, D., Weeranoppanant, N., Wongnate, T., & Chaiyen, P. (2021). Enzymes, in vivo biocatalysis, and metabolic engineering for enabling a circular economy and sustainability. *Chemical Reviews, 121*, 10367–10451.

Jahangeer, M., Rehman, M. U., Nelofer, R., Nadeem, M., Munir, B., Smułek, W., Jesionowski, T., & Qamar, S. A. (2024). Biotransformation of lignocellulosic biomass to value-added bioproducts: insights into bio-saccharification strategies and potential concerns. *Topics in Catalysis*, 1–22.

Jaiswal, N., & Jaiswal, P. (2024). Thermostable α-amylases and Laccases: Paving the way for sustainable industrial applications. *Processes, 12*, 1341.

Jameel, M. K., Mustafa, M. A., Ahmed, H. S., Mohammed, A. J., Ghazy, H., Shakir, M. N., Lawas, A. M., Mohammed, S. K., Idan, A. H., Mahmoud, Z. H., Sayadi, H., & Kianfar, E. (2024). Biogas: Production, properties, applications, economic and challenges: A review. *Results in Chemistry 7*, 101549.

John, N., Fathima, P., Harsha, V., Paul, N. M., & Nisha, P. (2024). Physical conversion of biomass: dewatering, drying, size reduction, densification, and separation. Handbook of Biomass, pp. 987–1013 Springer.

Joshi, M., & Manjare, S. (2024). Chemical approaches for the biomass valorisation: A comprehensive review of pretreatment strategies. *Environmental Science and Pollution Research, 31*, 48928–48954.

Kandasamy, S., Narayanan, M., Raja, R., Devarayan, K., & Kavitha, R. (2023). The current state of algae in wastewater treatment and energy conversion: A critical review. *Current Opinion in Environmental Science & Health, 33*, Article 100469.

Kennes, D., Abubackar, H. N., Diaz, M., Veiga, M. C., & Kennes, C. (2016). Bioethanol production from biomass: Carbohydrate versus syngas fermentation. *Journal of Chemical Technology & Biotechnology, 91*, 304–317.

Kiss, A. A., & Smith, R. (2020). Rethinking energy use in distillation processes for a more sustainable chemical industry. *Energy, 203*, Article 117788.

Klemeš, J. J., Varbanov, P. S., Walmsley, T. G., & Jia, X. (2018). New directions in the implementation of Pinch Methodology (PM). *Renewable and Sustainable Energy Reviews, 98*, 439–468.

Krishna Rao, C., Sahoo, S. K., & Yanine, F. F. (2024). IoT enabled Intelligent Energy Management System employing advanced forecasting algorithms and load optimization strategies to enhance renewable energy generation. *Unconventional Resources, 4*, Article 100101.

Kumar, B., & Verma, P. (2020). Enzyme mediated multi-product process: A concept of bio-based refinery. *Industrial Crops and Products, 154*, Article 112607.

Lanucara, S., Praticò, S., Pioggia, G., Di Fazio, S., & Modica, G. (2024). Web-based spatial decision support system for precision agriculture: A tool for delineating dynamic management unit zones (MUZs). *Smart Agricultural Technology, 8*, Article 100444.

Li, T., Wang, J., Chen, H., Li, W., Pan, P., Wu, L., Xu, G., & Chen, H. (2023). Performance analysis of an integrated biomass-to-energy system based on gasification and pyrolysis. *Energy Conversion and Management, 287*, Article 117085.

Lin, H.-F., Mansir, I. B., Ameen, H. F. M., Cherif, A., Abdulwahab, A., Dahari, M., Lin, H., Aly, A. A., & Nasr, S. (2023). Economic, environmental and multi objective optimization of a clean tri-generation system based co-firing of natural gas and biomass: An emergy evaluation. *Process Safety and Environmental Protection, 173*, 289–303.

Lu, H., Xia, C., Chinnathambi, A., Nasif, O., Narayanan, M., Shanmugam, S., Chi, N. T. L., Pugazhendhi, A., On-Uma, R., & Jutamas, K. (2023). Evaluation of cadmium tolerance and remediated efficacy of wild and mutated Enterobacter species isolated from potassium nitrate (KNO_3) processing unit contaminated soil. *Chemosphere, 311*, Article 136899.

Luo, L., Cristofari, C., & Levrey, S. (2023). Cogeneration: Another way to increase energy efficiency of hybrid renewable energy hydrogen chain–A review of systems operating in cogeneration and of the energy efficiency assessment through exergy analysis. *Journal of Energy Storage, 66*, Article 107433.

Lutzu, G. A., Usai, L., Ciurli, A., Chiellini, C., Di Caprio, F., Pagnanelli, F., Parsaeimehr, A., Malina, I., Malins, K., & Fabbricino, M. (2024). Engineering strategies of microalgal cultivation for potential jet fuel production–A critical review. *Journal of Environmental Chemical Engineering, 12*, Article 113886.

Maitlo, G., Ali, I., Mangi, K. H., Ali, S., Maitlo, H. A., Unar, I. N., & Pirzada, A. M. (2022). Thermochemical conversion of biomass for syngas production: Current status and future trends. *Sustainability, 14*, 2596.

Mandley, S. J., Daioglou, V., Junginger, H. M., van Vuuren, D. P., & Wicke, B. (2020). EU bioenergy development to 2050. *Renewable and Sustainable Energy Reviews, 127*, Article 109858.

Mani, A., Narayanan, M., & Rajinikanth, V. (2024). Neurodegenerative marine algae bioactive compounds: A viable cure to treat amyotrophic lateral sclerosis (ALS): A Review. *Dubai Medical Journal 7*, 201–217–201–217.

Megía, P. J., Vizcaíno, A. J., Calles, J. A., & Carrero, A. (2021). Hydrogen production technologies: From fossil fuels toward renewable sources. *A Mini Review. Energy & Fuels, 35*, 16403–16415.

Mishra, R. K., Kumar, D. J. P., Narula, A., Chistie, S. M., & Naik, S. U. (2023). Production and beneficial impact of biochar for environmental application: A review on types of feedstocks, chemical compositions, operating parameters, techno-economic study, and life cycle assessment. *Fuel, 343*, Article 127968.

Mohamed Almazrouei, S., Dweiri, F., Aydin, R., & Alnaqbi, A. (2023). A review on the advancements and challenges of artificial intelligence based models for predictive maintenance of water injection pumps in the oil and gas industry. *SN Applied Sciences, 5*, 391.

Mohan, D., Pittman, C. U., Jr., & Steele, P. H. (2006). Pyrolysis of wood/biomass for bio-oil: A critical review. *Energy & Fuels, 20*, 848–889.

Mohan, R., Narayanan, M., & Rajinikanth, V. (2024). Cancer region segmentation in pre-processed breast ultrasound image using VGG16 Based UNet/SegNet. In *2024 9th International Conference on Communication and Electronics Systems (ICCES)*. IEEE, pp. 1–6.

Mohanasundari, C., Anbalagan, S., Srinivasan, K., Chinnathambi, A., Salmen, S. H., Meganathan, V., & Narayanan, M. (2023). Evaluation of antibacterial efficacy of various solvent extracts of Evolvulus alsinoides and Mucuna pruriens against multidrug resistant (MDR) pathogenic bacteria. *Applied Nanoscience*, 1–11.

Mondejar, M. E., Avtar, R., Diaz, H. L. B., Dubey, R. K., Esteban, J., Gómez-Morales, A., Hallam, B., Mbungu, N. T., Okolo, C. C., Prasad, K. A., She, Q., & Garcia-Segura, S. (2021). Digitalization to achieve sustainable development goals: Steps towards a smart green planet. *Science of the Total Environment, 794*, Article 148539.

Nahak, B., Preetam, S., Sharma, D., Shukla, S., Syväjärvi, M., Toncu, D.-C., & Tiwari, A. (2022). Advancements in net-zero pertinency of lignocellulosic biomass for climate neutral energy production. *Renewable and Sustainable Energy Reviews, 161*, Article 112393.

Nair, L. G., & Verma, P. (2025). Harnessing carbon potential of lignocellulosic biomass: advances in pretreatments, applications, and the transformative role of machine learning in biorefineries. *Bioresources and Bioprocessing, 12.*

Nair, L. G., Agrawal, K., & Verma, P. (2022a). An insight into the principles of lignocellulosic biomass-based zero-waste biorefineries: A green leap towards imperishable energy-based future. *Biotechnology and Genetic Engineering Reviews, 38*, 288–338.

Nair, L. G., Agrawal, K., & Verma, P. (2022b). An overview of sustainable approaches for bioenergy production from agro-industrial wastes. *Energy Nexus, 6*, Article 100086.

Narayanan, M. (2023). Origination, fate, accumulation, and impact, of microplastics in a marine ecosystem and bio/technological approach for remediation: A review. *Process Safety and Environmental Protection, 177*, 472–485.

Narayanan, M. (2024a). Biorefinery products from algal biomass by advanced biotechnological and hydrothermal liquefaction approaches. *Discover Applied Sciences, 6*, 146.

Narayanan, M. (2024b). Evaluation of antibacterial (Antibiofilm) activity potential of ZnONPs coated on wound dressing cloth. *Dubai Medical Journal 7*, 149–159–149–159

Narayanan, M. (2025). An evaluation of antibacterial, antioxidant, and biocompatibility (hemocompatibility) nature of green synthesized ZnONPs: an in-vitro approach. *Dubai Medical Journal*, 1–11–11–11.

Narayanan, M., & Ma, Y. (2024). Recent progress on conservation and restoration of soil fertility for horticulture. *Chemosphere*, 142599.

Narayanan, M., & Rajinikanth, V. (2025). Effects of bioactive compounds from marine algae on cancer-related inflammation: A review. *Medical Oncology, 42*, 1–18.

Narayanan, M., Ayyandurai, M., & Rajinikanth, V. (2024a). Exosomes: A fluid biopsy source for clinical interventions of noncommunicable diseases treatment: A Review. *Dubai Medical Journal 7*, 39–54–39–54.

Narayanan, M., Deepika, M., Ma, Y., Nasif, O., Alharbi, S.A., Srinivasan, R., & Natarajan, D. (2021a). Phyto-fabrication, characterization, and biomedical activity of silver nanoparticles mediated from an epiphytic plant Luisia tenuifolia Blume. *Applied Nanoscience*, 1–11.

Narayanan, M., Mohan, R., & Rajinikanth, V. (2024b). Solar cell defect detection using deep-learning segmentation with two-fold training. In *2024 9th International Conference on Communication and Electronics Systems (ICCES).* IEEE, pp. 168–172.

Narayanan, M., Vijay, A., Kandasamy, S., Nasif, O., Alharbi, S. A., Srinivasan, R., & Kavitha, R. (2021b). Phytochemical profile and larvicidal activity of aqueous extract of Ocimum americanum against mosquito vectors. *Applied Nanoscience*, 1–13.

Ndukwu, M. C., Horsfall, I. T., Ubouh, E. A., Orji, F. N., Ekop, I. E., & Ezejiofor, N. R. (2021). Review of solar-biomass pyrolysis systems: Focus on the configuration of thermal-solar systems and reactor orientation. *Journal of King Saud University–Engineering Sciences, 33*, 413–423.

Negi, S., Chai, J.-Y., Tjhin, A. C. T., & Pan, S.-Y. (2025). Electro-anaerobic digestion as carbon–neutral solutions. *Chemical and Biological Technologies in Agriculture, 12*, 64.

Ngabala, F. J., & Emmanuel, J. K. (2024). Potential substrates for biogas production through anaerobic digestion-an alternative energy source. *Heliyon, 10*, Article e40632.

Nguyen, T., Nguyen, H., & Nguyen Gia, T. (2024). Exploring the integration of edge computing and blockchain IoT: Principles, architectures, security, and applications. *Journal of Network and Computer Applications, 226*, Article 103884.

Nnabuife, S. G., Hamzat, A. K., Whidborne, J., Kuang, B., & Jenkins, K. W. (2025). Integration of renewable energy sources in tandem with electrolysis: A technology review for green hydrogen production. *International Journal of Hydrogen Energy, 107*, 218–240.

Nunes, L. J. (2024). Exploring the present and future of biomass recovery units: Technological innovation, policy incentives and economic challenges. *Biofuels, 15*, 375–387.

Olabi, A. G., Elsaid, K., Obaideen, K., Abdelkareem, M. A., Rezk, H., Wilberforce, T., Maghrabie, H. M., & Sayed, E. T. (2023). Renewable energy systems: Comparisons, challenges and barriers, sustainability indicators, and the contribution to UN sustainable development goals. *International Journal of Thermofluids, 20*, Article 100498.

Olguin-Maciel, E., Singh, A., Chable-Villacis, R., Tapia-Tussell, R., & Ruiz, H. A. (2020). Consolidated bioprocessing, an innovative strategy towards sustainability for biofuels production from crop residues: An overview. *Agronomy, 10*, 1834.

Osman, A. I., Chen, Z., Elgarahy, A. M., Farghali, M., Mohamed, I. M., Priya, A., Hawash, H. B., & Yap, P. S. (2024). Membrane technology for energy saving: Principles, techniques, applications, challenges, and prospects. *Advanced Energy and Sustainability Research, 5*, 2400011.

Pandey, A., & Sharma, Y. C. (2024). Advancements in biomass valorization in integrated biorefinery systems. *Biofuels, Bioproducts and Biorefining, 18*, 2078–2090.

Pandey, V., Sircar, A., Bist, N., Solanki, K., & Yadav, K. (2023). Accelerating the renewable energy sector through Industry 4.0: Optimization opportunities in the digital revolution. *International Journal of Innovation Studies, 7*, 171–188.

Paramasivam, G., Yadavali, S.P., Atchudan, R., Arya, S., & Sundramoorthy, A.K. (2024) Recent advances in the medical applications of two-dimensional MXene nanosheets. *Nanomedicine, 19*, 2633–2654.

Parveen, B., Narayanan, M., & Rajinikanth, V. (2025). Empowering patient self-care in plantar hyperkeratotic/palmoplantar keratodermas eczema: A case report. *Dubai Medical Journal 8*, 42–47–42–47.

Paudel, P. P., Kafle, S., Park, S., Kim, S. J., Cho, L., & Kim, D. H. (2024). Advancements in sustainable thermochemical conversion of agricultural crop residues: A systematic review of technical progress, applications, perspectives, and challenges. *Renewable and Sustainable Energy Reviews, 202*, Article 114723.

Peng, W., Lü, F., Hao, L., Zhang, H., Shao, L., & He, P. (2020). Digestate management for high-solid anaerobic digestion of organic wastes: A review. *Bioresource Technology, 297*, Article 122485.

Poornima, S., Manikandan, S., Prakash, R., Deena, S. R., Subbaiya, R., Karmegam, N., Kim, W., & Govarthanan, M. (2024). Biofuel and biochemical production through biomass transformation using advanced thermochemical and biochemical processes–a review. *Fuel, 372*, Article 132204.

Qadir, S. A., Al-Motairi, H., Tahir, F., & Al-Fagih, L. (2021). Incentives and strategies for financing the renewable energy transition: A review. *Energy Reports, 7*, 3590–3606.

Radhakrishnan, N., & Narayanan, M. (2025). Diffuse pulmonary lesions due to invasive fungal infection in an immune-capable male: A case report. *Dubai Medical Journal., 8*(2), 1–8. https://doi.org/10.18502/DMJ-41

Rajendran, L. P., Raúl, L., Chen, M., Guerrero Andrade, J. C., Akhtar, R., Mngumi, L. E., Chander, S., Srinivas, S., & Roy, M. R. (2024). The 'peri-urban turn': A systems thinking approach for a paradigm shift in reconceptualising urban-rural futures in the global South. *Habitat International, 146*, Article 103041.

Rajinikanth, V., Mohan, R., & Narayanan, M. (2024a). Deep learning and features fusion for colorectal cancer detection from histopathology images. In *2024 9th International Conference on Communication and Electronics Systems (ICCES)*. IEEE, pp. 1406–1411.

Rajinikanth, V., Mohan, R., & Narayanan, M. (2024b). Parameter estimation of PEM fuel-cell using brownian butterfly algorithm. In *2024 International Conference on System, Computation, Automation and Networking (ICSCAN)*. IEEE, pp. 1–5.

Ramos, A., Monteiro, E., & Rouboa, A. (2022). Biomass pre-treatment techniques for the production of biofuels using thermal conversion methods–a review. *Energy Conversion and Management, 270*, Article 116271.

Rocco, M. V., Colombo, E., & Sciubba, E. (2014). Advances in exergy analysis: A novel assessment of the extended exergy accounting method. *Applied Energy, 113*, 1405–1420.
Rozina, Emmanuel, O., & Ezeji, T. C. (2024). Exploring the synergy of nanomaterials and microbial cell factories during biohydrogen and biobutanol production from different carbon sources. *Sustainable Chemistry for the Environment 6*, 100098.
Ryu, H., Lee, D., Shin, J., Song, M., Lee, S., Kim, H., & Kim, B.-I. (2023). A web-based decision support system (DSS) for hydrogen refueling station location and supply chain optimization. *International Journal of Hydrogen Energy, 48*, 36223–36239.
Sakheta, A., Nayak, R., O'Hara, I., & Ramirez, J. (2023). A review on modelling of thermochemical processing of biomass for biofuels and prospects of artificial intelligence-enhanced approaches. *Bioresource Technology, 386*, Article 129490.
Saleem, M. (2022). Possibility of utilizing agriculture biomass as a renewable and sustainable future energy source. *Heliyon, 8*, Article e08905.
Samoraj, M., Çalış, D., Trzaska, K., Mironiuk, M., & Chojnacka, K. (2024). Advancements in algal biorefineries for sustainable agriculture: Biofuels, high-value products, and environmental solutions. *Biocatalysis and Agricultural Biotechnology, 58*, Article 103224.
Sar, T., Harirchi, S., Yazdian, F., & Taherzadeh, M. J. (2023). Microorganisms used in biorefineries. *Biotic Resources*, 21–58
Sarker, S., Lamb, J. J., Hjelme, D. R., & Lien, K. M. (2019). A review of the role of critical parameters in the design and operation of biogas production plants. *Applied Sciences, 9*, 1915.
Sarker, T. R., Nanda, S., Meda, V., & Dalai, A. K. (2023). Densification of waste biomass for manufacturing solid biofuel pellets: A review. *Environmental Chemistry Letters, 21*, 231–264.
Scheelhaase, J., Maertens, S., & Grimme, W. (2021). Options for improving the EU emissions trading scheme (EU ETS) for aviation. *Transportation Research Procedia, 59*, 193–202.
Schipfer, F., Mäki, E., Schmieder, U., Lange, N., Schildhauer, T., Hennig, C., & Thrän, D. (2022). Status of and expectations for flexible bioenergy to support resource efficiency and to accelerate the energy transition. *Renewable and Sustainable Energy Reviews, 158*, Article 112094.
Shah, T. M., Khan, A. H., Nicholls, C., Sohoo, I., & Otterpohl, R. (2023). Using landfill sites and marginal lands for socio-economically sustainable biomass production through cultivation of non-food energy crops: An analysis focused on South Asia and Europe. *Sustainability, 15*, 4923.
Shahbaz, M., Ammar, M., Korai, R. M., Ahmad, N., Ali, A., Khalid, M. S., Zou, D., & Li, X. (2020). Impact of C/N ratios and organic loading rates of paper, cardboard and tissue wastes in batch and CSTR anaerobic digestion with food waste on their biogas production and digester stability. *SN Applied Sciences, 2*, 1–13.
Shao, C., Zhao, Y., & Qu, L. (2022). Recent advances in highly integrated energy conversion and storage system. *SusMat, 2*, 142–160.
Shi, Z., Ferrari, G., Ai, P., Marinello, F., & Pezzuolo, A. (2023). Artificial Intelligence for biomass detection, production and energy usage in rural areas: A review of technologies and applications. *Sustainable Energy Technologies and Assessments, 60*, Article 103548.
Singh, R., Dogra, S., Dixit, S., Vatin, N. I., Bhardwaj, R., Sundramoorthy, A. K., Perera, H. C. S., Patole, S. P., Mishra, R. K., & Arya, S. (2024). Advancements in thermoelectric materials for efficient waste heat recovery and renewable energy generation. *Hybrid Advances, 5*, Article 100176.
Singhania, R. R., Patel, A. K., Singh, A., Haldar, D., Soam, S., Chen, C.-W., Tsai, M.-L., & Dong, C.-D. (2022). Consolidated bioprocessing of lignocellulosic biomass: Technological advances and challenges. *Bioresource Technology, 354*, Article 127153.
Talari, G., Cummins, E., McNamara, C., & O'Brien, J. (2022). State of the art review of big data and web-based decision support systems (DSS) for food safety risk assessment with respect to climate change. *Trends in Food Science & Technology, 126*, 192–204.
Tarekegne, B. (2021). Centralized versus decentralized electrification pathways. *Affordable and Clean Energy*, 117–126.
Thaha, A. N., Ghamari, M., Jothiprakash, G., Velusamy, S., Karthikeyan, S., Ramesh, D., & Sundaram, S. (2025). High impact biomass valorization for second generation Biorefineries

in India: Recent developments and future strategies for sustainable circular economy. *Biomass, 5*, 16.

Thanh, N. C., Narayanan, M., Saravanan, M., Chinnathambi, A., Alahmadi, T. A., Brindhadevi, K., Sharma, A., & Pugazhendhi, A. (2023a). Hibiscus rosa-sinensis as a potential hyperaccumulator in metal contaminated magnesite mine tailings. *Chemosphere, 339*, Article 139738.

Thanh, N. C., Narayanan, M., Saravanan, M., Chinnathambi, A., Alharbi, S. A., Brindhadevi, K., Sharma, A., & Pugazhendhi, A. (2023b). Bio/phyremediation potential of Leptospirillum ferrooxidans and Ricinus communis on metal contaminated mine sludge. *Chemosphere, 339*, Article 139739.

Thirumalaivasan, N., Nangan, S., Kanagaraj, K., & Rajendran, S. (2024). Assessment of sustainability and environmental impacts of renewable energies: Focusing on biogas and biohydrogen (Biofuels) production. *Process Safety and Environmental Protection, 189*, 467–485.

Thrän, D., Adetona, A., Borchers, M., Cyffka, K.-F., Daniel-Gromke, J., & Oehmichen, K. (2025). Potential contribution of biogas to net zero energy systems–A comparative study of Canada and Germany. *Biomass and Bioenergy, 193*, Article 107561.

Tshikovhi, A., & Motaung, T. E. (2023). Technologies and innovations for biomass energy production. *Sustainability, 15*, 12121.

Vaish, S., Sharma, N. K., & Kaur, G. (2022). A review on various types of densification/briquetting technologies of biomass residues. *IOP conference series: materials science and engineering*, p. 012019. IOP Publishing.

Varghese, S.M., Srihari, R.S., Anagha, M.O., & Rakhi, R.B. (2025). Transition metal Oxide–decorated titanium carbide MXene electrodes for high-energy supercapacitors with an expanded potential windo. *Batteries and Supercaps*, 2500304.

Vassiliadis, V. S., Mappas, V., Espaas, T. A., Dorneanu, B., Isafiade, A., Möller, K., & Arellano-Garcia, H. (2024). Reloading process systems engineering within chemical engineering. *Chemical Engineering Research and Design.*

Vijayakumarr, K., Maziz, M. N. H., & Narayanan, M. (2025). Classification of Benign/Malignant digital mammogram images using deep learning scheme. In *2025 International Conference on Frontier Technologies and Solutions (ICFTS)*, pp. 1–6.

Vinestock, T., Short, M., Ward, K., & Guo, M. (2024). Computer-aided chemical engineering research advances in precision fermentation. *Current Opinion in Food Science, 101196.*

Wakeel, M., Hayat, T., Shah, N. S., Iqbal, J., Khan, Z. U. H., Shah, G. M., & Rasool, A. (2023). Biogas energy resources in Pakistan status, potential, and barriers. *Utilities Policy, 84*, Article 101643.

Wang, Q., Li, Y., & Li, R. (2025). Integrating artificial intelligence in energy transition: A comprehensive review. *Energy Strategy Reviews, 57*, Article 101600.

Williams, C. L., Westover, T. L., Emerson, R. M., Tumuluru, J. S., & Li, C. (2016). Sources of biomass feedstock variability and the potential impact on biofuels production. *BioEnergy Research, 9*, 1–14.

Woźniak, A., Kuligowski, K., Świerczek, L., & Cenian, A. (2025). Review of Lignocellulosic biomass pretreatment using physical, thermal and chemical methods for higher yields in bioethanol production. *Sustainability, 17*, 287.

Xu, H., Ou, L., Li, Y., Hawkins, T. R., & Wang, M. (2022). Life cycle greenhouse gas emissions of biodiesel and renewable diesel production in the United States. *Environmental Science and Technology, 56*, 7512–7521.

Zabaniotou, A. (2018). Redesigning a bioenergy sector in EU in the transition to circular waste-based Bioeconomy-A multidisciplinary review. *Journal of Cleaner Production, 177*, 197–206.

Zafar, M. H., Langås, E. F., & Sanfilippo, F. (2024). Exploring the synergies between collaborative robotics, digital twins, augmentation, and industry 5.0 for smart manufacturing: A state-of-the-art review. *Robotics and Computer-Integrated Manufacturing 89*, 102769.

Zaidi, S. M. N. B. S. W., Shirin, L., Hemalatha, S., & Narayanan, M. (2025). Automatic detection of happy/sad face images with DL-AN analysis. In *2025 International Conference on Frontier Technologies and Solutions (ICFTS)*, pp. 1–6.

Zheng, J.-L., Zhu, Y.-H., Sun, G.-T., Dong, Y.-Y., & Zhu, M.-Q. (2022). Bio-oil gasification for production of the raw gas as ammonia syngas. *Fuel, 327*, Article 125029.

Chapter 15
Advancements in Cellulosic Ethanol: Production Technologies, Commercial Challenges, and Strategic Solutions

Vaishnavi Kashyap, Karan Arya, Tanishq, Aditya Sharma, Priya Kumari, Parul Bali, and Ravi Kant Bhatia

Abstract Cellulosic ethanol has emerged as a key component of next-generation biofuels, providing a sustainable alternative to fossil fuels while overcoming the limitations of first-generation ethanol derived from food crops. Cellulosic ethanol, which is made from lignocellulosic biomass such as agricultural residues, forestry byproducts, and dedicated energy crops, takes advantage of abundant non-edible feedstocks, reducing competition with food supply chains. This chapter examines the technological advances driving cellulosic ethanol production, with a focus on pretreatment innovations, enzymatic hydrolysis, microbial fermentation, and process integration. It highlights advances in consolidated bioprocessing, metabolic engineering of robust microbes, and energy-efficient separation methods that improve yields while lowering costs. Despite these advances, commercialization still faces significant challenges, such as high capital investment, enzyme costs, feedstock variability, and complex logistics. The chapter examines case studies of operational biorefineries and the economic, environmental, and policy barriers that have slowed their widespread deployment. It also investigates strategic solutions for increasing competitiveness, such as biorefinery integration, lignin and co-product valorization, supportive policy frameworks, and circular bioeconomy approaches. This chapter emphasizes cellulosic ethanol's potential to significantly contribute to global decarbonization goals, energy security, and rural development by linking technological innovation with strategic planning.

Keywords Cellulosic ethanol · Lignocellulosic biomass · Pretreatment technologies · Enzymatic hydrolysis · Consolidated bioprocessing (CBP) · Techno-economic challenges

V. Kashyap · K. Arya · Tanishq · A. Sharma · R. K. Bhatia (✉)
Department of Biotechnology, Himachal Pradesh University, Summer Hill, Shimla, India
e-mail: ravibiotech07@gmail.com

P. Kumari · P. Bali
Department of Microbiology, Himachal Pradesh University, Summer Hill, Shimla, India

P. Verma (ed.), *Sustainable Practices in Biorefinery*,
https://doi.org/10.1007/978-981-95-6071-4_15

15.1 Introduction

For thousands of years, humanity has relied on the natural world for warmth, light, and sustenance. Early civilizations survived by burning wood, dried grasses, and other plant matter the very first biofuels, the original "fuels of life." Yet it was not until the late nineteenth century that the seeds of the modern biofuel revolution were sown. In the 1890s, Rudolf Diesel unveiled his remarkable invention, the diesel engine (Samil, 2007). In a vision far ahead of its time, Diesel imagined his engine running not on fossil fuels but on vegetable oils such as peanut oil (Chaudhary et al., 2025). The 1970s brought turmoil as oil crises shook global economies and exposed the fragility of energy security. It was during this decade that the word "biofuel" entered our modern vocabulary, denoting fuels derived not from fossil reserves but from life itself plants, algae, and biomass (Jeswani et al., 2020; Timilsina & Shrestha, 2011). Governments responded with bold initiatives. Brazil launched the Proálcool Program in 1975, turning sugarcane into a national energy resource. In 1978, the U.S. Department of Energy began the Aquatic Species Program, envisioning algae as a future fuel (Maheshwari et al., 2020). South Africa pioneered biodiesel from sunflower oil in 1979, establishing the continent's first commercial biodiesel plant by 1987. In India, innovation also surged: ethanol-blended fuels were explored as early as 1975, with the Indian Oil Corporation conducting vehicle trials by 1980. The first pilot program for 5% ethanol blending began in 2001, followed by the ambitious National Mission on Biofuels in 2003 (Jiménez-Islas et al., 2021), which emphasized non-edible oilseeds like Jatropha to reduce fossil fuel dependence and empower rural communities.

This marked the dawn of second-generation biofuels. Among them, cellulosic ethanol emerged as the most promising produced not from food crops but from agricultural residues, forest waste, and energy grasses (Kumar et al., 2020). Cleaner than gasoline or diesel, it generates fewer carbon emissions, negligible sulfur, and reduced particulate matter (Mukherjee & Arkalji, 2025). In 2009, India codified its ambitions with the National Policy on Biofuels, targeting 20% ethanol and biodiesel blending by 2017 (Azadi et al., 2017). A revised policy in 2018 expanded the focus to second- and third-generation biofuels, including algae, aiming for 20% ethanol blending in petrol and 5% biodiesel blending in diesel by 2030. By 2025, India has reached a remarkable milestone, achieving 19.6% ethanol blending and emerging as the world's third-largest producer of biofuels (Puri, 2025). This achievement, driven by scientific innovation and collective commitment, has not only reduced dependence on fuel imports but also cut greenhouse gas emissions and strengthened rural livelihoods. The journey of biofuels is, therefore, more than a tale of technology and policy it reflects humanity's evolving harmony with nature. It illustrates how, by drawing energy from life itself, we can build a future that is sustainable, equitable, and inspiring.

15.2 Cellulosic Ethanol

A transformative form of biofuel is emerging—rooted in the very structure of plants. Unlike conventional ethanol, which relies on the sugars and starches of food crops such as corn and sugarcane, cellulosic ethanol is derived from non-food biomass often considered agricultural or industrial waste (Chundawat et al., 2011). This includes crop residues like corn stover, sugarcane bagasse, and wheat straw; forestry by-products such as sawdust, wood chips, and timber remnants (Rathour et al., 2023a, 2023b); dedicated energy crops like switchgrass, miscanthus, kenaf, and giant reed; and even the organic fraction of municipal solid waste. However, converting this material into fuel is complex. Cellulose, the structural framework of plants, is highly resistant an evolutionary triumph in durability (Fortuin et al., 2025). Unlocking its energy requires advanced pretreatment, hydrolysis, and fermentation (Bhatt et al., 2018). With the aid of specialized enzymes and engineered microbes, this once formidable challenge is becoming increasingly viable. The potential of cellulosic ethanol is immense. It transforms residues and non-food crops into clean-burning fuel without competing with food resources (Nielsen et al., 2020), while achieving up to 90% lower greenhouse gas emissions compared to petrol. By utilizing locally available biomass, it strengthens energy security, reduces reliance on oil imports, and revitalizes rural economies (Chauhan et al., 2025).

15.2.1 Generations of Ethanol

First-generation ethanol, produced from food crops, is commercially established but fraught with drawbacks—competition with food supplies, water stress, and land degradation (Shrestha et al., 2011). While it offers modest emission reductions compared to petrol, its sustainability is limited. Cellulosic ethanol, by contrast, is derived from residues, wild grasses, and woody biomass resources that do not threaten food security. It enables deeper greenhouse gas cuts, can grow on marginal lands, and even aids soil restoration (Gupta & Tuohy, 2013a, 2013b). Although cost and large-scale deployment remain hurdles, it embodies innovation with the power to create livelihoods, secure energy futures, and guide humanity toward a cleaner, more sustainable balance with nature. A comparative analysis of first and second generation biofuels is summarised in Table 15.1.

First-generation ethanol, while simpler and cheaper to produce, comes with a troubling dilemma such as diverting food crops for fuel, and offering only modest environmental gains. In contrast, cellulosic ethanol, drawn from the inedible remnants of plants, holds far greater promise (Hirani et al., 2018). It offers cleaner emissions and deeper sustainability. Yet, the path forward is not without challenge, costs remain high, and the science is still evolving (Azadi et al., 2017).

Table 15.1 Benefits of cellulosic ethanol compared with 1st generation ethanol

	1st Generation ethanol	2nd Generation ethanol
Source	Food crops- Competes with food supply	Non-food biomass- Uses agricultural waste or other wild crops
Examples	Corn, sugarcane, and wheat	Crop residues, grasses (Jatropha), and wood
Environmental	Greenhouse emission reduction by 20–40% compared to gasoline	Greenhouse emission reduction by almost 90%
	Requires arable land which may cause deforestation	Can be grown on marginal lands or use existing waste lands
	High water usage	Low water usage overall
	May cause soil degradation such as overproduction of corn crop	Less likely as perennial crops improve soil and prevent erosion
Economic	Low production cost (mature technology and infrastructure)	Higher production cost (complex process, however it is scaling up, R&D in progress)
	Has a commercially established global market	Commercially has an emerging market which is improving with innovation
	Limited job opportunities in farming and ethanol plants	Does have scope for jobs in farming, R&D, collection, and bio refineries
	Globally it is heavily subsidized	At the moment it is supported through R&D grants and renewable fuel standards

15.2.2 Production Processes for Cellulosic Ethanol

Cellulosic ethanol is a renewable biofuel that offers a more sustainable alternative to both gasoline and first-generation biofuels, which are derived from food crops. Unlike conventional ethanol, it is produced from cellulosic materials such as agricultural residues (e.g., rice straw, maize stover) and other lignocellulosic resources (Rathour et al., 2023a, 2023b). The process begins with the collection of plant waste, collectively referred to as cellulosic biomass, which is primarily composed of cellulose, hemicellulose, and lignin (Rathour et al., 2025). To release fermentable sugars, the biomass undergoes pretreatment, which may be thermal, chemical, or enzymatic. This step breaks down the rigid plant cell walls, making cellulose fibers more accessible. The cellulose is then subjected to enzymatic hydrolysis, converting it into simple sugars, which can subsequently be fermented into ethanol as depicted in Fig. 15.1 (Gupta et al., 2013). This pathway allows cellulosic ethanol to utilize non-food resources, reducing competition with food supplies while offering significant environmental benefits.

For the pretreated biomass, special carbohydrate-binding proteins known as lignocellulose sap proteins (often referred to as specialty enzymes) are used so that complicated carbs like cellulose and hemicellulose can be hydrolysed and fermentable sugars are extracted (Suri et al., 2022). Fermentation tanks are adept at receiving the sugar solution and the yeast or other microorganisms that are to be added. These

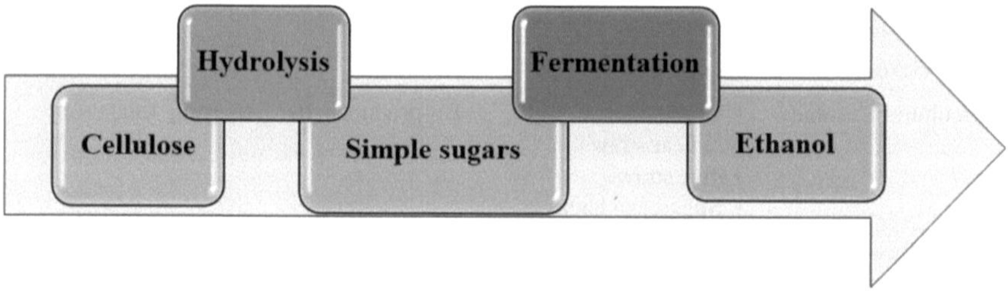

Fig. 15.1 Schematic diagram of cellulosic ethanol production

microorganisms utilize the carbohydrates and produce ethanol and carbon dioxide. It is a fermentation process that takes days to complete and is part of the process of turning corn and sugarcane into ethanol (Dwivedi et al., 2022). The ethanol that is mixed with the fermentation mixture undergoes distillation so that water and other impurities can be removed. Recycled plant material not required for other uses can instead be utilized for the more efficient and less polluting processes with the purified cellulosic ethanol that can be integrated with gasoline, reducing greenhouse gas emissions.

15.2.3 Feedstock Sources

Maize, sugarcane, and sugar beet are the most common traditional crops used for bioethanol production. However, their large-scale use is limited because of their primary role as food and feed. For example, starch from agricultural commodities, particularly maize, accounts for over 99% of global ethanol production (Saini et al., 2015). Yet, the heavy reliance on these food crops raises concerns regarding food security and resource competition. Agricultural residues such as sorghum straw, millet straw, and maize stalks represent nearly 75% of the potential lignocellulosic resources available from fields (Nassir & Al-Sahlany, 2021). These residues, along with wheat straw, rice bran, rice straw, corn stover, and sugarcane bagasse, form the basis of cellulosic ethanol, classified as a second-generation biofuel (Neha, 2013).

Unlike starch-based ethanol, which can be produced through relatively straightforward hydrolysis, lignocellulosic biomass is far more resistant to degradation and demands advanced pretreatment and conversion strategies (Chauhan et al., 2025). In such processes, cellulose and hemicellulose are deconstructed into fermentable sugars, which are then fermented into ethanol using well-established techniques adapted from first-generation systems (Nanda et al., 2018). Beyond agricultural residues, woody biomass serves as another important feedstock, with sawdust, wood chips, and other forestry by-products offering significant potential as shown in Table 15.2 (Vohra et al., 2014). Dedicated energy crops like switchgrass and

Table 15.2 Cellulosic ethanol sources with examples and categories

Feedstock sources	Examples	Remarks
Agricultural Residues	• Corn stover • Wheat straw • Rice straw • Sugarcane bagasse	By-products after harvesting food crops
Forestry Residues	• Wood chips • Sawdust • Bark • Logging waste	Leftover from timber and paper industries
Energy Crops	• Switchgrass • Miscanthus • Poplar • Willow	Grown specifically for biofuel production

miscanthus are also under intensive research and development for large-scale deployment due to their high productivity and resilience (Bušić et al., 2018). Altogether, these resources underscore the promise of cellulosic ethanol as a sustainable fuel pathway—minimizing reliance on food crops, valorizing waste streams, and providing a scalable alternative to address rising global energy demands.

15.2.4 Pretreatment Methods

Pretreatment essentially opens up the rigid structure of plant cell walls, enabling enzymes—biological catalysts—to access and break them down into simple sugars (Beig et al., 2021). Since different biomasses vary in composition, they require distinct pretreatment methods, including physical, chemical, and biological approaches, to effectively disrupt lignin and hemicellulose. A single method alone is often insufficient for optimal results (Baruah et al., 2018).

15.2.4.1 Physical Pretreatment

Mechanical methods such as chipping, grinding, hammer and ball milling, compression milling, and agitation bead milling reduce particle size, decrease cellulose crystallinity, lower polymerization, and increase surface area, thereby improving enzyme accessibility (Bhatia et al., 2020). Other techniques—γ-radiation, ultrasound, electron beam irradiation, pulsed electric fields, UV, and microwave heating—further enhance digestibility by disrupting cell walls, reducing polymerization, and partially depolymerizing lignin. Liquid Hot Water (LHW) pretreatment, one of the most widely adopted, employs high-pressure saturated steam to hydrolyze hemicellulose. Sudden decompression then disrupts fibers, improving cellulose accessibility (Rana et al., 2019). Efficiency depends on temperature, particle size, moisture, and residence time. LHW can remove up to 80% of hemicellulose, enhance enzymatic digestibility, and produce prehydrolysates with fewer fermentation inhibitors, while reducing the need for neutralization and extensive size reduction (Beig et al., 2021; Rathoure et al., 2025).

15.2.4.2 Chemical Pretreatment

This method involves milling biomass, pre-soaking it in water, and treating it with an acid solution at controlled temperatures for a defined time. After treatment, the mixture is filtered to separate liquids from solids, followed by washing or neutralization of solids before enzymatic hydrolysis (Rathoure et al., 2025). The effectiveness of acid pretreatment depends on hydrogen ion concentration, as stronger acids with lower pKa values exhibit higher hydrolytic efficiency. Sulfuric acid (H_2SO_4) and phosphoric acid (H_3PO_4) are commonly used due to their cost-effectiveness and efficiency in hydrolyzing lignocellulosic biomass (Zhou et al., 2012). Concentrated acid pretreatment typically employs sulfuric acid (65–86% w/v), hydrochloric acid (41% w/w), or phosphoric acid (85% w/w) under mild conditions of 30–60 °C and low pressure, using dried and pulverized biomass (5–10% moisture).

In recent years, salts such as iron (III) chloride ($FeCl_3$) and calcium chloride ($CaCl_2$) have been explored as alternatives in biomass pretreatment (Bhatia et al., 2020). These salts hydrolyze in water to generate strong acidic environments, facilitating rapid hemicellulose removal. For example, treatment of olive tree wastes with $FeCl_3$ (0.26 M) at 152.6 °C for 30 min achieved 100% hemicellulose removal, with saccharification yielding 36.6 g glucose per 100 g biomass (Amin et al., 2017). Similarly, a combined $CaCl_2$–microwave pretreatment applied to maize stover demonstrated promising results. At optimal conditions (162.1 °C, 12 min), glucose recovery reached 65.5%, outperforming steam-exploded corn stover (1.5 MPa, 5 min) (Godin et al., 2016). Acid- and salt-assisted pretreatments serve as versatile and highly effective methods for disrupting lignocellulosic biomass. However, optimizing process conditions remains essential to balance sugar yield, energy requirements, cost efficiency, and environmental sustainability.

15.2.4.3 Biological Pretreatment

Biological pretreatment offers an eco-friendly and sustainable route for processing lignocellulosic biomass into cellulosic ethanol. This approach harnesses microorganisms, primarily fungi—such as white-rot, brown-rot, and soft-rot species—as well as certain bacteria, to degrade lignin and hemicellulose, which shield cellulose fibers in plant cell walls (Saritha et al., 2012; Nair et al., 2022). The goal is to increase cellulose accessibility for enzymatic hydrolysis by selectively removing or modifying these protective polymers through natural enzyme-mediated reactions. Typically, biological pretreatment is conducted under mild operating conditions, including ambient temperatures (25–30 °C), slightly acidic pH (4.5–6.0), and aerobic environments (Beig et al., 2021). In practice, biomass is moistened, inoculated with microbial cultures, and incubated to facilitate microbial growth. During incubation, the organisms secrete ligninolytic and hemicellulolytic enzymes that progressively disrupt lignin and open up the biomass matrix (Amin et al., 2017). Although this process is highly sustainable, requiring minimal energy and avoiding toxic chemicals, it is comparatively slow, often taking several days to weeks for substantial lignin degradation. Nevertheless, biological pretreatment remains a promising low-cost and environmentally friendly alternative, especially when combined with physical or chemical methods to balance efficiency with sustainability (Chauhan et al., 2025).

15.3 Bioethanol Production

Lignocellulosic bioethanol production relies on agricultural residues, forestry by-products, and dedicated energy crops rich in cellulose, hemicellulose, and lignin. The process begins with pretreatment to overcome biomass recalcitrance and enhance enzyme accessibility. Subsequently, cellulose and hemicellulose are hydrolyzed into fermentable sugars via enzymatic or acid hydrolysis, while lignin is generally utilized for energy recovery (Dwivedi et al., 2022). The liberated sugars are then fermented into ethanol by microorganisms, followed by distillation and dehydration to achieve fuel-grade ethanol. As a second-generation biofuel, lignocellulosic ethanol significantly reduces greenhouse gas emissions, avoids direct competition with food crops, and contributes to a circular bioeconomy, offering a sustainable alternative to fossil fuels and food-based ethanol (Carriquiry et al., 2011).

15.3.1 Fermentation

Fermentation represents a critical stage in cellulosic ethanol production, where fermentable sugars from hydrolyzed lignocellulosic biomass are converted into ethanol under anaerobic conditions. This step enables the transformation of agricultural and forestry residues into renewable fuels, aligning with global energy and climate goals (Kambam & Henson, 2010). Fermentation can be conducted in batch, fed-batch, or continuous modes, with fed-batch operation in stirred-tank bioreactors being the most widely applied at industrial scale due to its ability to maintain favorable conditions for microbial growth and ethanol productivity. The primary aim is to efficiently convert both hexose sugars (e.g., glucose) and pentose sugars (e.g., xylose, arabinose) derived from cellulose and hemicellulose into ethanol and carbon dioxide (Saritha et al., 2012).

Successful fermentation requires robust microorganisms capable of co-fermenting C6 and C5 sugars, tolerating pretreatment-derived inhibitors, and maintaining high ethanol yields as shown in Fig. 15.2 and summarised in Table 15.3. Advances

$$\underset{\text{Pentose}}{C_5H_{10}O_5} \xrightarrow{\textbf{Fermentation}} \underset{\text{Ethanol}}{5C_2H_5OH} + \underset{\text{Carbon Dioxide}}{5CO_2}$$

$$\underset{\text{Hexose}}{C_6H_{12}O_6} \xrightarrow{\textbf{Fermentation}} \underset{\text{Ethanol}}{2C_2H_5OH} + \underset{\text{Carbon Dioxide}}{2CO_2}$$

Fig. 15.2 Simplified ethanol production from hexoses and pentoses during the fermentation stage

Table 15.3 Microorganisms used for the production of various fermentable products from different substrates

Organism	Sugar utilized	Type of product formed	Fermentation technique
Saccharomyces cerevisiae	Glucose	Ethanol	Separate Hydrolysis and Fermentation (SHF)
Escherichia coli (engineered)	Glucose, Xylose, Arabinose	Ethanol	Simultaneous Saccharification and Fermentation (SSF)
Pichia stipites	Xylose	Ethanol	Separate Hydrolysis and Fermentation (SHF)
Zymomonas mobilis	Glucose, Fructose, Sucrose	Ethanol	Simultaneous Saccharification and Co-Fermentation (SSCF)
Clostridium thermocellum	Cellulose	Ethanol, Acetate, Lactate	Simultaneous Saccharification and Co-Fermentation (SSCF)
Thermoanaerobacterium saccharolyticum	Xylose, Glucose	Ethanol, Acetate	Consolidated Bioprocessing (CBP)

in metabolic engineering and microbial strain development continue to address these challenges, solidifying fermentation as the cornerstone of cost-effective and sustainable second-generation bioethanol production.

15.3.2 *Distillation and Purification*

After fermentation of lignocellulosic biomass, the resulting broth contains **ethanol**, **water**, **unfermented sugars**, **microbial cells**, and other by-products. To obtain **fuel-grade ethanol**, it must undergo a series of downstream processes, primarily **distillation and dehydration** (Nhien et al., 2021). Distillation is the most common and essential method for separating ethanol from the fermentation broth. It exploits the difference in boiling points between **ethanol (78.37 °C)** and **water (100 °C)**. In a distillation column, the mixture is heated, causing ethanol to vaporize first. The ethanol vapor is then condensed back into liquid form, achieving ethanol concentrations of **90–95%** (Bušić et al., 2018). Distillation is highly efficient and widely recognized in industry, but it has some limitations such as **volatile by-products** with boiling points similar to ethanol may remain after distillation, process is **energy-intensive and costly**, involving repeated vaporization and condensation., ethanol and water form an **azeotrope** at ~95.6% ethanol and 4.4% water, making complete separation impossible with conventional distillation (Ebrahimiaqda & Ogden, 2017).

However, to produce **anhydrous ethanol (>99% purity)** suitable for fuel applications, additional dehydration methods are employed such as a**zeotropic Distillation**—Involves adding a third component (e.g., benzene, cyclohexane) to break the ethanol–water azeotrope and enable water separation, **Molecular Sieves**—Synthetic zeolites with micropores selectively adsorb water, allowing production of > 99% pure ethanol (Nimangre et al., 2021), **Membrane-Based Processes (Pervaporation)**—Special membranes separate water from ethanol at the molecular level, offering energy efficiency, **Vacuum Distillation**—Reduces pressure to lower boiling points, thereby saving energy while improving separation efficiency. For non-fuel applications (e.g., beverages, pharmaceuticals), high ethanol concentrations are not required, making repeated distillation unnecessary and uneconomical. Research efforts have also focused on developing **alternatives to energy-intensive distillation** for bioethanol purification (Chandra et al., 2018).

15.4 Technological Challenges in Cellulosic Ethanol Production

Lignocellulosic biomass can be transformed into bioethanol via two different approaches i.e. biochemical or thermochemical conversion. Both routes involve degradation of the recalcitrant cell wall structure of lignocellulose into fragments of lignin, hemicellulose and cellulose (Broda et al., 2022). The cellulosic biochemical fermentation centers primarily on the complex nature of lignocellulose biomass which is the raw material for the producing cellulosic ethanol. It is mainly composed of cellulase, hemicellulose and lignin (Klose & Paës, 2023). These components are tightly intertwined by strong chemical bonds forming highly recalcitrant matrix that resists breakdown (Ibrahim et al., 2017).

This problem is resolved by pretreating the lignocellulose which aim to disrupt the biomass structure and reduce cellulose crystallinity. However, this step is challenging as lignin restricts enzyme access and can irreversibly bind enzyme reducing hydrolysis efficiency. Following pretreatment hydrolyzing cellulose and hemicellulose into fermentable sugars require efficient enzymes (Queiroz et al., 2022). The crystalline nature of cellulose and accessibility issue limit enzymatic action and thus sugar yield. Following are the challenges discussed in detail that one faces during cellulosic ethanol production.

15.4.1 High Cost of Enzymes for Hydrolysis

Biocatalysts such as cellulases and hemicellulases play a crucial role in the enzymatic hydrolysis of lignocellulosic biomass, enabling the release of fermentable sugars for ethanol production. The economic feasibility of bioethanol production is strongly linked to the efficiency and cost-effectiveness of this enzymatic step (Krassnitzer et al., 2023). Among all components of the bioethanol production chain, enzyme cost remains one of the most debated and unresolved issues. Some researchers argue that high enzyme costs are a major barrier to large-scale biofuel commercialization (Daniel & Piotr, 2012), while others believe costs will decline with technological innovation and process optimization. A further challenge is that publicly available data on enzyme pricing are scarce, making transparent assessment difficult (Zhu & Pan, 2022).

Reported estimates of enzyme costs for ethanol production vary significantly, ranging from $0.10/gal to $0.40/gal, depending on factors such as feedstock type, enzyme loading rate, and ethanol yield (Dutta et al., 2010; Kazi et al., 2010). This wide variability complicates robust techno-economic analyses (TEA), thereby limiting policymakers, investors, and researchers from making well-informed, data-driven decisions. To address this, a bottom-up techno-economic model for enzyme production was proposed, wherein costs are estimated from individual process steps and inputs rather than relying on broad assumptions or historical averages. Additionally, process innovations such as steam explosion pretreatment have been introduced. In this method, biomass is subjected to high-pressure steam, and upon sudden pressure release, the lignocellulosic matrix becomes more accessible to enzymatic attack. This enhances hydrolysis efficiency by cellulases produced by fungi such as *Trichoderma reesei* (Klein-Marcuschamer et al., 2012).

15.4.2 Understanding the Economic Challenge of the Enzymes

The cost of enzymes remains a major barrier in lignocellulosic bioethanol production, as it significantly increases the overall cost of the final product. Lignocellulosic biomass has a complex and recalcitrant structure that resists enzymatic breakdown (Rathoure et al., 2025). Consequently, large quantities of enzymes are required to efficiently hydrolyze cellulose and hemicellulose into fermentable sugars, thereby inflating costs. Moreover, the industrial production of enzymes itself is an expensive process, further contributing to the economic challenge. A techno-economic model revealed that the cost of enzyme production for ethanol ranges from $0.68 to $1.47 per gallon, which is much higher than earlier assumptions (Klein-Marcuschamer et al., 2012). The efficiency of enzymatic hydrolysis is strongly influenced by factors such as biomass composition and complexity, enzyme source, pretreatment method, and enzyme cocktail formulation. Under suboptimal conditions, enzyme efficiency declines, requiring even greater enzyme loading and further escalating costs.

15.4.3 Inefficiencies of Feedstock Pretreatment

Pretreatment is the first and essential step in the bioconversion of lignocellulosic biomass to ethanol. It disrupts the complex structure of lignocellulose by breaking cross-linkages between structural polymers, separating carbohydrates from lignin, and reducing hydrogen bonding between cellulose chains. This leads to decreased cellulose crystallinity and a lower degree of polymerization, thereby enhancing enzyme accessibility (Nair et al., 2023; Zhang et al., 2017). Pretreatment improves the surface area, porosity, and digestibility of biomass, ultimately increasing fermentable sugar yield and ethanol production (Broda et al., 2022). Several pretreatment methods, such as steam explosion, dilute acid, and alkaline treatment, operate under high temperature, pressure, or strong chemicals. Although effective, these methods result in high operational costs, equipment corrosion, and reduced sustainability (Li et al., 2022). Furthermore, they may degrade carbohydrates, particularly hemicellulose, leading to lower sugar recovery, reduced ethanol yield, and additional purification requirements (Rathoure et al., 2025). Feedstocks with high crystallinity or low surface area often resist enzymatic and microbial attack, and insufficient pretreatment hampers hydrolysis, thereby lowering product yield (Mankar et al., 2021).

Feedstock variability—such as differences in lignin content, hemicellulose composition, and harvesting practices—further complicates pretreatment, making it difficult to optimize conditions for heterogeneous biomass blends (Cowan et al., 2023). For lignin-rich feedstocks, wet oxidation is a suitable method that uses oxygen or air as a catalyst and water or hydrogen peroxide as a medium, generating fewer inhibitory furan derivatives compared to other methods (Zhou et al., 2012). However, the high cost of oxygen and pressure-resistant equipment limits its widespread use (Awogbemi & Von Kallon, 2022). Harsh pretreatments often generate inhibitory by-products such as furfural, 5-HMF, acetic acid, and phenolics, which negatively affect fermentation, enzymatic hydrolysis, and downstream processes (Hong et al., 2021). In contrast, biological pretreatment employing ligninolytic microbes (fungi, bacteria) or their enzymes offers a mild and eco-friendly approach to reducing recalcitrance. However, the long operation time remains a significant drawback (Broda et al., 2022).

15.4.4 Low Sugar Yield Due to Biomass Recalcitrance

Biomass recalcitrance refers to the **natural resistance of plant cell walls to deconstruction and conversion into fermentable sugars**, primarily due to their complex structural and chemical composition (Singhania et al., 2022). This resistance applies

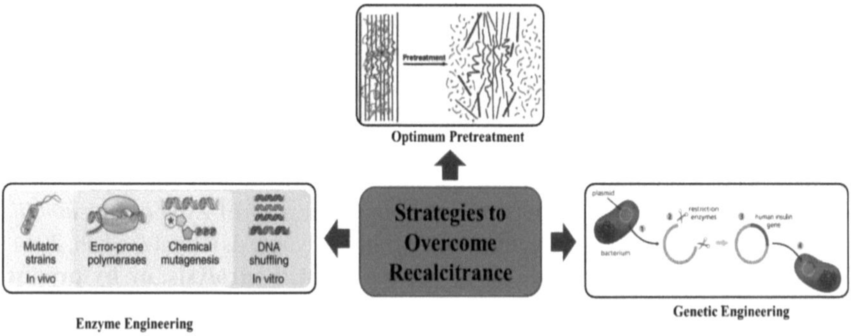

Fig. 15.3 A schematic representation of strategies employed to overcome recalcitrance

to **mechanical, physical, chemical, and biological deconstruction strategies**, making it a central challenge in bioethanol production. The plant cell wall is a **heterogeneous network** of cellulose, hemicellulose, and lignin (Zhu & Pan, 2022). These polymers are tightly interconnected, creating strong **physical and chemical barriers** to enzymatic hydrolysis. The variability in cell wall composition among plant species, tissues, and environmental conditions further influences the degree of recalcitrance, complicating biomass processing strategies (Chaudhari et al., 2023).

Lignin content is a major contributor to recalcitrance. Lignin surrounds and embeds cellulose and hemicellulose, thereby **blocking enzymatic access** to polysaccharides (Saritha et al., 2012). Additionally, lignin can bind to hydrolytic enzymes, reducing their effectiveness and necessitating **harsher or energy-intensive pretreatments** to enhance enzyme accessibility (Wikandari et al., 2019). To overcome recalcitrance, **pretreatment optimization** is crucial. Methods such as **dilute acid and hydrothermal pretreatment** have shown promise in enhancing sugar release and improving downstream fermentation (Straathof, 2023).). Beyond pretreatment, **biotechnological strategies** are increasingly important. Genetic engineering enables the development of plant varieties with **reduced lignin content** or modified cell wall architecture, thereby improving saccharification efficiency (Rathoure et al., 2025). Likewise, **enzyme engineering** can be used to design tailored enzyme cocktails with enhanced specificity, stability, and efficiency, making biomass deconstruction more **cost-effective and sustainable as depicted in Fig. 15.3**.

15.4.5 Microbial Inhibition During Fermentation

Microbial inhibition during fermentation refers to the **suppression of microbial growth and metabolic activity** caused by inhibitory factors within the fermentation vessel. This phenomenon reduces **fermentation efficiency, ethanol yield, and product quality**, making it a major challenge in lignocellulosic bioethanol production (Czatzkowska et al., 2020; Rathoure et al., 2025). Several mechanisms contribute to microbial inhibition such as **microbial antagonism** occurs when one microbial species inhibits another through **resource competition, secretion of inhibitory compounds, or environmental modifications**. For example, *Pediococcus* isolates from cucumber brines were shown to inhibit *Lactobacillus plantarum*, delaying acidification and disrupting fermentation (Hong et al., 2021). Accumulation of end-products such as **ethanol, organic acids, and other metabolites** can impair microbial metabolism. Ethanol disrupts the membrane integrity of *Zymomonas mobilis*, causing leakage of essential cofactors and inhibiting glycolysis (Baral & Shah, 2014).

Toxic compounds generated during **pretreatment, hydrolysis, or by-product accumulation** hinder fermentation. For instance, medium-chain fatty acids (octanoic, decanoic, and dodecanoic acids) inhibit *Saccharomyces cerevisiae*, leading to cell death and fermentation arrest (Vohra et al., 2014). Similarly, pretreatment-derived inhibitors like **furans, phenolics, and weak acids** in lignocellulosic hydrolysates suppress microbial growth and ethanol yield (Mussatto et al., 2010). Unwanted microorganisms or byproducts introduced during fermentation can outcompete ethanol-producing microbes, lowering yield and efficiency. To mitigate these challenges, **detoxification strategies** for lignocellulosic hydrolysates, process optimization, and the use of **antimicrobial agents** are applied (Zhu & Pan, 2022). However, antimicrobial treatments may also hinder the desired microbial strains, highlighting the need for **selective inhibitors, engineered tolerant strains, and adaptive evolution approaches** to sustain robust fermentation (Vasić et al., 2021).

15.4.6 Scaling up from Lab to Industrial Production

Transitioning the cellulosic ethanol fermentation process from laboratory to industrial scale poses significant scientific, engineering, and economic challenges. A critical hurdle lies in reactor design, as scaling up introduces physical and biological complexities not observed at bench scale (Alvarado-Morales et al., 2010). In laboratory fermenters, precise control over mixing, mass transfer, and environmental conditions ensures consistent performance. However, in large-scale industrial reactors, achieving uniform mixing and sufficient oxygen transfer becomes challenging (Pérez-Pimienta et al., 2020). Poor mixing can create substrate gradients, local pH fluctuations, and uneven microbial growth, all of which negatively affect ethanol yield. Additionally, the larger impeller sizes and higher agitation rates needed at scale may generate shear forces that damage sensitive microorganisms (Zhu & Pan, 2022).Another issue is the accumulation of phenolic compounds released during pretreatment, which are difficult to remove at industrial scale and can inhibit microbial fermentation (Tse et al., 2021). Furthermore, large-scale reactors are more vulnerable to microbial contamination, and maintaining consistent yield, productivity, and product quality becomes increasingly difficult due to non-uniform process dynamics and environmental variability (González-Gloria et al., 2022). To address these issues, computational fluid dynamics (CFD) has emerged as a powerful tool in reactor design. CFD supports fluid flow, heat and mass transfer, and mixing simulations, enabling optimization of reactor performance across scales. It is particularly valuable in designing advanced reactor systems such as simultaneous saccharification and fermentation (SSF) and membrane bioreactors, where process integration can enhance efficiency and sustainability (Freitas et al., 2017). Overall, careful reactor design aided by advanced modeling is essential for overcoming scale-up challenges and ensuring the commercial viability of cellulosic ethanol production.

15.5 Economic Challenges in Commercialization

Cellulosic ethanol has a lot of potential to be used as a sustainable biofuel. Cellulosic ethanol is sometimes referred to as a "second-generation biofuel" with significant sustainability potential. But, a number of economic, technical and policy barriers prevent its commercialization, which limits its wide spread adoption (Carriquiry et al., 2011). Some of the barriers are depicted in Fig. 15.4 and also discussed below.

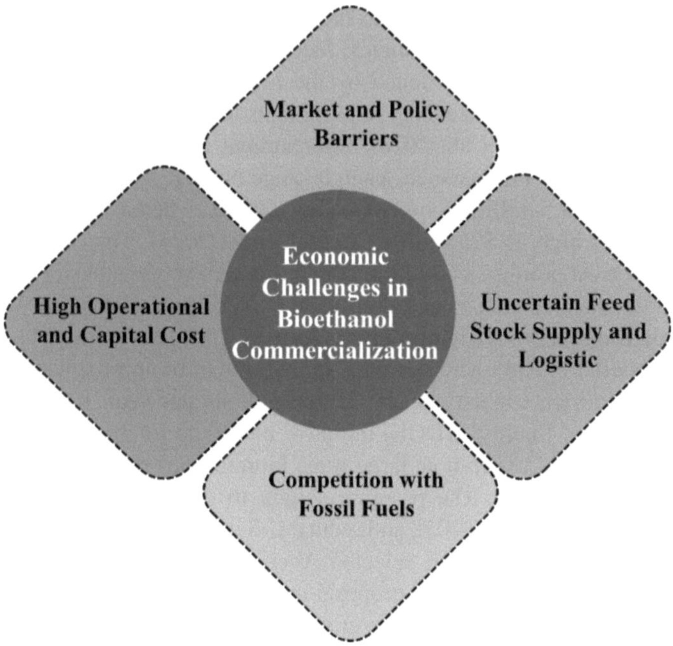

Fig. 15.4 Schematic diagram for challenges faced during commercialization

15.5.1 High Operational & Capital Cost in Cellulosic Ethanol Productions

One of the major cost barriers in cellulosic ethanol production is the need for multiple pretreatment steps and enzymatic hydrolysis, both of which substantially increase capital expenditure (CapEx) and operational costs (OpEx). The common feedstocks—such as corn stover, straw, and woody biomass—have high lignin and cellulose content, making them more structurally recalcitrant than starch-based substrates (Afedzi et al., 2025). As a result, processing requires intensive pretreatment and large enzyme inputs, both of which are expensive. The thermal energy demand is also considerably higher. Pretreatment and distillation in lignocellulosic ethanol production can consume 15–20 MJ/L ethanol, nearly double that of starch-based ethanol (Gnansounou, 2010). In addition, specialized equipment, complex feedstock supply chains, and repeated processing steps drive costs for cellulosic ethanol plants to be 2–3 times higher than conventional corn ethanol facilities.

Recent techno-economic studies show that producing ethanol from sugarcane bagasse, pretreated in multiple stages, costs $3.83–$4.90 per gallon, significantly higher than corn-based ethanol (Yamakawa et al., 2023). Although scaling up cellulosic ethanol plants can lower costs per liter, investor confidence remains weak due to uncertainties in government policies, feedstock logistics, and market stability. Operating costs are further burdened by the high price of enzymes required for hydrolysis and the substantial energy requirements for pretreatment, distillation, and waste handling (Nielsen et al., 2020). Pretreatment alone contributes 11–27% of total production costs. For instance, a single-stage hot water pretreatment requires a CapEx of around $4.5 million for a 2,000 t/day facility, whereas dilute acid pretreatment can cost as high as $25 million (Ceaser et al., 2024). Thus, while cellulosic ethanol holds great promise as a sustainable biofuel, the cost-intensive pretreatment and hydrolysis steps remain a central obstacle to its commercial competitiveness.

Abengoa Bioenergy—Hugoton Plant (Kansas, USA) case study: The Abengoa Biorefinery, built on a 385-acre site with an investment of approximately USD 685 million, had a design capacity of 25 million gallons per year. It was part of the U.S. Department of Energy's (DOE) initiative under the Energy Policy Act (EPA) of 2005, which aimed to promote large-scale biorefineries producing ethanol from lignocellulosic feedstocks. The program sought to make cellulosic ethanol cost-competitive with gasoline by 2012 and reduce U.S. petroleum consumption by 20% within a decade. In 2007, DOE selected Abengoa and five other companies for funding support. Abengoa's initial proposal included a grain-to-ethanol integration, but in 2009, this was revised to exclude grain ethanol and incorporate a steam-driven turbine to make the plant more energy self-sufficient. Although Abengoa was eligible under Sect. 932 of the EPA, DOE initially denied its loan guarantee since only Part One of the application process had been completed. By 2011, DOE approved a USD 132.4 million loan guarantee for the project. The Hugoton plant was designed to convert 300,000 tons of agricultural residues annually into 23 million gallons of ethanol. However, it never achieved commercial-scale performance due to technical and operational challenges. By 2015, the plant was shuttered amid Abengoa's bankruptcy proceedings. In 2021, the same site was repurposed, and a renewable diesel facility was established, marking a shift from cellulosic ethanol to alternative renewable fuels.

15.5.2 Competition with Fossil Fuel and Food-Based Biofuels

It becomes difficult to commercialize cellulosic ethanol when we compare it with fossil fuels & food-based biofuels. The cost of production of cellulosic ethanol is unable to compete with low production cost of gasoline. Like, straw-based ethanol produced by complex pretreatment and dilute acid by hydrolysis was seen to be almost 4.5 times more expensive than gasoline (Bhatt et al., 2018). Ethanol is twice as costly as gasoline when produced with softwood feedstock. Ethanol is price sensitive. It depends on subsidies and oil prices. Therefore, it's economic commercialisation depends on it. A study analysed these ethanol revenue scenarios:

(a) **E5 + subsidy (5% Ethanol + government Subsidies)**

Ethanol price = Gasoline price + Subsidy - incentive margin distribution cost.It is profitable since ethanol use is encouraged due to subsidy. Ethanol has high octane and it reduces emissions when mixed with gasoline in 5% quantity. This reduces carbon credits and attracts buyers due to subsidies, compatible with pre-existing infrastructure.

(b) **E5 Without Subsidy**

Without subsidy, the ethanol revenus drops largely. This shows the reality that without government subsidies commercializing cellulosic ethanol is not economically viable.

(c) **E85** (85% ethanol + 15% gasoline)

The pricing of ethanol is generally linked to two-thirds of gasoline's price, with adjustments for margin incentives and distribution costs. However, E85 fuel, which contains about 83% ethanol, delivers 27–33% less energy per gallon compared to gasoline, resulting in lower mileage and reduced consumer appeal (Aui et al., 2021). Without government subsidies, cellulosic ethanol becomes costlier, leading to lower revenues and significant commercialization losses. Discounts used to attract buyers further squeeze margins, and once removed, consumers naturally gravitate toward cheaper fossil fuels. In contrast, food-based biofuels benefit from well-established infrastructure, reliable supply chains, and lower operating costs, enabling them to generate more revenue than cellulosic ethanol under current market conditions (Chaudhary et al., 2025).

The economics of ethanol are thus highly policy-dependent, with subsidies, blending mandates, and tax incentives playing a critical role in determining profitability. Any shifts in government support directly impact revenues, often making marketing and distribution unprofitable. According to the U.S. Department of Energy (2007), the estimated production cost of cellulosic ethanol was USD 2.20 per gallon, nearly 2–3 times higher than corn ethanol and frequently costlier than gasoline (then priced above USD 4.00 per gallon). A major contributor to these expenses was enzyme cost, which added approximately USD 0.40 per gallon for cellulosic ethanol, compared to just USD 0.03 per gallon for corn ethanol (Sirjohn et al., 2025).

POET-DSM Project Liberty, Emmetsburg, USA, Case Study

Project liberty was launched in 2014 in Emmetsburg, low, USA to commercialise cellulosic ethanol from corn stover. It costed around $275 million for construction which was very costly as compared to a corn-based ethanol plant. It had high cost of operation, lots of energy required for enzyme pre-treatment. Even after production of ethanol, selling was difficult since fossil fuels were inexpensive and cellulosic ethanol had high cost along with lack of proper marketing. In 2017–2019, EPA granted "small refinery exemptions" allowing some refineries to skip adding certain volume of cellulosic ethanol or any renewable fuels to gasoline thus reducing further demand for cellulosic ethanol. POET then stopped commercial production at Project Liberty by 2019 and shifted to research and development and shut down in 2020.

15.5.3 Uncertain Feedstock Supply Chain and Logistics

The most critical factor determining the success of cellulosic ethanol commercialization is the supply and logistics of feedstock. Lignocellulosic feedstocks are scattered, seasonal, low in bulk density, and lack a universal logistical model (Afedzi et al., 2025). This creates major challenges in continuous availability, as agricultural residues are not produced year-round and are not uniformly distributed. Logistics are highly sensitive to feedstock characteristics (Zhu & Pan, 2022). For example, a reduction in bulk density from 96 to 48 kg/m^3 increases costs by USD 15.47 per tonne, while improving density can reduce costs by USD 6.78 per tonne. Similarly, boosting harvest yields from 2.7 to 4.5 t/ha lowers logistics costs by USD 7.74 per tonne (Wendt et al., 2018). The inherently low bulk density of lignocellulosic biomass means transporting large volumes over long distances yields relatively small usable quantities, sharply increasing logistics costs (Daniel & Piotr, 2012).

Plant location and supply chain design significantly influence economics. Centralized biorefineries benefit from economies of scale and lower per-litre processing costs, but require massive feedstock volumes transported to a single site, raising logistics expenses. Conversely, decentralized plants, located near farms, reduce transportation costs and ensure easier access to feedstock, though they may operate at smaller scales (Slade et al., 2009). Storage is another major issue. Biomass may degrade over time due to moisture and microbial activity, leading to material losses and added risk. Enhanced collection technologies can reduce delivered costs of switchgrass from USD 80.64/Mg to 71.16/Mg, with transportation alone accounting for

USD 15.42/Mg (Hess et al., 2024; Li et al., 2022). Thus, efficient logistics planning, densification technologies, and improved storage infrastructure are essential for reliable, cost-effective feedstock supply.

DuPont Cellulosic Ethanol Plant, USA, Case Study: The plant launched in 2015 with 30 million gallons /year capacity. It had nearly 200 farmers within 35-mile radius of DuPont's Nevada, selling their corn stoves to DuPont. Farmers get $30–45 per bale of stover and the nutrient loss was valued at 4.92 per bale. So net value would be:—bale cost- nutrient loss. This causes an economic uncertainty. The plant required approx. 500 farmers to run at full capacity but DuPont was at the risk of under supply. If the farmer number is increase, then only supply chain would be expanded. The plant shut in 2017, sold to Verbio North America in 2018. In 2021, it was redeveloped to produce renewable natural gas from corn stover.

15.5.4 Market and Policy Barriers

The commercialization of cellulosic ethanol faces significant market and policy bottlenecks. Its economic viability is largely policy-driven, relying heavily on subsidies, blending mandates, and tax credits (Brown, 2018). Uncertainty in government mandates undermines investment confidence, while delays in policy implementation introduce market risks. Cellulosic ethanol's competitiveness becomes feasible only when petroleum prices exceed ~ USD 191 per barrel or under stringent carbon pricing frameworks (Das, 2020). Without dependable policy support, projects exhibit negative Net Present Values (NPVs) and high default probabilities (Carriquiry et al., 2011). Market saturation is another challenge. In many regions, gasoline is already blended with 5–10% ethanol, which represents the current infrastructure limit. Without raising blend limits, the market for ethanol remains capped. Higher ethanol blends (E15–E85) would require new infrastructure, including special engines, pumps, and retailer investments (Ebadian et al., 2020).

Governments also face higher costs in promoting high blends compared to maintaining low-blend usage (Afedzi et al., 2025). Policy underperformance has already hindered commercialization. For instance, under the U.S. Renewable Fuel Standard (RFS), the 2020 target of 10.5 billion gallons of cellulosic ethanol was drastically reduced to only 510 million gallons, less than 5% of the original mandate (Stewart et al., 2023). Frequent policy revisions and delayed support mechanisms create an unstable investment climate, discouraging long-term capital deployment (Jiménez-Islas et al., 2021). Thus, stable, consistent, and forward-looking policy frameworks are critical to unlock large-scale cellulosic ethanol commercialization and enable it to compete with conventional fuels.

Beta Renewables Crescentino plant, Italy case study: Beta Renewables, whose parent company was M&G (Mossi & Ghisolfi) run many businesses like biofuel production, plastics etc. The biofuel company used PROESA technology which used low temperature and low steam pretreatment for cellulosic ethanol production. Beta launched its 1st commerical plant in 2012 with 75 million litres per year capacity and began shipping of ethanol in 2013. But in 2017, the plastic company of M&G in Texas faced problems like cost overruns and a hurricane hit which led to heavy debts on M&G that it entered bankruptcy. So, even though Beta renewables were not the reason for its downfall, it faced huge financial crisis, thus shutting down in 2017.

15.6 Strategies for Successful Commercialization

15.6.1 Economic and Policy Measures

Global biofuel production increased from 64 billion liters in 2007 to 145 billion liters in 2017, positioning biofuels as a central strategy for decarbonizing transportation (Ebadian et al., 2020). Despite their environmental benefits, cellulosic ethanol faces major economic hurdles, including high pretreatment and capital costs, making it nearly 60% more expensive than corn-based ethanol (Edenhofer et al., 2014). The lack of standardization in facility design, equipment, and operations further discourages large-scale investments. To counter these challenges, governments worldwide have implemented supportive policies, including blending mandates, tax incentives, low-carbon fuel standards, public funding, and R&D grants as summarised in Table 15.4 (Aui et al., 2021).

Tax incentives have been particularly instrumental in reducing production costs and encouraging investment. The Energy Tax Act of 1978 introduced investment tax credits for renewable energy (Su et al., 2015). The Volumetric Ethanol Excise Tax Credit (VEETC) under the Energy Policy Act of 2005 and the Energy Independence and Security Act of 2007 provided a \$0.45/gallon ethanol blending credit, administered by the IRS (Hochman et al., 2017). Complementary programs included the Small Ethanol Producer Credit (\$0.10/gallon), the Cellulosic Biofuel Producer Credit (\$0.46/gallon, 2009–2011), and the Special Depreciation Allowance, which enabled a 50% deduction on new cellulosic biofuel plant investments (Yacobucci, 2011). Internationally, Germany's Renewable Energy Sources Act (EEG, 2000) pioneered feed-in tariffs for renewable energy, setting a precedent for global policy design (Su et al., 2015).

In the U.S., public funding has been vital in bridging the so-called "Valley of Death." Programs include the USDA's Biomass Crop Assistance Program (BCAP) and Rural Energy for America Program (REAP), along with DOE's \$3.7 billion investment (1970–2011) through the Loan Guarantee Program and Cellulosic Ethanol Reserve Auction (Su et al., 2015; Yacobucci, 2011). The 2009 American Clean Energy and Security Act (ACES) pledged \$190 billion for clean energy, while President Obama's 2012 All-of-the-Above Energy Strategy launched a \$2 billion initiative supporting the Biomass Program, BRDI, SBIR, and STTR. Other countries also introduced strong policy frameworks. Brazil's Pro-Alcool program reduced production costs via R&D (Das, 2020). The EU Horizon 2020 and Framework Programmes (FP6) allocated €20 million to biorefineries using organic residues (Su

Table 15.4 Global policies to support commercialization of bioethanol

Country/ region	Policy/program	Tax incentives	Subsidies/financial support	R&D/ infrastructure support	References
India	National Policy on Biofuels (NPB) 2018	Tax credits, advance depreciation for 2G ethanol, differential pricing over 1G ethanol	₹50,000 million Viability Gap Funding (VGF) for 2G ethanol plants; subsidized power and water	R&D on advanced biofuels, conversion technologies, and non-food feedstock	Das (2020); Raj et al. (2021); Mankar et al. (2021)
USA	Renewable Fuel Standard (RFS2); Energy Independence and Security Act (EISA) 2007	VEETC: $0.45/gallon tax credit (until 2011); excise tax exemptions	Federal grants, loan guarantees, and blending mandates	Mandatory CI reduction of 60% for cellulosic ethanol; DOE funding for feedstock and process R&D	Bracmort (2015); Aui et al. (2021)
Canada	EcoENERGY for Biofuels; Agriculture Bioproducts Innovation Program (ABIP)	Variable tax incentives based on profitability	Capital cost contributions for biofuel plants (ecoABC)	Multiyear R&D program on biomass, bioproducts, and processing	Das (2020);
Brazil	RenovaBio; Proálcool	Carbon credit trading (CBIOs), tax incentives for flex-fuel vehicles	Blending mandates (27% ethanol in gasoline); price support for lignocellulosic ethanol	Government-led R&D in fermentation and biomass utilization	Raj et al. (2021)
European union (EU)	RED Directive 2009/28/EC; CAP (Common Agricultural Policy)	Tax exemptions under Directive 2003/96/EC	CAP subsidies for energy crops including lignocellulosic biomass	R&D for lifecycle GHG reduction, sustainable biomass use	Zahraee et al. (2024)
Germany	GHG-based biofuel quota system	Full tax exemption until 2009; post-2009 linked to GHG savings	Incentives based on verified emission reduction (6% target by 2025)	R&D on high-yield non-food crops and advanced conversion tech	Mussatto et al. (2010)
France	Finance Act 2019	Tax exemptions for biofuels (excluding palm oil)	Blending mandates (8.2% by 2020); incentives for waste biomass	Support for regional bio-refineries using residual lignocellulosic feedstock	Raj et al., (2021)

(continued)

Table 15.4 (continued)

Country/ region	Policy/program	Tax incentives	Subsidies/financial support	R&D/ infrastructure support	References
Argentina	Biofuels Law 26,093	Tax incentives for domestic biodiesel and ethanol producers only	Accelerated depreciation for capital investment	R&D on sugarcane residue and other domestic feedstock	Das (2020)
Philippines	Biofuels Act 2006 (RA9367)	VAT exemption on biofuel raw materials	Price guarantees for domestic production; blending mandates (10% ethanol)	R&D encouragement on domestic bio-resources for 2G ethanol	Su et al. (2015)

et al., 2015). India introduced Viability Gap Funding (VGF) of ₹50,000 million for second-generation (2G) biorefineries (Zhou et al., 2021). Canada's ecoABC program (2007–2011) supported biofuel plants based on agricultural feedstocks (Das, 2020).

15.6.2 Carbon Credits

Governments and regulatory bodies worldwide have increasingly adopted market-based mechanisms to drive decarbonization. Under cap-and-trade systems, regulators set a cap on total greenhouse gas (GHG) emissions and issue permits (carbon credits) that authorize specific emission allowances. Companies emitting less than their permitted quota can sell surplus credits to firms exceeding their limits, thereby creating financial incentives for emission reductions. Similarly, carbon offset credits, each representing one metric ton of CO_2 (or equivalent GHG) reduced or removed, are generated through renewable energy, reforestation, or carbon capture projects (Gupta, 2024). In transportation, Low Carbon Fuel Standards (LCFS) are emerging as powerful tools to reduce emissions by targeting fuel carbon intensity rather than blending mandates. Implemented in California, Oregon, and British Columbia, these policies reward fuels with lower carbon intensity than petroleum-based alternatives by granting additional carbon credits, which in turn increase their market value (Rinke Dias de Souza et al., 2021).

Several countries have also introduced biofuel-linked carbon reduction frameworks. Germany and Sweden enforce GHG reduction quotas in transportation, with Germany mandating a 6% cut in fuel-related emissions by 2025, supported by biofuel quotas linked to lifecycle emission savings. Brazil's RenovaBio program seeks to reduce transport-related carbon emissions by 10% by 2028, creating a dedicated carbon credit market that issues tradable CBio certificates for verified GHG reductions. Meanwhile, the Columbia-Labrie Act of 2016 introduced a direct carbon tax on fossil fuels, penalizing high-emission energy sources (Das, 2020; Ebadian et al., 2020). Together, these instruments—cap-and-trade, carbon taxes, LCFS, and biofuel quotas—demonstrate a diversified policy toolkit aimed at balancing emissions reduction targets with market-driven incentives.

15.6.3 Renewable Fuel Standard (RFS)

The Renewable Fuel Standard (RFS), established under the Energy Policy Act of 2005 and expanded by the Energy Independence and Security Act (EISA) of 2007, mandates a minimum annual volume of biofuels in the U.S. transportation fuel supply. The required renewable fuel volumes were set to rise from 9 billion gallons in 2008 to 36 billion gallons by 2022 (Lark et al., 2022). Specifically, the RFS aimed for 100 million gallons of cellulosic biofuel in 2010, scaling up to 16 billion gallons by 2022, representing roughly 44% of the total mandate. Under EISA 2007, advanced biofuels are defined as fuels derived from non-corn feedstocks with a minimum 50% reduction in life cycle greenhouse gas (GHG) emissions compared to conventional gasoline (Bracmort, 2015; Su et al., 2015).

The RFS framework incorporates detailed compliance mechanisms for fuel suppliers, including a tracking system using Renewable Identification Numbers (RINs), which enables credit verification and trading (Posen et al., 2015). The policy also includes provisions for small refineries and mechanisms for general waivers in special cases. To support adoption, various incentives were introduced, such as a \$0.51 per gallon tax credit for blended ethanol and a \$0.54 per gallon import tariff, which stimulated both supply and demand (Chen et al., 2021). Between 2010 and 2017, mandated renewable fuel content levels ranged from 8 to 11%, with fuels categorized into four groups based on feedstock type and carbon intensity (CI) reductions. For cellulosic biofuels, the required CI reduction is at least 60% relative to petroleum-based fuels, accounting for indirect land-use GHG emissions (Das, 2020).

15.6.4 Supply Chain Optimization

Biomass collection, inventory control, biorefinery operations, biofuel storage, and end-product distribution are the five main elements of a traditional cellulosic biofuel supply chain (CBSC). These factors have been the subject of extensive research on the design and optimization of CBSCs. (Ge and others, 2021). A strong and well-designed supply chain that guarantees steady feedstock availability, lowers expenses, and lessens environmental impact is essential for the efficient production of lignocellulosic bioethanol. Modular logistics hubs, integrated preprocessing depots, and local biomass sourcing are important tactics that lower transportation distances, increase bulk density, and stabilize seasonal supply (Duku et al., 2011; Lamers et al., 2015).

Cost-effective collecting, storage, and distribution networks can be designed with the use of mathematical modeling and optimization techniques including mixed-integer programming, linear programming, and metaheuristic algorithms (Zahraee et al., 2024). Real-time monitoring of feedstock quality, moisture, and degradation is made possible by integrating digital tools like IoT sensors, artificial intelligence, and data analytics. This improves operational resilience and decision-making (Guo et al., 2020). Working together with farmers, cooperatives, and the forestry industry ensures a steady supply of biomass and for the co-location of processing plants and biorefineries. Overall, the foundation of a scalable lignocellulosic bioethanol economy is supply chain optimization, which combines logistical effectiveness, economic feasibility, and environmental sustainability.

15.6.5 Localised Biomass Collection and Pre-Processing

Local biomass sourcing and preprocessing can reduce costs and carbon footprints, support sustainable bioenergy, and stimulate rural economies by creating jobs and utilizing idle agricultural resources (Duku et al., 2011). Integrated Biomass Logistical Centers (IBLCs) often adapted from food or feed facilities enhance operational efficiency by sharing labor, equipment, and storage across diverse feedstocks, thereby increasing flexibility and throughput (Guo et al., 2020). Utilizing mixed, local, and seasonal feedstocks helps stabilize supply, reduce price volatility, improve conversion efficiency, and ultimately lower ethanol production costs (Dessbesell et al., 2017).

Despite these benefits, challenges persist, including high capital investment, feedstock variability, and inconsistent quality. Modular preprocessing depots address these issues by performing size reduction, moisture control, densification, blending, partial pretreatment, and fractionation, yielding cost savings through optimized equipment use, integrated processing steps, and improved logistics (Lamers et al., 2015). The adoption of digital technologies such as AI, IoT sensors, and data analytics enhances feedstock monitoring, preprocessing optimization, and supply chain resilience. Furthermore, biomass supply chain (BSC) design and operations are increasingly optimized using mathematical models like linear programming (LP), nonlinear programming (NLP), mixed-integer linear programming (MILP), mixed-integer nonlinear programming (MINLP), and evolutionary algorithms such as Genetic Algorithms. Advanced hybrid and metaheuristic methods, including Tabu Search and Simulated Annealing, integrated with simulation and mixed-integer programming, support strategic decision-making and improve overall system performance (Zahraee et al., 2024).

15.6.6 Partnerships with Agricultural and Forestry Sector

The efficient production and commercialization of cellulosic ethanol rely on a well-structured and resilient supply chain, which can be significantly enhanced through strategic collaboration with the agriculture and forestry sectors (Awogbemi & Von Kallon, 2022). Crop residues, forest residues, and dedicated energy crops form the primary sources of lignocellulosic biomass. Partnering with farmers, landowners, and cooperatives helps reduce biomass transportation costs, ensures sustainable feedstock availability, and bridges research with practical implementation for a forest-based circular bioeconomy (Dessbesell et al., 2017). Integrated biorefineries that co-produce ethanol alongside high-value co-products-such as electricity, lignin, organic acids, and biogas can improve economic returns and overall process efficiency (Afedzi et al., 2025). Collaborative innovation in areas such as pretreatment, enzymatic hydrolysis, and fermentation accelerates the development of cost-effective technologies, while supportive policies and market incentives mitigate investment risks and promote stakeholder alignment (Raj et al., 2021). Ultimately, fostering robust partnerships with the agriculture and forestry sectors not only stabilizes biomass supply chains but also contributes to environmental conservation, rural development, and the transition to a sustainable bioenergy economy.

15.6.7 Market Development

Commercializing **cellulosic ethanol,** a second-generation biofuel derived from lignocellulosic biomass, requires addressing multiple demand-side barriers, including **blending mandates, infrastructure for high-ethanol blends, flex-fuel vehicles, consumer awareness, and corporate sustainability,** to enable scale-up and integration into transportation fuels (Hochman et al., 2017). Additionally, **social considerations** such as public acceptance, community involvement, land use, food security, and rural livelihoods must be incorporated alongside policy, economic, and environmental factors to ensure sustainable and equitable bioethanol development (Afedzi et al., 2025).

15.6.7.1 Blending Mandates and Infrastructure for E85/Flex-Fuel Vehicles

Biofuel blending mandates play a crucial role in promoting ethanol integration in the transport sector. For instance, Canada mandates 5% renewable content, the U.S. RFS requires 8–11%, and Brazil's RenovaBio targets 27% ethanol blending (Mussatto et al., 2010). Other countries have adopted similar policies: Argentina (12%), Colombia (10%), France (8.2%), Indonesia (5%), Germany (2.8%), and the

UK targeted 10% by 2020 under Directive 2009/28/EC (Das, 2020). India is considering a 20% blending target (Ebadian et al., 2013).High-ethanol blends such as E85 (85% ethanol, 15% gasoline) require both vehicle compatibility and upgraded infrastructure. Flex-fuel vehicles (FFVs) from manufacturers like Ford, Chrysler, and GM can operate on E85, requiring ethanol-resistant components, larger fuel tanks, and alcohol sensors (Mussatto et al., 2010). Infrastructure enhancements, including multi-blend dispensers, have been supported by programs such as the USDA's REAP, which funded blender pump installations with a target of 10,000 pumps by 2015. These initiatives, combined with manufacturer incentives, are essential to enable the widespread adoption of cellulosic ethanol and its integration into existing transport fuel systems (Green et al., 2024).

15.6.8 Consumer Awareness and Corporate Sustainability Commitments

Consumer awareness and corporate sustainability commitments are pivotal drivers for the successful commercialization of cellulosic ethanol. Educating consumers about its environmental benefits-such as reduced greenhouse gas emissions and decreased reliance on fossil fuels-can significantly enhance market demand and social acceptance (Mussatto et al., 2010). Targeted education campaigns and transparent communication addressing technical concerns, including fuel infrastructure compatibility and vehicle performance, help mitigate skepticism and foster adoption (Searle et al., 2014).

At the same time, corporate sustainability initiatives reinforce market confidence and stimulate investment in supply chain development. Companies that integrate cellulosic ethanol into their fuel procurement policies and commit to carbon reduction goals signal long-term support for the biofuel market (Ebadian et al., 2020). Firms actively engaging in sustainability reporting and leveraging carbon credit mechanisms further incentivize production scale-up while aligning commercial interests with broader environmental objectives (Edenhofer et al., 2014; Gupta, 2024). Promoting consumer awareness and embedding sustainability commitments within corporate strategies are essential for overcoming social and economic barriers, accelerating the adoption of cellulosic ethanol, and integrating it effectively into the transportation fuel sector.

15.7 Conclusion

The development of cellulosic ethanol has advanced significantly in recent years, driven by innovations in pretreatment methods, enzyme engineering, microbial fermentation, and process integration. Modern pretreatment technologies, including steam explosion, ionic liquids, and organosolv processes, have improved the efficiency of lignocellulosic biomass deconstruction while minimizing inhibitors. Enzyme cocktails with enhanced specificity and thermostability, along with engineered microbes capable of co-fermenting pentoses and hexoses, have substantially increased yields. Furthermore, advances in consolidated bioprocessing (CBP) and integration of hydrolysis with fermentation have reduced costs and streamlined production. Despite these technological breakthroughs, large-scale commercialization faces persistent challenges such as high capital investment, variable feedstock quality, complex supply chains, and the energy-intensive nature of downstream processing. Policy uncertainties and market competitiveness with cheaper fossil fuels further constrain deployment. However, strategic solutions are emerging, including biorefinery concepts that valorize lignin and co-products, techno-economic optimization, and carbon credit incentives that enhance profitability. Collaborations between industry, academia, and government are fostering knowledge transfer and innovation to close the gap between laboratory success and industrial-scale implementation. Looking forward, digitalization, artificial intelligence, and metabolic engineering will further optimize processes and resource efficiency. By addressing economic, technological, and policy barriers through integrated strategies, cellulosic ethanol can transition from a niche technology to a mainstream renewable fuel. Ultimately, its sustainable deployment has the potential to decarbonize transport, reduce dependence on fossil fuels, and contribute meaningfully to a global bio-based circular economy.

References

Afedzi, A. E. K., Afrakomah, G. S., Gyan, K., Khan, J., Seidu, R., Baidoo, T., & Parakulsuksatid, P. (2025). Enhancing economic and environmental sustainability in lignocellulosic bioethanol production: key factors, innovative technologies, policy frameworks, and social considerations. *Sustainability, 17*(2), 499.

Alvarado-Morales, M., Abd Hamid, M. K., Sin, G., Gernaey, K. V., Woodley, J. M., & Gani, R. (2010). A model-based methodology for simultaneous design and control of a bioethanol production process. *Computers & Chemical Engineering, 34*(12), 2043–2061.

Amin, F. R., Khalid, H., Zhang, H., Rahman, S. U., Zhang, R., Liu, G., & Chen, C. (2017). Pretreatment methods of lignocellulosic biomass for anaerobic digestion. *AMB Express, 7*(1), 72.

Aui, A., Wang, Y., & Mba-Wright, M. (2021). Evaluating the economic feasibility of cellulosic ethanol: A meta-analysis of techno-economic analysis studies. *Renewable and Sustainable Energy Reviews, 145*, Article 111098.

Awogbemi, O., & Von Kallon, D. V. (2022). Pretreatment techniques for agricultural waste. *Case Studies in Chemical and Environmental Engineering, 6*, Article 100229.

Azadi, P., Malina, R., Barrett, S. R., & Kraft, M. (2017). The evolution of the biofuel science. *Renewable and Sustainable Energy Reviews, 76*, 1479–1484.

Baral, N. R., & Shah, A. (2014). Microbial inhibitors: Formation and effects on acetone-butanol-ethanol fermentation of lignocellulosic biomass. *Applied Microbiology and Biotechnology, 98*(22), 9151–9172.

Baruah, J., Nath, B. K., Sharma, R., Kumar, S., Deka, R. C., Baruah, D. C., & Kalita, E. (2018). Recent trends in the pretreatment of lignocellulosic biomass for value-added products. *Frontiers in Energy Research, 6*, 141.

Beig, B., Riaz, M., Naqvi, S. R., Hassan, M., Zheng, Z., Karimi, K., & Chi, N. T. L. (2021). Current challenges and innovative developments in pretreatment of lignocellulosic residues for biofuel production: A review. *Fuel, 287*, Article 119670.

Bhatia, S. K., Jagtap, S. P., Bedekar, A. A., Bhatia, R. K., Patel, A. K., Pant, D., Banu, J. R., Rao, C. V., Kim, Y. J., & Yung-Hun, Y. (2020). Recent advancement in lignocellulosic biomass pretreatment and deteoxificaion: Effect of key factors, technological improvements and challenges. *Bioresource Technology*. https://doi.org/10.1016/j.biortech.2019.122724

Bhatt, A.K., Bhatia, R.K., Thakur, S., Rana, N., Sharma, V., Rathour, R.K. (2018). Fuel from waste: a review on scientific solution for waste management and environment conservation. *Prospects of Alternative Transportation Fuels*. Pp. 205–233.

Bracmort, K. (2015). *The renewable fuel standard (RFS): Cellulosic biofuels*. Congressional Research Service.

Broda, M., Yelle, D. J., & Serwańska, K. (2022). Bioethanol production from lignocellulosic biomass challenges and solutions. *Molecules, 27*(24), 8717.

Brown, T. R. (2018). Price uncertainty, policy, and the economic feasibility of cellulosic biorefineries. *Biofuels, Bioproducts and Biorefining, 12*(3), 485–496.

Bušić, A., Marđetko, N., Kundas, S., Morzak, G., Belskaya, H., Ivančić Šantek, M., & Šantek, B. (2018). Bioethanol production from renewable raw materials and its separation and purification: A review. *Food Technology and Biotechnology, 56*(3), 289–311.

Carriquiry, M. A., Du, X., & Timilsina, G. R. (2011). Second generation biofuels: Economics and policies. *Energy Policy, 39*, 4222–4234.

Ceaser, R., Montané, D., Constantí, M., & Medina, F. (2024). Current progress on lignocellulosic bioethanol including a technological and economical perspective. *Environment, Development and Sustainability*, 1–46.

Chandra, R., Castillo-Zacarias, C., Delgado, P., & Parra-Saldívar, R. (2018). A biorefinery approach for dairy wastewater treatment and product recovery towards establishing a biorefinery complexity index. *Journal of Cleaner Production, 183*, 1184–1196.

Chaudhari, Y.B., Várnai, A., Sørlie, M., Horn, S.J., & Eijsink, V.G. (2023). Engineering cellulases for conversion of lignocellulosic biomass. *Protein Engineering, Design and Selection, 36*, gzad002.

Chaudhary, A., Rathour, R. K., Solanki, P., Mehta, P., Pathania, S., Walia, A., Baadhe, R. R., & Bhatia, R. K. (2025). Emerging Technological Updates and hybrid systems in Biomass to biofuels and bioenergy: A roadmap for circular bioeconomy. *Renewable Energy, 122714*,. https://doi.org/10.1016/j.renene.2025.122714

Chauhan, S., Solanki, P., Putatunda, C., Walia, A., Keprate, A., Bhatt, A. K., Thakur, V. K., & Bhatia, R. K. (2025). Recent advancements in biomass to bioenergy management and carbon capture through artificial intelligence integrated technologies to achieve carbon neutrality. *Sustainable Energy Technologies and Assessments, 73*, Article 104123. https://doi.org/10.1016/j.seta.2024.104123

Chen, L., Debnath, D., Zhong, J., Ferin, K., VanLoocke, A., & Khanna, M. (2021). The economic and environmental costs and benefits of the renewable fuel standard. *Environmental Research Letters, 16*(3), Article 034021.

Chundawat, S. P., Beckham, G. T., Himmel, M. E., & Dale, B. E. (2011). Deconstruction of lignocellulosic biomass to fuels and chemicals. *Annual Review of Chemical and Biomolecular Engineering, 2*(1), 121–145.

Czatzkowska, M., Harnisz, M., Korzeniewska, E., & Koniuszewska, I. (2020). Inhibitors of the methane fermentation process with particular emphasis on the microbiological aspect: A review. *Energy Science & Engineering, 8*(5), 1880–1897.

Daniel, K.M., & Piotr, O.P. (2012). The challenge of enzyme cost in the production of lignocellulosic biofuels. *Biotechnology and Bioengineering, 109*(4).

Das, S. (2020). The national policy of biofuels of India–A perspective. *Energy Policy, 143*, Article 111595.

Dessbesell, L., Xu, C., Pulkki, R., Leitch, M., & Mahmood, N. (2017). Forest biomass supply chain optimization for a biorefinery aiming to produce high-value bio-based materials and chemicals from lignin and forestry residues: A review of literature. *Canadian Journal of Forest Research, 47*(3), 277–288.

Rinke Dias de Souza, N., Colling Klein, B., Ferreira Chagas, M., Cavalett, O., & Bonomi, A. (2021). Towards comparable carbon credits: harmonization of LCA models of cellulosic biofuels. *Sustainability, 13*(18), 10371.

Duku, M. H., Gu, S., & Hagan, E. B. (2011). A comprehensive review of biomass resources and biofuels potential in Ghana. *Renewable and Sustainable Energy Reviews, 15*(1), 404–415.

Dutta, A., Dowe, N., Ibsen, K. N., Schell, D.J., & Aden, A. (2010). An economic comparison of different fermentation configurations to convert corn stover to ethanol using Z. mobilis and Saccharomyces. *Biotechnology Progress, 26*(1), 64–72.

Dwivedi, D., Rathoure, R. K., Sharma, V., Rana, N., Bhatt, A. K., & Bhatia, R. K. (2022). Co-fermentation of forest pine needle waste biomass hydrolysate into bioethanol. *Biomass Conversion and Biorefinery*. https://doi.org/10.1007/s13399-022-02896-1.

Ebadian, M. (2013). *Design and scheduling of agricultural biomass supply chain for a cellulosic ethanol plant*. The University of British Columbia (Canada).

Ebadian, M., van Dyk, S., McMillan, J. D., & Saddler, J. (2020). Biofuels policies that have encouraged their production and use: An international perspective. *Energy Policy, 147*, Article 111906.

Ebrahimiaqda, E., & Ogden, K. L. (2017). Simulation and cost analysis of distillation and purification step in production of anhydrous ethanol from sweet sorghum. *ACS Sustainable Chemistry & Engineering, 5*(8), 6854–6862.

Edenhofer, O., Pichs-Madruga, R., Sokona, Y., Farahani, E., Kadner, S., Seyboth, K., et al. (2014). Summary for policymakers. In *Climate change 2014: Mitigation of climate change. Contribution of Working Group III to the Fifth Assessment Report of the Intergovernmental Panel on Climate Change*. Cambridge University Press.

Fortuin, J., Hoffmeester, L. J., Minnaar, L. S., & den Haan, R. (2025). Advancing cellulose utilization and engineering consolidated bioprocessing yeasts: Current state and perspectives. *Applied Microbiology and Biotechnology, 109*(1), 43.

Freitas, H. F. S. D., Olivo, J. E., & Andrade, C. M. G. (2017). Optimization of bioethanol in silico production process in a fed-batch bioreactor using non-linear model predictive control and evolutionary computation techniques. *Energies, 10*(11), 1763.

Ge, Y., Li, L., & Yun, L. (2021). Modeling and economic optimization of cellulosic biofuel supply chain considering multiple conversion pathways. *Applied Energy, 281*, Article 116059.

Gnansounou, E. (2010). Production and use of lignocellulosic bioethanol in Europe: Current situation and perspectives. *Bioresource Technology, 101*(13), 4842–4850.

Godin, B., Nagle, N., Sattler, S., Agneessens, R., Delcarte, J., & Wolfrum, E. (2016). Improved sugar yields from biomass sorghum feedstocks: Comparing low-lignin mutants and pretreatment chemistries. *Biotechnology for Biofuels, 9*(1), 251.

González-Gloria, K. D., Rodríguez-Jasso, R. M., Saxena, R., Sindhu, R., Ali, S. S., Singhania, R. R., & Ruiz, H. A. (2022). Bubble column bioreactor design and evaluation for bioethanol production using simultaneous saccharification and fermentation strategy from hydrothermally pretreated lignocellulosic biomass. *Biochemical Engineering Journal, 187*, Article 108645.

Green, Y. (2024). The application of ethanol fuel: Taking the United States as an example. *Biological Evidence, 14*.

Guo, X., Voogt, J., Annevelink, B., Snels, J., & Kanellopoulos, A. (2020). Optimizing resource utilization in biomass supply chains by creating integrated biomass logistics centers. *Energies, 13*(22), 6153.

Gupta, V.K. and Tuohy, M.G. (2013). Biofuel technologies. In: Biofuel Technologies: Recent Developments. Springer Berlin Heidelberg. https://doi.org/10.1007/978-3-642-34519-7.

Gupta, V.K., & Tuohy, M.G. (2013). Biofuel technologies. *Biofuel Technologies: Recent Developments. Springer Berlin Heidelberg.* https://doi.org/10.1007/978-3-642-34519-7.

Gupta, K. (2024). Carbon credits and offsetting: Navigating legal frameworks, innovative solutions, and controversies. *International Journal for Multidisciplinary Research.* https://doi.org/10.36948/ijfmr.2024.v06i02.17370

Hess, J. R., & Tumuluru, J. S. (2024). Biomass supply chain logistics: Challenges and technological advancements. In *Handbook of biorefinery research and technology: biomass logistics to saccharification* (pp. 3–24). Springer, Netherlands.

Hirani, A. H., Javed, N., Asif, M., Basu, S.K., & Kumar, A. (2018). A review on first-and second-generation biofuel productions. *Biofuels: greenhouse gas mitigation and global warming: next generation biofuels and role of biotechnology*, 141–154.

Hochman, G., Traux, M. & Zilberman, D. (2017). US biofuel policies and markets. In *Handbook of Bioenergy Economics and Policy: Volume II: Modeling Land Use and Greenhouse Gas Implications*, pp. 15–38.

Hong, J. W., Gam, D. H., Kim, J. H., Jeon, S. J., Kim, H. S., & Kim, J. W. (2021). Process development for the detoxification of fermentation inhibitors from acid pretreated microalgae hydrolysate. *Molecules, 26*(9), 2435.

Ibrahim, M. F., Ramli, N., Bahrin, E. K., & Abd-Aziz, S. (2017). Cellulosic biobutanol by Clostridia: Challenges and improvements. *Renewable and Sustainable Energy Reviews, 79*, 1241–1254.

Jeswani, H. K., Chilvers, A., & Azapagic, A. (2020). Environmental sustainability of biofuels: A review. *Proceedings of the Royal Society a: Mathematical, Physical and Engineering Sciences, 476*, 20200351.

Jiménez-Islas, D., Perez-Romero, M., Ventura-Cruz, I., & Flores-Romero, M. (2021). Development of biofuels research in South Africa. *International Journal of Energy Economics and Policy, 11*, 99–105.

Kambam, P. K. R., & Henson, M. A. (2010). Engineering bacterial processes for cellulosic ethanol production. *Biofuels, 1*(5), 729–743.

Kazi, F.K., Fortman, J., Anex, R., Kothandaraman, G., Hsu, D., Aden, A., & Dutta, A. (2010). Techno-economic analysis of biochemical scenarios for production of cellulosic ethanol (No. NREL/TP-6A2–46588). National Renewable Energy Lab.(NREL), Golden, CO (United States).

Klein-Marcuschamer, D., Oleskowicz-Popiel, P., Simmons, B. A., & Blanch, H. W. (2012). The challenge of enzyme cost in the production of lignocellulosic biofuels. *Biotechnology and Bioengineering, 109*(4), 1083–1087.

Klose, H., & Paës, G. (2023). Understanding plant cell wall recalcitrance for efficient lignocellulose processing. *Frontiers in Plant Science, 14*, 1284658.

Krassnitzer, P., Wenger, J., & Stern, T. (2023). Techno-economic learning in biorefinery research; a meta-level perspective of three exemplary cases. *Biofuels, Bioproducts and Biorefining, 17*(6), 1736–1756.

Kumar, B., Bhardwaj, N., Agrawal, K., Chaturvedi, V., & Verma, P. (2020). Current perspective on pretreatment technologies using lignocellulosic biomass: An emerging biorefinery concept. *Fuel Processing Technology*, 199.

Lamers, P., Roni, M. S., Tumuluru, J. S., Jacobson, J. J., Cafferty, K. G., Hansen, J. K., Kenney, K., Teymouri, F., & Bals, B. (2015). Techno-economic analysis of decentralized biomass processing depots. *Bioresource Technology, 194*, 205–213.

Lark, T. J., Hendricks, N. P., Smith, A., Pates, N., Spawn-Lee, S. A., Bougie, M., & Gibbs, H. K. (2022). Environmental outcomes of the US renewable fuel standard. *Proceedings of the National Academy of Sciences, 119*(9), Article e2101084119.

Li, Y., Tao, L., Nagle, N., Tucker, M., Chen, X., & Kuhn, E. M. (2022). Effect of feedstock variability, feedstock blends, and pretreatment conditions on sugar yield and production costs. *Frontiers in Energy Research, 9*, Article 792216.

Maheshwari, P., Haider, M. B., Yusuf, M., Klemeš, J. J., Bokhari, A., Beg, M., Al-Othman, A., Kumar, R., & Jaiswal, A. K. (2022). A review on latest trends in cleaner biodiesel production:

Role of feedstock, production methods, and catalysts. *Journal of Cleaner Production, 355*, Article 131588.

Mankar, A. R., Pandey, A., Modak, A., & Pant, K. K. (2021). Pretreatment of lignocellulosic biomass: A review on recent advances. *Bioresource Technology, 334*, Article 125235.

Mukherjee, A. and Arkalji, C. (2025). Energy Transition and Global South Cooperation: Case of Biofuels. ORF America Research Paper No. 33.

Mussatto, S. I., Dragone, G., Guimarães, P. M., Silva, J. P., Carneiro, L. M., Roberto, I. C., Vicente, A., Domingues, L., & Teixeira, J. A. (2010). Technological trends, global market, and challenges of bio-ethanol production. *Biotechnology Advances, 28*(6), 817–830.

Nair, L. G., Agrawal, K., & Verma, P. (2022). An overview of sustainable approaches for bioenergy production from agro-industrial wastes. *Energy Nexus, 6*(March), Article 100086.

Nair, L. G., Agrawal, K., & Verma, P. (2023). Organosolv pretreatment: An in-depth purview of mechanics of the system. *Bioresources and Bioprocessing, 10*(1), 50.

Nanda, S., Rana, R., Sarangi, P.K., Dalai, A.K., & Kozinski, J. A. (2018). A broad introduction to first-, second-, and third-generation biofuels. In *Recent advancements in biofuels and bioenergy utilization* (pp. 1–25). Singapore: Springer Singapore.

Nassir, T. H., & Al-Sahlany, S. (2021). Bioethanol production from agricultural wastes by Zymomonas mobilis and used in vinegar production. *Journal of Microbiology, Biotechnology and Food Sciences, 11*(3), e3709–e3709.

Neha Patni, S.G. (2013). Wheat as a Promising Substitute of Corn for Bioethanol Production. *SciVerse Science Direct*.

Nhien, L. C., Van Duc Long, N., & Lee, M. (2021). Novel heat-integrated hybrid distillation and adsorption process for coproduction of cellulosic ethanol, heat, and electricity from actual lignocellulosic fermentation broth. *Energies, 14*(12), 3377.

Nielsen, F., Galbe, M., Zacchi, G., & Wallberg, O. (2020). The effect of mixed agricultural feedstocks on steam pretreatment, enzymatic hydrolysis, and cofermentation in the lignocellulose-to-ethanol process. *Biomass Conversion and Biorefinery, 10*(2), 253–266.

Nimangre, L. S., Patil, P. P., Sankpal, P. S., & Patil, S. V. (2021). Ethanol production, purification, and analysis techniques. *International Journal of Creative Research Thoughts, 9*(7), 1234–1245.

Pérez-Pimienta, J. A., Papa, G., Gladden, J. M., Simmons, B. A., & Sanchez, A. (2020). The effect of continuous tubular reactor technologies on the pretreatment of lignocellulosic biomass at pilot-scale for bioethanol production. *RSC Advances, 10*(31), 18147–18159.

Posen, I. D., Griffin, W. M., Matthews, H. S., & Azevedo, I. L. (2015). Changing the renewable fuel standard to a renewable material standard: Bioethylene case study. *Environmental Science & Technology, 49*(1), 93–102.

Puri, H.S. (2025). India looking at increasing ethanol blending with petrol to over 20 pc. The Hindu.

Queiroz, S. S., Jofre, F. M., Mussatto, S. I., & Felipe, M. D. G. A. (2022). Scaling up xylitol bioproduction: Challenges to achieve a profitable bioprocess. *Renewable and Sustainable Energy Reviews, 154*, Article 111789.

Raj, T., Chandrasekhar, K., Kumar, N., Banu, R., Yoon, J., Bhatia, S., Yang, Y., Varjani, S., & Kim, S. (2021). Recent advances in commercial biorefineries for lignocellulosic ethanol production: Current status, challenges and future perspectives. *Bioresource Technology , Article, 126292,*. https://doi.org/10.1016/j.biortech.2021.126292

Rana, N., Sharma, V., Rathour, R. K., Ahuja, V., Bhatia, R. K., & Bhatt, A. K. (2019). Utilization of corn cob waste for xylanase production by newly isolated *Bacillus pumilus* XRL5 and its application in saccharification of lignocellulosic biomass. *Trends in Carbohydrate Research, 3*, 22–32.

Rathour, R.K., Devi, M., Dahiya, P., Sharma, N., Kaushik, N., Kumari, D., Kumar, P., Baadhe, R.R., Walia, A., Bhatt, A.K., Bhatia, R.K. (2023). Recent Trends, Opportunities and Challenges in Sustainable Management of Rice Straw Waste Biomass for Green Biorefinery. *Energies*. https://doi.org/10.3390/en16031429

Rathour, R. K., Behl, M., Dhashmana, K., Sakhuja, D., Ghai, H., Sharma, N., & Bhatia, R. K. (2023b). Non-food crops derived lignocellulose biorefinery for sustainable production of biomaterials, biochemicals and bioenergy: A review on trends and techniques. *Industrial Crops and Products, 204*, Article 117220.

Rathoure, R.K., Behl, M., Sakhuja, D., Kumar, N., Chauhan, N., Bhatt, A.K., Bhatia, R.K. (2025). Recent updates in biomass pretreatment techniques for a sustainable biofuel industry: a comprehensive review. *Waste Biomass Valor* (2025). https://doi.org/10.1007/s12649-025-03016-6 IF-2.78.

Saini, J.K., Saini, R., & Tewari, L. (2015). Lignocellulosic agriculture wastes as biomass feedstocks for second-generation bioethanol production: concepts and recent developments. *3 Biotech, 5*(4), 337–353.

Saritha, M., Arora, A., & Lata. (2012). Biological pretreatment of lignocellulosic substrates for enhanced delignification and enzymatic digestibility. *Indian journal of microbiology, 52*(2), 122–130.

Searle, S., Sanchez, F.P., Malins, C. and German, J. (2014). Technical barriers to the consumption of higher blends of ethanol. *The International Council on Clean Transportation.*

Shrestha, P., Pometto III, A.L., Khanal, S.K. and van Leeuwen, J. 2011. Second-generation biofuel production from corn-ethanol industry residues. *In: Sustainable Bioenergy and Bioproducts: Value Added Engineering Applications*, pp. 71–87. London: Springer London.

Singhania, R. R., Patel, A. K., Raj, T., Tsai, M. L., Chen, C. W., & Dong, C. D. (2022). Advances and challenges in biocatalysts application for high solid-loading of biomass for 2nd generation bio-ethanol production. *Catalysts, 12*(6), 615.

Sirjohn, N., Bhatia, R. K., & Kumar, P. (2025). Bioalcohol Production: Fermenting Nature's Bounty into Liquid Gold. In Microbial Biofuel (pp. 9–50). CRC Press.

Slade, R., Bauen, A., & Shah, N. (2009). The commercial performance of cellulosic ethanol supply-chains in Europe. *Biotechnology for Biofuels, 2*(1), 3.

Smil, V. (2007). The two prime movers of globalization: History and impact of diesel engines and gas turbines. *Journal of Global History, 2*, 373–394.

Stewart, D. W., Cortés-Peña, Y. R., Li, Y., Stillwell, A. S., Khanna, M., & Guest, J. S. (2023). Implications of biorefinery policy incentives and location-specific economic parameters for the financial viability of biofuels. *Environmental Science & Technology, 57*(6), 2262–2271.

Straathof, A. J. (2023). Modelling of end-product inhibition in fermentation. *Biochemical Engineering Journal, 191*, Article 108796.

Su, Y., Zhang, P., & Su, Y. (2015). An overview of biofuels policies and industrialization in the major biofuel producing countries. *Renewable and Sustainable Energy Reviews, 50*, 991–1003.

Suri, P., Dwivedi, D., Rathour, R.K., Rana, N., Sharma, V., Bhatia, R.K., & Bhatt, A.K. (2022). Enhanced C-5 sugar production from pine needle waste biomass using Bacillus sp. XPB-11 mutant and its biotransformation to bioethanol. *Biomass Conversion and Biorefinery, 12*(9), 3663–3672.

Timilsina, G. R., & Shrestha, A. (2011). How much hope should we have for biofuels? *Energy, 36*, 2055–2069.

Tse, T. J., Wiens, D. J., & Reaney, M. J. (2021). Production of bioethanol—A review of factors affecting ethanol yield. *Fermentation, 7*(4), 268.

Vasić, K., Knez, Ž, & Leitgeb, M. (2021). Bioethanol production by enzymatic hydrolysis from different lignocellulosic sources. *Molecules, 26*(3), 753.

Vohra, M., Manwar, J., Manmode, R., Padgilwar, S., & Patil, S. (2014). Bioethanol production: Feedstock and current technologies. *Journal of Environmental Chemical Engineering, 2*(1), 573–584.

Wendt, L. M., Smith, W. A., Hartley, D. S., Wendt, D. S., Ross, J. A., Sexton, D. M., & Kenney, K. L. (2018). Techno-economic assessment of a chopped feedstock logistics supply chain for corn stover. *Frontiers in Energy Research, 6*, 90.

Wikandari, R., Sanjaya, A.P., Millati, R., Karimi, K., & Taherzadeh, M.J. (2019). Fermentation inhibitors in ethanol and biogas processes and strategies to counteract their effects. In *Biofuels:*

alternative feedstocks and conversion processes for the production of liquid and gaseous biofuels (pp. 461–499). Academic Press.

Yacobucci, D. B. (2011). Biofuels incentives: A summary of federal programs. *International Journal of Energy, Environment and Economics, 19*(1/2), 133.

Yamakawa, C. K., Rojas, S. T., Herrera, W. E., Rossell, C. E., Maciel, M. R. W., & Maciel Filho, R. (2023). Recovery and characterization of cellulosic ethanol from fermentation of sugarcane bagasse. *Chemical Engineering Research and Design, 196*, 568–576.

Zahraee, S. M., Shiwakoti, N., & Stasinopoulos, P. (2024). Metaheuristic optimization of the agricultural biomass supply chain: Integrating strategic, tactical, and operational planning. *Energies, 17*(16), 4040.

Zhang, H., Wu, S., & Xie, J. (2017). Evaluation of the effects of isolated lignin on enzymatic hydrolysis of cellulose. *Enzyme and Microbial Technology, 101*, 44–50.

Zhou, S., Zhang, Y., & Dong, Y. (2012). Pretreatment for biogas production by anaerobic fermentation of mixed corn stover and cow dung. *Energy, 46*(1), 644–648.

Zhou, Y., Searle, S., & Anup, S. (2021). *Techno-economic analysis of cellulosic ethanol in India using agricultural residues.* International Council on Clean Transportation.

Zhu, J. Y., & Pan, X. (2022). Efficient sugar production from plant biomass: Current status, challenges, and future directions. *Renewable and Sustainable Energy Reviews, 164*, Article 112583.

Chapter 16
Lignino-Cellulolytic Enzymes and Their Biotechnological Applications in Biomass Waste Management

Aafreen Khan, Simant Giri Goswami, Gaurishankar Jaiswal, and Harit Jha

Abstract Bacteria and fungi produce enzymes that naturally depolymerize lignin and cellulose and are considered to be important in converting plant waste to useful and environment-friendly products. The enzymes break down challenges such as cellulose and lignin that exist within the wood and the agricultural production wastes. They develop an environmental friendly biopulping process and biobleaching of pulp and papers, by necessitating lesser harmful chemicals and less power. They recycle their waste material by recycling textile waste into new materials and thus promoting sustainable fashion in the textile industry. They, also, are important in biofuels production whereby biomass wastes that are not used as foodstuffs are converted to sugars and fermented to generate clean energy like bioethanol. Also, these enzymes enhance the nutrient level of livestock feed because they enhance the nutritional accessibility of nutrients to livestock. Although the enzyme-based alternatives still have certain problems of cost and efficiency, further research continues to make the alternatives more feasible and affordable. All things being equal, cellulose and lignin-degrading enzymes offer great potential to manage biomass waste in a responsible manner and produce a more environmentally friendly future.

Keywords Biopulping · Biobleaching · Wastes · Ligninolytic enzymes

16.1 Introduction

16.1.1 Lignocellulosic Biomass and Its Global Significance

Lignocellulosic biomass is the richest source of renewable energy in the world. This is mainly furnished by 3 relevant polymers which are lignin, cellulose, and hemicellulose. Polysaccharide hemicellulose takes the form of heteropolysaccharide

A. Khan · S. G. Goswami · G. Jaiswal · H. Jha (✉)
Department of Biotechnology, Guru Ghasidas Vishwavidyalaya (A Central University), Bilaspur, Chhattisgarh, India
e-mail: haritjha74@gmail.com

P. Verma (ed.), *Sustainable Practices in Biorefinery*,
https://doi.org/10.1007/978-981-95-6071-4_16

network and binds to cellulose filaments and lignin (Kumar et al., 2016b). Taken in combination, these components lend immunity to microbial invasion, which also adds to the difficulty of converting biomass into anything useful. Lignocellulosic biomass is forest by-product, agricultural waste, and external organic waste that forms nearly 60 percent of total biomass annually. The enormous potent application of lignocellulosics provide untapped sustainable source of value-added chemicals, biodegradable plastics, and bio-energy (Bhatia et al., 2023b).

However, more frequent reliance on agrarian, external, and agro-industrial biomass wastes has also imposed an extra burden on the environment. These wastes result in the increased pollution, a rise in the landfills, and indirect but severe health issues (Sankaran et al., 2021b). Such amounts of biomass waste require the adequate safeguarding developed with the help of the appropriate waste management and metal-sustained technologies in the long term. The nations have grown less favorable to old-fashioned ways of disposing wastes like open burning of solid waste that has adverse impact on the quality of air and the environment. Therefore, the waste process can be transformed into a system to recover resources and create value by implementing the use of innovative biotechnological methods grounded on microbial and enzyme-subsystems (Xia et al., 2021b). Enzymes of lignino-cellulolytic nature (the enzyme consortium that acts synergistically to decompose lignin and polysaccharides) are highly important in this action. Such enzymes may also facilitate bioconversion of the broad form of biomass to simpler components, thereby simplifying operations in many fields such as biofuels, pulp and paper manufacturing, textile processing and animal nutrition (Del Mar Contreras-Gámez et al., 2022). Its high catalytic efficiency, sustained activity, and green factors render it pillars in the transformation towards a circular bio-economies.

The mechanistic understanding and process optimization of the enzymes of lignino-cellulolytic nature are essential in the development of biomass use and mitigation of environmental residues (Ethaib et al., 2020).

16.1.2 Lignocellulosic Biomass's Composition, Abundance, and Resistance

Lignocellulosic biomass (LB) is the most abundant renewable dry mass on the planet, and it can be used as the building block of a large number of bioproducts, including biofuels (Chukwuma et al., 2020a, 2020b; Kumar et al., 2020a, 2020b). The three chief biopolymers comprising this extremely complex natural product, namely cellulose, hemicelluloses, and lignin are intricately organized and are not easily degraded by enzymes (Zoghlami & Paës, 2019b; Nair & Verma, 2025).

The most abundant organic polymer is cellulose, which has a weight ranging between 40–60% of lignocellulosic biomass by dry weight. It is a homopolymer made by a 1, 4-glycosidic bond that contains beta-D-glucopyranose units. The lignocellulosic matrix stores these units in highly long (500–1400 D-glucose units) chains that are continuously arranged in a fibrillar and microfibrillar forms. In this structure, glucose is less susceptible to hydrolytic action by enzymes, and as a consequence, some cellulolytic enzymes can hardly digest it chemically or naturally (Jayasekara & Ratnayake, 2019). Among the most uncommon aspects in terms of lignin-carbohydrate complex (LCC) resistance, the degree of polymerization (DP) of cellulose can be identified. Nevertheless, its individual influence has yet to be studied, as changes in DP can be accompanied by simultaneous changes in other structural parameters, including the crystallinity and porosity (Chukwuma et al., 2020c).

Unlike the other phytomass fractions, hemicelluloses are an anomeric and heterophasic group of branching polysaccharides that constitute about 20–35 percent of the total plant biomass. Combinations of hemicelluloses, which are composed of different monosaccharides, namely xylans, xyloglucans, mannans, glucomannans, etc., in contrast to cellulose, to which only glucose can be bound, are referred to as hemicelluloses. They are more prone to cleavage by diluted acids, bases, or hemicellulase enzymes because their DP is significantly lower than cellulose, usually in the 100–200 range, and they are not produced naturally (Chukwuma et al., 2020c). One of the difficulties in processing lignocellulosic biomass is the covalent bond between lignin and hemicellulose, often mediated by ferulic acids, which hinders the release of fermentable sugars (Zoghlami & Paës, 2019a, 2019b). In a similar manner, hemicelluloses constitute a physical protective barrier that limits access to the underlying cellulose (Jayasekara & Ratnayake, 2019).

Lignin is a complex heterogenous polymer composed of three or four different monomeric units, and the relative proportions of these monomers vary depending on the plant species. It is defined by being hydrophobic and cross-rigid, providing structural stability to plants. The enzymatically resistant and structurally heterogenous nature of lignin often restrict its use to energy production (Chukwuma et al., 2020c). It's strong association with cellulose and hemicellulose forms a stiff lignocellulosic matrix that serves as a protective barrier and lowers enzymatic accessibility and conversion efficiency (Nair et al., 2022a; Zoghlami & Paës, 2019a, 2019b).

The recalcitrance of LB to enzymatic conversion, is explained by both structural and chemical considerations. Crystallinity and degree of polymerization of cellulose, specific face dimension of cellulose, biomass harvesting volume and extent, and the particle size are examples of structural variables. The concentration or composition of lignin, hemicelluloses, and acetyl groups can be modulated chemically (Chukwuma et al., 2020c). One crucial discovery in the enzymatic degradation of lignocelluloses is that hemicelluloses and/or lignin must be changed or removed in order to increase enzyme accessibility to hemicelluloses and/or cellulose (Zoghlami & Paës, 2019a, 2019b). This highlights that the role of lignin is more than just structural support; it acts as a "lignin guard," effectively prevent enzyme access to the easily digestible polysaccharides (Jayasekara & Ratnayake, 2019). Such a protective hedge effect implies that efficient lignocellulose transformation requires substantial modifications or removal of lignin prior to any meaningful deconstruction of cellulose and hemicellulose (Benatti & Polizeli, 2023). Consequently, the research studies in this field are now directed to the development of lignin-modifying enzymes/pretreatment processes that directly operate on the lignin or lignin-hemicellulose. These techniques are generally both efficient and cost effective. Overcoming the primary protective barrier is necessary to maximize the profitability of the lignocellulosics biorefineries (Kumar et al., 2016b).

Lignocellulosic biomass feedstocks include a variety of sources such as agricultural residues, forestry wastes, dedicated energy crops, and industrial by-products (Chukwuma et al., 2020c; Nair et al., 2022b). These can be divided into three categories: virgin biomass (like straws), adequate energy biomass (like sugarcane bagasse and stover), forestry wastes (such timber and paper industry waste), and energy crops (like switchgrass and miscanthus) (Zoghlami & Paës, 2019a, 2019b). An estimated 181.5 billion tons of lignocellulosic biomass is produced worldwide annually (Jayasekara & Ratnayake, 2019). Although the total available biomass is vast, only about 8.2 billion tons is utilized, with the majority coming from timber, livestock-related residues, and grasslands, totaling around 7 billion tons (Benatti & Polizeli, 2023). A large portion of the world's biomass includes agro-residues, estimated at approximately 1.2 billion tons annually. Some of the examples include rice straw, which accounts for around 370–520 million tons per year and sugarcane bagasse with estimated worldwide production to 279 million tons on a per year basis (Kumar et al., 2016b) (Table 16.1).

Table 16.1 Lignocellulosic biomass sources are distributed widely throughout the world, and each source has unique characteristics of supply of biomass as well as its composition

Biomass type	Specific examples	Global production/availability estimates	Morbidity range (L % dry weight)
Agricultural waste	Sugarcane bagasse, rice straw, Corn stover	2.8 billion tons (total agricultural residues), 250–380 million tons (rice straw), 239 million metric ton (sugarcane bagasse) Chukwuma et al. (2020c)	The ratio of composition is as follows: Cellulose 40–60%, Hemicellulose 20–35%, Lignin 15–30% Chukwuma et al. (2020c)
Forest residues	Paper mill slash, Saw mill wastes, Wood biomass	The allocation 5.3 billion tons (forest/agriculture/grasses), 1.3 billion tons (forests) Chukwuma et al. (2020c) Zoghlami and Paës (2019a, 2019b)	Index of cellulose: 40–60, Index of hemicellulose: 20–35, Index of lignin: 15–30 Chukwuma et al. (2020c)
Energy crops	Switchgrass, Elephant grass, miscanthus, poplar	AF biomass, produced on biomass (Chukwuma et al., 2020 c)	A cellulose content of 40–60%, hemicellulose 20–35% and lignin 15–30% Chukwuma et al. (2020c)
Industrial waste	Municipal solid wastes, Waste pulp mill and waste lumber mill	Significant quantities Chukwuma et al. (2020c) Zoghlami and Paës (2019a, 2019b)	Differs much by origin

16.2 Lignino-Cellulolytic Enzymes: Classification, Sources, and Mechanisms

Lignocellulolytic enzymes are innovative biocatalysts able to degrade complex structures of lignin and cellulose into physically simpler compounds that can be broken down further into many useful end products. The preferred enzymes are mostly extracellular, secreted proteins acting on insoluble substances by microbes (Chukwuma et al., 2020c). These are broadly classified into two major classes: the ligninolytic enzymes, which are classified under the oxidoreductase enzyme family, and the hydrolytic enzymes that are categorized as the hydrolase family of enzymes (Chukwuma et al., 2020c). In order to digest lignocellulosic biomass fully several enzyme systems should work in cooperation (Sweeney & Xu, 2012).

Lignin and cellulose-retarding enzymes produced by bacteria and fungi are now essential not only to guard the environment but also in transforming plant waste into useful products. These enzymes are responsible to digest insoluble materials such as lignin and cellulose found in wood and agriculture waste produced by plants. The coordinated action of a series of hydrolytic/oxidative enzymes makes lignocellulosic biomass susceptible to the enzymatic breakdown (Grgas et al., 2023).

16.2.1 Enzyme Processes of Oxidation and General Categories of Lignin-Degrading Enzymes (Ligninolytic Enzymes)

Ligninolytic enzymes are highly specific in the degradation of lignin, which is a highly complex and recalcitrant aromatic polymer. Their mode of degradation is predominantly an oxidative rather than hydrolytic, a difference created by the complexity of the structure of lignin, with its carbon–carbon and ether linkages (Martínez et al., 2018). In contrast to the stereospecific cleavage of carbohydrates, ligninolytic enzymes exhibit lower substrate specificity, as the irregular stereochemistry of lignin is not precisely recognized by the protein active site. These enzymes start the depolymerization of lignin through a cascade of oxidative reactions that leads to generation of unstable intermediate products. The oxidative character of lignin breakdown is a fundamental design principle that is crucial for the development of efficient enzymatic solutions (Chukwuma et al., 2020c). This indicates that lignin-degrading enzyme development must focus the electron transfer process, whereas strategies based on water-mediated bond cleavage is not effective for deconstructing the complex lignin polymer. This suggest that oxidative pretreatments of lignin may be beneficial in enhancing its susceptibility to subsequent enzymatic degradation (Jha, 2019).

Peroxidases: Peroxidases are a major family of enzymes, which oxidize lignin or other phenolic molecules with hydrogen peroxide (H_2O_2) as co-substrate and in most cases using mediators. Their catalytic action has been associated with catalyzing oxidations, which are expected to generate reactive ions (like Mn^{III+}) or free radicals (like phenoxyl and aryl cation radicals) that directly target lignin (Chukwuma et al., 2020c).

Lignin Peroxidase (LiP): Secreted mostly by secondary metabolic processes of white-rot fungi, it is a strong oxidant that has high-redox potential and low optimum pH (Kato et al., 2024). LiP has a special natural tendency to form cation radicals by withdrawing an electron from an aromatic molecule that isn't phenolic. After that, the radicals go through a number of processes, including ring-opening, cleavage of aryl ether bonds and aliphatic side chains, benzylic alcohol oxidation, and lignin polymer breakdown (Chukwuma et al., 2020c).

Manganese Peroxidase (MnP): This secreted peroxidase is one of the most important enzymes, mainly occurring in basidiomycetes fungi capable of degrading lignin, catalyzes the oxidation of Mn^{2+} to Mn^{3+}, a highly reactive form (Kato et al., 2024). A number of phenolic compounds in the lignin structure will be oxidized by the generated Mn^{3+}, which will then act as a diffusible mediator (Chukwuma et al., 2020c; Sahadevan et al., 2016).

Versatile Peroxidase (VP): VP contains all of the features mentioned above characteristic of LiP and MnP. It is able to oxidize Mn^{2+}, methoxybenzenes as well as a broad variety of other non-phenolic lignin model derivatives. Due to this extended substrate spectrum, VP is of great interest to be used in bioremediation and industrial applications (Blasi et al., 2023).

Dye-decolorizing Peroxidase (DyP): Classical LiP, MnP, and VP enzymes are not related to the DyP enzymes, which are a distinct superfamily of heme peroxidases that are usually bacterial and fungal. The DyP enzymes can oxidize high-redox-potential anthraquinone dyes and model lignin compounds and can also operate efficiently under lower pH (Blasi et al., 2023).

Laccase: Laccases are multi-copper oxidases that are commonly found in bacteria, fungi, and plants. They are capable of catalyzing the one-electron oxidation of a wide range of substrates, such as simple phenolic compounds as well as complex aromatics, and can reduce molecular oxygen (O_2) to water through a four-electron transfer. Laccases can depolymerize lignin, leading to the release of phenolic compounds that can serves as nutrients for microorganisms. These enzymes have been noted to be particularly resilient and stable and in most of the cases, are secreted extracellularly by fungi during secondary metabolism, with their substrate affinity and specificity often being affected by the pH conditions (Chukwuma et al., 2020c).

16.2.2 *Mechanisms and Synergistic Action of Cellulolytic Enzymes*

The hydrolysis of cellulose requires a complex set of enzyme-cellulases. Their process involves the hydrolytic breakage of the cellulose polymer's 1,4-glycosidic linkages, which ultimately yields glucose, cellobiose, and cello-oligosaccharides

(Chukwuma et al., 2020c; Agrawal et al., 2023). The biosphere's biological recycling of cellulose relies heavily on enzymatic transformation, which has great promise for a variety of industrial uses (Jayasekara & Ratnayake, 2019). The hydrolysis of cellulose is completely and efficiently carried out by interaction of three major types of cellulases in a synergistic manner (Chukwuma et al., 2020c).

Endoglucanases (EC 3.2.1.4): These are enzymes that initiate the breakdown of cellulose by breaking the present 1, 4-glycosidic bonds in the amorphous region of the polymer. The production of new chain ends in this process makes cellulose more accessible for further enzymatic digestion (Chukwuma et al., 2020c).

Exoglucanases (Cellobiohydrolases, EC 3.2.1.74/91): Following the activity of endoglucanases, exoglucanases acts progressively on the reducing and/or non-reducing ends of cellulose chains. To break crystalline cellulose, they break down cellobiose molecules, which are glucose disaccharides (Chukwuma et al., 2020c).

Beta-glucosidases (EC 3.2.1.21): These enzymes break cellobiose and other cello-oligosaccharides to glucose monomers by completing the hydrolysis process. Avoiding product inhibition is crucial because cellobiose may make exoglucanases and endoglucanases inactive if they are not converted to glucose (Chukwuma et al., 2020c).

Cellulases are not a single enzyme; rather multiple types are required to achieve the synergy that enables breakdown of cellulose (Chukwuma et al., 2020c). This mean that a single type of enzyme cannot break down cellulose efficiently and there is a need to break down cellulose in a cocktail style (Angural et al., 2020). This synergistic effect is a direct impact of the complex structure of cellulose having a crystalline, amorphous part, and long polymeric chains with directional opposite ends (Zoghlami & Paës, 2019a, 2019b). Industrial applications that necessitate complete cellulose degradation cannot depend solely on isolated enzymes. Instead, they require the use of highly efficient enzyme cocktails that are often customized to match specific biomass feedstocks (Angural et al., 2020). Although this introduces complexity to the production and cost of the enzyme, it is essential aspect to the process (Sweeney & Xu, 2012).

16.2.3 Hemicellulases or Multicellulose-Degrading Enzymes Are Necessary for a Variety of Hydrolytic Processes and Auxiliary Enzymes

A broad class of enzymes known as hemicellulases breaks down hemicellulose into simple sugars and release acetic acid from its acetyl groups (Chukwuma et al., 2020c). Hemicellulose degradation is critical to liberate fermentable sugars and to avoid the potential effect of these components to hinder the cellulase activity and form a structural barrier that limits the access of the enzyme to cellulose (Zoghlami & Paës, 2019a, 2019b). Since hemicellulose is heterogeneous and complex, it's complete breakdown requires a more diverse and extensive set of enzymes compared to the relatively uniform cellulose polymer (Juturu & Wu, 2012). Successful degradation depends on the synergistic interactions of several hemicellulases (Chukwuma et al., 2020c).

Xylanases (EC 3.2.1.8): These are significant enzymes that break down xylan into D-xylose, xylobiose, and xylo-oligosaccharides. Xylanases consist of:

- **Endoxylanases (EC 3.2.1.8)**: They break the β-1, 4 bond in the backbone of the xylan in a completely random manner.
- **Exoxylanases (EC 3.2.1.37)**: After hydrolysis of β-1, 4 linkages at the non-reducing xylan ends through xylanases (EC 3.2.1.37) produces xylooligosaccharides.

Xylosidases: These enzymes release monomeric xylose by hydrolyzing the xylooligosaccharides and xylobiose.

Adding Enzymes: Allowing the main-chain enzymes to operate freely, there are a variety of other enzymes necessary to sever the various side chains in hemicelluloses. These are alpha-L-arabinofuranosidases, alpha-4-O-methyl glucuronidases, and esterases (acetyl xylan esterase and feruloyl xylan esterase).

The degradation of hemicellulose promotes the basic process of lignocellulose degradation. This is the breakdown of hemicellulose not only produces desirable sugars but also alleviates inhibition on cellulases, enhancing their activity (Yamaguchi et al., 2019). This linkage shows the interdependence of lignocellulosic deconstruction, indicating the deconversion of one component makes the other one more easy to break. In multi-enzymatic systems developed to degrade lignocellulose, the optimization of hemicellulases is as important as optimizing cellulases and ligninases. Their significance is not limited to the transformation of hemicellulose itself but plays a significant role in the process efficiency overall as well as the total production of fermentable sugars of all the biomass. This provides further rationale for employing comprehensive enzyme blends in the industrial conversion processes (Juturu & Wu, 2012) (Table 16.2).

16.2.4 Synergistic Enzymatic Degradation Process of Lignocellulosic Biomass

The figure below (Hsin et al., 2025b), Flowchart 1, demonstrates that lignocellulosic biomass is successively and cooperatively broken down by enzymes with delignification and lignin modification being the initial and often rate-limiting steps (Andlar et al., 2018). One of the examples includes the ligninolytic enzymes which use the oxidative mechanism to degrade the highly recalcitrant lignin polymer: peroxidases, laccases (Chukwuma et al., 2020c). Since lignin constitutes a protective block that impairs the ability of enzymes to reach cellulose and hemicelluloses, this is a necessary step (Mehta & Chelike, 2024). Degradation of lignin also renders the polysaccharides more accessible to enzymatic attack (Resch et al., 2013).

Table 16.2 Names and types of lignino-cellulolytic enzymes

Enzyme class	Substrate target	Enzymes	Function	Primary producers
Hydrolytic enzymes	Cellulose	Endoglucanases, Exoglucanases, 1Beta- glucosidases	Breaking down of cellulose in glucose	Various microbes
	Hemicellulose	Xylanases	Mitigation of xylan to xylooligosaccharides and xylose	Yeasts and different microorganisms Chukwuma et al. (2020c) Zoghlami and Paës (2019a, 2019b) Juturu and Wu (2012)
Oxidative enzymes	Lignin	Laccases, Manganese Peroxidases (MnP) and Lignin Peroxidases (LiP)	Oxidative and depolymerization of the lignin structures	White-rot fungi Kato et al., (2024)

Hemicellulose components are then subjected to hydrolytic treatments after lignin modification, and the polysaccharides are degraded into simpler sugars. The heterogeneous hemicellulose is broken down by these enzymes into several monosaccharide forms, including mannose, arabinose, and xylose (Chukwuma et al., 2020c; Zoghlami & Paës, 2019a, 2019b). Hemicellulose breakdown is crucial for the release of fermentable sugars as well as for breaking down the physical barrier and reducing the inhibition of cellulase activity (Fig. 16.1).

And lastly, cellulases attack the cellulose polymer. The process results in synergistic activity of several cellulase enzyme components and is a step that hydrolyzes the 1, 4 β-glycosidic bonds of cellulose (Chukwuma et al., 2020c). This process monomeric units of glucose. The resultant fermentable sugars, relying mostly on xylose and glucose, can be utilized in a series of biotechnological processes, such as the production of various kinds of biochemicals and biofuels (Paul & Dutta, 2017). This multi-step mechanism highlights the complexity of the enzymatic apparatus required for effective lignocellulose valorization (Verma et al., 2020).

16.3 Biotechnology Applied in Managing Waste of Biomass

Utilization of the lignocellulolytic enzymes in a broad biotechnological platform includes biopulping, biobleaching, textile treatment, biofuel production, and production of foodstuff and animal feed. Biopulping is an enzyme-based pretreatment that delignifies fibers and uses less harsh chemicals and energy-intensive processes in

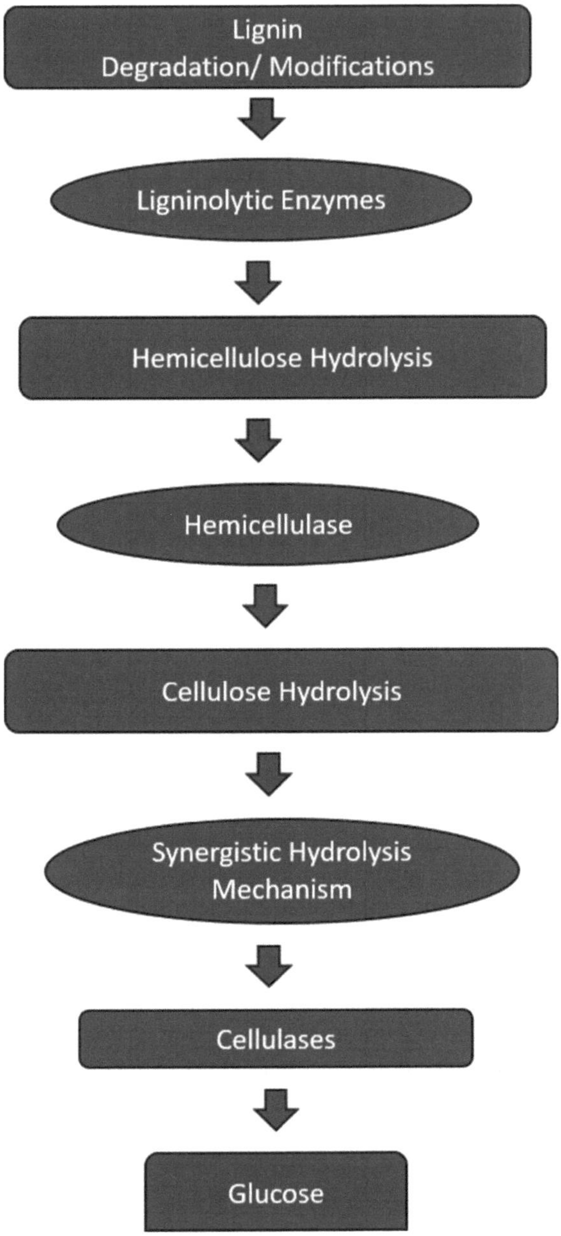

Fig. 16.1 Visual illustration of the lignocellulosic biomass synergistic enzymatic degradation pathway

the pulp and paper industry (Jha & Patil, 2013). Biobleaching involves the use of enzymes, i.e., xylanases and laccases, to remove any remaining lignin chromophores to allow whitening pulp using an environment friendly process (Kumar et al., 2020a, 2020b; Kazeem et al., 2017). Enzymatic treatments are useful in the textile industry to degrade dyes as well as the modification of fibers to improve the quality of fabrics and reducing environmental impact of textile processing. In biofuel production, enzymatic hydrolysis is a key part of turning cellulose and hemicellulose into fermentable sugar as part of the second-generation bioethanol and other energy carriers. Moreover, by enzymatic transformation, agro-industrial residues become enhanced animal feed in terms of their digestibility and availability of nutrients.

These applications although useful have face hurdles at industrial scale, which includes, enzyme cost of production, operation stability, and scalability (Abena & Simachew, 2024). The economic viability of the technology would depend on the ability to produce a high-yield enzyme system and to increase enzyme stability in the industrial environment. These bottlenecks can be addressed to ensure biotechnological intervention in biomass waste transformation to ecofriendliness and to a circular economy (Ndochinwa et al., 2024).

16.3.1 Biobleaching and Biopulping in Pulp and Paper Industry

The paper and pulp industry closely depends on energy-consuming processes (chemicals) which are used in pulping and bleaching, leading to high pollution loads into the environment (Jha & Patil, 2013). Less environmentally harmful alternatives are biobleaching and biopulping by using lignocellulolytic enzymes (Barapatre & Jha, 2016; Jha et al., 2002).

16.3.1.1 Fungal Pretreatment of Wood Chips

Bio pulping refers to the process in which wood chips are pretreated with lignin-degrading fungi, followed by conventional pulping method (Akhtar, 1994). The purpose of this fungal pretreatment is to make the existing pulping methods more efficient, and at the same time minimizing its harmful environmental impacts (Kumar et al., 2020a, 2020b).

The path to the detailed process is generally multi-staged:

1. **Wood Preparation**: Preparation stage starts with the process of turning the wood into the chip with the manageable size usually between 1/8 and 3/4 inch. Not only this uniform chipping make it easier to handle but also the surface area available on a substrate is increased, making the substrate more accessible to biological or chemical treatment. Adequate moisture content, normally ranging from 55 to 65 percent of the wood's total body weight is also essential. The presence of high

levels of water in the substrate renders it soft and increases the availability of nutrients, thereby providing the best conditions in which the fungi can multiply. The fungi then secrete enzymes which work on the thick material (dentine-like material), ensuring its breakdown. Combining the size of the chip and content of moisture will be the basis of successful bioprocessing (Akhtar, 1994).

2. **Decontamination**: Decontaminating wooden chips serves to eliminate naturally occurring, competitive bacteria and fungus, most often through the use of steam. This will make sure the chosen biopulping fungus can easily colonize on the chips without being hindered (Akhtar, 1994).
3. **Inoculation**: A selected fungus is inoculated on the wood chips after steaming and cooling by spraying it with a dilute inoculum of a particular fungus, which is often supported by a nutrient adjuvant such as corn steep liquor, molasses, or yeast extract (Akhtar, 1994).
4. **Incubation**: After inoculation the wood chips are moved to a warm and moist environment that stimulates initiation of fungal growth. Overall, this stage takes one to four weeks and can be undertaken in aerated piles or in managed bioreactor systems. The wet condition, elevated temperatures, and availability of oxygen make the environment suitable for the fungi. In this process, lignin-degrading fungi form an intricate net of hyphae which initially covers the surface of the chip, and then infiltrates its internal structure. Such progressive colonization allows the fungi to penetrate lignin-rich areas and facilitate the active biodegradation (Akhtar, 1994).
5. **Fungal Activity**: The lignin-degrading pathway in white-rot fungi, which selectively eliminates lignin and extractives from the wood cell wall, this step is crucial for biopulping process (Ethaib et al., 2020; Kato et al., 2024). These chips become softer as a result, which facilitates their separation. Hemicellulases, such as xylanases, break down the hemicellulose component and make it easier for the remaining lignin-destroying agents to penetrate the pulp, whereas ligninases like laccase, lignin peroxidase, manganese peroxidase, and versatile peroxidase break down the lignin component (Akhtar, 1994).
6. **Pulping**: These chips are then pulped, and often broken up more easily during refining process (Akhtar, 1994).

Key factors for fungi employed in commercial biopulping include their preference for lignin and hemicellulose, their low activity on cellulose, comparatively fast growth rate, capacity to grow on both soft and hardwoods, nonallergenic nature, and their quick sporulation rate to guarantee an adequate supply of inocula. Some of the commonly used fungi are: *Trametes versicolor*, *Phanerochaete chrysosporium*, and *Ceriporiopsis subvermispora* (Kumar et al., 2020a, 2020b).

16.3.1.2 Environmental and Economic Advantages of Biopulping

There are a number of economic and ecological benefits available when we compare the biopulping techniques to the conventional ones:

Fungal pretreatment prior to mechanical pulping has the potential to reduce energy use during refining by 20 to 30% (Akhtar, 1994). This translates to large savings in the costs of energy, in a chip-pile system could run between 9 and 20 dollars per ton of pulp or even up to 50 dollars per ton with increased mill throughput.

Less Use of Chemicals: Biopulping does not require excessive chemicals used in the pulping industry and thereby, contributes to less environmental pollution (Kumar et al., 2020a, 2020b). It lowers the content of pitch (extractives) and toxicity of effluents (Akhtar, 1994). Biopulping inherently decreases the formation of toxic by-products by reducing the need for harsh chemicals during bleaching (Kumar et al., 2020a, 2020b).

Biopulping Technology Offers Improved Pulp and Paper Quality: Biopulping has been found to enhance the paper strength properties that is, tensile index, burst index, and folding endurance. It also helps to make cleaner pulp and at times gives a brighter final pulp (Kumar et al., 2016b).

Enhanced Mill Capacity: Biobleaching or enzyme pulp bleaching is a biodegradable alternative to the traditional chemical pulp bleaching which involves the reduction of lignin and hemicellulose in pulp by the utilization of enzymes like laccases, xylanases, and peroxidases. Through lignin modification and partial degradation of hemicellulose enzymes, it increased pulp brightness and did not destroy the integrity of cellulose. It consumes less harsh chemicals and therefore lowers the creation of toxic compounds such as Adsorbable Organic Halides (AOX) and the environment costs minimal. Moreover, biobleaching has less energy demands and thus more mills can manage a lot of pulp as well as extract products more efficiently. These enhancements carry with them a lot of economic benefits in terms of saving energy and offering efficiency in processing that helps in lowering the cost of operation besides improving the quality of pulp (Akhtar et al., 1993). Altogether, the enzymatic pulp bleaching is a sustainable and financially feasible solution to the production of modern paper.

16.3.1.3 Bio Bleaching/Enzymatic Pulp Bleaching

Biobleaching involves the use of enzymes to reduce or replace conventional chlorine-based biobleaching chemicals, it reduces the formation of toxic chlorinated organic compounds, collectively referred as adsorbable organic halides (AOX) (Kumar et al., 2016b).

Important enzymes and their action in biobleaching are:

1. **Xylanases**: During pulp pre-bleaching the main objective is to partially break down lignin and hemicellulose in order to make the pulp receptive to further chemical bleaching. The enzymes most commonly used include xylanases because they are able to selectively degrade xylan, which is one of the key constituents of hemicelluloses. These xylanases are usually cellulase-free in order to sustain pulp strength because additional breakdown of undesired cellulose can

occur. Also, xylanases that are thermostable should be used, since, in fact, industrial bleaching is frequently performed at high temperatures and these enzymes can be retained in this temperature regime. Cellulase-free thermostable xylanases can also enhance the pulp brightness, chemical penetrability, and pulp quality as a whole, selectively targeting hemicellulose while minimizing the reasoning for using harsh chemicals, advancing the sustainability, and reducing costs of the process (Bajar et al., 2020).

Mechanism: Although cutting down lignin is not a direct effect, xylanases improve pulp bleachability by degrading the xylan network that physically forms a barrier around lignin (Bajar et al., 2020; Kadam et al., 2022). This process allows the pulp to be more susceptible to further chemical bleach reagents such as chlorine dioxide (ClO_2) and liberates more lignin during the wash-off phase (Kumar et al., 2016b).

Efficacy: Xylanase treatment can result in a 2.0% ISO increase in pulp brightness and/or a 15 percent reduction in requirement of chlorine-based bleach chemicals (Bajar et al., 2020). It can also reduce ClO_2 and NaOH rate by 20 and 10 percent, respectively, and minimize AOX formation within a bleach plant effluent by 20–25 percent. This results in a lower bleaching cost; some sources claim that the cost of bleaching hardwood core pulp went down by nearly 89 percent (Kadam et al., 2022; Tolan & Guenette, 1997). Treating pulps with xylanase does not seem to have any adverse effect on pulp properties in relation to pulp strength characteristics nor does it produce any adverse effect on brightness stability (Tolan & Guenette, 1997).

2. **Laccases**: Laccases comprise a group of oxidative enzymes found mainly in fungi and a few bacteria which are central to the biodegradation of lignin. During pulp bleaching, these enzymes can work directly on the lignin, and the colored products, which support brown color of pulp, and destroy their complex polymer constitution. Laccase oxidizes both phenolic and non-phenolic lignin compounds, lowering the chromophores, hence increasing pulp brightness, but without harsh chemical oxidants. They do not only enhance the visual quality of the pulp but they can also help in environmental sustainability as they reduce the generation of toxic chlorinated by-products of the chemical bleaching process. The bleaching method to incorporate laccases is especially beneficial in delivering eco-friendly, high-quality paper, and at the same time both decreasing the usage of chemicals and lowering the operational expenses (Kadam et al., 2022).

Mechanism: To eliminate pulp lignin in the following alkaline extraction, laccase mediator systems (LMS) oxidize it. Laccase is able to oxidize lignin although it often requires low-molecular-weight phenoxy synthetic/natural mediators (such as ABTS or HBT) to enhance its oxidation potential. Pulp fibers can also be grafted by the phenol radical produced by laccase and this influences the solubility and removal of the lignin (Moldes & Vidal, 2010).

Efficacy: Laccase treatment can be used to make paper bright and reduce kappa number, suggesting lignin removal or modification (Moldes & Vidal, 2010). Laccase and xylanase used in synergistic biobleaching save 28.6 percent H_2O, increasing pulp viscosity by 6.7 percent, and improving the brightness by 3 ISO to wheat straw pulp. Notably, in contrast to conventional chlorine-based processes, Totally Chlorine Free (TCF) biobleaching processes with laccase and xylanase do not leave any measurable amount of AOX in their effluent, thus showing low environmental impact (Xu et al., 2013).

3. **Manganese peroxidases (MnP)**: The other important enzyme is manganese peroxidase (MnP), which initiates delignification by using Mn^{2+} as cofactors to oxidize the lignin structures that result in brighter pulp (Bajpai, 2004). Lignin is found to be modified by these enzymes in a cooperative manner and does not destroy cellulose in them; hence they are preferred in eco-friendly and affordable bleaching. When pulp is treated with ligninolytic enzymes, the results of enhancement in both the visual and physical appearance of the paper are observed, and a reduction of the toxic byproduct like Adsorbable Organic Halides (AOX) is generated, which ensures a sustainable industrial activity (Bajpai, 2004; Kadam et al., 2022).

Mechanism: MnP acts as a diffusible redox shuttle to oxidize phenolic compounds through the catalysis of the peroxide-dependent oxidation of Mn(II) to Mn(III) (Chukwuma et al., 2020c; Sahadevan et al., 2016). The MnP treatment may make no direct contribution to its solubilization, but more or less oxidizes the lignin in the pulp, making the residual lignin more accessible to alkali extraction. This oxidation has the ability to make an object susceptible to peroxide bleaching due to demethoxylation and o-quinones or o-carbonyls generating (Sahadevan et al., 2016).

Efficacy: Pure manganese peroxidase (MnP) can drastically enhance the quality of pulp in terms of brightening by 5–15 points and at the same time, reducing the lignin percentage, as shown by the decrease in the kappa number of 6 points (Jeffries & Viikari, 1996b).

16.3.1.4 Coming Problems, Difficulties, and Opportunities

Despite the possible advantages, there are obstacles via which enzymatic pulping and bleaching may be adopted on a large scale in the industry. The relevant enzymes had not been as readily available or commercially viable earlier on exploration (Kumar et al., 2016b). Current setbacks have incorporated the use of highly priced enzymes, inconsistent enzyme activity due to the mill unique factors (pH, temperature, and raw material), as well as the fact that more investigations are required to come up with more powerful enzyme systems that can devise cleanly surveyed substitute routes to traditional bleaching agents (Kumar et al., 2016b). Such engineering challenges as far as a sustained cleaning, inoculation, and maintenance of optimal temperature and moisture in large chip piles occur when the process of biopulping is scaled up to about the scale of 200–2000 tons/day (Akhtar et al., 1993). These technological and financial obstacles will have to be addressed by further research on optimal processes and cost-cutting methods of enzyme manufacturing as well as enzyme engineering (Walia et al., 2017).

16.3.2 Sustainable Manufacturing Enzymatic Processing of Textiles

The use of intensive chemical treatment is a longstanding tradition in the textile industry; the processes of bleaching, dyeing, and finishing use large volumes of water and energy producing toxic wastewater. These effluents contain dyes and salts with the presence of residual chemicals that are hazardous to the environment (Ribul et al., 2021). Enzyme-based processing is considered as an alternative to conventional techniques, allowing for operations under less harsh conditions. This method can be conducted at standard environmental temperatures and pH, utilizing low temperatures and minimizing the use of harsh chemicals. Cellulases improve cellulose softening and bio-polishing of fabrics, laccases contribute to decolorization and bleaching of dye, and amylases eliminate a starch-based sizing formulation. This allows manufacturers of fabrics to use a smaller amount of chemicals, consume less water and energy, and avoid polluting the environment but still retain or enhance the quality of the fabric (Ren & Guan, 2025).

16.3.2.1 Enzymatic Desizing

The initial processing of textiles is the process of desizing, which entails removal of sizing agents that have been deposited on warp yarns to secure them during weaving. This is a pretreatment to move the fabric to further stages of finishing and dyeing (Ribul et al., 2021).

Mechanism: A process is performed to remove this desizing using some enzymes known as amylase. They break down the starch molecules into shorter chains of glucose polymers (maltose) and dextrins that can be washed off easily from a piece of fabric. Specifically, alpha-amylase will be used to metabolize amylose to glucose, whereas amylopectin will be converted to 50% glucose and maltose (Ren & Guan, 2025).

Advantages: Enzymatic desizing consumes less energy, process water, and caustic agents since the operation is carried out in low temperatures (30–60 C and optimal pH of 5.5–6.5). It provides renewable effluents with low pollutant levels to ensure a stable size removal devoid of weakening the cloth (Ren & Guan, 2025).

16.3.2.2 Biostoning/Biopolishing Cellulases Used in Denim Finishing

In denim finishing, cellulase enzymes are widely applied in order to receive the required aesthetic effect and to improve fabric quality as the mechanical means of finish such as stone washing (Heikinheimo et al., 2000).

Biostoning: By using cellulases, the process generates a worn-stained or even stone-washed look in denim garments (Heikinheimo et al., 2000).

Mechanism: Cellulases come into action and abrasion is carried out on the surface of cotton at a microscale on exposed cellulose fibers. This has the desired washed-out or faded appearance as it fades away surface fuzz and the indigo dye. This effect can be changed by mechanical agitation as well as the addition of neutral or acidic cellulases. Endoglucanases are excellent color removers in the untapped hydrolyzes (Heikinheimo et al., 2000).

Biostoning has a few benefits over pumice stone washing, such as the avoidance of damage done to fabrics and the loss of strength, avoidance of damage done to the laundry machines, avoidance of solid wastes and sewage issues, and augmented efficiency. It also reduces the water consumed and energy requirements as it functions at moderate temperatures and pH values (*A New Approaches in Community Science (Volume-1)*, 2023).

Bio-Polishing: Liquid cellulases could be used in postspinning polishing of cotton textiles to flatten agitating fibers on the cotton fabric surfaces to generate cotton fabric with a smoother finish, soft-pile fabric, better drape, and hence greater color highlight (Ribul et al., 2021). This improves dimensional stability of low-shrinkage and low-strength cellulosic fabrics (Heikinheimo et al., 2000).

16.3.2.3 Laccases as Combined Surface Finishing and Textile Dyeing

Laccases have gained interest in the textile dyeing and finishing industry as an eco-friendly alternative to chemical processing, particularly in terms of changing the characteristics of the fabric and decontaminating effluents (Bhatt, 2022).

Mechanism: Laccases oxidize a wide range of aromatic substances, such as synthetic and natural dyes and pigments, with their degradation or alteration (Bhatt, 2022). They too are able to generate the oxidation of flavonoids that yield quinones which may be polymerized and grafted onto cotton surfaces to give color (Kim et al., 2007b).

Advantages: Laccases can be employed to bleach fabrics and in traditional cotton bleaching, consequently increasing whiteness. They suggest a greener solution to the finishing of denim, whereby the indigo dye is bleached off using oxidation, thereby eliminating use of chemicals when bleaching the denim. Laccases can be used to increase fixation of dyes on wool, thereby saving time and dye, and can be used to decolorize wool of azo dyes. Their use mitigates pollution through the substitution of toxic chemicals, retic water and energy demands, and leads to more environmentally sustainable processes, such as anti-shrinking wool products (Bhatt, 2022).

16.3.2.4 Ecologically Neutral Trend in Enzyme Applications in the Textile Processing

The use of enzymatic processing in the textile industry results in certain meaningful environmental benefits:

Less use of water: Vast quantities of water are subsequently saved due to the lessened number of rinse procedures required by enzymatic preparations (Ren & Guan, 2025). By enzymes such as catalase, for example, excess hydrogen peroxide left over by bleaching is efficiently degraded, thus eliminating the long wash-up routines (Ribul et al., 2021).

Energy Savings: Since the enzyme works at moderated temperatures, low temperatures, and neutral pH, energy required to perform the process is also reduced radically (Ren & Guan, 2025).

Less Use of Chemicals: Harsh substances (i.e., alkalis, detergents, and chlorine-based bleaching chemicals, which are commonly used in the normal textile production) are substituted by enzymes (Ribul et al., 2021). The consumption of biodegradable enzymes will help manufacturers to limit the ecological impact, the release of hazardous by-products to the water, and create a safer working environment (Bhatt, 2022). This is an increasingly frequent shift in line with the increasing need to have green processes in the production process (Guo et al., 2025).

16.3.2.5 Top Priorities and Scope of Novelty

Enzymatic processing of textiles has a number of advantages, but there are some barriers to its intensive application. These are the initial expenditures that are incurred using enzyme technology and process optimization, and some companies are reluctant to switch the traditional process due to fears of scalability and consistency (Ren & Guan, 2025). As pH, temperature, and reaction time are significantly affected by enzyme efficiency and may vary across textile mills, specific solutions and process optimization must be developed. Though efforts to reduce the cost of enzymes in microbial enzyme production are still being carried out, enzyme manufacturing and stabilization may be too costly as well (Ren & Guan, 2025). In addition, not every enzyme can be used on every textile type, or necessitating the use of a multi-enzyme blend to be able to achieve the desired performance on difficult matrices or impurities (Torres et al., 2012).

16.3.3 Lignocellulolytic Enzymes, Energy Production

One promising feedstock of the renewable energy to produce biofuels, such as biogas (biomethane), bioethanol, and biohydrogen, is lignocellulosic biomass. The process normally involves a pretreatment of materials, fermentation, and a conversion process by enzyme (saccharification) (Chukwuma et al., 2020b).

16.3.3.1 The Biological Digestion of Carbohydrate Called Saccharification

Enzymatic digestion is utilized in biofuel production to convert lignocellulosic biomass into fermentable mono or oligosaccharides using lignocellulolytic enzymes (Chukwuma et al., 2020b). This methodology is favored compared to chemical hydrolysis because it has milder operating conditions, less energy issues as well as only a small amount of inhibitors formed (Benatti & Polizeli, 2023b).

Process: Cellulases hydrolyze the source material by cleaving the 1, 4-bonds in chains of cellulose to obtain glucose, cellobiose, and oligosaccharides. Xylan undergoes initial hydrolysis into xylo-oligosaccharides through the action of xylanases. These xylo-oligosaccharides are further converted into xylose monomers by hemicellulases. The ability of the hydrolytic enzymes to get to cellulose and hemicellulose can thus be enhanced by converting lignin into aromatic molecules through ligninases (Kato et al., 2024).

Yield Enhancement: Before enzymatic digestion, LCB is most importantly pretreated in order to improve the accessibility of the structure to enzymes (Chukwuma et al., 2020b). This would involve the removal of lignin and hemicellulose, crystallinity of cellulose, and the porosity increase. An example is that a 90% efficiency of enzymatic hydrolysis in 24 h can be reached with steam explosion pretreatment of poplar chips, where only 15% of enzymatic hydrolysis occurs in an untreated poplar chip (Juturu & Wu, 2012). Biological pretreatment procedures, such as enzymatic pretreatment, are more popular due to low energy costs, chemical-free operation, and economic benefits (Barapatre & Jha, 2016; Dinca et al., 2024b).

Factors That Affect Efficiency: Efficiency depends on the source of the enzyme, properties of the substrate, and reaction factors (temperature, pH) (Dinca et al., 2024b). At solids loadings above 20 percent w/w in enzyme hydrolysis, high sugar and ethanol concentrations can be achieved, reducing energy requirements and distillation costs, but can also cause water constraint and increased viscosity, a mass-conversion limiting factor. During pretreatment, inhibitors may also inhibit enzyme activity and yield of sugar (e.g., phenolic compounds, furans, acetic acid) (Chen & Liu, 2016). Non-ionic surfactants, e.g., polyethylene glycol (PEG), may enhance the convertibility of LCB over 30% by altering cellulose surface properties and reduction of enzyme loading (Chukwuma et al., 2020c).

16.3.3.2 Fermentation of Bioethanol, Biogas, and Biohydrogen Production

Bacteria are used to convert the released sugars into a range of biofuels after saccharification.

Bioethanol Production

Fermentation: Fermentation of glucose, mainly cellulose by yeasts (e.g., *Saccharomyces cerevisiae*) or bacteria is performed to produce ethanol (Saini et al.,

2015). Up to 30% of hemicellulose pentoses, like xylose, can be fermented by yeasts like *Candida shehatae* (Beluhan et al., 2023).

Strategies

- **Separate Hydrolysis Fermentation (SHF) Fermentation**: When working with lignocellulosic biomass, fermentable monosaccharide sugars in cellulose and hemicellulose have to be first phytotransformed and the end product fermented by microorganisms. Under the Separate Hydrolysis and Fermentation (SHF) method, the processes are separated. To begin with, the biomass can be broken down into sugars by first using enzymes (e.g., cellulases and hemicellulases) in conditions near the optimal enzyme activity (e.g., increased temperatures). Fermentable sugars undergo a conversion to ethanol through the action of yeast, which is performed under controlled conditions to ensure consistency and efficacy. By separating the processes of hydrolysis and fermentation into distinct steps, it becomes feasible to optimize each phase specifically. This methodological separation enhances the conversion efficiency and ultimately increases the yield of ethanol produced, making the process more effective and productive (Beluhan et al., 2023).
- **Simultaneous Saccharification and Fermentation (SSF)**: It is a process in which fermentation and hydrolysis occur concurrently in the same reactor. Consequently, the inhibition of the cellulase products available as a result of this immediate sugar adsorption is minimized, the consequent enzyme rate of hydrolysis is accelerated, the content of enzyme is reduced, and the product yield and process duration are cut short (Beluhan et al., 2023).
- **Direct Microbial Conversion (DMC)**: The process that combines enzyme production, hydrolysis, and fermentation into one step, making the process simple and cost effective (Beluhan et al., 2023).

Processed sugarcane bagasse, rice straw, and corn cob have all so far produced yields of ethanol of 86% ± 2 when *Candida magnoliae* was used in the process (Beluhan et al., 2023). New methods have increased the conversion yields to nearly 92 percent of the ideal conversion (Madhavan et al., 2011; Kang et al., 2014b).

Biogas or Biomethane Production

- **Process**: The transformation of lignocellulosic biomass into biogas (mostly methane) occurs through a multi-step biological process termed as anaerobic digestion, where lignocellulosic biomass is acted upon by a consortia of microbes, the sequence of which includes: hydrolysis, acidogenesis, acetogenesis, and methanogenesis (Chukwuma et al., 2020b).
- **Enzymatic Pretreatment**: Enzymatic pretreatment is the most friendly heading on increasing the yield of biogas. This enhances biogas production and LCB that is prepared to become more bioavailable (Chukwuma et al., 2020b).
- **Increase**: A 19 percent and 13 percent rise in biogas were attained when sugar beet pulp and wasted hops were enzymatically treated, respectively (Chukwuma et al.,

2020b). There was an increase of 135 and 76 percent in cumulative biogas production in the acid-treated agave mezcal bagasse and untreated material, respectively (Hernández-López et al., 2025).

Biohydrogen Production

- **Process**: An enzymolysis is used in the first phase to convert pretreated lignocellulosic materials into monosaccharides, which are in turn fermented to H_2 (Chen et al., 2013).
- **Yield Enhancement**: Hydrolysis can be enhanced by ensuring effective removal of the inhibitors along with interception of sugar build-up (an impediment to hydrolysis). Technologies such as SSF and simultaneous saccharification and co-fermentation (SSCF) are already considered viable alternatives due to direct utilization of hydrolyzed products by fermentative microorganisms, keeping the concentrations of monosaccharides low and increasing efficiency. Combinations of pretreatments are also effective to enhance digestibility and H_2 yield, e.g., ammonia and diluted sulfuric acid pretreatment of rice straw resulted in a high H2 yield (Chen et al., 2013).

16.3.3.3 Challenges and Opportunity of the Biofuel Production

Lignocelluloses biofuels production is plagued with the following difficulties:

- **Expensive Pretreatment**: Biomass pretreatment is a costly process of biogas or biofuel production, thus making it a major challenge when large-scale processes are to be implemented. It requires specialized equipment, chemicals, and energy-demanding processes (Bajpai, 2024).
- **Enzyme Price and Productivity**: Cellulase enzymes are very expensive, and when used in the wrong setting, they hamper cost-effective production of biofuel (Sharada et al., 2009).
- **Biomass Recalcitrance**: The compact and rigid nature of LCB, especially the lignin content makes it harder to qualify the enzymes in hydrolyzing cellulose to release sugars leading to low yields (Zoghlami & Paës, 2019a, 2019b).
- **Formation of Inhibitors**: Pretreatment procedures have been found to produce inhibitors of enzyme activity that adversely affect the yield of monosaccharides (Chen & Liu, 2016).
- **Scale-up and Supply Chain**: Supply chains of biomass are irregular in nature, saccharification is complex, and its technology and scale-up issues cause high capital and operating cost, thereby hindering commercialization (Cheah et al., 2020b).
- **Process Complexity**: Complexity of the Process Technological investigations and analyses have shown that process complexity is a big negative issue that prevents scale-up (Cheah et al., 2020b).

A more vigorous and efficient system of enzyme production and a more efficient conversion capability of biomass process and integration can be realized. The research efforts concentrate on the diversification of the sources of feedstock, analysis of the overall costs, and optimization of operating parameters (Cheah et al., 2020b). In order to reduce dependency on fossil fuels and restrict greenhouse gas emissions toward a more environmentally friendly and renewable energy future, lignocellulosic biomass can be transformed into biofuels (Beluhan et al., 2023).

16.3.4 Digestibility and Nutritional Value of Animal Feed Production

Lignocellulosic biomass, especially agricultural residues like straw, presents significant potential as a sustainable component in animal feed, enhancing both digestibility and nutrient content. However, its lignin and fiber content do restrict the livestock's ability to use cellulose and hemicellulose (Ajila et al., 2012). To surmount these limitations and acquire digestibility and nutritional quality, animal feeds are increasingly complemented by exogenous lignocellulolytic enzymes (Sridar, 2017b).

16.3.4.1 Cellulases and Hemicellulases Functional Insights

Cellulases: These have the effect of digesting cellulose into glucose making the nutrients more readily available by hydrolyzing complex fibers. This boosts the absorption of nutrients, improves feed efficiency, and optimal growth of the animal (Imran et al., 2016; Wenk & Boessinger, 1993). Cellulases are particularly useful to herbivores, the food of which contains large amounts of fibrous material. They also catalyze the fermentation process of the ruminant in the rumen, therefore, improving nutrient utilization and increasing milk yield (Ashaolu et al., 2024b).

- **Mechanism**: Cellulases target 1, 4-glycosidic linkages and cellulose, which are tough plant fibers, and break them down into cellobiose and glucose. The animal can readily absorb these simple sugars. Cellulases in ruminants are used in conjunction with how fiber is broken down using the inherent microbial enzymes found in rumen that increase the rate of digestion (Imran et al., 2016).
- **Advantages**: Optimal body growth and growth efficiency, due to better nutrient absorption, is achieved by the use of cellulases in livestock, especially herbivores that feed off high fiber diets. Cellulases in rumen enhance fermentation effectiveness in big animals because, in ruminants, fermentation enhances nutrient use and has the potential to dramatically boost milk production in dairy livestock (Imran et al., 2016; Wenk & Boessinger, 1993).

Hemicellulases: Hemicellulases, namely pectinase, beta-glucanase, beta-mannanase, xylanase, and arabinoxylanase, aim at hemicellulose, which is one of the key components of feed sources such as soybean meal. The enzymes remove the heteropolysaccharides, thereby decreasing the viscosity of the digest and liberation of the nutrient bound to insoluble structural components. Hemicellulases break down complex carbohydrates to oligosaccharides and monosaccharides, rendering them digestible (more creatively, accessible) to monogastric animals (Jayasekara & Ratnayake, 2019; Wang et al., 2023). Xylanase and beta-glucanase supplements not only make xylans and beta-glucans more easily digestible but also boost the energy content of hemicellulose-enriched feed and the overall growth rates and feed ratio (Wang et al., 2023).

- **Mechanism**: They are enzymes (hemicellulases) that break down heteropolysaccharides, thus lowering the viscosity of the digest and freeing nutrients chelated to insoluble structural components of the diets (Wang et al., 2023). This destroys complex carbohydrates into oligosaccharides or monosaccharides which are easily broken down by animals with monogasts (Wang et al., 2023).
- **Advantages**: xylanases and beta-glucanases supplementation enhance the intake of arabinoxylans and beta-glucans present in the diet (Wang et al., 2023). Hemicellulases have the possibility to raise the available energy content of hemicellulose-rich foodstuffs (Wang et al., 2023).

16.3.4.2 A Few More Benefits of Broad Spectrum of Exogenous Enzyme Additives

There are numerous other advantages of exogenous enzymes beyond breaking down feed and freeing nutrients so they can be absorbed. These advantages are:

- **Enhanced Feed Conversion Rates**: Enzymes boost the rate of feed conversion into animal products or animals raised (e.g., milk, eggs) (Imran et al., 2016).
- **Cost Savings**: Enzymes increase fiber digestibility and nutrient absorption and enable livestock producers to extract more energy out of less feed, and thus eliminate the overall feeding cost.
- **Enhanced Gut Health**: By stabilizing feed consistency, enzymes can promote gut health and the digestion and absorption process, perhaps halting the growth of pathogens that cause disease (Imran et al., 2016).
- **Lowering Environmental Burden**: Increased feed efficiency can reduce dietary concentrations of certain nutrients, which will reduce nutrient excretion into the environment (Wang et al., 2023). Thus, pollutants such as phosphate, nitrogen, and ammonia are reduced, limiting the eutrophication and acidification potential of manure (Ajila et al., 2012).
- **Bioactive Compounds**: Bioactive peptides are a product of enzymatic digestion of protein in diets; they enhance the immune system, increase resistance to disease, and quicken recovery during an infection (Jayasekara & Ratnayake, 2019; Juturu & Wu, 2012).

16.3.4.3 Other Challenges Ahead Strategic Directions

Although promising, there are some issues that surround the use of exogenous enzymes in animal feed:

- **Formulation/Stability**: The enzymes used in animal feeds are susceptible to changes in the environment, which cause variability in the performance of the product and changes in animal performance. Stability of the enzymes during storage and at high temperatures during pelleting processes is also a challenge because a lack of protection can degrade the enzyme effectiveness in the digestive system of the animal. Liquid enzyme products tend to expire faster (Bedford & Partridge, 2010).
- **Cost/Equipment**: Use of liquid enzyme after the pellet increases maintenance and operational cost due to additional installations at the feed mill (Bedford & Partridge, 2010).
- **Fragile Efficacy**: Studies concerning exogenous fibrolytic enzymes in ruminants have inconclusively yielded both ineffective and even adversely affecting enzyme mixtures on digestion (Wang et al., 2023).
- **Knowledge Gaps**: The exact mechanism by which white-rot fungi break down lignin to improve digestion in ruminants is not well understood, and there is a dearth of information on the fungal strains utilized in different research as well as consistent growth conditions (Kadam et al., 2022).

The next field of study should focus on improving fungal strains with respect to selective lignin breakdown by optimizing cultures and gene expression (Van Kuijk et al., 2014). The growing body of knowledge in the field of enzyme discovery and engineering is also making rudimentarily thermostable enzymes a possibility, which can survive temperatures and time under conditioning that would normally require a coating to avoid deactivation (Bedford & Partridge, 2010). To fully tap the potential of exogenous enzymes in enhancing production of ruminants and to assuage the concerns of the customers regarding growth promoters and antibiotics, these problems will have to be eliminated (Ajila et al., 2012).

16.4 Impacts to the Environment and Visions on Sustainable Development

16.4.1 Enzymatic Treatment of Waste Biomass Reduces Pollution

Using ligninolytic enzymes in bioprocesses lowers pollution in two ways: by replacing harsh chemicals with biodegradable catalysts that may eliminate xenobiotics and clean textile effluents (Van Kuijk et al., 2014). Cleaner wastewater properties result from the effective decolorization of the dyes utilizing the immobilized enzymes

(Paul & Dutta, 2017b). The enzymatic treatment of lignocellulosic waste is used to valorize waste and provides circular economy models because this waste is converted to resources (Kumar et al., 2016a). Biomass waste in general, in terms of municipal and industrial, is dealt with the help of microbial and enzymatic interventions and the resultant products are diversified, eliminating dependency on landfills (Sankaran et al., 2021b). This substitution of chemical by enzymatic reaction removes another source of greenhouse gases associated with the acidic treatment of the conventional biomass (Bhatia et al., 2023b).

16.4.2 The Problems with Enzyme to Be Applied and the Adaptation of Industrial Enzyme

Despite these advantages, enzyme applications are facing challenges that do not allow other already known enzyme properties to be used, such as the cost of the enzyme, production yield limitations, and limited or a lack of performance under industrial processing conditions (Angural et al., 2020; Son & Ravindran, 2011). The variety of modes used to carry out the storage, handling, and delivery of enzymes must be optimized in order to preserve their activities and guarantee consistency of the process (Liu et al., 2025). Future work since 2020 focuses on engineering more stability into the enzymes, decreasing the cost of producing them, as well as increased substrate specificity, and is performed through use of synthetic biology and metagenomics (Mehta & Chelike, 2024b). It is essential to fill these technological loopholes to allow the industry to be adopted widely.

16.4.3 Human Resources and Health Policies, Economic Incentives, and the Future

Government regulations in the field of sustainable production, waste disposal, and reduction of greenhouse gases encourage the invention of enzyme-based biotechnologies (Abena & Simachew, 2024). Economic implications of enzyme integration have shown that it can result in reducing operations costs through less chemical and effluent cost treatment, but costs are competitive when enzyme prices are lowered and process optimization is achieved (Bhatia et al., 2023b). That biotechnology is aligned with the frameworks of circular bioeconomy contributes to sustainability and resource efficiency, and is enabled by continued technological innovation (Kumar et al., 2016a).

16.5 New Trends and New Enzyme Systems

16.5.1 LPMO Discovery and Engineering

The discovery of Lytic Polysaccharide Monooxygenase (LPMOs) brought about a new paradigm in oxidative enzymes capable of oxidatively cleaving glycosidic bonds in crystalline polysaccharides to vastly improve the efficiency of enzymatic hydrolysis when used in conjunction with cellulases (Bonnen et al., 1994). There is the challenge to reconsider the paradigms of the LPMO actions and optimum process parameters because this family of enzymes also uses hydrogen peroxide as a co-substrate (Ethaib et al., 2020). Industrial opportunities to apply LPMOs in enzyme mixtures are on the horizon, but issues surrounding enzyme stability and regulation of reactive oxygen species during processing are still outstanding (Mehta & Chelike, 2024b).

16.5.2 Enzymes of Extremophiles and Thermostable Variants

In extremophilic organisms, thermostable and non-pH-sensitive enzymes are produced, which make them more adaptable to industrial practice, which requires extreme conditions of operating (Salas-Nuñez et al., 2024). Structural and functional studies allow the engineering of such enzymes in order to obtain increased catalytic activity and robustness (Bien-Cuong et al., 2009b). Case studies reveal the enhancements in the biofuel yields and efficiencies of biomass degradation by the use of thermostable cellulases, which thereby confirms their industrial uses.

16.5.3 Technology Radicals Unrelated to the Common Context of Biomass Conversion

In addition, ligninolytic enzymes have new uses such as in biosensors, analytical chemistry, and production of bioactive molecules (Benatti & Polizeli, 2023). The sensitive detection of environmental pollutants and biomolecules can be carried out with the use of biosensors where laccase and peroxidases can be used (Moldes & Vidal, 2010). Bioproducts such as bioplastics utilize enzyme-mediated conversion of lignocellulosic biomass intermediates into bioproducts using biomass to products (Del Mar Contreras-Gámez et al., 2022b). Integration with synthetic biology develops metabolic engineering strategies toward the bio-optimal synthesis of bioproducts (Tyagi et al., 2013).

16.6 Combining Multi-Enzymatic Processes in Waste Management of Biomass

16.6.1 Synergistic Consortia of Enzymes to Facilitate High Efficiency in Biomass Conversion

Enhancement of the synergistic effects to improve biomass degradation can be achieved by mixing cellulases, hemicellulases, and ligninolytic enzymes into enzyme consortia with complementary and sequential activity (Grgas et al., 2023b). More complex biomass structures can be broken down in a multi-step catalyzed process that allows maximum substrate conversion (Mehta & Chelike, 2024b).

16.6.2 Single-Step Biorefinery Consolidated Bioprocessing

Consolidated bioprocessing has the promise of carrying out enzyme production, hydrolysis, and fermentation in the same organism or co-cultures making a bioprocess less complex and less expensive (Zoghlami & Paës, 2019d). Combining these functions is, however, inefficient to metabolic balance; to achieve this, we have to have strain engineering and bioprocess development areas (Mehta & Chelike, 2024b). The CBP development complies with sustainability objectives, because of the reduction of steps involved in the process, and increases overall efficiency (Bonnen et al., 1994).

16.6.3 Residual Biomass and Waste Valorization Feedback

Secondary valorization can occur with the use of post-harvest residues (e.g., spent agro-residues after mushroom or enzyme harvest) to drive the cyclic utilization of resources and improved resource recovery (Kumar et al., 2016b). The value-added potential is further manifested by recovery of antioxidative phenolic compounds contained in such residues (Moreno et al., 2014). These waste streams are then converted into a bio-management regime which encourages environmental management and reduction in waste (Xia et al., 2021b).

16.7 Summary and Outlook

Lignin-cellulolytic enzymes shall be important catalyst in sustainable use and value addition of ligno-cellulolytic biomass waste. The very recalcitrant nature of LCB, mostly as a structural obstacle by lignin, requires viable pretreatment methodologies in order to increase its enzyme-attackable nature. Fungi and bacteria are the most common microorganisms used as sources of these enzymes, and their reproducibility, good yield, and flexibility to the various conditions are important factors determining industrial up-scalability.

Applications of these enzymes are changing many industries:

Pulp and Paper: Chemical-free biopulping with lignin-degrading fungi can cut energy costs (20–30 percent) and reduce operations chemical costs, strengthen pulp and paper, and eliminate environmental risks. When used in synergy (xylanases + laccase or H_2O_2), biobleaching yields significant savings on classic chlorine-bearing chemicals (up to 15% with xylanase, 28.6% with laccase/H_2O_2 hybrid), and eradicates toxic AOX emissions, making the result whiter and stronger with a lighter carbon footprint.

Textiles: Enzymes can be used as a desizing agent (amylases), in denim, to bio-stone the denim (cellulase) and bio-polish denim (cellulase), and to or desizing and dyeing in denim (laccases). The applications save water, energy, use less intense chemicals, and end products are of superior fabric material, and provide a greener manufacturing paradigm.

Biofuels: The enzymatic conversion of LCB into fermentable sugars to be used in the production of bioethanol, biogas, and biohydrogen relies on the lignocellulolytic enzymes. Efficient enzymatic hydrolysis and fermentation processes (such as SSF) are essential in maximizing sugar production and biofuel production, and pretreatment methods play a vital role in this aspect. Although much has been advanced (e.g., 90% hydrolysis activity in pretreated poplar chips, 86% yields of ethanol against agricultural waste, 135% increase in biogas generation), there is still a need to overcome relatively high pretreatment costs, enzyme performance, as well as scale-up.

Animal Feed: Cellulases and hemicellulases, when added as supplements to high-fiber animal feeds, can dramatically improve the digestibility of nutrients in these feeds and their nutritional value, leading to increased feed efficiency, decreased production cost, and a favorable impact on the environment via reduced excretion of nutrients.

All such applications are characterized by the global shift toward a circular bioeconomy, in which biomass waste is used to produce valuable goods, eliminating fossil raw materials consumption and minimizing pollution of the environment. The entire potential of lignino-cellulolytic enzymes to play a significant part in a sustainable future is currently limited by technical and financial obstacles that must be overcome by additional advancements in enzyme engineering, process design, and feedstock expansion research and development.

References

Abena, T., & Simachew, A. (2024). A review on xylanase sources, classification, mode of action, fermentation processes, and applications as a promising biocatalyst. *Biotechnologia, 105*(3), 273–285. https://doi.org/10.5114/bta.2024.141806

Agrawal, K., Nair, L. G., Chaturvedi, V., & Verma, P. (2023). Designing microbial cellulases using genetic engineering approach: A promising strategy towards zero-waste cellulosic biorefinery. *Biocatalysis and Agricultural Biotechnology, 52*(July), Article 102830. https://doi.org/10.1016/j.bcab.2023.102830

Ajila, C. M., Brar, S. K., Verma, M., Tyagi, R. D., Godbout, S., & Valéro, J. R. (2012). Bio-processing of agro-byproducts to animal feed. *Critical Reviews in Biotechnology, 32*(4), 382–400. https://doi.org/10.3109/07388551.2012.659172

Akhtar, M. (1994). Biomechanical pulping of Aspen wood chips with three strains of *Ceriporiopsis subvermispora. Hfsg, 48*(3), 199–202. https://doi.org/10.1515/hfsg.1994.48.3.199

Akhtar, et al. (1993). Biomechanical pulping of loblolly pine chips with selected white-rot fungi. *Holzforchung, 47,* 36–40.

Andlar, M., Rezić, T., Marđetko, N., Kracher, D., Ludwig, R., & Šantek, B. (2018). Lignocellulose degradation: An overview of fungi and fungal enzymes involved in lignocellulose degradation. *Engineering in Life Sciences, 18*(11), 768–778. https://doi.org/10.1002/elsc.201800039

Angural, S., Gupta, N., Warmoota, R., Kumar, A., Kumar, D., & Sondhi, S. (2020). Lignolytic and hemicellulolytic enzyme cocktail production from Bacillus tequilensis LXM 55 and its application in pulp biobleaching. *Bioprocess and Biosystems Engineering, 43*(12), 2219–2229. https://doi.org/10.1007/s00449-020-02407-4

Ashaolu, T. J., Malik, T., Soni, R., Prieto, M. A., & Jafari, S. M. (2024). Extremophilic microorganisms as a source of emerging enzymes for the food industry: a review. *Food Science & Nutrition, 13*(1). https://doi.org/10.1002/fsn3.4540

Bajar, S., Bishnoi, N. R., & Singh, A. (2020). Exploration of low-cost agro-industrial waste substrate for cellulase and xylanase production using Aspergillus heteromorphus. *Applied Water Science, 10*(6). https://doi.org/10.1007/s13201-020-01236-w

Bajpai, P. (2004). Biological bleaching of chemical pulps. *Critical Reviews in Biotechnology, 24*(1), 1–58. https://doi.org/10.1080/07388550490465817

Bajpai, P. (2024). Challenges in the engineering of lignocellulolytic enzymes. https://doi.org/10.1016/B978-0-443-21492-9.00013-6.

Barapatre, A., & Harit, J. (2016). Decolourization and biological treatment of pulp and paper mill effluent by lignin-degrading fungus aspergillus flavus strain F10. *International Journal of Current Microbiology and Applied Sciences, 5,* 19–32. https://doi.org/10.20546/ijcmas.2016.505.003.

Barapatre, A., & Jha, H. (2016). Decolourization and biological treatment of pulp and paper mill effluent by lignin-degrading fungus aspergillus flavus strain F10. *International Journal of Current Microbiology and Applied Sciences, 5*(5), 19–32. https://doi.org/10.20546/ijcmas.2016.505.003

Bedford, M. R., & Partridge, G. G. (2010). *Enzymes in Farm Animal Nutrition.* CABI. https://doi.org/10.1079/9781845936747.0000.

Beluhan, S., Mihajlovski, K., Šantek, B., & Ivančić Šantek, M. (2023). The production of bioethanol from lignocellulosic biomass: Pretreatment methods, fermentation, and downstream processing. *Energies, 16*(19), 7003. https://doi.org/10.3390/en16197003

Benatti, A. L. T., & Polizeli, M. L. T. M. (2023). Lignocellulolytic biocatalysts: The main players involved in multiple biotechnological processes for biomass valorization. *Microorganisms, 11*(1), 162. https://doi.org/10.3390/microorganisms11010162

Bhatia, L., Jha, H., Sarkar, T., & Sarangi, P. K. (2023). Food waste utilization for reducing carbon footprints towards sustainable and cleaner environment: A review. *International Journal of Environmental Research and Public Health, 20*(3), 2318. https://doi.org/10.3390/ijerph20032318

Bhatt, P. (2022). *Industrial applications of microbial enzymes*. CRC Press.

Bien-Cuong, D., Thi-Thu, D., Berrin, J., Haltrich, D., Kim-Anh, T., Sigoillot, J., & Yamabhai, M. (2009). Cloning, expression in Pichia pastoris, and characterization of a thermostable GH5 mannan endo-1,4-β-mannosidase from Aspergillus Niger BK01. *Microbial Cell Factories, 8*(1). https://doi.org/10.1186/1475-2859-8-59

Blasi, A., Verardi, A., Lopresto, C. G., Siciliano, S., & Sangiorgio, P. (2023). Lignocellulosic agricultural waste valorization to obtain valuable products: An overview. *Recycling, 8*(4), 61. https://doi.org/10.3390/recycling8040061

Bonnen, A. M., Orth, A. B., & Anton, L. H. (1994). Lignin-degrading enzymes of the commercial button Mushroom, *Agaricus bisporus. Applied and Environmental Microbiology, 60*(3), 960–965. https://doi.org/10.1128/aem.60.3.960-965.1994

Cheah, W. Y., Sankaran, R., Show, P. L., Ibrahim, T. N. B. T., Chew, K. W., Culaba, A., & Chang, J. (2020). Pretreatment methods for lignocellulosic biofuels production: Current advances, challenges and future prospects. *Biofuel Research Journal, 7*(1), 1115–1127. https://doi.org/10.18331/brj2020.7.1.4

Chen, H. Z., & Liu, Z. H. (2016). Enzymatic hydrolysis of lignocellulosic biomass from low to high solids loading. *Engineering in Life Sciences, 17*(5), 489–499. https://doi.org/10.1002/elsc.201600102

Chen, R., Wang, Y. Z., Liao, Q., Zhu, X., & Xu, T. F. (2013). Hydrolysates of lignocellulosic materials for biohydrogen production. *BMB Reports, 46*(5), 244–251. https://doi.org/10.5483/bmbrep.2013.46.5.038

Chukwuma, O. B., Rafatullah, M., Tajarudin, H. A., & Ismail, N. (2020a). Lignocellulolytic enzymes in biotechnological and industrial processes: A review. *Sustainability, 12*(18), 7282. https://doi.org/10.3390/su12187282

Chukwuma, O., Rafatullah, M., Tajarudin, H., & Ismail, N. (2020b). Lignocellulolytic enzymes in biotechnological and industrial processes: A review. *Sustainability, 12*, 7282. https://doi.org/10.3390/su12187282

del Mar C-Gámez, M., Galán-Martín, Á., & Seixas, N., et al. (2023). Deep eutectic solvents for improved biomass pretreatment: Current status and future prospective towards sustainable processes. *Bioresource Technology, 369*, 128396. https://doi.org/10.1016/j.biortech.2022.128396

Dinca, M., Ferdes, M., Paraschiv, G., & Zabava, B. (2024). Enzymatic pretreatment of lignocellulosic biomass for biogas production—review. *Engineering for Rural Development, 23*. https://doi.org/10.22616/erdev.2024.23.tf181

Ethaib, S., Zubaidi, S. L., Omar, R., Siti Mazlina, M. K., & Dayang Radiah, A. B. (2020). Toward sustainable processes of pretreatment technologies of lignocellulosic biomass for enzymatic production of biofuels and chemicals: A review. *BioResources, 15*(4), 10063–10088. https://doi.org/10.15376/biores.15.4.ethaib

Grgas, D., Rukavina, M., Bešlo, D., Štefanac, T., Crnek, V., Šikić, T., Habuda-Stanić, M., & Landeka Dragičević, T. (2023). The bacterial degradation of lignin—a review. *Water, 15*(7), 1272. https://doi.org/10.3390/w15071272

Guo, X., Wu, X., Wang, B., Liu, F. (2025). Biopulping, biobleaching, and deinking. https://doi.org/10.1016/B978-0-443-21903-0.00019-9.

Heikinheimo, L., Buchert, J., Miettinen-Oinonen, A., & Suominen, P. (2000). Treating denim fabrics with Trichoderma Reesei Cellulases. *Textile Research Journal, 70*, 969–973. https://doi.org/10.1177/004051750007001106

Hernández-López, R., Moreno-Andrade, I., Barragán-Huerta, B. E., Estrada-Arriaga, E. B., & Garzón-Zúñiga, M. A. (2025). Biogas production from *Agave durangensis* Mezcal Bagasse pretreated using chemical processes. *Fermentation, 11*(7), 399. https://doi.org/10.3390/fermentation11070399

Hsin, K., Lee, H., Huang, Y., Lin, G., Lin, P., Lin, Y. J., & Chen, P. (2025). Lignocellulose degradation in bacteria and fungi: Cellulosomes and industrial relevance. *Frontiers in Microbiology, 16*. https://doi.org/10.3389/fmicb.2025.1583746

Imran, M., Nazar, M., Saif, M., Khan, M. A., Sanaullah, Vardan, M., & Javed, O., (2016). Role of enzymes in animal nutrition: A review. *PSM Veterinary Research, 01*(2), 38–45.

Jayasekara, S., & Ratnayake, R. (2019). Microbial cellulases: An overview and applications. In *Cellulose*. https://doi.org/10.5772/intechopen.84531

Jeffries, T. W., & Viikari, L. (1996). Enzymes for pulp and paper processing. In *ACS symposium series*. https://doi.org/10.1021/bk-1996-0655.

Jha, H., & Patil, M. (2013). Biopulping of sugarcane bagasse and decolorization of Kraft liquor by the Laccase produced by Klebsiella Aerogenes NCIM 2098. *Malaysian Journal of Microbiology, 9*, 301–307.

Jha, H. (2019). Fungal diversity and enzymes involved in lignin degradation. In R. Naraian (Ed.) *Mycodegradation of lignocelluloses. Fungal biology*. Springer, Cham. https://doi.org/10.1007/978-3-030-23834-6_3.

Juturu, V., & Wu, J. (2013). Insight into microbial hemicellulases other than xylanases: A review. *Journal of Chemical Technology & Biotechnology., 88*, 353–363. https://doi.org/10.1002/jctb.3969

Kadam, A. A., Saratale, G. D., Ghodake, G. S., Saratale, R. G., Shahzad, A., Magotra, V. K., Kumar, M., Palem, R. R., & Sung, J.-S. (2022). Recent advances in the development of Laccase-based biosensors via nano-immobilization techniques. *Chemosensors, 10*(2), 58. https://doi.org/10.3390/chemosensors10020058

Kang, Q., Appels, L., Tan, T., & Dewil, R. (2014). Bioethanol from lignocellulosic biomass: Current findings determine research priorities. *The Scientific World Journal, 2014*, 1–13. https://doi.org/10.1155/2014/298153

Kato, H., Miura, D., Kato, M., & Shimizu, M. (2024). Metabolic mechanism of lignin-derived aromatics in white-rot fungi. *Applied Microbiology and Biotechnology, 108*(1). https://doi.org/10.1007/s00253-024-13371-4

Kazeem, M. O., Baharuddin, A. S., Shah, U. K. M., & Abdulrahman, N. A. (2017). Prospecting agro-waste cocktail: Supplementation for cellulase production by a newly isolated thermophilic B. Licheniformis 2D55. *Applied Biochemistry and Biotechnology, 182*(4), 1318–1340. https://doi.org/10.1007/s12010-017-2401-z

Kim, S., Moldes, D., & Cavaco-Paulo, A. (2007). Laccases for enzymatic colouration of unbleached cotton. *Enzyme and Microbial Technology, 40*(7), 1788–1793. https://doi.org/10.1016/j.enzmictec.2007.01.002

Kumar, A., Gautam, A., & Dutt, D. (2016a). Biotechnological transformation of lignocellulosic biomass into industrial products: An overview. *Advances in Bioscience and Biotechnology, 07*(03), 149–168. https://doi.org/10.4236/abb.2016.73014

Kumar, V., Marín-Navarro, J., Shukla, P. (2016b). Thermostable microbial xylanases for pulp and paper industries: trends, applications and further perspectives. *World Journal of Microbiology and Biotechnology 32*. https://doi.org/10.1007/s11274-015-2005-0.

Kumar, A., Gautam, A., & Dutt, D. (2020a). Bio-pulping: An energy saving and environment-friendly approach. *Physical Sciences Reviews, 5*(10). https://doi.org/10.1515/psr-2019-0043

Kumar, B., Bhardwaj, N., Agrawal, K., Chaturvedi, V., & Verma, P. (2020b). Current perspective on pretreatment technologies using lignocellulosic biomass: An emerging biorefinery concept. *Fuel Processing Technology, 199*(July 2019). https://doi.org/10.1016/j.fuproc.2019.106244

Kushwaha, R., Kesarwani, P., Kushwaha, A. (2023). Bio-stoning: Heighten the appearance of denim garment through application of cellulase enzyme. https://doi.org/10.22271/ed.book.2560.

Liu, M., Xiao, R., Li, X., Zhao, Y., & Huang, J. (2025). A comprehensive review of recombinant technology in the food industry: Exploring expression systems, application, and future challenges. *Comprehensive Reviews in Food Science and Food Safety, 24*(2). https://doi.org/10.1111/1541-4337.70078

Madhavan, A., Srivastava, A., Kondo, A., & Bisaria, V. S. (2011). Bioconversion of lignocellulose-derived sugars to ethanol by engineered Saccharomyces cerevisiae. *Critical Reviews in Biotechnology, 32*(1), 22–48. https://doi.org/10.3109/07388551.2010.539551

Martínez, A. T., Ruiz-Dueñas, F. J., Camarero, S., & Martínez, M. J. (2018). *Chapter 8. Biological lignin degradation* (pp. 199–225). Royal society of chemistry. https://doi.org/10.1039/9781788010351-00199

Mehta, P., & Chelike, D. K. (2024). Utilizing fungal biodegradation for valorisation of lignocellulosic waste biomass and its diverse applications. *Applied Research, 3*(4). https://doi.org/10.1002/appl.202300119

Moldes, D., & Vidal, T. (2011). New possibilities of Kraft pulp Biobleaching with Laccase and sulfonated mediators. *Process Biochemistry, 46*, 656–660. https://doi.org/10.1016/j.procbio.2010.11.005

Moreno, A. D., Ibarra, D., Alvira, P., Tomás-Pejó, E., & Ballesteros, M. (2014). A review of biological delignification and detoxification methods for lignocellulosic bioethanol production. *Critical Reviews in Biotechnology, 35*(3), 342–354. https://doi.org/10.3109/07388551.2013.878896

Nair, L. G., Agrawal, K., & Verma, P. (2022a). An insight into the principles of lignocellulosic biomass-based zero-waste biorefineries: A green leap towards imperishable energy-based future. *Biotechnology and Genetic Engineering Reviews, 38*(2), 288–338. https://doi.org/10.1080/02648725.2022.2082223

Nair, L. G., Agrawal, K., & Verma, P. (2022b). An overview of sustainable approaches for bioenergy production from agro-industrial wastes. *Energy Nexus, 6*(March), Article 100086. https://doi.org/10.1016/j.nexus.2022.100086

Nair, L. G., & Verma, P. (2025). Harnessing carbon potential of lignocellulosic biomass: advances in pretreatments, applications, and the transformative role of machine learning in biorefineries. *Bioresources and Bioprocessing, 12*(1). https://doi.org/10.1186/s40643-025-00935-z

Ndochinwa, G. O., Odiba, A. S., Nwagu, T. N., Okoro, N. O., Amadi, O. C., Moneke, A. N., Nnamchi, C. I., & Wang, Q.-Y. (2024). New advances in protein engineering for industrial applications: Key takeaways. *Open Life Sciences, 19*(1). https://doi.org/10.1515/biol-2022-0856

Paul, S., & Dutta, A. (2018). Challenges and opportunities of lignocellulosic biomass for anaerobic digestion. *Resources, Conservation and Recycling., 130*, 164–174. https://doi.org/10.1016/j.resconrec.2017.12.005

Ren, Z., & Guan, X. (2025). Evaluating the environmental and easy-care benefits of diacetate fiber blended textiles: Implications for sustainability in the textile industry. *Research Journal of Textile and Apparel*. https://doi.org/10.1108/rjta-07-2024-0109

Resch, M. G., Decker, S. R., Himmel, M. E., Bayer, E. A., Donohoe, B. S., Baker, J. O., & Beckham, G. T. (2013). Fungal cellulases and complexed cellulosomal enzymes exhibit synergistic mechanisms in cellulose deconstruction. *Energy & Environmental Science, 6*(6), 1858. https://doi.org/10.1039/c3ee00019b

Ribul, M., Lanot, A., Tommencioni Pisapia, C., Purnell, P., Mcqueen-Mason, S. J., & Baurley, S. (2021). Mechanical, chemical, biological: Moving towards closed-loop bio-based recycling in a circular economy of sustainable textiles. *Journal of Cleaner Production, 326*, Article 129325. https://doi.org/10.1016/j.jclepro.2021.129325

Sahadevan, L. D. M., Misra, C. S., & Thankamani, V. (2016). Characterization of lignin-degrading enzymes (LDEs) from a dimorphic novel fungus and identification of products of enzymatic breakdown of lignin. *3 Biotech, 6*(1). https://doi.org/10.1007/s13205-016-0384-z

Saini, A., Aggarwal, N. K., Sharma, A., & Yadav, A. (2015). Actinomycetes: A source of Lignocellulolytic enzymes. *Enzyme Research, 2015*, Article 279381. https://doi.org/10.1155/2015/279381

Salas-Nuñez, L. F., Barrera-Ocampo, A., Caicedo, P. A., Cortes, N., Osorio, E. H., Villegas-Torres, M. F., & González Barrios, A. F. (2024). Machine learning to predict enzyme-substrate interactions in elucidation of synthesis pathways: A review. *Metabolites, 14*(3), 154. https://doi.org/10.3390/metabo14030154

Sankaran, R., Markandan, K., Deepanraj, B., Khoo, K. S., Ashokkumar, V., Cheng, C. K., & Show, P. L. (2021). The expansion of lignocellulose biomass conversion into bioenergy via nanobiotechnology. *Frontiers in Nanotechnology, 3*. https://doi.org/10.3389/fnano.2021.793528

Sharada, R., Swathi, K., Venkateswar, S., AnandRao, M., & Narsi, R. M. (2009). Optimization of cultural conditions for cellulase production by Aspergillus Niger (MTCC 2196) using submerged fermentation. *Biosciences Biotechnology Research Asia, 6*(1), 289–292.

Son, J.-H., & Ravindran, V. (2011). Feed enzyme technology: Present status and future developments. *Recent Patents on Food, Nutrition & Agriculturee, 3*(2), 102–109. https://doi.org/10.2174/2212798411103020102

Sridar, M. (2017). Scope of exogenous enzymes in enhancing ruminant productivity. *Journal of Dairy Veterinary & Animal Research, 5*(2). https://doi.org/10.15406/jdvar.2017.05.00137

Sweeney, M. D., & Xu, F. (2012). Biomass converting enzymes as industrial biocatalysts for fuels and chemicals: Recent developments. *Catalysts, 2*(2), 244–263. https://doi.org/10.3390/catal2020244

Tolan, J. & Guenette, M. (2007). Using enzymes in pulp bleaching: Mill applications. https://doi.org/10.1007/BFb0102078

Torres, C., Negro, C., Fuente, E., Blanco, A. (2012). Enzymatic approaches in the paper industry for pulp refining and biofilm control. *Applied Microbiology and Biotechnology, 96,* 327–44. https://doi.org/10.1007/s00253-012-4345-0

Tyagi, V. K., Lo, S.-L., Appels, L., & Dewil, R. (2014). Ultrasonic treatment of waste sludge: A review on mechanisms and applications. *Critical Reviews in Environmental Science and Technology, 44*(11), 1220–1288. https://doi.org/10.1080/10643389.2013.763587

van Kuijk, S. J. A., Sonnenberg, A. S. M., Baars, J. J. P., Hendriks, W. H., & Cone, J. W. (2015). Fungal treated lignocellulosic biomass as ruminant feed ingredient: A review. *Biotechnology Advances, 33*(1), 191–202. https://doi.org/10.1016/j.biotechadv.2014.10.014

Verma, N., Bansal, M. C., & Kumar, V. (2020). Valorization of waste biomass in fermentative production of cellulases: A review. *Waste and Biomass Valorization, 12*(2), 613–640. https://doi.org/10.1007/s12649-020-01048-8

Walia, A., Guleria, S., Mehta, P., Chauhan, A., & Parkash, J. (2017). Microbial xylanases and their industrial application in pulp and paper biobleaching: a review. *3 Biotech, 7*(1), 11. https://doi.org/10.1007/s13205-016-0584-6

Wang, J., Jiang, Q., Cai, M., Huang, Z., Roubik, H., Yang, K., Sun, P., & Wang, Y. (2023). Solid-state fermentation of soybean meal with edible mushroom mycelium to improve its nutritional. *Antioxidant Capacities and Physicochemical Properties. Fermentation, 9*(4), 322. https://doi.org/10.3390/fermentation9040322

Wenk, C., & Boessinger, M. (1993). *Enzymes in animal nutrition: Proceedings of the 1st Symposium, Kartause Ittingen, Switzerland, October 13–16.*

Xia, Q., He, S., Li, T., Yao, Y., Chen, C., Li, J., Hu, L., Zhou, Y., Yao, Y., & Pan, X. (2021). A strong, biodegradable and recyclable lignocellulosic bioplastic. *Nature Sustainability, 4*(7), 627–635. https://doi.org/10.1038/s41893-021-00702-w

Xu, G., Wang, X., & Hu, J. (2013). Biobleaching of wheat straw pulp using Laccase and Xylanase. *BioResources, 8*(3). https://doi.org/10.15376/biores.8.3.3181-3188

Yamaguchi, A., Shirai, M., Mimura, N., & Sato, O. (2019). Cascade utilization of biomass: Strategy for conversion of cellulose, hemicellulose, and lignin into useful chemicals. *ACS Sustainable Chemistry & Engineering, 7*(12), 10445–10451. https://doi.org/10.1021/acssuschemeng.9b00786

Zoghlami, A., & Paës, G. (2019). Lignocellulosic biomass: Understanding recalcitrance and predicting hydrolysis. *Frontiers in chemistry, 7*, 874. https://doi.org/10.3389/fchem.2019.00874

Zoghlami, A., & Paës, G. (2019). Lignocellulosic biomass: Understanding recalcitrance and predicting hydrolysis. *Frontiers in Chemistry, 7*. https://doi.org/10.3389/fchem.2019.00874

Chapter 17
A Detailed Overview of the Role of Nanotechnology in Biofuel Production

Farhana Yasmin, Ritushree Roy, Abu Barkat Md. Gulzar, and Pranab Behari Mazumder

Abstract The growing global demand for sustainable energy has intensified interest in biofuels as an environmentally friendly alternative to fossil fuels. However, conventional biofuel production faces challenges related to low conversion efficiencies, high operational costs, and limited environmental concerns. This chapter explores the application of nanotechnology in revolutionizing biofuel generation, highlighting its challenges through innovative applications. It examines the integration of various nanomaterials in improving product yield across first to fourth-generation biofuels. This chapter also outlines the benefits of nanotechnology and its emerging innovations. Despite these promising advances, critical challenges are also highlighted, along with future research directions focusing on green synthesis. Overall, this chapter underscores nanotechnology as a game-changer in sustainable biofuel production, potentially reshaping the global energy system.

Keywords Nanotechnology · Biofuel production · Renewable energy · Sustainability · Green energy · Biofuel generation

F. Yasmin · R. Roy · A. B. Md. Gulzar · P. B. Mazumder (✉)
Plant and Microbial Molecular Biology Laboratory, Department of Biotechnology, Assam University, Silchar, Assam, India
e-mail: pbmazumder65@gmail.com

F. Yasmin
e-mail: farhanayasmin886@gmail.com

R. Roy
e-mail: ritushree345@gmail.com

A. B. Md. Gulzar
e-mail: gulzar.hussain282@gmail.com

P. Verma (ed.), *Sustainable Practices in Biorefinery*,
https://doi.org/10.1007/978-981-95-6071-4_17

17.1 Introduction

The rise in oil consumption, the variation in the global price of petroleum, the reduction of fossil fuel, and the adverse environmental consequences have gradually increased the need for sustainable and renewable energy sources (Kumar et al., 2020b; Umbach, 2010). Biofuels, an alternative substitute for fossil fuels, generated from biological materials which include microalgae, agricultural and domestic residues, and lignocellulosic biomass obtained directly from plants, animal wastes, and agricultural leftovers, have become a promising substitute since they can lower greenhouse gas emissions and dependency on non-renewable resources (Arya et al., 2021; Mahapatra et al., 2021). As a result, there is a significant amount of ongoing research conducted in the field of biofuel, and it is also predicted that, by 2030, biofuel will account for 4–7% of global energy consumption (Abdelfattah et al., 2018). First-generation biofuels are derived from feedstocks and are responsible for the bioethanol and biodiesel production. These techniques use large volumes of feedstocks such as vegetable and animal fats and sucrose from sugar cane or starch from corn for biodiesel and bioethanol production, respectively. However, the widespread usage of essential feedstocks limits the use of first-generation biofuels. As a result, new technologies have been developed for the production of biofuel using non-edible plant biomass and agricultural residues. Biofuels production from such biomass is known as second-generation biofuels (Kumar et al., 2020a). On the other hand, a potential source of biofuels production is the utilization of microbial biomass as substrate; this is called third-generation biofuels. There is also a fourth generation, consisting of biofuel from the bio-engineered plants, trees, and algae, which function as a carbon-capturing and storing source (Chanu et al., 2023; Ho et al., 2014; Karthik et al., 2023; Renzaho et al., 2017; Saha et al., 2019). However, conventional biofuel methods for production frequently meet challenges, such as low conversion efficiency, high costs, competition with food resources, scalability, and other environmental risks (Devi et al., 2023; Negi et al., 2023).

In this regard, nanotechnology has attained a lot of interest because of its possibility to revolutionize the biofuel industry and to overcome the limitations of conventional biofuel generation. Since each biofuel generation faces technical and economic challenges. Nanotechnology, with its ability to operate at the nanoscale level, offers revolutionary solutions for improving biofuel production's efficiency, scalability, and sustainability throughout all generations (Singh et al., 2020a, 2020b, 2020c). In nanotechnology, materials are altered or modified at the nanoscale level, usually less than 100 nm, leading to unique physical and chemical properties that can accelerate various processes in biofuel production pathways (Singh et al., 2020a, 2020b, 2020c). In biofuel production processes, the integration of nanomaterials, such as carbon nanotubes, magnetic nanoparticles, core–shell nanoparticles, hybrid nanoparticles, metal oxide, and non-metal oxide nanoparticles, has been shown to improve catalytic activity, biomass conversion efficiency, and product yield (Islam & Ahmed, 2025; Rai et al., 2016). Figure 17.1 highlights the different types of nanoparticles used in biofuel production utilizing various feedstocks. Moreover, nanotechnology

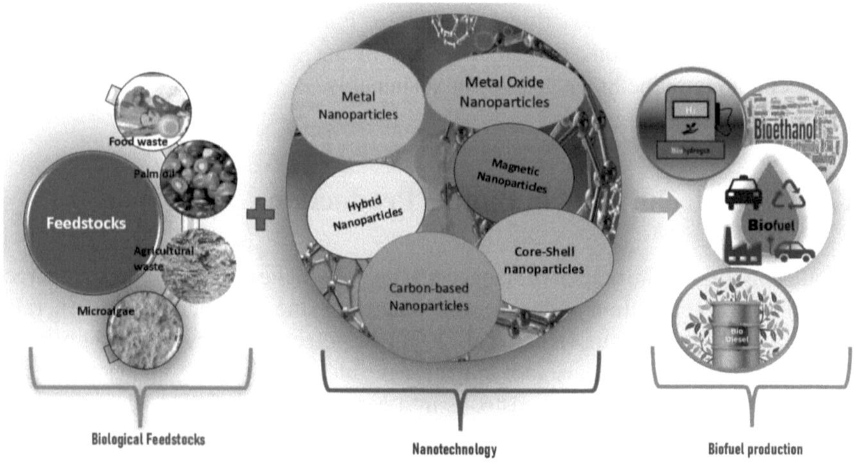

Fig. 17.1 Nanotechnology-based biofuel production from various biodegradable feedstock sources

has tremendous potential to achieve a cost-effective and process-efficient biofuel industry (Nizami & Rehan, 2018).

For instance, compared to conventional biodiesel production catalysts, nanocatalysts, have shown a higher surface-to-volume ratio, increased catalytic activity, specificity, resistance to saponification, and reusability, which thereby lowers energy input and reaction times (Kazemi Shariat Panahi et al., 2024). In algal biofuel production, nanotechnology has facilitated more efficient growth, harvesting, lipid extraction, lipid content, and biofuel processing, addressing some of the major technical bottlenecks of conventional algal production and enhancing the prospect for commercializing algae-based production (Ali et al., 2024; Pattarkine & Pattarkine, 2012; Thanigaivel et al., 2023). Additionally, nanotechnology-based pretreatment of lignocellulosic biomass has improved the breakdown of complex polymers like cellulose and lignin, increasing the amount of fermentable sugars accessible for bioethanol production (Hussain et al., 2024).

However, the application of nanotechnology in biofuel production overcomes high production costs, enhances the separation and purification process, conversion rate, improves product quality, and reduces technical barriers, allowing for the recycle, recovery and reuse of resources, yet it comes with several critical challenges (Awogbemi & Kallon, 2024a; Rai et al., 2016). Key concerns regarding nanoparticle toxicity, environmental accumulation, scalability of nanomaterial production, technical limitations, and lack of comprehensive regulatory frameworks need to be critically addressed to ensure sustainable advancement and progress in the field (Kumar et al., 2023).

The goal of this chapter is to explore the multifaceted role of nanotechnology in revolutionizing biofuel production. It will delve into its growing applications of nanoparticles in biofuel production technologies, recent innovations, potential benefits, and its associated critical challenges. Furthermore, it will also focus on future research directions to guide the significant and impactful integration of nanotechnology in the bioenergy sector sustainably.

17.2 Nanotechnology in Biofuel Production

Nanotechnology is the branch of science that deals with the design, synthesis, characterization, and application of devices and materials at the nanometre scale, generally between 1 and 100 nm (nm) (Khan et al., 2022). Nanotechnology is increasingly being recognized as a revolutionary tool in the renewable energy sector, and especially in the conversion of biological feedstocks into eco-friendly biofuel. Its incorporation into biofuel production processes can potentially overcome numerous technical and economic barriers traditionally associated with bioenergy systems (Kazemi Shariat Panahi et al., 2024). By leveraging the unique physicochemical properties of materials at the nanoscale, including high surface area-to-volume ratios, enhanced reactivity, catalytic activity, thermal stability, and tunable electronic properties (Osman et al., 2023). Researchers and scientists can improve the efficiency, yield, and sustainability of biofuel production from a variety of sources, including lignocellulosic biomass, vegetable and fruit waste, algae, microbial culture, natural plant products, municipal waste and agricultural waste, making them ideal for improving key processes in biofuel, such as biomass pretreatment, fermentation, transesterification, and combustion efficiency (Rai et al., 2016). In general, nanotechnology significantly accelerates the production of biofuels by enhancing conversion efficiency, reducing environmental risks, and facilitating the development of economically viable and sustainable energy sources (Khujamberdiev & Cho, 2025). Different types of nanoparticles/nanocatalysts used in biofuel production are discussed below.

17.2.1 Carbon-Based Nanoparticles

Carbon-based nanoparticles (CBNs) such as graphene, graphene oxide (GO), and carbon nanotubes (CNTs) have become valuable materials because of their excellent thermal conductivity, high mechanical strength, chemical stability, and high surface area (Khujamberdiev & Cho, 2025; Nair & Verma, 2025a). The major breakthroughs started with the finding of multi-walled CNTs by Sumio Iijima in 1991 and single-layer graphene by Novoselov in 2004, opening up diverse applications ranging from industrial materials to biomedical applications. In the energy application, these nanomaterials have also proven beneficial in the improvement of biodiesel performance through better combustion efficiency and emission reduction (Hoa et al., 2017). The oxygen-rich functional groups in graphene and GO enhance solubility and reactivity, besides increasing brake thermal efficiency (BTE) and decreasing NOx emissions.

Yet, their use is limited by drawbacks such as high production costs and agglomeration, necessitating strategies such as ultrasonication or surfactant stabilization for uniform dispersion (Khujamberdiev & Cho, 2025; Rodoshi Khan & Bin Rashid, 2024) Likewise, CNTs, particularly MWCNTs and SWCNTs, enhance engine efficiency and minimize toxic emissions in biodiesel formulations, but are limited by low solubility and potential clogging of fuel pathways if not effectively functionalized. Despite these challenges, recent work on low-cost synthesis and stabilization processes serves to underscore the increasing importance of CBNs in the development of clean fuel technology (Arya et al., 2021b; Khujamberdiev & Cho, 2025).

17.2.2 Magnetic Nanoparticles

Enzymes like lipases and cellulases are crucial in the production of biofuels, specifically in the hydrolysis of lignocellulosic biomass (LCB). Magnetic nanoparticles (MNPs) have been found to be extremely efficient in immobilizing enzymes, increasing their stability, reusability, and separation from reaction mixtures (Arya et al., 2021; Thanigaivel et al., 2023). Enzyme coating on nanomaterial-supported matrices not only enhances enzyme efficiency but also facilitates repeated use, thereby making the process economical. MNPs such as $CaSO_4/Fe_2O_3–SiO_2$ have also been effectively applied to biodiesel production in Jatropha curcas, producing up to 94% yields under ideal conditions. Upon repeated application, inactivation of nanoparticles gradually occurs because nanoparticle pores become blocked by reaction media deposits, both surface area and catalytic activity decreasing (Dunmade et al., 2024). The same application of MnO_2 nanoparticles in bioethanol production from sugarcane leaves has indicated improved enzyme binding and ethanol yield. Furthermore, calcium-doped magnetic ferrites also enhanced soybean oil biodiesel yield considerably. Iron-based nanoparticles like Fe_3O_4 and nano zero-valent iron in bioH_2 and biogas production were found to enhance microbial growth and enzymatic activity and greatly enhance gas yields (Muhammad & Badshah, 2019). High-performance nanocomposites such as reduced graphene oxide with polyaniline (rGO/PANI) and functionalized Fe_3O_4 have proven to show great electron transfer in bioelectrocatalysis, extending the application of nanoparticles even further in enzymatic biofuel cells (Arya et al., 2021). In general, MNPs greatly improve the different stages of biofuel production, and therefore, they are pivotal enablers in enhancing the efficiency of conversion, enzyme operation, and long-term sustainability in bioenergy uses (Kim & Lee, 2016).

17.2.3 Metal-Based Nanoparticles

Metal-based nanoparticles such as TiO_2, Al_2O_3, ZnO, and CeO_2 have been found to be useful additives in biodiesel due to their high surface area and catalytic activity, improving combustion efficiency, fuel stability, and emissions control. TiO_2 is an oxygen donor, enhancing oxidation stability and minimizing CO and HC emissions, whereas Al_2O_3 enhances brake thermal efficiency but at high levels can raise viscosity. ZnO increases thermal stability and is synergistic with other additives, although its restricted solubility necessitates the use of dispersion aids. CeO_2, due to its capability for oxygen storage, facilitates complete combustion and minimizes soot, although long-term deposition can be engine-wear hazardous. Hybrid blends of the nanoparticles exhibit better engine performance and lower NOx emissions (Khujamberdiev & Cho, 2025). Also, metal-oxide nanoparticles such as CaO, Fe_3O_4, SiO_2, and ZnO are effective catalysts in biofuel production, particularly in transesterification reactions, greatly enhancing the yield of biodiesel. Methods such as the sol–gel process enable accurate regulation of nanoparticle formation, which improves their catalytic activity and compatibility with different feedstocks like jatropha, algae, and waste cooking oil, ultimately enabling cleaner and more efficient production of biofuel (Dunmade et al., 2024; Thanigaivel et al., 2023).

17.2.4 Hybrid Nanoparticles

Hybrid nanoparticles created through the integration of materials such as TiO_2-CuO, TiO_2-Al_2O_3, and GO-CNTs provide synergistic benefits in biodiesel usage through improved thermal conductivity, efficiency of combustion, and decreased emissions (Borthakur, 2025). These multipurpose composites take advantage of the individual properties of the constituents to provide enhanced engine performance under different operation conditions. For instance, TiO_2-Al_2O_3 improves thermal stability and combustion, whereas GO-CNT hybrids establish stable blends of biodiesel with greatly decreased pollutant emission. Nonetheless, avoiding agglomeration during synthesis is essential to preserve their efficacy (Khujamberdiev & Cho, 2025). Novel materials like Ag@MOF-801, a silver hybridized metal–organic framework, exhibited significant transesterification catalytic performance while minimizing energy consumption (Alduhaish et al., 2022). On the same note, composites with ZnO, Al_2O_3, and TiO_2 offer increased thermal and oxidative stability, crucial to biodiesel's functionality. Hybrid nanofluids such as Al_2O_3-SiO_2 in diesel–biodiesel blends have also indicated heightened brake thermal efficiency and lower fuel usage. Even with such advantages, issues like dispersion stability, risk of engine component buildup, and cost-effectiveness in large quantities are significant areas for further research (Jabraeili et al., 2021; Khujamberdiev & Cho, 2025).

17.2.5 Core–Shell Nanoparticles

Core–shell nanoparticless are biphasic structures with a well-defined inner core and an external shell composed of materials other than the core, like metals, elements, or biomolecules. In contrast to homogeneous nanocomposites, core–shell NPs show evident segregation between core and shell phases and can be bimetallic or trimetallic. Such structures possess special properties in biodiesel synthesis because of well-controlled size, shape, and surface chemistry (Jones et al., 2024; Khatami et al., 2018). A good example is the hierarchically porous $CaSO_4/Fe_2O_3$-SiO_2 core–shell nanostructure, prepared under mild solvothermal conditions with ethanol–water media, $NaNO_3$ etchant, and CH_3COONa as a reducing agent. The material proved highly efficient in the production of biodiesel from Jatropha curcas and methanol with a yield of 94% under the optimal conditions (Changmai et al., 2021). It exhibited superior dispersion, simple separation from the reaction mixture without filtration or centrifugation, and preserved catalytic activity through nine cycles. These observations emphasize the promise of such green, reusable core–shell architectures in furthering biodiesel synthesis with both superior process efficiency and performance (Teo et al., 2019).

17.3 Applications of Nanotechnology-Based Biofuel Production

Biofuel, a sustainable source of energy, acts as an alternative to traditional fossil fuel and has significant applications in diverse field globally. Its synthesis and production are accelerated by the augmentation of various types of nanoparticles/nanocatalysts. Thus, the contribution of nanotechnology results in the production of eco-friendly and sustainable biofuel. Below are some of the most widely produced biofuels.

17.3.1 Biodiesel

Biodiesel, a biodegradable, non-toxic, and renewable fuel alternative to fossil fuels, is derived from vegetable oils, animal fats, microbial sources, or recycled cooking grease through a chemical process called transesterification (Abusweireh et al., 2022). During transesterification, triglycerides (fats and oils) react with methanol, in the presence of a catalyst, to produce FAMEs, which is fatty acid methyl esters, the chemical name for biodiesel, along with glycerol as a by-product (Zhong et al., 2020). However, the conventional production of biodiesel has several limitations, including high energy input, slow reaction kinetics, and poor catalyst reusability. Nanotechnology, which involves manipulating materials at the nanoscale, presents a revolutionary solution to these issues by improving catalyst efficiency, reducing reaction time, enhancing biodiesel yields, and enabling feedstock purification and versatility (Nizami & Rehan, 2018). Nanotechnology primarily enhances the fermentation and transesterification processes of first-generation biofuels (Zhang et al., 2019). Metal oxides such as MgO, CeO_2, TiO_2, ZnO, and Al_2O_3 are examples of nanocatalysts that increase biodiesel production by minimizing reaction temperatures, combustion inefficiencies, reducing toxic gas emissions, and thus, optimizing their energy effectiveness (Mofijur et al., 2024; Rajak et al., 2022; S, 2019; Srinivasan et al., 2021). Recent developments in biodiesel production have yielded composite-based heterogeneous nanocatalysts like Ag@MOF-801 by introducing metal–organic frameworks (MOFs) hybridized with nanoparticles like silver (Ag). This hybrid technique increases catalytic efficiency during transesterification, simultaneously reducing the energy needed to produce biodiesel (Alduhaish et al., 2022). For the production of biodiesel, several additional technologies have also been introduced, such as pyrolysis, microwave irradiation, and Emulsification. Leveraging pyrolysis to generate bio-oil high in fatty acids that can be subsequently converted to biodiesel, incorporating nanoparticles into pyrolysis is becoming increasingly common for waste cooking oils and agricultural residues. Using co-pyrolysis and advanced catalysts, such as nanocatalysts, can improve fuel quality and yield sustainability (Su et al., 2022; Xiong et al., 2023). Moreover, when direct transesterification is challenging because of the distinctive features of oil, particularly when encountering high viscosity, microemulsions are especially helpful because they provide a functional route for specific feedstocks, and the combination of nanoparticles with microemulsions can significantly shorten reaction times and reduce the required reaction temperature (Bin Rashid, 2023; Mishra & Goswami, 2018). In recent years, nanomaterials with immobilized enzymes, such as lipase, have gathered interest in producing biodiesel by immobilizing the enzyme on nanoparticles to improve its stability, activity, and reusability (Wei et al., 2023). Algae-based third-generation substrates are preferable for biodiesel production owing to the elevated energy content, oil content, and low pollution emission. Therefore, nanoparticle integration in microalgae cultivation for biodiesel production includes promoting microalgal growth, enhancing lipid production, light harvesting, photosynthesis enhancement, and microalgae harvesting (Bin Rashid & Hayashi, 2023). According to Wang et al., magnetic flocculants such as CTAB-decorated Fe_3O_4 nanoparticles have also been shown to increase the biodiesel production when incubated with *Chlorella ellipsoidea.* It evaluates their harvesting ability; as a result, 96% of the microalgae were harvested at a particle dose of 120 mg/L with a 10 min reaction time of particles and microalgae (Wang et al., 2014). Various nanoparticles utilized in biodiesel production are shown in Table 17.1.

17.3.2 Biohydrogen

Conventional methods of biohydrogen production, such as photofermentation, dark fermentation, microbial electrolysis process or photocatalysis, have been responsible for the production of cost-effective, sustainable, and renewable hydrogen, yet struggle with low hydrogen yields, expensive pretreatment procedures, protracted lag phase, and release of toxic intermediates (Arya et al., 2021). Therefore, there is a need to overcome the consequences by the application of nanoparticles/catalysts due to their

Table 17.1 Application of various types of nanoparticles in biofuel production

Types of biofuel	Nanoparticles	Feedstocks/substrates/inoculum	Summary of reaction conditions/notable yield	References
Biodiesel	Mo-Zr/CS	Waste *Gallus domesticus* shells	The transesterification reaction results in 90.1% yield in 3 h. 10Mo-Zr/CS catalyst is efficiently recovered and sustains a yield of over 70% after three consecutive reuses	(Mansir et al., 2018)
	Fe_2O_3/Chitosan	*Candida antarctica* lipase B/Palm oil	>64% of its relative activity at 85 °C, after 14 days of storage retains >59% of its activity, 93.7% yield was observed after 7 times regeneration. Microwave-assisted transesterification results in 70.2% biodiesel yield recovery	(Kamel Ariffin & Idris, 2022)
	Fe_3O_4/ZnMg(Al)O	Microalgae	Temperature-65 °C, duration-3 h, under optimum conditions, the yield reaches up to 94%. An 82% yield was observed after 7 times of reuse	(Chen et al., 2018)
	CFA-ZnO	Cooking oil	Temperature-140 °C, Time interval-3 h, methanol: oil = 12:1. At optimum temperature, biodiesel yield was 83.17% with 0.5 wt% catalyst load. Reuse up to 4 successive cycles generated 98.14 wt% biodiesel yield	(Yusuff et al., 2021)
	Heterogeneous catalyst LaTiO3	Wild mustard seed oil	Temperature-80 °C, alcohol: oil = 4:1, catalyst-100 mg, reaction time-60 min. Biodiesel yield was 92.21%, and An 87% yield was observed after 8 times of reuse	(Rezania et al., 2022)

(continued)

Table 17.1 (continued)

Types of biofuel	Nanoparticles	Feedstocks/substrates/inoculum	Summary of reaction conditions/notable yield	References
	$MgO/MgFe_2O_4$	Sunflower oil	Temperature -110 °C, methanol: oil-12:1, catalyst concentration– 4 wt.%, reaction time-4 h, under a fuel ratio of 1.5, biodiesel yield was up to 91.2%. An 82.4% biodiesel yield was observed after 5 consecutive cycles	(Alaei et al., 2018)
Biohydrogen	TiO_2	Purple non-sulfur bacterial-*Rhodobacter sphaeroides*/Malate	In presence of 60 µg/mL concentration of TiO_2, production rate was increased by 1.54 folds and duration by 1.88 folds. Under photofermentation, H_2 yield was 1900 mL/L with malate conversion of 63.27%	(Pandey et al., 2015)
	$CoCu_{0.2}Fe_{1.8}O_4$	*Clostridium* sensu stricto*1*/Glucose	Anaerobic sludge; temperature-37 °C, Higher H_2 yield 212.25 ml/g glucose observed at 300 mg/L concentration of $CoCu_{0.2}Fe_{1.8}O_4$	(Li et al., 2022)
	$NiCo_2O_4$	*Bacillus subtilis* and *Rhodobacter* sp./Rice straw	Employing *Bacillus subtilis* and *Rhodobacter* sp., conversion of rice-straw combined with NPs produced a hydrogen yield of 2978 ml/L from a total of 51.7 g/L of sugar hydrolyzate. Enhance microbial growth	(Srivastava et al., 2021)
	NiO	Glucose and xylose	In 20 mg/L Ec-NiO-NP, the total H_2 production and H_2 yield were 4842.19 mL/L and 101.45 mL/g substrate, respectively. H_2 production and H_2 yield 47.29% and 37.78% higher compared to control without NPs	(Zhang et al., 2021)
	Fe^0	Biochar/grass	Along with the grass, a combination of biochar-Fe^0 NP produces an H_2 yield of 50.6 mL/g-dry grass, when compare to control, it is 89.8% higher and reduces the lag phase	(Yang & Wang, 2019)

(continued)

Table 17.1 (continued)

Types of biofuel	Nanoparticles	Feedstocks/substrates/inoculum	Summary of reaction conditions/notable yield	References
Bioethanol	NiO	Waste potato peels/*S. cerevisiae* BY4743/glucose	Temperature-30 °C, rotation-120 rpm, duration-24 h, Addition of NiO NP increases ethanol production up to 59.96%, improved productivity by 145% and reduced acetic acid concentration by 110%	(Sanusi et al., 2021)
	MgO and Fe_2O_3	Engineered *Synechocystis* sp. PCC 6803/ Potato Waste	The NADPH regeneration enhanced by the addition of NPs and increases bioethanol production up to 5,100 mg/L on a 5 L scale	(Velmurugan & Incharoensakdi, 2019)
	ZnO	*Fusarium oxysporum*/Rice straw	Maximum ethanol yield of 0.0359 g/g was observed at a dosage of 200 mg/L ZnO NP	(Gupta & Chundawat, 2020)
	Fe_3O_4	*S. cerevisiae* BY4743/ Potato peel waste	Fe_3O_4 at 0.01 wt% glucose utilization of 99.95% yield 0.26 g/g ethanol, produce ethanol of 0.22 g/L/h	(Sanusi et al., 2019)
	NiO	*Pichia kudriavzveii* IFM 53,048 / Banana waste	NiO at 0.01 wt% glucose utilization of 99.95%, yield 0.27 g/g bioethanol and produce bioethanol of 0.23 g/L/h^{-1} and fermentation efficiency is of 51.28%	(Nduka et al., 2024)
Biogas (Methane)	Ni	Poultry litter	On adding NP to the substrate, CH_4 production was enhanced by 38.4%, i.e., 368 mL CH_4/g VS, and on higher NP concentration reduces H_2S	(Hassanein et al., 2019)
Biogas (Methane)	nZVI and Fe_2O_3	Waste-activated sludge	On addition of 10 mg/g TSS nZVI and 100 mg/ g TSS Fe_2O_3 increases methane production by 120% and 117% as compared to the control respectively and reduces H_2S	(Wang et al., 2016)

(continued)

Table 17.1 (continued)

Types of biofuel	Nanoparticles	Feedstocks/substrates/inoculum	Summary of reaction conditions/notable yield	References
Biogas (Methane)	NiO	Wastewater bacteria(*Providencia alcalifaciens* and *Alcaligenes aquatilis*) and Aquatic Macrophytes (*Pistia stratiotes*) biomass	2 ppm NiO + 3.4 gm of *Pistia stratiotes* increases the production by 87.91% as compare to control	(Wang et al., 2016)
Biogas and methane	NiO, CoO, and Fe_3O_4	Sewage sludge	Optimum dosage of combined NPs(1 mg/l NiO, 1 mg/l CoO, and 10 mg/l Fe_3O_4) produces biogas of 43.90% and methane of 62.85%, and also reduces H_2S to a maximum of 52.57%	(Gran et al., 2022)
Biobutanol	ZnO	*Clostridium saccharoperbutylacetonicum*/ sugarcane molasses/glucose	After inoculum initiation, 80 g/l of glucose yields a maximum of 10.59 g/l butanol	(Abel et al., 2022)

distinctive physical and chemical characteristics such as enhanced electroconductivity, stability, catalytic features, crystalline nature, adsorption capacity, and a high surface-to-volume ratio and also for its O_2 scavenging features in the production of biohydrogen, moreover offer promising approaches to boost yields, enhance enzyme activity, and enable the effective conversion of biomass (Karthikeyan & Velvizhi, 2024; Yildirim & Ozkaya, 2024). In recent years, the application of several metals (Zn, Ag, Co, Au, Cu, Fe, Ni) and metal oxides (Fe_2O_3, NiO, Fe_3O_4, and TiO_2) nanoparticles has been explored enormously in biohydrogen production (Khan et al., 2021; Lin et al., 2016; Mohanraj et al., 2016; Rambabu et al., 2021; Taherdanak et al., 2015; Wu et al., 2017). Implementing nanoparticles produced by low-cost and green synthesis methods while employing a versatile range of organic waste, such as sludge from sewage, food, agricultural, and forestry and industrial waste, for producing renewable hydrogen and the utilization of organic waste may be one of the most viable and sustainable choices (Karthikeyan & Velvizhi, 2024; Yang & Wang, 2018). Gadhe et al. (2012a, 2015b) studied the impact of co-addition of Fe_2O_3 and NiO NP on bioH_2 production from dairy wastewater and complex distillery wastewater and observed a maximum H_2 yield of about 17.2 mmol/g COD, and specific H_2 production rate of 47.67 mmol/g VSS.d, at concentration of 50 mg Fe_2O_3/L, and 10 mg NiO/L, respectively utilizing dairy wastewater. In distillery wastewater, maximum yield and specific H_2 production rate were observed at 8.83 mmol/g COD, and 18.14 mmol/g VSS.d, respectively, with the combined addition of 200 mg/L of Fe_2O_3 and 5 mg/L NiO NPs. Rambabu et al. studied the use of NiO and CoO nanoparticles for enhancing bioH_2 production from rice mill wastewater, where hydrogen yield increased by 109% for NiO and 90% for CoO NP with a dosage of 1.5 ml/L of each nanoparticle (Rambabu et al., 2021). On the other hand, Beckers et al. explored the impacts of Iron nanoparticles encapsulated in porous SiO_2 for biohydrogen production, obtaining a yield of 11.46 mmol/g COD at a dosage of 135 mg/L utilizing glucose as a feedstock (Beckers et al., 2013). The application of various nanoparticles in biohydrogen production is mentioned in Table 17.1.

17.3.3 Bioethanol

Unlike fossil fuels, bioethanol is liquid, renewable, biodegradable, and non-toxic burning biofuel derived from renewable biomass, such as edible and non-edible feedstocks, food waste, agricultural residues, industrial waste, and municipal waste (Prabhu et al., 2021). As a result, it offers an eco-friendly and sustainable alternative to petroleum derivatives (Nair et al., 2022). Despite its potential, conventional bioethanol production has certain drawbacks, such as low conversion efficiencies, high energy inputs, low enzyme stability, substrate inhibition, and low reusability. Therefore, to overcome these issues, the application of nanoparticles with high octane number, evaporation enthalpy, and flammability throughout a wide temperature range has revolutionized bioethanol production by offering innovative solutions that enhance conversion efficiency, reduce production and yield costs, and improve sustainability (Bosu et al., 2022). In bioethanol production, nanoparticles have been proven to increase the efficiency of pretreatment, enzyme hydrolysis, and fermentation of substrates (Ndaba et al., 2025). It is considered the most widely used biofuel globally because of these advantages. Many research efforts have delved into the deployment of magnetic nanoparticles to improve bioethanol production. In terms of quantity, algae-based bioethanol holds enormous potential and has proven to be an ideal source of bioethanol production. According to Sharma et al. (2015), bioethanol was produced by synthesizing ZnO NP utilizing the microalga *Chlorella vulgaris*, which obtained a bioethanol yield of 13.2 ± 0.5 wt% (Sharma & Ghose, 2015). Several studies have shown the effectiveness of nanoparticles in producing bioethanol utilizing plant extract and microbes as substrates. According to Rekha and Saravanathamizhan (2021), 53.7% ethanol was produced by synthesizing iron oxide NPs using *Spinacia oleracea* leaves extract for the production of bioethanol from corncob (Rekha & Saravanathamizhan, 2021). The association between metal and metal-oxide nanoparticles in heterogeneous catalysis provides an unraveled catalytic performance that has been an area of concern in biological research. Sarma and Saha (2025) reported the use of Fe-ZnO NPs for the production of bioethanol from wasted *Camellia sinensis* leaves which resulting in 75% of bioethanol yield. In another study, Iyyappan et al. (2023) used 15 μg/L of NiO NPs from *Kluyveromyces marxianus* efficiently deploy biopretreated elephant grass and produced about 14.65 g/L of bioethanol. Besides this, Nanoparticles offer several other benefits over broader nanomaterials when utilized to ameliorate bioethanol production shown in Table 17.1.

17.3.4 Other Biofuels

Besides the most widely explored biofuels like biodiesel, biohydrogen, and bioethanol, there are several other biofuels that have gained interest due to their significant potential in the production of sustainable energy. Among those are biogas, biobutanol, bio-oil, etc. Biogas is an alternative to traditional fuels such as firewood, LPG, and burning charcoal, which is composed mainly of methane, CO_2, and trace elements of other gases. Biogas production mostly relies on the anaerobic digestion of organic matter, such as vegetables and fruit waste, sewage sludge, manure waste, dairy waste, and poultry manure, resulting in the production of sustainable energy, reducing greenhouse gas emissions, and also helps in waste management (Arif et al., 2018). Incorporation of nanotechnology can significantly increase the production of biogas by increasing the efficiency of anaerobic digestion, boosting microbial growth, reducing H_2S, enhancing methane production, acting as a bio-stimulant, and purifying biogas, eventually leading to an increase in biogas yield (Manikandan et al., 2023). Another emerging biofuel is biobutanol, a sustainable liquid fuel alternative to conventional gasoline and diesel, produced through the acetone-butanol-ethanol (ABE) fermentation process with the help of *Clostridium* sp. (Rozina et al., 2024).

However, its large-scale production encounters several limitations that can be overcome with the aid of Nanotechnology. Nanotechnology offers potential approaches to significantly accelerate biomass breakdown during fermentation, minimize reaction time, enhance enzyme efficiency, and obtain cost-effective products, resulting in the production of sustainable biobutanol (Zarea et al., 2025). Some examples in Table 17.1 highlight the contribution of nanotechnology in biogas and biobutanol production.

17.4 Innovations in Nanotechnology-based biofuel production

Along with enhancing existing biofuel production techniques, researchers are now looking into completely novel nano-enabled strategies for biofuel production. Cutting-edge work is exploring how multi-functional nanocatalysts or hybrid nanocatalysts such as metal-based nanobiocatalysts, carbon-based nanobiocatalysts, silica-based nanobiocatalysts, and polymeric nanobiocatalysts can be used to perform multiple functions, thus enhancing the production process, reducing the production cost, reducing processing steps, increasing recyclability, and improving biofuel quality (Awogbemi & Kallon, 2024b). Another breakthrough in nanotechnology-based biofuel production is the immobilization of enzymes in nanoporous matrices, which permits selective exchange of substrates and products. In order to synthesize nanobiocatalysts with potential stability and activity, various nanostructured materials can act as carriers, such as nanofibers, nanoporous carriers, and nanocomposites (Ayub et al., 2023). Utilizing advanced nanostructured materials can also enhance fuel cell performance by facilitating better electron and proton transport in bioethanol and biodiesel production. It may also enhance fuel characteristics, optimize engine efficiency, and reduce toxic gas emissions (Khanna et al., 2019). Recent innovation in green synthesis of nanoparticles, which may be plant-based synthesis using photochemical, microorganism-mediated synthesis, or products from food and agricultural waste (Osman et al., 2024). Use of green synthesis nanoparticles in biofuel processing stages, benefits over conventional methods, and their effect have been shown in Table 17.2. Other novel strategies paving the way in nanoparticles for sustainable biofuel production include integration of magnetic nanoparticles in catalyst recovery, nanosensors in real-time monitoring of fuel quality and purity, use of nano-additives and nano-emulsions in improving biofuel performance, nanocomposites in improving the stability and energy density of biofuels, etc. (Parra et al., 2025). Continued research and innovation in nanotechnology are anticipated to further optimize biofuel separation, purification, and recovery and to accelerate the shift to more sustainable energy sources.

Table 17.2 A comparative overview of green nanoparticles synthesis over traditional approaches

Processing stages	Conventional approaches	Green nanoparticles synthesis and their usage	Effects	References
Catalyst synthesis	Catalyst synthesizes chemically, e.g., CaO via calcination	Green synthesis of nanoparticles using natural plant extracts, algal biomass, and microbes such as bacteria and fungi	Energy efficient, cost-effective, eco-friendly, eliminate waste, reduce toxicity	(Osman et al., 2024; Rozina et al., 2024)
Transesterification (Biodiesel)	Chemically produced homogeneous catalysts (KOH, NaOH)	Green-synthesized TiO_2, Fe_3O_4, or ZnO NPs used as reusable heterogeneous nanocatalysts	Enhance biodiesel yield, reaction time increases, reusable up to 7–8 cycles	(Pramanik et al., 2023)
Fermentation (Bioethanol)	Microbial fermentation with a restricted turnover of input resources	Phyto-synthesized Ag or ZnO NPs enhance enzyme and microbial activity	Enhance metabolic activity, increase substrate uptake, and improve ethanol yield	(Gupta & Chundawat, 2020)
Pretreatment of lignocellulosic biomass	Acid or alkali pretreatment	Green-synthesized SiO_2 or ZnO NPs, helping enzymetic hydrolysis	Ecofriendly, enhance cellulose breakdown	(Zhang et al., 2023)
Biohydrogen production	Anaerobic digestion	Green-synthesized Ag, Pd, Fe or FeO using microbes facilitates redox reaction	Increase Dark fermentation efficiency, enhance electron transfer, microbial yield, and enhance hydrogen yield	(Dogmaz & Cavas, 2023; Karthikeyan & Velvizhi, 2024)

(continued)

Table 17.2 (continued)

Processing stages	Conventional approaches	Green nanoparticles synthesis and their usage	Effects	References
Algal biomass harvesting	Centrifugation and flocculation	Green-synthesized iron-based nanoparticles (e.g., iron oxide and Fe_2O_3 NPs) separates the algal biomass	High algal recovery, low energy input, reusable nanoparticles	(Yildirim & Ozkaya, 2023)
End-product purification	Distillation and washing	Nanoadsorbents (e.g., Graphene Oxide or activated carbon NPs) from green method purifying biofuels	Selective removal of glycerol, crude methyl esters, water, and other contamination, high fuel purity	(Fadhil et al., 2012)

17.5 Potential Benefits of Nanotechnology in Biofuel Production

Nanotechnology offers a reframing potential in biofuel production by increasing yield, enhancing enzyme immobilization, catalyst recovery, lowering production costs, boosting process efficiency across various biofuel types, including biodiesel, bioethanol, biohydrogen, etc., and enabling sustainability. According to current research trends, nanotechnology seems to have potential benefits in various key areas of biofuel production. The application of nano-catalysts with their high surface area-to-volume ratio, flexible properties, and improved sites of activation allows for enhancing catalytic conversion efficiency of biofuel production via processes such as transesterification, hydrolysis, and fermentation. Nanocatalysts are suitable for a sustainable and large-scale production of biofuel since they are effective with a wide range of raw materials, such as waste oils and non-edible biomasses (Singh et al., 2020a, 2020b, 2020c). Moreover, the field of nanotechnology provides a promising alternative to conventional pre-treatment technologies for lignocellulosic biomass, enabling economically viable, efficient, and environmentally friendly solutions. Utilizing highly valuable nanomaterials such as Carbon nanotubes, nanofibers, nanosheets, carbon dots, porous and graphitic nanocarbons can be used for the pretreatment of lignocellulosic biomass for biofuel production by enhancing enzyme performance, reducing toxicity, enabling reusability, and stability (Zhang et al., 2023). Nanotechnology also helps to improve the separation and purification of biofuel by-products using magnetic nanoparticles and other sophisticated nanomaterial-based porous membranes and filtrates, thus enhancing the yield and quality of the products sustainably (Yadav et al., 2022). In addition to biofuel recovery, nanoparticles are also employed as fuel additives to boost the overall engine performance, fuel combustion efficiency, and reduce toxic gas emissions. For example, Mofijur et al. (2024) incorporate TiO_2 NPs, reducing smoke emission by 32.98%, CO by 30% and hydrocarbons by 28.68% and also highlighting their positive impact on engine parameters like brake thermal efficiency, heat release rate, and encouraging cleaner combustion (Mofijur et al., 2024). Nanoparticle formulation on microalgae (a third-generation biofuel substrate) is used to overcome the challenges in cultivation, and lipid extraction is energy-intensive. Thus, nano-additives act as a prominent innovation to optimize the cultivation and harvesting of microalgae along with nutrient utility and CO_2 fixation. Besides this, the application of nanoparticles can also assist in biofuel extraction by algae conversion and enhancement of biofuel combustion (Hossain et al., 2019). Furthermore, nanotechnology can be employed to minimize waste produced during biofuel production or recycle waste, and can aid in converting by-products of biofuel production into other valuable fuel. One such example is the conversion of low-value glycerol into high-value fuels, such as methanol and ethanol (Mehejabin et al., 2024).

17.6 Challenges and Limitations

Production of biofuel may advance to the innovative stage with the application of nanotechnology, which has vast potential to improve biofuel efficiency, yield, reduce the amount of energy consumption, and accelerate the conversion of biological feedstocks into biofuels to lower toxic gases emission, minimize carbon footprint, and environmental impacts as well as mass production of sustainable and eco-friendly biofuel. Nonetheless, its incorporation is confronted by a number of other notable challenges and constraints that need to be critically examined, including environmental and human health, scalability, ethical, and regulatory issues in the production of biofuels. One of the major nanotechnology-based biofuel production challenges is nanoparticle toxicity, where their incorporation induces various cytotoxic effects on humans, and the long-term stability of heavy metal-based nanoparticles can be detected to accumulate in water bodies and soil, disrupting the ecosystem, and leading to the possibility of interfering with the plant and microbial systems. Moreover, inhalation and ingestion of nanoparticles and their by-products and waste material release can cause chronic health diseases in humans, such as respiratory disorders and cancer. Long-term exposure can damage DNA, too. Significant economic limitations also exist due to the use of nanomaterials, as they can increase biofuel production and operational costs, making large-scale production less likely with a lack of advanced technologies and expansion of infrastructure. The economic viability of nanotechnology-based biofuels production can be frequently challenged by the demand for expensive feedstocks, sophisticated technologies, and large-scale infrastructure adoption. Furthermore, due to the lack of standardized guidelines, safety policies for nanoparticle use and disposal hinder the validation of their effectiveness. Thus, well-established policies and comprehensive regulatory frameworks are of great concern to manage the risk of nanomaterials in biofuel production and to create sustainable energy pathways.

17.7 Future Research Directions

Scientists and researchers are focused on developing advanced nanomaterials that can leverage their unique characteristics, such as high surface area-to-volume ratio, varied shape and size, and increase reaction and enzyme activity to produce safer, cleaner, more cost-effective nanomaterials and innovative process designs. Research has now prioritized interdisciplinary collaboration to overcome barriers such as nanoparticles recovery, reducing nanotoxicity, process scalability and compatibility, and to address regulatory and technical gaps for safe deployment of consistent application of nanoparticles in sustainable biofuel production. The future of biofuel production relies on recent discoveries of nanobiocatalysts and nanostructured membranes that employ carbon-based nanomaterials to provide more effective approaches to the biofuel industry by optimizing the kinetics of the reactions, engine efficiency, and minimizing pollutant emissions. However, innovation in green synthesis and biodegradable nanoparticles offers promising alternatives to conventional biofuel production. Recent use of green-synthesized nanomaterials, such as plant extracts, algae biomass, and microbial biomass, in emerging biofuel pathways such as biodiesel production, biohydrogen production, and carbon recycling, to reduce carbon footprints, minimize waste by-products, and release of hazardous chemicals to further prevent nanoparticles toxicity and environmental accumulation. Ultimately, advancing green nanotechnology for capturing CO_2 and storage in biofuel production can significantly reduce the long-term environmental impact as well as eliminate the risk of bioaccumulation and toxicity of nanomaterials in humans and the ecosystem. Furthermore, innovations in green technology require not only technical innovation but also economic analysis and policy support to ensure eco-friendly, sustainable, and responsible implementation. Finally, for further research work, it is crucial to analyze the life cycle, cost-benefits, and safety evaluation when using nanotechnology for large-scale biofuel production.

17.8 Conclusion

In today's world, high energy demand is creating a massive problem. However, the production of biofuel possesses immense potential for a paradigm shift in the worldwide energy source, offering a sustainable alternative that encourages the recycling and reuse of resources, by-products, and end-products. Conventional biofuel production exhibits numerous technical barriers; as a result, emerging nanotechnology offers a promising solution for lowering the costs of biofuel production and addressing environmental issues. Various forms of nanoparticles/noncatalysts with their distinctive characteristics have been effectively applied to improve biofuel production from different substrates. Moreover, recent innovation highlights that nanoparticles can be synthesized from different organic substance such as plant extract, algal biomass, and microbial culture by green synthesis Therefore, in light of the challenges and future opportunities, the best course of action is to act as responsible risk reducers by minimizing pollution and global warming by exploiting green biofuels to create a self-sustainable and eco-friendly nation in the field of green energy.

Acknowledgements We would like to acknowledge the DBT-Electronic Library Consortium (DeLCON) of the Ministry of Science and Technology, Government of India, for providing access to research articles. We are also thankful to UGC-SAP for providing Laboratory Infrastructure to the Department of Biotechnology, Assam University, Silchar.

References

Abdelfattah, M. S. H., Abu-Elyazeed, O. S. M., Abd El mawla, E., & Abdelazeem, M. A. (2018). On biodiesels from castor raw oil using catalytic pyrolysis. *Energy, 143*, 950–960. https://doi.org/10.1016/j.energy.2017.09.095

Abel, S., Tesfaye, J., Gudata, L., Nagaprasad, N., Subramanian, K., Mani, M., Shanmugam, R., Dwarampudi, L. P., Roy, A., Stalin, B., & Krishnaraj, R. (2022). Biobutanol preparation through sugar-rich biomass by *Clostridium saccharoperbutylacetonicum* conversion using ZnO nanoparticle catalyst. *Biomass Conversion and Biorefinery*. https://doi.org/10.1007/s13399-022-02424-1

Abusweireh, R. S., Rajamohan, N., & Vasseghian, Y. (2022). Enhanced production of biodiesel using nanomaterials: A detailed review on the mechanism and influencing factors. *Fuel, 319*, Article 123862. https://doi.org/10.1016/j.fuel.2022.123862

Alaei, S., Haghighi, M., Toghiani, J., & Rahmani Vahid, B. (2018). Magnetic and reusable MgO/MgFe2O4 nanocatalyst for biodiesel production from sunflower oil: Influence of fuel ratio in combustion synthesis on catalytic properties and performance. *Industrial Crops and Products, 117*, 322–332. https://doi.org/10.1016/j.indcrop.2018.03.015

Alduhaish, O. M., Shaik, M. R., & Adil, S. F. (2022). Photo-induced preparation of Ag@MOF-801 composite based heterogeneous nanocatalyst for the production of biodiesel. *Catalysts, 12*(5), 533. https://doi.org/10.3390/catal12050533

Ali, H. E. A., El-fayoumy, E. A., Soliman, R. M., Elkhatat, A., Al-Meer, S., Elsaid, K., Hussein, H. A., Zul Helmi Rozaini, M., & Azmuddin Abdullah, M. (2024). Nanoparticle applications in Algal-biorefinery for biofuel production. *Renewable and Sustainable Energy Reviews, 192*, 114267. https://doi.org/10.1016/j.rser.2023.114267

Arif, S., Liaquat, R., & Adil, M. (2018). Applications of materials as additives in anaerobic digestion technology. *Renewable and Sustainable Energy Reviews, 97*, 354–366. https://doi.org/10.1016/j.rser.2018.08.039

Arya, I., Poona, A., Dikshit, P. K., Pandit, S., Kumar, J., Singh, H. N., Jha, N. K., Rudayni, H. A., Chaudhary, A. A., & Kumar, S. (2021). Current trends and future prospects of nanotechnology in biofuel production. In *Catalysts* (Vol. 11, Issue 11). https://doi.org/10.3390/catal11111308

Awogbemi, O., & Kallon, D. V. Von. (2024a). Recent advances in the application of nanomaterials for improved biodiesel, biogas, biohydrogen, and bioethanol production. *Fuel, 358*(PB), 130261. https://doi.org/10.1016/j.fuel.2023.130261

Awogbemi, O., & Von Kallon, D. V. (2024b). Recent advances in the application of nanomaterials for improved biodiesel, biogas, biohydrogen, and bioethanol production. *Fuel, 358*, Article 130261. https://doi.org/10.1016/j.fuel.2023.130261

Ayub, J., Saeed, M. U., Hussain, N., Zulfiqar, I., Mehmood, T., Iqbal, H. M. N., & Bilal, M. (2023). Designing robust nano-biocatalysts using nanomaterials as multifunctional carriers—expanding the application scope of bio-enzymes. *Topics in Catalysis, 66*(9–12), 625–648. https://doi.org/10.1007/s11244-022-01657-8

Beckers, L., Hiligsmann, S., Lambert, S. D., Heinrichs, B., & Thonart, P. (2013). Improving effect of metal and oxide nanoparticles encapsulated in porous silica on fermentative biohydrogen production by *Clostridium butyricum*. *Bioresource Technology, 133*, 109–117. https://doi.org/10.1016/j.biortech.2012.12.168

Bin Rashid, A. (2023). Utilization of nanotechnology and nanomaterials in biodiesel production and property enhancement. *Journal of Nanomaterials, 2023*, 1–14. https://doi.org/10.1155/2023/7054045

Bin Rashid, A., & Hayashi, Y. (2023). Utilization of nanotechnology and nanomaterials in biodiesel production and property enhancement. *Journal of Nanomaterials, 2023*. https://doi.org/10.1155/2023/7054045

Borthakur, P. P. (2025). Nanoparticle enhanced biodiesel blends: Recent insights and developments. *Hybrid Advances, 10*, Article 100442. https://doi.org/10.1016/j.hybadv.2025.100442

Bosu, S., Pooja, R. P., & Rajasimman, M. (2022). Role of nanomaterials in enhanced ethanol production through biological methods—Review on operating factors and machine learning applications. *Fuel, 320*, Article 123905. https://doi.org/10.1016/j.fuel.2022.123905

Changmai, B., Rano, R., Vanlalveni, C., & Rokhum, S. L. (2021). A novel Citrus sinensis peel ash coated magnetic nanoparticles as an easily recoverable solid catalyst for biodiesel production. *Fuel, 286*, Article 119447. https://doi.org/10.1016/j.fuel.2020.119447

Chanu, N. B., Singh, A. B., & Chandrakumar Singh, M. (2023). Microwave assisted catalysis for biofuel production. In *Bioenergy Engineering* (pp. 427–445). Elsevier. https://doi.org/10.1016/B978-0-323-98363-1.00016-8

Chen, Y., Liu, T., He, H., & Liang, H. (2018). Fe3O4/ZnMg(Al)O magnetic nanoparticles for efficient biodiesel production. *Applied Organometallic Chemistry, 32*(5). https://doi.org/10.1002/aoc.4330

Devi, A., Bajar, S., Sihag, P., Sheikh, Z. U. D., Singh, A., Kaur, J., Bishnoi, N. R., & Pant, D. (2023). A panoramic view of technological landscape for bioethanol production from various generations of feedstocks. *Bioengineered, 14*(1), 81–112. https://doi.org/10.1080/21655979.2022.2095702

Dogmaz, S., & Cavas, L. (2023). Biohydrogen production via green silver nanoparticles synthesized through biomass of *Ulva lactuca* bloom. *Bioresource Technology, 379*, Article 129028. https://doi.org/10.1016/j.biortech.2023.129028

Dunmade, I. S., Daramola, M. O., & Iwarere, S. A. (Eds.). (2024). *Sustainable Engineering*. Springer International Publishing. https://doi.org/10.1007/978-3-031-47215-2

Fadhil, A. B., Dheyab, M. M., & Abdul-Qader, A.-Q.Y. (2012). Purification of biodiesel using activated carbons produced from spent tea waste. *Journal of the Association of Arab Universities for Basic and Applied Sciences, 11*(1), 45–49. https://doi.org/10.1016/j.jaubas.2011.12.001

Gadhe, A., Sonawane, S. S., & Varma, M. N. (2015a). Enhancement effect of hematite and nickel nanoparticles on biohydrogen production from dairy wastewater. *International Journal of Hydrogen Energy, 40*(13), 4502–4511. https://doi.org/10.1016/j.ijhydene.2015.02.046

Gadhe, A., Sonawane, S. S., & Varma, M. N. (2015b). Influence of nickel and hematite nanoparticle powder on the production of biohydrogen from complex distillery wastewater in batch fermentation. *International Journal of Hydrogen Energy, 40*(34), 10734–10743. https://doi.org/10.1016/j.ijhydene.2015.05.198

Gran, S., Motiee, H., Mehrdadi, N., & Tizghadam, M. (2022). Impact of metal oxide nanoparticles (NiO, CoO and Fe3O4) on the anaerobic digestion of sewage sludge. *Waste and Biomass Valorization, 13*(11), 4549–4563. https://doi.org/10.1007/s12649-022-01816-8

Gupta, K., & Chundawat, T. S. (2020). Zinc oxide nanoparticles synthesized *using Fusarium oxysporum* to enhance bioethanol production from rice-straw. *Biomass and Bioenergy, 143*, Article 105840. https://doi.org/10.1016/j.biombioe.2020.105840

Hassanein, A., Lansing, S., & Tikekar, R. (2019). Impact of metal nanoparticles on biogas production from poultry litter. *Bioresource Technology, 275*, 200–206. https://doi.org/10.1016/j.biortech.2018.12.048

Ho, D. P., Ngo, H. H., & Guo, W. (2014). A mini review on renewable sources for biofuel. *Bioresource Technology, 169*, 742–749. https://doi.org/10.1016/j.biortech.2014.07.022

Hoa, L., Vestergaard, M., & Tamiya, E. (2017). Carbon-based nanomaterials in biomass-based fuel-fed fuel cells. *Sensors, 17*(11), 2587. https://doi.org/10.3390/s17112587

Hossain, N., Mahlia, T. M. I., & Saidur, R. (2019). Latest development in microalgae-biofuel production with nano-additives. *Biotechnology for Biofuels, 12*(1), 125. https://doi.org/10.1186/s13068-019-1465-0

Hussain, A., Parveen, F., Saxena, A., & Ashfaque, M. (2024). A review of nanotechnology in enzyme cascade to address challenges in pre-treating biomass. *International Journal of Biological Macromolecules, 270*, Article 132466. https://doi.org/10.1016/j.ijbiomac.2024.132466

Islam, M. S., & Ahmed, A. S. (2025). Biofuel Production: A Nanotechnological Approach. *Premier Journal of Science, 9*, 1–10. https://doi.org/10.70389/PJS.100072

Iyyappan, J., Pravin, R., Al-Ghanim, K. A., Govindarajan, M., Nicoletti, M., & Baskar, G. (2023). Dual strategy for bioconversion of elephant grass biomass into fermentable sugars using *Trichoderma reesei* towards bioethanol production. *Bioresource Technology, 374*, Article 128804. https://doi.org/10.1016/j.biortech.2023.128804

Jabraeili, M., Pourdarbani, R., Najafi, B., & Nematollahzadeh, A. (2021). Modelling the effects of Al2O3-SiO2 nanocomposite additive in biodiesel-diesel fuel on diesel engine performance using hybrid ANN-ABC. *Acta Technologica Agriculturae, 24*(1), 20–26. https://doi.org/10.2478/ata-2021-0004

Jones, C. F., Resina, L., Ferreira, F. C., Sanjuan-Alberte, P., & Esteves, T. (2024). Conductive core-shell nanoparticles: Synthesis and applications. *The Journal of Physical Chemistry C, 128*(27), 11083–11100. https://doi.org/10.1021/acs.jpcc.4c02012

Kamel Ariffin, M. F., & Idris, A. (2022). Fe2O3/Chitosan coated superparamagnetic nanoparticles supporting lipase enzyme from *Candida Antarctica* for microwave assisted biodiesel production. *Renewable Energy, 185*, 1362–1375. https://doi.org/10.1016/j.renene.2021.11.077

Karthik, V., Periyasamy, S., Varalakshmi, V., Pauline, J. M. N., & Suganya, R. (2023). Biofuel: A prime eco-innovation for sustainability. In *Environmental Sustainability of Biofuels* (pp. 267–284). Elsevier. https://doi.org/10.1016/B978-0-323-91159-7.00006-0

Karthikeyan, B., & Velvizhi, G. (2024). A state-of-the-art on the application of nanotechnology for enhanced biohydrogen production. *International Journal of Hydrogen Energy, 52*, 536–554. https://doi.org/10.1016/j.ijhydene.2023.04.237

Kazemi Shariat Panahi, H., Hosseinzadeh-Bandbafha, H., Dehhaghi, M., Orooji, Y., Mahian, O., Shahbeik, H., Kiehbadroudinezhad, M., Kalam, M. A., Karimi-Maleh, H., Salehi Jouzani, G., Mei, C., Guillemin, G. G., Nizami, A.-S., Wang, Y., Gupta, V. K., Lam, S. S., Pan, J., Kim, K.-H., Peng, W & Tabatabaei, M. (2024). Nanotechnology applications in biodiesel processing and production: A comprehensive review. *Renewable and Sustainable Energy Reviews, 192*, 114219. https://doi.org/10.1016/j.rser.2023.114219

Khan, I., Anburajan, P., Kumar, G., Yoon, J., Bahuguna, A., de Moura, A. G. L., Pugazhendhi, A., Kim, S., & Kang, S. (2021). Comparative effect of silver nanoparticles (AgNPs) derived from actinomycetes and henna on biohydrogen production by *Clostridium beijerinckii* (KTCC1737). *International Journal of Energy Research, 45*(12), 17269–17278. https://doi.org/10.1002/er.6076

Khan, Y., Sadia, H., Ali Shah, S. Z., Khan, M. N., Shah, A. A., Ullah, N., Ullah, M. F., Bibi, H., Bafakeeh, O. T., Khedher, N. B., Eldin, S. M., Fadhl, B. M., & Khan, M. I. (2022). Classification, synthetic, and characterization approaches to nanoparticles, and their applications in various fields of nanotechnology: A review. *Catalysts, 12*(11), 1386. https://doi.org/10.3390/catal1211 1386

Khanna, K., Jamwal, V. L., Gandhi, S. G., Ohri, P., & Bhardwaj, R. (2019). Metal resistant PGPR lowered Cd uptake and expression of metal transporter genes with improved growth and photosynthetic pigments in *Lycopersicon esculentum* under metal toxicity. *Scientific Reports, 9*(1), 5855. https://doi.org/10.1038/s41598-019-41899-3

Khatami, M., Alijani, H., Nejad, M., & Varma, R. (2018). Core@shell nanoparticles: Greener synthesis using natural plant products. *Applied Sciences, 8*(3), 411. https://doi.org/10.3390/app 8030411

Khujamberdiev, R., & Cho, H. M. (2025). Synthesis and characterization of nanoparticles in transforming biodiesel into a sustainable fuel. *Molecules, 30*(6), 1352. https://doi.org/10.3390/mol ecules30061352

Kim, Y.-K., & Lee, H. (2016). Use of magnetic nanoparticles to enhance bioethanol production in syngas fermentation. *Bioresource Technology, 204*, 139–144. https://doi.org/10.1016/j.biortech. 2016.01.001

Kumar, B., Bhardwaj, N., Agrawal, K., Chaturvedi, V., & Verma, P. (2020). Current perspective on pretreatment technologies using lignocellulosic biomass: An emerging biorefinery concept. *Fuel Processing Technology*, 199(July 2019). https://doi.org/10.1016/j.fuproc.2019.106244

Kumar, B., Bhardwaj, N., & Verma, P. (2020b). Microwave assisted transition metal salt and orthophosphoric acid pretreatment systems: Generation of bioethanol and xylo-oligosaccharides. *Renewable Energy, 158*, 574–584. https://doi.org/10.1016/j.renene.2020. 05.006

Kumar, S., Tirlangi, S., Kumar, A., Imran, M., Pillai HP, J. S., Kumar Koshariya, A., Sathish, T., Ubaidullah, M., Ayub, R., Minnam Reddy, V. R., AlAbdulaal, T. H., Algarni, H., Maiz, F., & Shkir, M. (2023). A review on the contribution of nanotechnology for biofuel production from algal biomass: A bridge to the reduction of carbon footprint. *Sustainable Energy Technologies and Assessments, 60*, 103498. https://doi.org/10.1016/j.seta.2023.103498

Li, W., Zhang, J., Yang, J., Zhang, J., Li, Z., Yang, Y., & Zang, L. (2022). Comparison of copper and aluminum doped cobalt ferrate nanoparticles for improving biohydrogen production. *Bioresource Technology, 343*, Article 126078. https://doi.org/10.1016/j.biortech.2021.126078

Lin, R., Cheng, J., Ding, L., Song, W., Liu, M., Zhou, J., & Cen, K. (2016). Enhanced dark hydrogen fermentation by addition of ferric oxide nanoparticles using *Enterobacter aerogenes*. *Bioresource Technology, 207*, 213–219. https://doi.org/10.1016/j.biortech.2016.02.009

Mahapatra, S., Kumar, D., Singh, B., & Sachan, P. K. (2021). Biofuels and their sources of production: A review on cleaner sustainable alternative against conventional fuel, in the framework of the food and energy nexus. *Energy Nexus, 4*, Article 100036. https://doi.org/10.1016/j.nexus. 2021.100036

Manikandan, S., Krishnan, R. Y., Vickram, S., Subbaiya, R., Kim, W., Govarthanan, M., & Karmegam, N. (2023). Emerging nanotechnology in renewable biogas production from biowastes: Impact and optimization strategies—a review. *Renewable and Sustainable Energy Reviews, 181*, Article 113345. https://doi.org/10.1016/j.rser.2023.113345

Mansir, N., Teo, S. H., Rashid, U., & Taufiq-Yap, Y. H. (2018). Efficient waste *Gallus domesticus* shell derived calcium-based catalyst for biodiesel production. *Fuel, 211*, 67–75. https://doi.org/ 10.1016/j.fuel.2017.09.014

Mehejabin, F., Musharrat, A., Ahmed, S. F., Kabir, Z., Khan, T. M. Y., & Saleel, C. A. (2024). Sustainable biofuel production utilizing nanotechnology: Challenges and potential solutions. *GCB Bioenergy, 16*(10). https://doi.org/10.1111/gcbb.70001

Mishra, V. K., & Goswami, R. (2018). A review of production, properties and advantages of biodiesel. *Biofuels, 9*(2), 273–289. https://doi.org/10.1080/17597269.2017.1336350

Mofijur, M., Ahmed, S. F., Ahmed, B., Mehnaz, T., Mehejabin, F., Shome, S., Almomani, F., Chowdhury, A. A., Kalam, M. A., Badruddin, I. A., & Kamangar, S. (2024). Impact of nanoparticle-based fuel additives on biodiesel combustion: An analysis of fuel properties, engine performance, emissions, and combustion characteristics. *Energy Conversion and Management: X, 21*, Article 100515. https://doi.org/10.1016/j.ecmx.2023.100515

Mohanraj, S., Anbalagan, K., Rajaguru, P., & Pugalenthi, V. (2016). Effects of phytogenic copper nanoparticles on fermentative hydrogen production by *Enterobacter cloacae* and *Clostridium acetobutylicum*. *International Journal of Hydrogen Energy, 41*(25), 10639–10645. https://doi.org/10.1016/j.ijhydene.2016.04.197

Muhammad, A., & Badshah, M. (2019). *Magnetic nanoparticles: Eco-friendly application in biofuel production* (pp. 109–129). https://doi.org/10.1007/978-3-030-16439-3_7

Nair, L. G., Agrawal, K., & Verma, P. (2022). An overview of sustainable approaches for bioenergy production from agro-industrial wastes. *Energy Nexus, 6*(March), Article 100086. https://doi.org/10.1016/j.nexus.2022.100086

Nair, L. G., & Verma, P. (2025). Harnessing carbon potential of lignocellulosic biomass: advances in pretreatments, applications, and the transformative role of machine learning in biorefineries. *Bioresources and Bioprocessing*, 12(1). https://doi.org/10.1186/s40643-025-00935-z

Ndaba, B., Rama, H., Bingwa, N., & Roopnarain, A. (2025). Unravelling the role of nanoparticles during bioethanol production: A review on pretreatment, hydrolysis and fermentation. *Fuel, 396*, Article 135336. https://doi.org/10.1016/j.fuel.2025.135336

Nduka, F. O., Onwurah, I. N. E., Obeta, C. J., Nweze, E. J., Nkwocha, C. C., Ujowundu, F. N., Eje, O. E., & Nwigwe, J. O. (2024). Effect of nickel oxide nanoparticles on bioethanol production by *Pichia kudriavzveii* IFM 53048 using banana peel waste substrate. *Environmental Technology, 45*(16), 3283–3302. https://doi.org/10.1080/09593330.2023.2215450

Negi, P., Singh, Y., Yadav, A., Singh, N. K., Sharma, A., & Singh, R. (2023). Challenges and future opportunities of nanoparticle applications to various biofuel generation processes—a review. *Proceedings of the Institution of Mechanical Engineers, Part E: Journal of Process Mechanical Engineering, 237*(3), 1085–1099. https://doi.org/10.1177/09544089221145485

Nizami, A.-S., & Rehan, M. (2018). Towards nanotechnology-based biofuel industry. *Biofuel Research Journal, 5*(2), 798–799. https://doi.org/10.18331/BRJ2018.5.2.2

Osman, A. I., Elgarahy, A. M., Eltaweil, A. S., Abd El-Monaem, E. M., El-Aqapa, H. G., Park, Y., Hwang, Y., Ayati, A., Farghali, M., Ihara, I., Al-Muhtaseb, A. H., Rooney, D. W., Yap, P.-S., & Sillanpää, M. (2023). Biofuel production, hydrogen production and water remediation by photocatalysis, biocatalysis and electrocatalysis. *Environmental Chemistry Letters, 21*(3), 1315–1379. https://doi.org/10.1007/s10311-023-01581-7

Osman, A. I., Zhang, Y., Farghali, M., Rashwan, A. K., Eltaweil, A. S., Abd El-Monaem, E. M., Mohamed, I. M. A., Badr, M. M., Ihara, I., Rooney, D. W., & Yap, P.-S. (2024). Synthesis of green nanoparticles for energy, biomedical, environmental, agricultural, and food applications: A review. *Environmental Chemistry Letters, 22*(2), 841–887. https://doi.org/10.1007/s10311-023-01682-3

Pandey, A., Gupta, K., & Pandey, A. (2015). Effect of nanosized TiO2 on photofermentation by *Rhodobacter sphaeroides* NMBL-02. *Biomass and Bioenergy, 72*, 273–279. https://doi.org/10.1016/j.biombioe.2014.10.021

Parra, R., Chicaiza-Ortiz, C., Herrera-Feijoo, R. J., Arellano-Yasaca, D. V., Lee, L.-C., Supe-Tulcan, R. X., & Marti-Herrero, J. (2025). Advancements of biohydrogen production based on anaerobic digestion: Technologies, substrates, and future prospects. *Sci, 7*(2), 52. https://doi.org/10.3390/sci7020052

Pattarkine, M. V., & Pattarkine, V. M. (2012). *Nanotechnology for algal biofuels* (pp. 147–163). https://doi.org/10.1007/978-94-007-5110-1_8

Prabhu, N., Karthikadevi, S., & Gajendran, T. (2021). Comprehensive review of the prospectives and development for the production of bioalcohols using nanoparticles. In *Nanomaterials* (pp. 379–391). Elsevier. https://doi.org/10.1016/B978-0-12-822401-4.00005-2

Pramanik, A., Chaudhary, A. A., Sinha, A., Chaubey, K. K., Ashraf, M. S., Basher, N. S., Rudayni, H. A., Dayal, D., & Kumar, S. (2023). Nanocatalyst-based biofuel generation: An update, challenges and future possibilities. *Sustainability, 15*(7), 6180. https://doi.org/10.3390/su15076180

Rai, M., Dos Santos, J. C., Soler, M. F., Franco Marcelino, P. R., Brumano, L. P., Ingle, A. P., Gaikwad, S., Gade, A., & Da Silva, S. S. (2016). Strategic role of nanotechnology for production of bioethanol and biodiesel. *Nanotechnology Reviews, 5*(2), 231–250. https://doi.org/10.1515/ntrev-2015-0069

Rajak, U., Ağbulut, Ü., Veza, I., Dasore, A., Sarıdemir, S., & Verma, T. N. (2022). Numerical and experimental investigation of CI engine behaviours supported by zinc oxide nanomaterial along with diesel fuel. *Energy, 239*, Article 122424. https://doi.org/10.1016/j.energy.2021.122424

Rambabu, K., Bharath, G., Thanigaivelan, A., Das, D. B., Show, P. L., & Banat, F. (2021). Augmented biohydrogen production from rice mill wastewater through nano-metal oxides assisted dark fermentation. *Bioresource Technology, 319*, Article 124243. https://doi.org/10.1016/j.biortech.2020.124243

Rekha, B., & Saravanathamizhan, R. (2021). Catalytic conversion of corncob biomass into bioethanol. *International Journal of Energy Research, 45*(3), 4508–4518. https://doi.org/10.1002/er.6119

Renzaho, A. M. N., Kamara, J. K., & Toole, M. (2017). Biofuel production and its impact on food security in low and middle income countries: Implications for the post-2015 sustainable development goals. *Renewable and Sustainable Energy Reviews, 78*, 503–516. https://doi.org/10.1016/j.rser.2017.04.072

Rezania, S., Mahdinia, S., Oryani, B., Cho, J., Kwon, E. E., Bozorgian, A., Rashidi Nodeh, H., Darajeh, N., & Mehranzamir, K. (2022). Biodiesel production from wild mustard (*Sinapis Arvensis*) seed oil using a novel heterogeneous catalyst of LaTiO3 nanoparticles. *Fuel, 307*, Article 121759. https://doi.org/10.1016/j.fuel.2021.121759

Rodoshi Khan, N., & Bin Rashid, A. (2024). Carbon-based nanomaterials: A paradigm shift in biofuel synthesis and processing for a sustainable energy future. *Energy Conversion and Management: X, 22*, Article 100590. https://doi.org/10.1016/j.ecmx.2024.100590

Emmanuel, O., & Ezeji, T. C. (2024). Exploring the synergy of nanomaterials and microbial cell factories during biohydrogen and biobutanol production from different carbon sources. *Sustainable Chemistry for the Environment*, *6*, 100098. https://doi.org/10.1016/j.scenv.2024.100098

Ganesan, S., Arunkumar, T., Munuswamy, D., Appavu, P., & Devarajan, Y. (2019). Effect of egr & nanoparticles on performance and emission characteristics of a diesel engine fuelled with palm biodiesel and diesel blends. *Journal of Oil Palm Research, 31*(1), 130–137. https://doi.org/10.21894/fjopr.2018.0065

Saha, S., Sharma, A., Purkayastha, S., Pandey, K., & Dhingra, S. (2019). Bio-plastics and Biofuel. In *Plastics to Energy* (pp. 365–376). Elsevier. https://doi.org/10.1016/B978-0-12-813140-4.00014-5

Sanusi, I. A., Faloye, F. D., & Gueguim Kana, E. B. (2019). Impact of various metallic oxide nanoparticles on ethanol production by *Saccharomyces cerevisiae* BY4743: Screening, kinetic study and validation on potato waste. *Catalysis Letters, 149*(7), 2015–2031. https://doi.org/10.1007/s10562-019-02796-6

Sanusi, I. A., Suinyuy, T. N., & Kana, G. E. B. (2021). Impact of nanoparticle inclusion on bioethanol production process kinetic and inhibitor profile. *Biotechnology Reports (Amsterdam, Netherlands), 29*, Article e00585. https://doi.org/10.1016/j.btre.2021.e00585

Sarma, S., & Saha, R. (2025). Production and characterization of bioethanol from spent *Camellia sinensis* leaves using heterogeneous nanocatalysts. *Biomass Conversion and Biorefinery*. https://doi.org/10.1007/s13399-025-06523-7

Sharma, R. K., & Ghose, R. (2015). Synthesis of zinc oxide nanoparticles by homogeneous precipitation method and its application in antifungal activity against *Candida albicans*. *Ceramics International, 41*(1), 967–975. https://doi.org/10.1016/j.ceramint.2014.09.016

Singh, D., Sharma, D., Soni, S. L., Sharma, S., Kumar Sharma, P., & Jhalani, A. (2020a). A review on feedstocks, production processes, and yield for different generations of biodiesel. *Fuel, 262*, Article 116553. https://doi.org/10.1016/j.fuel.2019.116553

Singh, N., Dhanya, B. S., & Verma, M. L. (2020b). Nano-immobilized biocatalysts and their potential biotechnological applications in bioenergy production. *Materials Science for Energy Technologies, 3*, 808–824. https://doi.org/10.1016/j.mset.2020.09.006

Singh, V., Yadav, V. K., & Mishra, V. (2020). *Nanotechnology: An application in biofuel production* (pp. 143–160). https://doi.org/10.1007/978-981-13-9333-4_6

Srinivasan, S. K., Kuppusamy, R., & Krishnan, P. (2021). Effect of nanoparticle-blended biodiesel mixtures on diesel engine performance, emission, and combustion characteristics. *Environmental Science and Pollution Research, 28*(29), 39210–39226. https://doi.org/10.1007/s11356-021-13367-x

Srivastava, N., Mohammad, A., Srivastava, M., Syed, A., Elgorban, A. M., Bahadur Pal, D., Mishra, P. K., Yoon, T., & Gupta, V. K. (2021). Biogenic enabled in-vitro synthesis of nickel cobaltite nanoparticle and its application in single stage hybrid biohydrogen production. *Bioresource Technology, 342*, Article 126006. https://doi.org/10.1016/j.biortech.2021.126006

Su, G., Ong, H. C., Mofijur, M., Mahlia, T. M. I., & Ok, Y. S. (2022). Pyrolysis of waste oils for the production of biofuels: A critical review. *Journal of Hazardous Materials, 424*, Article 127396. https://doi.org/10.1016/j.jhazmat.2021.127396

Taherdanak, M., Zilouei, H., & Karimi, K. (2015). Investigating the effects of iron and nickel nanoparticles on dark hydrogen fermentation from starch using central composite design. *International Journal of Hydrogen Energy, 40*(38), 12956–12963. https://doi.org/10.1016/j.ijhydene.2015.08.004

Teo, S. H., Islam, A., Chan, E. S., Thomas Choong, S. Y., Alharthi, N. H., Taufiq-Yap, Y. H., & Awual, M. R. (2019). Efficient biodiesel production from *Jatropha curcus* using CaSO4/Fe2O3-SiO2 core-shell magnetic nanoparticles. *Journal of Cleaner Production, 208*, 816–826. https://doi.org/10.1016/j.jclepro.2018.10.107

Thanigaivel, S., Rajendran, S., Gnanasekaran, L., Chew, K. W., Tran, D. T., Tran, H.-D., Nghia, N. K., & Show, P. L. (2023). Nanotechnology for improved production of algal biofuels: A review. *Environmental Chemistry Letters, 21*(2), 821–837. https://doi.org/10.1007/s10311-022-01529-3

Umbach, F. (2010). Global energy security and the implications for the EU. *Energy Policy, 38*(3), 1229–1240. https://doi.org/10.1016/j.enpol.2009.01.010

Velmurugan, R., & Incharoensakdi, A. (2019). Metal oxide mediated extracellular NADPH regeneration improves ethanol production by engineered *Synechocystis sp.* PCC 6803. *Frontiers in Bioengineering and Biotechnology, 7*. https://doi.org/10.3389/fbioe.2019.00148

Wang, S.-K., Wang, F., Hu, Y.-R., Stiles, A. R., Guo, C., & Liu, C.-Z. (2014). Magnetic flocculant for high efficiency harvesting of microalgal cells. *ACS Applied Materials & Interfaces, 6*(1), 109–115. https://doi.org/10.1021/am404764n

Wang, T., Zhang, D., Dai, L., Chen, Y., & Dai, X. (2016). Effects of metal nanoparticles on methane production from waste-activated sludge and microorganism community shift in anaerobic granular sludge. *Scientific Reports, 6*(1), 25857. https://doi.org/10.1038/srep25857

Wei, H., Wang, Q., Zhang, R., Liu, M., & Zhang, W. (2023). Efficient biodiesel production from waste cooking oil by fast co-immobilization of lipases from *Aspergillus oryzae* and *Rhizomucor miehei* in magnetic chitosan microcapsules. *Process Biochemistry, 125*, 171–180. https://doi.org/10.1016/j.procbio.2022.12.025

Wu, W., Shan, G., Xiang, Q., Zhang, Y., Yi, S., & Zhu, L. (2017). Effects of humic acids with different polarities on the photocatalytic activity of nano-TiO2 at environment relevant concentration. *Water Research, 122*, 78–85. https://doi.org/10.1016/j.watres.2017.05.010

Xiong, M., Huang, J., He, X., Zhou, Z., Qu, X., Faisal, S., & Abomohra, A. (2023). Evaluation of bio-oil/biodiesel production from co-pyrolysis of corn straw and natural hair: A new insight towards energy recovery and waste biorefinery. *Fuel, 331*, Article 125710. https://doi.org/10.1016/j.fuel.2022.125710

Yadav, A. K., Purushotham, M., Gour, N. I., Gurnule, G. G., Choudhary, V. C., & Yadav, K. R. (2022). *Brief review on nanotechnology as an effective tool for production of biofuels*. 3–8. https://doi.org/10.4028/p-bdzjch

Yang, G., & Wang, J. (2018). Various additives for improving dark fermentative hydrogen production: A review. *Renewable and Sustainable Energy Reviews, 95*, 130–146. https://doi.org/10.1016/j.rser.2018.07.029

Yang, G., & Wang, J. (2019). Synergistic enhancement of biohydrogen production from grass fermentation using biochar combined with zero-valent iron nanoparticles. *Fuel, 251*, 420–427. https://doi.org/10.1016/j.fuel.2019.04.059

Yildirim, O., & Ozkaya, B. (2023). Effect of nanoparticles synthesized from green extracts on dark fermentative biohydrogen production. *Biomass and Bioenergy, 170*, Article 106707. https://doi.org/10.1016/j.biombioe.2023.106707

Yildirim, O., & Ozkaya, B. (2024). Enhancing fermentation yield for biohydrogen production using eco-friendly nickel and cobalt ferrite nanoparticles. *Biomass Conversion and Biorefinery*. https://doi.org/10.1007/s13399-024-05354-2

Yusuff, A. S., Bhonsle, A. K., Trivedi, J., Bangwal, D. P., Singh, L. P., & Atray, N. (2021). Synthesis and characterization of coal fly ash supported zinc oxide catalyst for biodiesel production using used cooking oil as feed. *Renewable Energy, 170*, 302–314. https://doi.org/10.1016/j.renene.2021.01.101

Zarea, M., Saady, N. M. C., Zendehboudi, S., Venkatachalam, P., Albayati, T. M., & Al-nayili, A. (2025). Nanomaterials in the fermentation of bioethanol and biobutanol: Strategies to improve process efficiency. In *Biomass Conversion through Nanomaterials* (pp. 309–354). Elsevier. https://doi.org/10.1016/B978-0-443-24748-4.00014-3

Zhang, Q., Xu, S., Li, Y., Ding, P., Zhang, Y., & Zhao, P. (2021). Green-synthesized nickel oxide nanoparticles enhances biohydrogen production of *Klebsiella sp.* WL1316 using lignocellulosic hydrolysate and its regulatory mechanism. *Fuel*, *305*, 121585. https://doi.org/10.1016/j.fuel.2021.121585

Zhang, R., Gao, H., Wang, Y., He, B., Lu, J., Zhu, W., Peng, L., & Wang, Y. (2023). Challenges and perspectives of green-like lignocellulose pretreatments selectable for low-cost biofuels and high-value bioproduction. *Bioresource Technology, 369*, Article 128315. https://doi.org/10.1016/j.biortech.2022.128315

Zhang, X., Yan, S., Tyagi, R. D., & Surampalli, R. Y. (2019). Biodiesel production by transesterification. In *Biodiesel Production* (pp. 27–52). American Society of Civil Engineers. https://doi.org/10.1061/9780784415344.ch03

Zhong, L., Feng, Y., Wang, G., Wang, Z., Bilal, M., Lv, H., Jia, S., & Cui, J. (2020). Production and use of immobilized lipases in/on nanomaterials: A review from the waste to biodiesel production. *International Journal of Biological Macromolecules, 152*, 207–222. https://doi.org/10.1016/j.ijbiomac.2020.02.258

Chapter 18
Hydrothermal Liquefaction: A Novel Biofuel Production Technique

Suchitra Rakesh

Abstract Hydrothermal liquefaction is an advanced technology that converts wet biomass feedstock into biofuel under high temperatures and pressures. Compared with other thermochemical methods, HTL facilitates the usage of wet biomass; hence, the cost of drying can be avoided. The various types of HTL processes, viz., batch, continuous, fast, and co-HTL, as well as their mechanism, are explained in the chapter. The chapter provides detailed insight into the factors affecting the HTL, like temperature, pressure, retention time, heating value, biomass-to-solvent ratio, and the effect of catalysts and solvents on HTL efficiency. The chapter also dealt with various biofuel products and their applications. Finally provides suggestions for future studies.

Keywords Hydrothermal liquefaction · Wet biomass · Biofuel · Biocrude · Biochar

18.1 Introduction

Biofuels have gained significant interest globally as they contribute majorly toward circular economy. In G20 summit, India marked significantly for self-sustainable biofuel market globally. Extraction of bio-compounds from lignocellulosic feedstock for biofuel production remains a significant challenge. Conventional extraction techniques usually fail to preserve the structural integrity and activity of the compounds. Hydrothermal liquefaction has recently emerged as an advanced technique based on the thermochemical transformation of biomass into high-value compounds. HTL converts the complex lignocellulosic organic biomass into simpler and high-value compounds, viz., polysaccharides, proteins and lipids, under high temperature and pressure (Schmidt et al., 2023). HTL is a sustainable and cost-efficient approach for extracting high-value compounds from lignocellulosic biomass (Deepika et al.,

S. Rakesh (✉)
Biofuel Research Laboratory, Department of Microbiology, Central University of Tamil Nadu, Thiruvarur, Tamil Nadu, India
e-mail: suchitrar@cutn.ac.in

P. Verma (ed.), *Sustainable Practices in Biorefinery*,
https://doi.org/10.1007/978-981-95-6071-4_18

2024). Many thermochemical conversion technologies include combustion, pyrolysis, gasification and hydrothermal liquefaction. Biomass with high moisture content is not preferred due to its low efficiency, as biomass can not be processed without drying for combustion, pyrolysis, and gasification (Mathanker et al., 2021). The hydrothermal process can perform the thermochemical conversion of biomass under high temperatures and pressure for disintegrating the lignocellulosic biomass into biofuel (Kumar et al., 2018). Hydrothermal processes are of three types depending on the range of temperature and pressure, i.e., HT carbonization, liquefaction and gasification. HTL process occurs with a pressure range of 2–25 MPa and temperature of 250–374 °C. The HTL produce a mixture of crude, aqueous phase products and solid residues, which can be further refined to biochemicals, bio-oil, biochar, and biogas. The biocrude yield from HTL can be improved by advanced HTL processes like batch, continuous, solvent, catalytic, fast or Co-HTL. HTL of biomass produces various high-value compounds with different reaction kinetics. Several studies recently highlighted the factors for enhancing the HTL yield, i.e., temperature, pressure, reaction time, solvent, etc. (Kumar et al., 2025).

This chapter explains the HTL process state-of-the-art. The chapter provides a clear introduction about the HTL process, type of feedstock, and further discusses the various types of HTL processes and their reaction mechanism involved. The second half of the chapter deals with factors influencing optimizing the HTL product recovery, like solvents, catalysts, temperature, pressure, etc. It also outlines the various HTL products and their application. Finally, it addresses the research gap and provides directions for future studies.

18.2 Feedstock for HTL Processing

High-energy-content feedstock selection is preferred for the hydrothermal liquefaction process for enhanced biofuel yield. The presence of sugars, starches, and fats in biomass is important to meet the specific fuel standards. Biomass with high ash content is not preferred as it increases the pollution during combustion. Other important factors for feedstock selection are low price and environmental sustainability. Both dry and wet biomasses are used directly in the HTL process.

Dry biomass feedstock

Lignocellulosic biomass comprises cellulose, hemicellulose and lignin in different proportions. Cellulose is the primary compound present in lignocellulosic biomass of plant cell walls (Woiciechowski et al., 2020; Kumar et al., 2020a, 2020b). The proportion of cellulose varies with the type of biomass; for example, woody biomass contains 40–45% cellulose, whereas paper pulp sludge comprises 50–60%. Various pretreatment methods like alkali, acid, or enzymatic hydrolysis, etc., can improve the recovery of cellulose (Nair et al., 2022a). The recovered cellulose from the biomass can be converted to biofuel via various biological or thermochemical processes

(Jayakumar et al., 2023). Hemicellulose is another important component of lignocellulosic biomass—hemicellulose is a heteropolymer of various monosaccharide units, which can be converted to biofuel after enzymatic hydrolysis. During biological conversion, acetic acid and furans of hemicelluloses degrade the quality of bio-oil and yield. Hence, the HTL process converts the hemicellulosic feedstock into biocrude, where it depolymerises into xylose and mannose. Its proportion also varies with the type of biomass, like woody biomass, which contains 25–35%, paper pulp sludge, 40–50%, etc. Lignin is a complex macromolecule responsible for plant cell wall rigidity, water resistance, binding capacity, etc. (Zhang et al., 2020). Plant-based biomass comprises huge amount of lignin, due to complex nature it required high amount of energy for breakdown. Lignin is well suitable for biofuel production as it reduces volatile compounds, and increases bio-oil heating value (Wang et al., 2017). Woody biomass comprises 25–35% lignin, whereas crops and herbs usually contain 10–25%. The cellulose and hemicellulose proportions in the biomass contribute to the biocrude yield during thermochemical conversions like hydrothermal liquefaction. In contrast, lignin-rich biomass has high energy content during biofuel conversion (Lopez et al., 2013). The chemical composition of various lignocellulosic biomasses is shown in Table 18.1.

Wet biomass

Wet biomass is highly preferred for the HTL process, as it does not require biomass drying before processing. Algal biomass is usually preferred for HTL feedstock due to its lipids, proteins, and carbohydrate composition. The composition of major

Table 18.1 Biochemical composition of lignocellulosic biomasses

Lignocellulosic biomass	Cellulose	Hemicelluloses	Lignin	Reference
Bagasse	30	35	18	Sarkar et al., (2012)
Barley straw	46.00	23.00	15.00	Zhu et al., (2015)
Cornstalk	34.34	27.55	21.81	Ma et al., (2011)
Corn stover	45.00	30.00	16.00	Mathanker et al., (2020)
Furniture sawdust	32.63	37.23	22.16	Jindal and Jha, (2016)
Oil palm shell	39.70	21.80	32.50	Mazaheri et al., (2013)
Peanut straw	36.56	20.37	18.36	Tian et al., (2020)
Palm kernel shell	24.50	22.90	33.50	Chan et al., (2014)
Rapeseed	51.3	17.3	44	Pei et al., (2016)
Rice straw	35.8	21.5	24.4	Imman et al., (2015)
Rice straw	46.33	31.09	10.17	Tian et al., (2020)
Rice straw	42.87	25.15	31.97	Younas et al., (2017)
Sugarcane bagasse	44	27	24	de Souza et al., (2013)
Soybean straw	42.39	22.05	18.93	Tian et al., (2020)
Sweet sorghum bagasse	36.9	17.8	19.5	Umagiliyage et al., (2015)

Table 18.2 Compounds formed during cellulose decomposition at varying temperatures

Temperature	Compounds formed
200–240 °C	Water soluble compounds like glucose, oligomers, etc
Above 240 °C	Non-glucose products, char, oil, and gas
240–270 °C	Complete disassociation of cellulose and maximum glucose
Above 270° to Maxi. 300 °C	Oil fraction increases
Above 300 °C	Oil yield started to decrease, char and gases started to increase

compounds, i.e., protein, lipids, and carbohydrates of algal biomass suitable for biofuel production is mentioned in Table 18.2. The lipid present in biomass usually enhances the oil recovery during the HTL process (Biller & Ross, 2011). Proteins can be transformed into aldehydes, amines and hydrocarbons via HTL process, thereby can be explored for biofuel production (Changi et al., 2015). Biofuels like ethanol or butanol can be achieved by protein fermentation. The carbohydrates can be converted to ethanol or hydrocarbons during fermentation or HTL, respectively (Singh et al., 2015). The biochemical components, i.e., carbohydrates, lipids, and proteins, account for the majority of the mass in the microalgal cell. The relative proportion of these components in microalgae depends on the type of species, their specific growth conditions, and growth phase. Microalgae comprise more proteins than lipids or carbohydrates. Under stress conditions, microalgal lipid content can be enhanced to more than 50%. Polar lipids are the main component of the cell membrane, whereas neutral lipids are stored intracellularly. The carbohydrates exist in the form of cellulose, starch, and polysaccharides. Polysaccharides comprise a significant fraction in most of the microalgae.

18.3 HTL Mechanism of Lignocellulosic Biomass as Feedstock

Agricultural and forest residues are the primary reservoir of lignocellulosic biomass. The lignocellulosic biomass majorly comprises lignin, cellulose and hemicelluloses, which vary among types of biomass. Cellulose is a homopolysaccharide formed by D-glucopyranoside units connected by β-glycosidic linkage in 1:4 proportions (De Jong & Van Ommen, 2014). Crystalline cellulose structures are insoluble in aqueous medium and require further hydrolysis and degradation, while non-crystalline structures are hydrolyzable (Tursi, 2019). During hydrothermal liquefaction, cellulose reacts with water at high temperatures, breaking its hydrogen bonds and weakening its crystallinity. Cellulose is hydrolyzed to monomeric units like glucose, fructose, etc., and the monomeric units are further degraded to simpler hydrocarbons. Based on the medium, the HTL is performed, i.e., acidic, basic, or neutral, the cellulosic hydrolysis and C–O–C bond cleavage differ (Yin & Tan, 2012). In acidic hydrolysis, the acidic proton and oxygen bond two glucose units and form a conjugated acid, forming two glucose units on cleavage of glycosidic bonds (Joksomovic & Markovic, 2007). In a basic medium, the breakage of the C–O–C bond occurs with an OH- attack on the anomeric carbon.

At the same time, due to the water, the glycosidic unit and water split simultaneously to form two units of glucose (Jin et al., 2014). In the catalytic hydrogenation, intermediates like erythrose, glyceraldehyde, etc., form stable C2-C3 alcohols (Hirano et al., 2020). Li et al., (2016) reported that the final composition of cellulosic HTL is comprised of a mixture of aldehydes, ketones, esters, and alcohols. The cellulose decomposition during the HTL process varies with temperature (Gao et al., 2012). The cellulose content of biomass decides the bio-oil yield after the HTL process, and it is observed that biomass with high cellulose content has higher bio-oil recovery.

Hemicellulose is composed of D-glucose, D-mannose, D-xylose, D-galactose, etc. Its poor structure is more water-resistant and reduces the crystallinity (Cao et al., 2017). Lignin has a complex structure of 3 different monomeric units, i.e., p-coumaryl alcohol, coniferyl alcohol, and sinapyl alcohol, connected by ether bonds and C–C linkages (Mathanker, 2020; Nair et al., 2022b). The basic phenylpropane units have low bond dissociation energy. Hence, monomeric units of lignin are formed in the presence of supercritical water from macromolecular units. These basic units form aromatics on further hydrolytic dissociation (Kang et al., 2011).

18.4 HTL Processes

Batch HTL

Batch-type autoclave-based bioreactors are well suited for laboratory-based research-level studies. Since it is batch type, controlling and monitoring factors are easier than in continuous flow systems (Basar et al., 2021). The reactor, after feeding the biomass, solvent and catalyst (if any), is sealed and set to the required temperature (200–400°C) and pressure (10–25 MPa) as per requirement with inert gas to the desired level. The uniform slurry will be prepared using a stirrer with a speed from 18 to 1300 rpm (Younas et al., 2017). After the desired time period is completed, the product will be collected and analyzed (Jasiunas et al., 2017). Some significant advantages of the batch HTL process are flexible reaction parameters adjustment, being well suited for small-scale production of high-value products, lower cost, and ease of cleaning with low maintenance charges (Holtze et al., 2022). It also ensures faster experimentation, easy testing with less waste generation (Castello et al., 2018). Due to its lower productivity and time-consuming nature, it limits its efficiency for large-scale production (Kumar et al., 2020a, 2020b). Hence, to overcome the challenges of large-scale production, continuous HTL processes are required.

Continuous HTL

Continuous stirred tank reactor (CSTR) is used for biomass conversion at high pressure and temperature, facilitating several reactions like hydrolysis, dehydration, decarboxylation, etc. Several modifications have been made so far. For example, the Reliance Company has made a continuous reactor with two CSTRs in series at a flow rate of 2–80 L/h. This reactor can process algal biomass, food waste, bio sludge, etc. (Ghadge et al., 2022). The important components of a continuous reactor are a heat exchanger, an electric heater, a high-pressure feed pump, a plug flow reactor, pressure and temperature control and a product collection unit (Anastasakis et al., 2018). Kristianto et al. (2019) improve the slurry concentration by dissolving lignin-rich biomass in water, ethanol, and isopropanol. Due to the complex biomass composition, phase separation, filtration problem, and high downstream processing during the continuous HTL process, efficient separation for biocrude and process efficiency are vital. Hence, to overcome such issues, advanced technologies, durable material selection, and process optimization are required to minimize the loss during continuous operation (Elliott et al., 2014). Operational complexity, sensitivity to feedstock variability and high capital expenditure are some drawbacks of continuous HTL reactors (Shahbeik et al., 2024).

Fast HTL

It's an advanced process of biomass conversion involving rapid cooling/heating, short duration, high temperature, and pressure. Fast HTL is commonly used for getting higher and better quality fuels from waste biomasses (Liu et al., 2023). One study used cow manure for fast HTL and achieved 21.32% biocrude yield (Conti et al., 2020). The less reaction time and high biomass loading make fast HTL a desired option (Gollakota et al., 2019). Compared with traditional HTL, fast HTL biocrude recovery and product quality will be high (Qian et al., 2017).

Co-solvent HTL

Co-solvent enhances the HTL efficiency as it facilitates the easy biomass breakdown. Solvents usually reduce the biomass viscosity, solubilize, and improve high-value compound recovery. The solvents will be selected based on the type of biomass used and the desired product recovery from HTL. Yerrayya et al., (2020) have reported that biocrude yield increases to 36.8% by using methanol as a cosolvent. Further catalytic HTL, along with co-solvents, gives the highest biocrude yield and conversion efficiency (Wang et al., 2018). Wu et al (2022) reported that combining co-solvents with catalysts improves the biocrude yield up to 67.35%. Ethanol/water mix during HTL improves the biomass conversion and biocrude yield drastically (Hu et al., 2020).

18.5 Factors Affecting HTL

There are various parameters that affect the HTL process, like temperature, retention time, pressure, heating rate, biomass-to-solvent ratio, type of solvent, and catalyst.

Temperature

Temperature is one of the important factors during the HTL process, as it decides the primary outcome from biomass conversion and the properties of the byproducts. As per the literature search, temperature ranges from 180–400 °C are preferred for the HTL process, depending on the type of biomass used. The temperature enhances the hydrolysis of cellulose, hemicelluloses and lignin. It further fragments and degrades the lignocellulosic biomass. The initial high temperature activates the endothermic process in HTL and provides the necessary energy for the breakage of bonds, and small compounds will be formed. Further rise in temperature leads to repolymerization by making new bonds and releasing energy (Akhtar & Amin, 2011). The temperature required for HTL mainly depends on the type and composition of biomass used. The other factors that also affect the temperature for HTL are the type of solvents and catalysts used, residence time, pressure, feed ratio, heating rate, etc. Minowa et al. (1998) reported that various compounds formed during cellulose decomposition at varying temperatures, as mentioned in Table 18.2.

Arturi et al., (2017) reported that during lignin liquefaction in the presence of catalyst and phenol, if the temperature raises from 280 °C to 300 °C the biocrude yield also significantly increases from 50.6% to 77%. However the oil yield reduces if the temperature rises above 310 °C. Zhu et al., (2015) reported that barley straw during HTL with K2 CO3 as catalyst produces maximum bio-oil at 300 °C, later with further increase it reduces. Also showed that with an increase in biochar, the oil yield reduces from 320–400 °C.

Pressure

Reactor pressure is another important parameter that needs to be considered for the HTL process. HTL process usually takes place above the boiling point of water since most solvents, viz., water, ethanol, methanol, and acetone, have a boiling point below 100 °C in atmospheric pressure conditions. The initial pressure in the reactor during HTL facilitates the phase conversion of solvent into vapor during sub and supercritical conditions; thereby, additional energy required for phase separation can be reduced (Yang et al., 2016). Under subcritical regions, at elevated temperatures of 330 °C or above, the pressure increases from 25 to 35 MPa, increasing water density as well (Chan et al., 2014). High solvent density facilitates more penetration and interaction of hydrolysis ions with the surface of cellulose, hemicelluloses and lignin. After reaching the supercritical condition, the pressure has little impact on bio-oil yield (Mathanker et al., 2020). Under supercritical conditions, an increase in pressure is not advised since this will raise the solvent density. This prevents C–C bond cleavage and, hence, the fragmentation of lignocellulosic materials (Akhtar & Amin, 2011). Kaur et al., (2019) reported that during the HTL process of oil palm biomass at 390 °C, the bio-oil yield gets reduced if the pressure rises from 25 to 30 MPa. Cantero et al., (2015) reported that a rise in pressure above the critical point reduces glucose's isomerisation to fructose.

In contrast, a decrease in pressure increases the formation of 5-HMF and hydrolysis of oligosaccharides. In the supercritical region, pressure does not influence the bio-oil yield, whereas, at 300 °C, the initial pressure increase from 2 to 4 MPa increases the bio-oil yield from 21 to 27% (Mathanker et al., 2020). Pressure plays a significant role in the recovery of gaseous products at a critical point, favoring the C2, C3 and C4 formation and reducing the H2 and CO2 yield (Kruse & Gawlik, 2003). High temperature during HTL, pressure is very important to maintain the single-phase system in the reactor.

Retention time

Retention time is the duration maintained in the reactor at a specified temperature. Retention time is the important factor during HTL that decides the overall outcome, i.e., biomass conversion, product recovery and composition. If the process starts with a low heating rate, reaching the final temperature will take more retention time. Hence, the overall time for biomass conversion and bio-oil formation will increase. At critical temperatures, hydrolysis occurs faster, reducing the need for more retention time. Recently, many researchers have reported the effect of retention time on various biomass resources. The pulp/paper sludge, at 280C during HTL, increases the bio-oil yield with an increase in retention time, whereas water-soluble organic compounds reduce (Xu & Lancaster, 2008). Ogi et al., (1985) found that during HTL of wood, the bio-oil yield decreases up to 180 min, whereas at o min, maximum oil was recovered. Hence, bio-oil yield decreases with increased retention time for the HTL process. Yang et al., (2016) reported the highest bio-oil yield with a 10-min retention period. The 10-min duration is enough to break down the biomass, and if the duration increases, the decomposition of bio-oil starts with the formation of lighter products and gases.

In contrast, many studies support longer retention time for increased bio-oil recovery. Yang et al., (2009) showed that birch powder for the HTL process increases the oil, gas and other water-soluble organics with an increase in retention time. Yim et al., (2017) reported that in the presence of catalysts at a supercritical point, the bio-oil increases with an increase in retention time. Hence, depending on the type of biomass and catalyst used for HTL, the retention time will vary accordingly for higher bio-oil yield.

Heating rate

It is defined as the rate of temperature rise per unit time. Most reactions occurring during the HTL process require a longer heating rate (Daniel et al., 2016). Very few studies highlight the importance of the heating rate on the HTL of agricultural biomasses. Other techniques of bio-oil recovery, like pyrolysis, have also pointed out their importance. The HTL of spruce wood with a heating rate of 66–179 °C min^{-1} at 350 °C shows an increase in bio-oil recovery with an increase in the heating rate (Tran et al., 2017). Zhang et al., (2009) used corn stover, aspen wood and grassland perennials for HTL and noticed that the heating rate significantly affects the lipid product yield. The hydrothermal liquefaction of sawdust produces more biocrude at the heating rate of 2 °C min^{-1} than 20 °C min^{-1} (Brand et al., 2014).

Biomass to solvent ratio

It is also known as the feed ratio since most HTL processes are conducted with water as solvent. Hence, it is also known as the biomass-to-water ratio. In a batch process, the feed ratio is represented as a biomass-to-water ratio, whereas pretreated concentrated slurry is used in a continuous system. Hence, biomass the biomass-to-solvent ratio is represented as reactor loading. The feed ratio is an important factor that decides the conversion rate and bio-oil yield. If the feed ratio is lower, the yield will be reduced as the carbon entering the system is low. Hence, it is not economical since heating involves expenditure as needed to raise the temperature to the desired level (Elliott et al., 2015). Akhtar et al., (2010) reported that HTL of empty palm fruit bunch increases the biomass conversion and bio-oil yield with an increase in feed ratio from 1:10 to 2:10 g mL^{-1}. Also, a further increase in feed ratio beyond 2:10 will drastically reduce the conversion rate and oil recovery. Many studies have supported the same by addressing the increase of feed concentration after a particular point decreases biomass conversion and oil yield. The solvents with good dissolution power facilitate easy biomass degradation and lead to higher conversion and bio-oil yield (Daniel et al., 2016). The higher reactor loading leads to reduce the gas fraction formation since high pressure will build up in the reactor (Wang et al., 2013).

Catalysts on HTL

Catalysts play an important role in the HTL process, enhancing bio-oil yield by facilitating faster biomass degradation. It also stops harmful secondary reactions like polymerization, cracking, etc. Two types of catalysts are used during the HTL process: homogeneous and heterogeneous.

Homogeneous catalysts, including hydroxides, carbonates, and acids, are widely used for the HTL process. The hydroxide and carbonates of alkali metals are commonly used with water medium to faster biomass degradation and high bio-oil yield. Tekin et al., (2012) used scotch pine wood with potassium tert-butoxide and KOH as a catalyst for the HTL process and found that bio-oil yield significantly increased in the presence of a catalyst at 300 °C. Khampuang et al. (Khampuang et al., 2015) studied the effect of catalysts in solvents other than water. They used corncobs for the HTL process with alkali in an ethanol solvent and noticed a steep rise in bio-oil yield with alkali. Alkali pretreatment of biomass significantly affects bio-oil yield compared to unpretreated cypress (Liu et al., 2014). The effect of various concentrations of K2 CO3 with a water ratio of 5:25 was reported with increased biomass degradation and oil recovery (Akhtar et al., 2010).

Heterogeneous catalysts are also widely used to enhance bio-oil recovery during the HTL process. The elements are used as their oxide, chloride or sulfate form as catalysts. Zhang et al., (2011) reported that paper mill sludge in the HTL process with homogeneous and heterogeneous catalysts did not significantly differ regarding elemental analysis and oil yield. De Caprariis et al., (2019) reported higher bio-oil yield and lower char with Fe powder as a catalyst. Ferric ions in Fe_2O_3 have a higher oxidation state, failing to enhance the bio-oil yield. Whereas, ferrous ions in Fe_3O_4 have good oxidation capacity, leading to degradation and dehydration of lignocellulosic biomass by dehydration of fructose and forming 5-HMF (Miyata et al., 2018).

18.6 HTL byproducts and applications

Bio-oil/biocrude

Recently, more attention has been given to sustainable biofuel production to meet the energy demand. Bio-oil can satisfy energy requirements due to its chemical composition and physical properties, such as viscosity, total acid number value, etc. Bio-oil from the HTL process is dark brown, with a high carbon number, highly viscous, low oxygen content, and a high HHV value. Bio-oil comprises aldehydes, ketones, phenolics, fatty acids, alcohols, saturated hydrocarbons, unsaturated hydrocarbons, and nitrogenous compounds (Mathanker et al., 2020). Compared to conventional fuels, bio-oil has high viscosity, water content and total acid number, making it a suitable choice for fuel (Yang et al., 2016; Zhu et al., 2014). The higher the TAN number of bio-oil, the more corrosive it is in nature, making it difficult to store. More viscosity also raises the difficulty in transporting the bio-oil. High water content reduces its combustion capacity. Hence, separating bio-oil to get various classes of fuels is very important for substituting it with conventional fuels (Taghipour et al., 2019). Pedersen et al., (2017) performed fractional distillation of biocrude obtained from HTL and confirmed the presence of various compounds like ketones, etc. Hence, bio-oil is suitable for producing biofuels. Biocrude is used not only to produce jet fuels but also to synthesize many important chemicals of industrial importance (Jiang et al., 2018; Tzanetis et al., 2017).

Char

Char is the solid by-product recovered using HTL. Char is also known as solid residue, biochar or hydrochar. Demirbas et al. (2000) have reported that biomass with high lignin content will yield higher char. He investigated that biomass with 41–48% lignin content produces 40–50% char, whereas biomass with 14–27%low lignin yields only 21–26% char. The char yield usually ranges from 5 to 60 wt% depending on the type and biomass composition (Chen et al., 2019). The yield also depends on HTL parameters like temperature, retention time, pressure, biomass-to-solvent ratio, and catalyst concentration. The char recovered from lignocellulosic biomass comprises carbon 55–78%, Hydrogen 4–6%, and oxygen 15–35% by weight (Hoekman et al., 2011). The char can be used for soil enhancement and as an adsorbent.

Due to its highly hydrophobic nature, it is resistant to humidity; allowing easy storage and handling (Liu et al., 2013). The char must go for pretreatment to eliminate the adverse effect on plant growth (Bargmann et al., 2014). The char recovered after HTL has a high calorific value, making it a suitable choice for energy applications like direct combustion or co-combustion with coal. It can also be explored further for energy storage, such as batteries, fuel cells, bio-capacitors, etc. (Liu et al., 2015). The HTL obtained char has less ash content compared to char from other methods. The inorganic minerals present in hemicelluloses are leached out during the HTL process. Hence, char is a cleaner fuel option. It avoids fouling, scaling, slagging, corrosion, water toxicity, and air during combustion (Smith et al., 2016). The char can be used as an adsorbent in wastewater treatment to remove heavy metals and other pollutants. Liu et al. (2009) reported that the char obtained from HTL of pinewood and rice husks has a maximum lead adsorption capacity of 2.40 and 4.25 mg/g, respectively.

Gases

The gas is not considered as important product of HTL, hence gas is either not analyzed or included with other byproducts (Neveux et al., 2014). The gas accounts for 5–15% of the total HTC product, greatly depends on the temperature used (Deniel et al., 2016). The gas yield will rise near the supercritical condition, due to the increased cracking of oil and char (Yang et al., 2009). The CO2 dominates up to 300–325 °C and on further rise in temperature CO fraction starts to increase (Brand et al., 2013).

Aqueous phase

The aqueous phase comprises 25–50% of the HTL yield (Panisko et al., 2015). The compounds commonly found aqueous phase are low molecular weight organic acids, sugars, ketones, phenolic compounds, etc. The major portion comprises of mixture of organic acids viz., propionic acid, formic acid, butanoic acid, glycolic acid, lactic acid, acetic acid and butenedioic acid. Methanol, glycol, ethylene glycol, propylene glycol, and catechol are the main alcohols and polyols present.

18.7 Challenges and Future Directions

The HTL is a promising process for producing biocrude from various biomass sources. The biomass composition is an important factor that decides the quality and quantity of biocrude. Further, there is a need to link HTL with biorefinery for high-value product recovery. Additionally, more research is required on the HTL process based on the type of biomass to improve the accuracy of kinetic models. Techno-economic feasibility is an unexplored area for large-scale biocrude production. The uncertainties and risks of large-scale HTL processes need to be evaluated. However, more elaborative research is required on the HTL process and operating parameters responsible for the quality and yield of biocrude. Future research also needs to target the industrial applications of HTL for sustainable biofuel production.

18.8 Conclusion

HTL is a promising process for converting various biomasses into liquid biofuels and chemicals. The type of biomass and HTL process parameters are used to decide the biocrude recovery and its characteristics. Advanced HTL processes like fast HTL and co-solvent HTL improve the biocrude yield and quality, reducing operational charges and energy consumption. Retention time, temperature, heating rate, and catalyst determine biomass's biocrude yield. The HTL has enormous potential to satisfy the future demand for renewable energy. More research must target pilot-scale facilities, parameter optimization, and standardizing more robust upgrading processes.

References

Akhtar, J., & Amin, N. A. S. (2011). A review on process conditions for optimum bio-oil yield in hydrothermal liquefaction of biomass. *Renewable and Sustainable Energy Reviews, 15*, 1615–1624.

Akhtar, J., Kuang, S. K., & Amin, N. S. (2010). Liquefaction of empty palm fruit bunch (EPFB) in alkaline hot compressed water. *Renewable Energy, 35*, 1220–1227.

Anastasakis, K., Biller, P., Madsen, R. B., Glasius, M., & Johannsen, I. (2018). Continuous hydrothermal liquefaction of biomass in a novel pilot plant with heat recovery and hydraulic oscillation. *Energies, 11*(10), 2695.

Arturi, K. R., Strandgaard, M., Nielsen, R. P., Søgaard, E. G., & Maschietti, M. (2017). Hydrothermal liquefaction of lignin in near-critical water in a new batch reactor: Influence of phenol and temperature. *Journal of Supercritical Fluids, 123*, 28–39.

Bargmann, I., Rillig, M., Kruse, A., Greef, J.-M., & Kücke, M. (2014). Effects of hydrochar application on the dynamics of soluble nitrogen in soils and on plant availability. *Journal of Plant Nutrition and Soil Science, 177*, 48–58.

Basar, I. A., Huan, L., Helene, C., Eric, T., & Cigdem, E. (2021). A review on key design and operational parameters to optimize and develop hydrothermal liquefaction of biomass for biorefinery applications. *Green Chemistry, 23*(4), 1404–1446.

Biller, P., & Ross, A. B. (2011). Potential yields and properties of oil from the hydrothermal liquefaction of microalgae with different biochemical content. *Bioresource technology, 102*(1), 215–225.

Brand, S., Hardi, F., Kim, J., & Suh, D. J. (2014). Effect of heating rate on biomass liquefaction: Differences between subcritical water and supercritical ethanol. *Energy, 68*, 420–427.

Brand, S., Susanti, R. F., Kim, S. K., Lee, H.-S., Kim, J., & Sang, B.-I. (2013). Supercritical ethanol as an enhanced medium for lignocellulosic biomass liquefaction: Influence of physical process parameters. *Energy, 59*, 173–182.

Cantero, D. A., Tapia, Á. S., Bermejo, M. D., & Cocero, M. J. (2015). Pressure and temperature effect on cellulose hydrolysis in pressurized water. *Chemical Engineering Journal, 276*, 145–154.

Cao, L., Zhang, C., Chen, H., Tsang, D., Luo, G., Zhang, S., & Chen, J. (2017). Hydrothermal liquefaction of agricultural and forestry wastes: State-of-the-art review and future prospects. *Bioresource Technology, 245*, 1184–1193.

Castello, D., Pedersen, T. H., & Rosendahl, L. A. (2018). Continuous hydrothermal liquefaction of biomass: A critical review. *Energies, 11*(11), 3165.

Chan, Y. H., Yusup, S., Quitain, A. T., Uemura, Y., & Sasaki, M. (2014). Bio-oil production from oil palm biomass via subcritical and supercritical hydrothermal liquefaction. *Journal of Supercritical Fluids, 95*, 407–412.

Changi, S. M., Faeth, J. L., Mo, N., & Savage, P. E. (2015). Hydrothermal reactions of biomolecules relevant for microalgae liquefaction. *Industrial & Engineering Chemistry Research, 54*(47), 11733–11758.

Chen, Y., Cao, X., Zhu, S., Tian, F., Xu, Y., Zhu, C., & Dong, L. (2019). Synergistic hydrothermal liquefaction of wheat stalk with homogeneous and heterogeneous catalyst at low temperature. *Bioresource Technology, 278*, 92–98.

Conti, F., Toor, S. S., Pedersen, T. H., Seehar, T. H., Nielsen, A. H., & Rosendahl, L. A. (2020). Valorization of animal and human wastes through hydrothermal liquefaction for biocrude production and simultaneous recovery of nutrients. *Energy Conversion and Management, 216*, Article 112925.

De Souza, A. P., Leite, D. C., Pattathil, S., Hahn, M. G., & Buckeridge, M. S. (2013). Composition and structure of sugarcane cell wall polysaccharides: Implications for second-generation bioethanol production. *Bioenergy Research, 6*(2), 564–579.

DeCaprariis, B., Bavasso, I., Bracciale, M. P., Damizia, M., De Filippis, P., & Scarsella, M. (2019). Enhanced bio-crude yield and quality by reductive hydrothermal liquefaction of oak wood biomass: Effect of iron addition. *Journal of Analytical and Applied Pyrolysis, 139*, 123–130.

Deepika, C., Mrinal, Pohrmen, C. B., Jaiswal, K. S., Sangmesh, B., Jaiswal, K. K., Ramasamy, A. P., & Jaiswal, A. K. (2024). Hydothermal liquefaction of wet microalgal biomass for biofuels and platform chemicals: advances and future prospects. *Discover Applied Sciences, 6*(5), 245.

DeJong, W., & Van Ommen, J. R. (2014). Biomass as a sustainable energy source for the future. In *Biomass as a sustainable energy source for the future* (vol. 9781118304, pp. 1–582). Wiley Hoboken, NJ, USA

Demirbas, A. (2000) Effect of lignin content on aqueous liquefaction products of biomass. *Energy Conversion Management, 41*, 1601–1607.

Déniel, M., Haarlemmer, G., Roubaud, A., Weiss-Hortala, E., Fages, J. (2016). Optimisation of bio-oil production by hydrothermal liquefaction of agro-industrial residues: Blackcurrant pomace (Ribes nigrum L.) as an example. *Biomass Bioenergy, 95*, 273–285.

Elliott, D. C., Hart, T. R., Neuenschwander, G. G., Rotness, L. J., Roesijadi, G., Zacher, A. H., & Magnuson, J. K. (2014). Hydrothermal processing of macroalgal feedstocks in continuous-flow reactors. *ACS Sustainable Chemistry & Engineering, 2*(2), 207–215.

Elliott, D., Biller, P., Ross, A. B., Schmidt, A. J., & Jones, S. B. (2015). Hydrothermal liquefaction of biomass: Developments from batch to continuous process. *Bioresource Technology, 178*, 147–156.

Gao, Y., Wang, X.-H., Yang, H.-P., & Chen, H.-P. (2012). Characterization of products from hydrothermal treatments of cellulose. *Energy, 42*, 457–465.

Ghadge, R., Nagwani, N., Saxena, N., Dasgupta, S., & Sapre, A. (2022). Design and scale-up challenges in hydrothermal liquefaction process for biocrude production and its upgradation. *Energy Conversion and Management: X, 14*, Article 100223.

Gollakota, A., & Savage, P. E. (2019). Biocrude production from fast and isothermal hydrothermal liquefaction of chitin. *Energy & Fuels, 33*(11), 11328–11338.

Hirano, Y., Miyataab, Y., Taniguchia, M., Funakoshia, N., Yamazakia, Y., Oginoa, C., & Kitaa, Y. (2020). Fe-assisted hydrothermal liquefaction of cellulose: Effects of hydrogenation catalyst addition on properties of water-soluble fraction. *Journal of Analytical and Applied Pyrolysis, 145*, Article 104719.

Hoekman, S. K., Broch, A., & Robbins, C. (2011). Hydrothermal carbonization (HTC) of lignocellulosic biomass. *Energy & Fuels, 25*, 1802–1810.

Holtze, C., & Boehling, R. (2022). Batch or flow chemistry?–a current industrial opinion on process selection. *Current Opinion in Chemical Engineering, 36*, Article 100798.

Hu, Y., Zicheng, G., Wenbin, L., & Chunbao, C. X. (2020). Alkali-catalyzed liquefaction of pinewood sawdust in ethanol/water co-solvents. *Biomass and Bioenergy, 134*, 105485.

Imman, S., Arnthong, J., Burapatana, V., Champreda, V., & Laosiripojana, N. (2015). Fractionation of rice straw by a single-step solvothermal process: Effects of solvents, acid promoters, and microwave treatment. *Renewable Energy, 83*, 663–673.

Jasiūnas, L., Pedersen, T. H., Toor, S. S., & Rosendahl, L. A. (2017). Biocrude production via supercritical hydrothermal co-liquefaction of spent mushroom compost and aspen wood sawdust. *Renewable Energy, 111*, 392–398.

Jayakumar, M., Gebeyehu, K. B., Abo, L. D., Tadesse, A. W., Vivekanandan, B., Sundramurthy, V. P., Bacha, W., Ashokkumar, V., & Baskar, G. (2023). A comprehensive outlook on topical processing methods for biofuel production and its thermal applications: Current advances, sustainability and challenges. *Fuel, 349*, 128690.

Jiang, W., Kumar, A., & Adamopoulos, S. (2018). Liquefaction of lignocellulosic materials and its applications in wood adhesives—a review. *Industrial Crops and Products, 124*, 325–342.

Jin, F., Wang, Y., Zeng, X., Shen, Z., Yao, G. (2014). Water under high temperature and pressure conditions and its applications to develop green technologies for biomass conversion. In F. Jin, (Ed.), *Application of hydrothermal reactions to biomass conversion. Green chemistry and sustainable technology*, Springer: Berlin/Heidelberg, Germany.

Jindal, M. K., & Jha, M. K. (2016). Hydrothermal liquefaction of wood: A critical review. *Reviews in Chemical Engineering, 32*(4), 459–488.

Joksimovic, G., & Markovic, Z. (2007). Investigation of the mechanism of acidic hydrolysis of cellulose. *Acta Agriculturae Serbica, 12*, 51–57.

Kang, S., Li, X., Fan, J., & Chang, J. (2011). Classified separation of lignin hydrothermal liquefied products. *Industrial and Engineering Chemistry Research, 50*, 11288–11296.

Kaur, R., Gera, P., Jha, M. K., & Bhaskar, T. (2019). Optimization of process parameters for hydrothermal conversion of castor residue. *Science of the Total Environment, 686*, 641–647.

Khampuang, K., Boreriboon, N., & Prasassarakich, P. (2015). Alkali catalyzed liquefaction of corncob in supercritical ethanol–water. *Biomass and Bioenergy, 83*, 460–466.

Kristianto, I., Limarta, S. O., Park, Y.-K., Ha, J.-M., Suh, D. J., Jeong, Y. & Jae, J. (2019). Hydrothermal liquefaction of concentrated acid hydrolysis lignin in a bench-scale continuous stirred tank reactor. *Energy & Fuels, 33*(7), 6421–6428.

Kruse, A., & Gawlik, A. (2003). Biomass conversion in water at 330 410 C and 30 50 MPa. Identification of key compounds for indicating different chemical reaction pathways. *Industrial & Engineering Chemistry Research, 42*, 267–279.

Kumar, A., Udugama, I. A., Gargalo, C. L., & Gernaey, K. V. (2020a). Why is batch processing still dominating the biologics landscape? Towards an integrated continuous bioprocessing alternative. *Processes, 8*(12), 1641.

Kumar, B., Bhardwaj, N., Agrawal, K., Chaturvedi, V., & Verma, P. (2020). Current perspective on pretreatment technologies using lignocellulosic biomass: An emerging biorefinery concept. *Fuel Processing Technology*, 199.

Kumar, J. M. S., Prakash, R., & Panneerselvam, P. (2025). Hydrothermal liquefaction−a sustainable technique for present biofuel generation: Opportunities, challenges and future prospects. *Fuel, 385,* 134141.

Kumar, M., Oyedun, A. O., & Kumar, A. (2018). A review on the current status of various hydrothermal technologies on biomass feedstock. *Renewable and Sustainable Energy Reviews, 81*, 1742–1770.

Li, Q., Liu, D., Hou, X., Wu, P., Song, L., & Yan, Z. (2016). Hydro-liquefaction of microcrystalline cellulose, xylan and industrial lignin in different supercritical solvents. *Bioresource Technology, 219*, 281–288.

Liu, D., Li, Q., Zhao, A., Song, L., Wu, P., & Yan, Z. (2015). Hydro-liquefaction of sawdust and its three components in supercritical ethanol with [BMIM]Cl/NiCl2 catalyst. *Chemical Engineering Journal, 279*, 921–928.

Liu, H.-M., Wang, F.-Y., & Liu, Y.-L. (2014). Alkaline pretreatment and hydrothermal liquefaction of cypress for high yield bio-oil production. *Journal of Analytical and Applied Pyrolysis, 108*, 136–142.

Liu, Q., Kong, G., Zhang, G., Cao, T., Wang, K., Zhang, X., & Han, L. (2023). Recent advances in hydrothermal liquefaction of manure wastes into value-added products. *Energy Conversion and Management, 292*, Article 117392.

Liu, Z., & Zhang, F.-S. (2009). Removal of lead from water using biochars prepared from hydrothermal liquefaction of biomass. *Journal of Hazardous Materials, 167*, 933–939.

Liu, Z., Quek, A., Hoekman, S. K., & Balasubramanian, R. (2013). Production of solid biochar fuel from waste biomass by hydrothermal carbonization. *Fuel, 103*, 943–949.

Lopez, F. A., Centeno, T. A., Garcia-Diaz, I., & Alguacil, F. J. (2013). Textural and fuel characteristics of the chars produced by the pyrolysis of waste wood, and the properties of activated carbons prepared from them. *Journal of Analytical and Applied Pyrolysis, 104*, 551–558.

Ma, S., Wang, H., Wang, Y., Bu, H., & Bai, J. (2011). Bio-hydrogen production from cornstalk wastes by orthogonal design method. *Renewable Energy, 36*(2), 709–713.

Mathanker, A., Das, S., Pudasainee, D., Khan, M., Kumar, A., & Gupta, R. (2021). A review of hydrothermal liquefaction of biomass for biofuels production with a special focus on the effect of process parameters, Cosolvents, and extraction solvents. *Energies, 14*(16), 4916.

Mathanker, A., Pudasainee, D., Kumar, A., & Gupta, R. (2020). Hydrothermal liquefaction of lignocellulosic biomass feedstock to produce biofuels: Parametric study and products characterization. *Fuel, 271*, Article 117534.

Mazaheri, H., Lee, K.T., & Mohamed, A. R. (2013). Influence of temperature on liquid products yield of oil palm shell via subcritical water liquefaction in the presence of alkali catalyst. *Fuel Processing Technology, 110*, 197–205.

Minowa, T., Zhen, F., & Ogi, T. (1998). Cellulose decomposition in hot-compressed water with alkali or nickel catalyst. *Journal of Supercritical Fluids, 13*, 253–259.

Miyata, Y., Yamazaki, Y., Hirano, Y., & Kita, Y. (2018). Quantitative analysis of the aqueous fraction from the Fe-assisted hydrothermal liquefaction of oil palm empty fruit bunches. *Journal of Analytical and Applied Pyrolysis, 132*, 72–81.

Nair, L. G., Agrawal, K., & Verma, P. (2022a). An insight into the principles of lignocellulosic biomass-based zero-waste biorefineries: A green leap towards imperishable energy-based future. *Biotechnology and Genetic Engineering Reviews, 38*(2), 288–338.

Nair, L. G., Agrawal, K., & Verma, P. (2022b). An overview of sustainable approaches for bioenergy production from agro-industrial wastes. *Energy Nexus, 6*(March), Article 100086.

Neveux, N., Yuen, A., Jazrawi, C., Magnusson, M., Haynes, B., Masters, A., Montoya, A., Paul, N., Maschmeyer, T., & de Nys, R. (2014). Biocrude yield and productivity from the hydrothermal liquefaction of marine and freshwater green macroalgae. *Bioresource Technology, 155*, 334–341.

Ogi, T., Yokoyama, S.-Y., Koguchi, K. (1985). Direct liquefaction of wood by catalyst. Part 1. Effects of pressure, temperature, holding time and wood/catalyst/water ratio on oil yield. *Journal of the Japan Petroleum Institute, 28*, 239–245.

Panisko, E., Wietsma, T., Lemmon, T., Albrecht, K., & Howe, D. (2015). Characterization of the aqueous fractions from hydrotreatment and hydrothermal liquefaction of lignocellulosic feedstocks. *Biomass and Bioenergy, 74*, 162–171.

Pedersen, T., Jensen, C., Sandström, L., & Rosendahl, L. (2017). Full characterization of compounds obtained from fractional distillation and upgrading of a HTL biocrude. *Applied Energy, 202*, 408–419.

Pei, Y., Li, Y., Zhang, Y., Yu, C., Fu, T., Zou, J.,... & Chen, P. (2016). G-lignin and hemicellulosic monosaccharides distinctively affect biomass digestibility in rapeseed. *Bioresource Technology, 203*, 325–333.

Qian, L., Wang, S., & Savage, P. E. (2017). Hydrothermal liquefaction of sewage sludge under isothermal and fast conditions. *Bioresource Technology, 232*, 27–34.

Sarkar, N., Ghosh, S. K., Bannerjee, S., & Aikat, K. (2012). Bioethanol production from agricultural wastes: An overview. *Renewable energy, 37*(1), 19–27.

Schmidt, A. R., Dresch, A. P., Junior, S. L. A., Bender, J. P., & Treichek, H. (2023). Applications of brewer's spent grain hemicelluloses in biorefineries: Extraction and value-added product obtention. *Catalysts, 13*(4), 755.

Shahbeik, H., Panahi, H. K. S., Dehhaghi, M., Guillemin, G. J., Fallahi, A., Hosseinzadeh-Bandbafha, H., Amiri, H., & et al. (2024). Biomass to biofuels using hydrothermal liquefaction: A comprehensive review. *Renewable and Sustainable Energy Reviews, 189,* 113976.

Singh, R., Chaudhary, K., Biswas, B., Balagurumurthy, B., & Bhaskar, T. (2015). Hydrothermal liquefaction of rice straw: Effect of reaction environment. *Journal of Supercritical Fluids, 104,* 70–75.

Smith, A., Singh, S., & Ross, A. B. (2016). Fate of inorganic material during hydrothermal carbonisation of biomass: Influence of feedstock on combustion behaviour of hydrochar. *Fuel, 169,* 135–145.

Taghipour, A., Ramirez, J. A., Brown, R. J., & Rainey, T. J. (2019). A review of fractional distillation to improve hydrothermal liquefaction biocrude characteristics; future outlook and prospects. *Renewable and Sustainable Energy Reviews, 115,* Article 109355.

Tekin, K., Karagöz, S., Bektas S. (2012). Hydrothermal liquefaction of beech wood using a natural calcium borate mineral. *The Journal of Supercritical Fluids, 72,* 134–139.

Tian, Y., Wang, F., Djandja, J. O., Zhang, S. L., Xu, Y. P., & Duan, P. G. (2020). Hydrothermal liquefaction of crop straws: Effect of feedstock composition. *Fuel, 265,* 116946.

Tran, K.-Q., Klemsdal, A. J., Zhang, W., Sandquist, J., Wang, L., & Skreiberg, Ø. (2017). Fast hydrothermal liquefaction of native and torrefied wood. *Energy Procedia, 105,* 218–223.

Tursi, A. (2019). A review on biomass: importance, chemistry, classification, and conversion. *Biofuel Research Journal, 6,* 962–979.

Tzanetis, K. F., Posada, J. A., & Ramirez, A. (2017). Analysis of biomass hydrothermal liquefaction and biocrude-oil upgrading for renewable jet fuel production: The impact of reaction conditions on production costs and GHG emissions performance. *Renewable Energy, 113,* 1388–1398.

Umagiliyage, A. L., Choudhary, R., Liang, Y., Haddock, J., & Watson, D. G. (2015). Laboratory scale optimization of alkali pretreatment for improving enzymatic hydrolysis of sweet sorghum bagasse. *Industrial Crops and Products, 74,* 977–986.

Wang, F., Chang, Z., Duan, P., Yan, W., Xu, Y., Zhang, L., Miao, J., & Fan, Y. (2013). Hydrothermal liquefaction of litsea cubeba seed to produce bio-Oils. *Bioresource Technology, 149,* 509–515.

Wang, S., Dai, G., Yang, H., & Luo, Z. (2017). Lignocellulosic biomass pyrolysis mechanism: A state-of-the-art review. *Progress in Energy and Combustion Science, 62,* 33–86.

Wang, W., Qi, Y., Meng, H., Han, W., Li, J., & Zhang, J. (2018). Catalytic liquefaction of municipal sewage sludge over transition metal catalysts in ethanol-water co-solvent. *Bioresource Technology, 249,* 361–367.

Woiciechowski, A. L., Neto, C. J. D., Vandenberghe, L. P. S., Neto, D. P. C., Sydney, A. C. N., Letti, L. A. J., Karp, S. G., Torres, L. A. Z. & Soccol, C. R. (2020). Lignocellulosic biomass: Acid and alkaline pretreatments and their effects on biomass recalcitrance–Conventional processing and recent advances. *Bioresource technology, 304,* 122848.

Wu, H., Shakeel, U., Zhang, Q., Zhang, K., Xia, X., & Jian, X. (2022). Ethanol-assisted hydrothermal liquefaction of poplar using Fe-Co/Al2O3 as catalyst. *Energies, 15*(9), 3057.

Xu, C., & Lancaster, J. (2008). Conversion of secondary pulp/paper sludge powder to liquid oil products for energy recovery by direct liquefaction in hot-compressed water. *Water Research, 42,* 1571–1582.

Yang, L., Nazari, L., Yuan, Z., Corscadden, K., Xu, C., & He, Q. (2016). Hydrothermal liquefaction of spent coffee grounds in water mediumfor bio-oil production. *Biomass and Bioenergy, 86,* 191–198.

Yang, Y., Gilbert, A., & Xu, C. (2009). Production of bio-crude from forestry waste by hydro-liquefaction in sub-/super-critical methanol. *AIChE Journal, 55,* 807–819.

Yerrayya, A., Shree Vishnu, A. K., Shreyas, S., Chakravarthy, S. R., & Vinu, R. (2020). Hydrothermal liquefaction of rice straw using methanol as co-solvent. *Energies, 13*(10), 2618.

Yim, S. C., Quitain, A. T., Yusup, S., Sasaki, M., Uemura, Y., & Kida, T. (2017). Metal oxide-catalyzed hydrothermal liquefaction of malaysian oil palm biomass to bio-oil under supercritical condition. *Journal of Supercritical Fluids, 120,* 384–394.

Yin, S., & Tan, Z. (2012). Hydrothermal liquefaction of cellulose to bio-oil under acidic, neutral and alkaline conditions. *Applied Energy, 92*, 234–239.

Younas, R., Hao, S., Zhang, L., & Zhang, S. (2017). Hydrothermal liquefaction of rice straw with NiO nanocatalyst for bio-oil production. *Renewable Energy, 113*, 532–545.

Zhang, B., von Keitz, M., & Valentas, K. (2009). Thermochemical liquefaction of high-diversity grassland perennials. *Journal of Analytical and Applied Pyrolysis, 84*, 18–24.

Zhang, L., Champagne, P., & Xu, C. (2011). Bio-crude production from secondary pulp/paper-mill sludge and waste newspaper via co-liquefaction in hot-compressed water. *Energy, 36*, 2142–2150.

Zhang, Y., Li, N., Chen, Z., Ding, C., Zheng, Q., Jindi, X., & Meng, Q. (2020). Synthesis of high-water-resistance lignin-phenol resin adhesive with furfural as a crosslinking agent. *Polymers, 12*(12), 2805.

Zhu, Y., Biddy, M. J., Jones, S. B., Elliott, D., & Schmidt, A. J. (2014). Techno-economic analysis of liquid fuel production from woody biomass via hydrothermal liquefaction (HTL) and upgrading. *Applied Energy, 129*, 384–394.

Zhu, Z., Toor, S. S., Rosendahl, L., Yu, D., & Chen, G. (2015). Influence of alkali catalyst on product yield and properties via hydrothermal liquefaction of barley straw. *Energy, 80*, 284–292.

Chapter 19
The Marketing of Sustainable Solution: Whether It is Market Driven or not?

Suryasneha Deb, Kaustav Purkayastha, and Sayak Das

Abstract Sustainable solutions are made up of many products, services, and systems designed to address environmental, social, and economic problems. This means effective implementation depends on market-oriented strategies as well as non-market interventions. Drawing on concepts such as the marketing mix (4Ps), stakeholder theory, institutional theory, and the triple bottom line, the chapter describes how organizations can adopt sustainable marketing through accountable product design, equitable pricing, ethical distribution, and honest communication. It contrasts business models founded on profit and consumer demand with those guided by public policy, civil society, and grassroots movements. Hybrid models are a promising means of delivering inclusive, scalable, and sustainable impact. Real-world examples from India and elsewhere illustrate these hybrid solutions in practice. The chapter also addresses issues like inadequate policy coordination, misleading claims of sustainability, and the intricacy of impact measurement. Also, it suggests future solutions like digital tracking platforms, blended finance, and inclusive governance. It states that sustainability works best where social efforts and market forces are blended, rather than in silos.

Keywords Sustainable solutions · Hybrid sustainability models · Market-driven and non-market approaches · Triple bottom line · Corporate social responsibility · Stakeholder

19.1 Introduction

Sustainability is the ability to meet the needs of the present generation without compromising the ability of future generations to meet their needs (John ORCID et al., n.d.). The idea is to achieve the middle ground between social welfare, environmental protection, and economic development, which is also known as the three

S. Deb · K. Purkayastha · S. Das (✉)
Department of Life Science and Bioinformatics, Har Gobind Khurana School of Life Sciences, Assam University, Silchar 788011, Assam, India
e-mail: sayak.das@aus.ac.in

P. Verma (ed.), *Sustainable Practices in Biorefinery*,
https://doi.org/10.1007/978-981-95-6071-4_19

pillars of sustainability (Ruggerio, 2021). Though "sustainability" has been around for centuries, it was officially elaborated in 1987 in a landmark report, Our Common Future, produced by the U.N.'s Brundtland Commission. The report emphasized that human environmental problems are holistic, rather than single-issue, in nature; therefore, to solve them best, one needs to develop integrated, long-term solutions that consider both people and the planet (Imperatives, 1987). Sustainable solutions are products, services, or systems, sometimes a combination, designed to reduce adverse impacts and maximize beneficial effects along environmental, economic, social, and ethical dimensions. Such solutions meet society's needs today, taking into account long-term well-being. Such activities go beyond current products; they may require changes in production processes, consumption patterns, or even the operation of entire systems. Whether incremental improvement or revolutionary innovation is needed, the objective remains the same: to create benefit than harm for all concerned (Petkoska et al., 2021). Genuine sustainable solutions are grounded on the collaboration of different stakeholders- firms, governments, communities, and consumers- and often require a shift in production and consumption patterns. Such solutions aim to create a positive and lasting impact that benefits humans and the environment at large (Charter & Tischner, 2017).

While sustainability offers the basis for long-term global resilience, it is through marketing that these sustainable solutions become visible, heard, and embraced in the marketplace (Peterson, 2021). Dr. Philip Kotler has defined marketing as "the science and art of exploring, creating, and delivering value to satisfy the needs of a target market at a profit" (Alić & Antunica, n.d.). Marketing identifies unmet needs and wants. This process segments the market and enables the company to position itself to address the needs and desires of various groups. It also considers the size of each market and how much profit it can generate. Accordingly, the company selects the segments it can serve best and develops the appropriate products and promotions for them (Kotler, 1994). Green product marketing is essential to facilitate a shift to environmentally and socially sustainable development. It serves the triple bottom line—economic, social, and environmental sustainability—by stimulating demand for sustainable products, driving innovation, and raising consumer awareness. Besides green product marketing, it shapes market behavior and business models, making sustainability operational and desirable (Danciu & Marketing, 2013).

19.2 Marketing as a Catalyst for Sustainable Transformation

Sustainable marketing best emerges as we put it within the framework of the classic marketing mix, that is, Product, Price, Place, and Promotion (Cătoiu et al., 2010). This enables the integration of sustainability in all the dimensions of functional marketing strategies and, therefore, equips organizations with the capability of serving economic goals, social justice, and environmental sustainability.

(a) ***Product: Sustainable Product Design and Development***

Sustainable marketing begins with the product development that is safe and beneficial to people and the planet. This includes the usage of eco-friendly resources, energy-efficient production processes, fair labor practices, and the design of products for durability, reuse, and recyclability (Sharma, 2024). Product innovation here is founded on "cradle-to-cradle" thinking, wherein every process in the product's lifecycle is assessed for its environmental footprint. In addition, companies are expected to avoid practices such as animal testing or using disadvantaged groups, and product policies must converge with overall social and responsibility commitments (Ahmad et al., 2018).

(b) ***Price: Fair and Transparent Pricing Mechanisms***

Sustainable pricing is based on fairness and long-term value creation rather than short-term profit maximization. Fair pricing is the fair exchange of the value delivered and the sacrifice made by the consumer, and no stakeholder should be deprived. This guarantees that exploitative rating practices built on scarcity, consumer ignorance, or uneven market power are prohibited (Nzegwu & Towolawi, 2024). Sustainable pricing may include environmental duties, such as carbon taxes or waste disposal charges, and support community causes through contributions or price subsidies for underrepresented groups. Transparency in communicating the pricing rationale is necessary to establish consumer confidence (Carter & Curry, 2010).

(c) ***Place: Ethical Distribution and Fair-Trade Practices***

The equity concept is extended to a distribution function, as sustainable marketing emphasizes inclusive access in a general sense and socially responsible logistics (Cosa, 2024). Distribution planning must try to reduce environmental degradation through efficient transportation, minimal packaging, and energy-efficient warehousing. Equitable trade is important to sustainable marketers, as supply chain relationships are governed by transparency, respect, and mutual benefit. This can include long-term partnerships with local suppliers, especially in the developing world, and adherence to certifications that guarantee ethical labor and environmental practices (Davies, 2003).

(d) ***Promotion: Responsible and Educative Communication***

The ethics of honesty, clarity, and intent of education walk through promotion strategies within sustainable marketing. Communication must reflect a company's honest commitment to sustainability, circumventing greenwashing or embroidered claims that misinform stakeholders. The promotion should depict both the functional aids and the environmental or social worth of the product, encouraging accountable consumption (Arora & Mishra, 2023). Additionally, sustainable marketers are engaged in reciprocal dialogue with customers and stakeholders, building a co-creation and rapid innovation culture. Public awareness campaigns and transparency also support a brand's credibility and commitment to long-term societal health (Sujanska & Nadanyiova, 2023).

The insistence of sustainable marketing arises from the intensifying global environmental crisis, spreading socio-economic inequalities, and the determined failure of conventional marketing strategies to drive widespread behavior change toward sustainability (Ambili, 2024). Despite growing awareness, unsustainable consumption remains the standard for most of the global population, with only a minority energetically participating in green consumerism. This stark reality is that the health of the planet continues to deteriorate, and progress toward attaining the United Nations Sustainable Development Goals (SDGs), particularly SDG 12 (Ensure sustainable consumption and production patterns) on responsible consumption and production, is worryingly off track (Belz & Peattie, 2012). Scientific evidence, such as warnings from the World Meteorological Organization, suggests we are approaching critical ecological thresholds. The swelling rate of extreme weather events, rising global temperatures, and widespread biodiversity loss signal the concrete consequences of unmanageable development pathways (Langsdorf et al., 2022).

Marketing is a powerful driver of consumption patterns and can play an important role in reversing these trends. However, conventional approaches to sustainability marketing, which typically take the form of altruistic appeals to "save the planet" or guilt-tripping, have failed in the broad marketplace (Gleim et al., 2023). As Lim (2022) suggests, these approaches do not resonate with the average consumer, who is most motivated by economic self-interest. This disconnect requires a new model of marketing that is goal-driven but consumer-focused (Lim & Rasul, 2022).

The Sustainability Pyramid, proposed by Lim, offers a convincing model that reorders sustainability priorities to first address economic value, followed by social and environmental dimensions (Lim & Rasul, 2022). This hierarchy admits that most consumers, particularly those in lower-income groups, will adopt sustainable alternatives if they see direct economic benefits, such as cost savings, efficiency, or durability. When economic value is proven, social and environmental value can be measured as added value, and thus open up a broader and more sustainable route to sustainable behavioral change (Lim, 2022). The need for organizations to embrace sustainable marketing practices is further compounded by increasing regulatory pressures due to legislation, changing consumer attitudes, and the need to protect their actions from environmental and reputational damage. This pressure is further increased by the increasing visibility of responsible consumers, who increasingly require greater transparency, accountability, and alignment with their values. Empirical evidence repeatedly shows that a high percentage of consumers, and young age groups in particular, are willing to pay a premium for ethically produced, ecologically sustainable, and socially responsible products (Vishnubhatla & Agashe, 2022).

Sustainable marketing is not an extra feature but an important imperative for modern business. Its urgency lies in addressing global and social challenges and creating new opportunities for growth, relevance, and resilience. It must be reinforced by cross-sector partnership, as highlighted by the triple helix model, hence all the sectors must work in a cycle to redesign the current system (Lim & Rasul, 2022).

19.3 Theoretical Foundations Guiding Sustainable Marketing Strategies

19.3.1 Stakeholder Theory and Sustainability

Over the past few decades, stakeholder theory has been a central paradigm in the changing role of business in society, particularly within the context of sustainability. Freeman (1984) first conceptualized the theory, which contends that the responsibility of a corporation goes beyond the shareholders (owners) to a broad range of stakeholders, including employees, customers, suppliers, communities, governments, NGOs, and even the environment (Lim & Rasul, 2022). This theoretical framework is in direct contrast to the neoclassical economic perspective, most notably supported by Friedman (Friedman 1970), that business has only one social responsibility: profits. In today's knowledge economy, corporations are under unprecedented analysis from various stakeholder groups (Hörisch et al., 2014). As Awa et al. (2024) highlight, these stakeholders are no longer mere witnesses but better-informed, vocal, and powerful influential players seeking that businesses respond to complex challenges, including climate change, inequality, public health, and ethical governance. They suggested a "Four-Stage Stakeholder Dialogue Ladder," which summarizes the evolution of engagement between businesses and stakeholders.

Companies communicate with their stakeholders in different ways depending on the extent of interaction they need from them. The most basic one is one-way communication, where the company communicates but does not expect any response. This will likely lead to shallow CSR practices intended to improve the image and not cause any alteration (Mohr & Nevin, 1990). A better method is two-way communication, where businesses open themselves to feedback and hear what stakeholders say. This allows them to refine their actions based on actual concerns (Jerman & Zavrsnik, 2012). A more sophisticated version is themed dialogue, where both parties discuss shared issues in a more structured manner, assisting in building understanding and generating ideas together (Lim & Rasul, 2022). Partnership and socializing are the most engaged forms. Stakeholders cooperate closely with the company to co-create value, shaping critical decisions, innovation, and day-to-day operations (Kosovych et al., 2022; Takahashi & Takahashi, 2022).

19.3.2 Institutional Theory and Market Influence in Sustainable Practice

Institutional theory provides a positive explanation of how and why companies embrace sustainable practices not just for market demand or profitability, but because of outside pressures to become legitimate, meet regulatory requirements, and address social norms (Bhuiyan et al., 2023). These external pressures generally fall into three areas: Coercive, Normative, and Mimetic (Skea et al., 2023).

- **Coercive Pressure**

Coercive Pressure debates the circumstances where powerful administrations (like buyers or governments) force others to track certain practices, usually using regulations or business contracts (Yue et al., 2023). For example, in the British dairy sector, retailers such as Tesco and Sainsbury's were found to employ coercive power over suppliers by authorizing sustainable practices like carbon audits and energy savings (Glover et al., 2014). Suppliers did so not because of explicit market demands, but to respect business with these powerful buyers. As in India, Tata Motors and Mahindra & Mahindra exercise their dominant supply chain position to drive sustainability downstream. Suppliers usually have to comply with environmental standards or implement energy-saving measures in order to retain their contracts. In either of the scenarios, coercive pressure is exerted by large companies that serve as gatekeepers, imposing sustainability terms that smaller partners have to abide by (Mani, 2017; Sarker et al., 2017).

- **Normative Pressure**

Normative pressure arises from the moral and societal expectations and norms that prompt the firms to behave correctly, even if it is not necessarily the law (Alziady & Enayah, 2019). For example, ITC Limited in India has water reclamation, reforestation, and solid waste management, with the dual goals of maximizing operating efficiency and meeting societal expectations for environmental responsibility (Nagano, 2023). In the same way, Infosys is famous for its green campuses and low-carbon footprint actions, further consolidating its image as a socially responsible corporate (P.D., 2016). Globally, Unilever has similarly adopted such normative pressures in its "Sustainable Living Plan," intending to lower its environmental footprint, and increase social value (Dhawan et al., 2010). These efforts make businesses attain legitimacy and goodwill if sustainability fails to bring instant profit.

- **Mimetic Pressure**

Mimetic pressure occurs when companies copy others' successful strategies to stay competitive or improve their legitimacy (Arranz et al., 2022). Infosys' success with energy-efficient infrastructure in India encouraged companies such as Wipro, TCS, and others in the IT segment to follow similar sustainable practices (Bhusankar & Kashyap, 2023; Publication & Monteiro, 2022). In the FMGG industry, Patanjali and Dabur have encouraged others to follow eco-friendly packaging and herbal branding, irrespective of whether all customers specifically demand it (Jadhav & Zaware, 2024). For sustainable solutions marketers, communication needs to be multi-layered: solutions cannot merely appeal to environmental ideals but also guarantee compliance, brand building, cost-effectiveness, and conventionality to prime institutional norms (Huang et al., 2022).

19.3.3 Triple Bottom Line Approach

The conversation about promoting sustainable solutions has increasingly identified the Triple Bottom Line (TBL) as a core conceptual model. First put forward by Elkington (1997), the TBL reframes organizational success by infusing three mutually supportive dimensions—People (social), Planet (environmental), and Profit (economic) (Zaharia & Zaharia, 2021). The classical one is a reaction to the increasing regulatory pressures, investor activism, and consumer demand for ethical responsibility, which leads organizations to rebalance their marketing narrative and value proposition (Svensson et al., 2018).

The Triple Bottom Line (TBL) model provides a broader and more balanced perspective on what it is for companies to be genuinely sustainable, with attention to three interrelated areas: the environment, society, and economic commitments, typically described as Planet, People, and Profit. The environmental dimension highlights how businesses can minimize their footprint on the world by consuming less, minimizing waste and emissions, and creating sustainable supply chains (Hong & Xiao, 2024). This has been a long-time priority for regulators and researchers and is now a significant sustainability initiative through eco-labels, green certifications like ISO 14001, and ESG standards (Prakash et al., 2023). In conjunction with this, the social dimension concerns how companies deal with people within the firm and society. This encompasses ethical labor practices, diversity and inclusion, community participation, and corporate philanthropy as a way to give back. The emergence of Corporate Social Responsibility (CSR) indicates how businesses are transcending mere transactions into deeper relationships underpinned by trust and mutual values (Tate & Bals, 2018). The third pillar—economic sustainability—calls for-profit to be all about. Instead of using the sole aim of short-term bottom-line profits, this process revolves around long-term value, quality governance, innovation, and shared prosperity of stakeholders (Majid & Koe, 2012). The financial crisis of 2008 exposed the danger of a lack of preparation. It encouraged enlarged attraction with financial theories likely to withstand time (Athreye et al., 2021). The TBL is not a thought experiment. Businesses currently apply functional tools such as the Global Reporting Initiative (GRI), the Dow Jones Sustainability Index, and Integrated Sustainability Assessment (ISA) to monitor and disclose their sustainability actions (Arribas et al., 2021; Mougenot & Doussoulin, 2023). Thus, the TBL demonstrates that sustainable marketing is not merely about keeping up with the market trend but influencing it to make business prosperity coincide with the happiness of people and the planet (Goh et al., 2020).

19.3.4 *Drivers of Sustainable Marketing*

19.3.4.1 Consumer Awareness and Demand

Consumer awareness is a key driver of demand generation for sustainable products and services. It allows consumers to make responsible decisions, promotes business accountability, and encourages a responsible consumption culture. In developed and emerging economies, greater awareness has shifted consumer expectations from product functionality to ethical sourcing, environmental stewardship, and social responsibility (Rhein & Schmid, 2020). Consequently, Indian and international brands are progressively adapting their strategies to the principles of conscious consumers (Ishak & Zabil, 2012). In India, the Tata Group provides a good example of consumer consciousness driving demand. Tata Tea's "Jaago Re" campaign was not about selling tea but about bringing civic consciousness to citizens and prompting them to cast their votes, resist corruption, and ask for improved governance. This successfully interconnected product identity and social empowerment (Menon et al., 2024). Outside India, brands like Patagonia and The Body Shop have created robust customer loyalty based on sustainability leadership. Patagonia's "Do not Buy This Jacket" campaign promoted less consumption, while The Body Shop has continued promoting cruelty-free and ethical sourcing, supporting their identification with conscious consumer values (Ganatra et al., 2021; Michel et al., 2019)—willingness to pay for ethical products. Recent reports based on Nielsen (2001) predict that 73% of consumers India, are willing to support environmentally responsible brands. This change has prompted Indian firms like Bisleri and Hindustan Unilever Limited to embrace biodegradable packaging amid increased consumer demand and changing regulations (Pareek, 2025; Raj et al., 2023). Thus, such brands that engage meaningfully with this awareness-driven demand are more likely to be relevant and sustainable in the long term.

19.3.4.2 Corporate Social Responsibility (CSR)

Corporate Social Responsibility (CSR) has become a keystone of business approach in modern times, on behalf of a corporation's everyday jobs beyond legal and economic necessities, to encompass ethics and voluntary contributions to society (Zaman et al., 2022). As defined by Archie B. Carroll, CSR encompasses four dimensions: economic, legal, ethical, and philanthropic responsibilities (Lagoudaki et al., 2024), each consisting of society's expectations of business at a specific period (Carroll & Laasch, 2020). One of the most relevant examples of pioneering CSR leadership is Cummins Engine Company, which in the 1970s became famous for contributing 5% of its pre-tax profits to community causes (Bowie, 2012). Similarly, IBM and Xerox embedded CSR in education and environmental initiatives that went beyond minimum compliance. Over the past decades, CSR has become a strategic imperative (Carroll, 2015). Companies like Unilever have rooted sustainability into their central business model through initiatives like the Unilever Sustainable Living Plan, a plan to improve health benefits, lower environmental footprints, and improve livelihoods throughout its value chain (Modreanu et al., 2022). In India, Infosys has provided CSR leadership in investing extensively in education, e-literacy, and rural development through the Infosys Foundation and aligning social initiatives with its corporate culture. Thus, CSR has evolved from corporate charity to a strategic role integral to business (Arora & Puranik, 2004). Not only is it about "doing good," but it is about stakeholder relationship management, constructing legitimacy, and helping businesses in a more complex world to be resilient and sustainable.

19.4 Market-Driven and Non-market-Driven Sustainable Solutions

Market-driven sustainability is an active fusion of economic sense with environmental and social mission. It shapes market intelligence, data analytics, and competitive marketing to reconcile sustainable actions with long-term organizational performance (Rastegar et al., 2024). Successful sustainability initiatives rely on comprehension of what people report and how they assess quality, price equity, and emotional value, typically described as "warm glow." Branding and positioning guarantee that customers gain both concrete advantages (product quality) and abstract satisfaction (warm glow) from purchasing sustainable products (Hult et al., 2023). Brands like Tesla, which combine luxury with clean technology, illustrate how sustainable products can be desirable (Maradin et al., 2022). At the same time, if reasonably priced, compared to less sustainable options, such products can appeal to a broader market without sacrificing competitiveness (Fig. 19.1).

Non-Market Sustainable Solutions refer to practices and structures that encourage environmental and social comfort outside the limitations of outdated market mechanisms. Contrary to market-driven approaches, which depend on pricing, competition, and consumer demand, non-market solutions are rooted in community collaboration, mutual assistance, knowledge sharing, and public or civil society support (Viti et al., 2022). These solutions tend to rise as a response to local requirements, especially where formal markets are out of reach or lacking, and they are usually led by values such as reciprocity, equity, and self-reliance rather than profit (Titumir et al., 2023). Notably, non-market mechanisms enable flexibility, inclusivity, and strong cultural fit, and they are particularly worth it in rural, marginalized, or resource-constrained contexts (Beumer et al., 2022). For instance, the System of Rice Intensification (SRI), which is practiced extensively in India and other developing countries, has been disseminated through farmer networks and NGO assistance instead of commercial routes (Barrett et al., 2022).

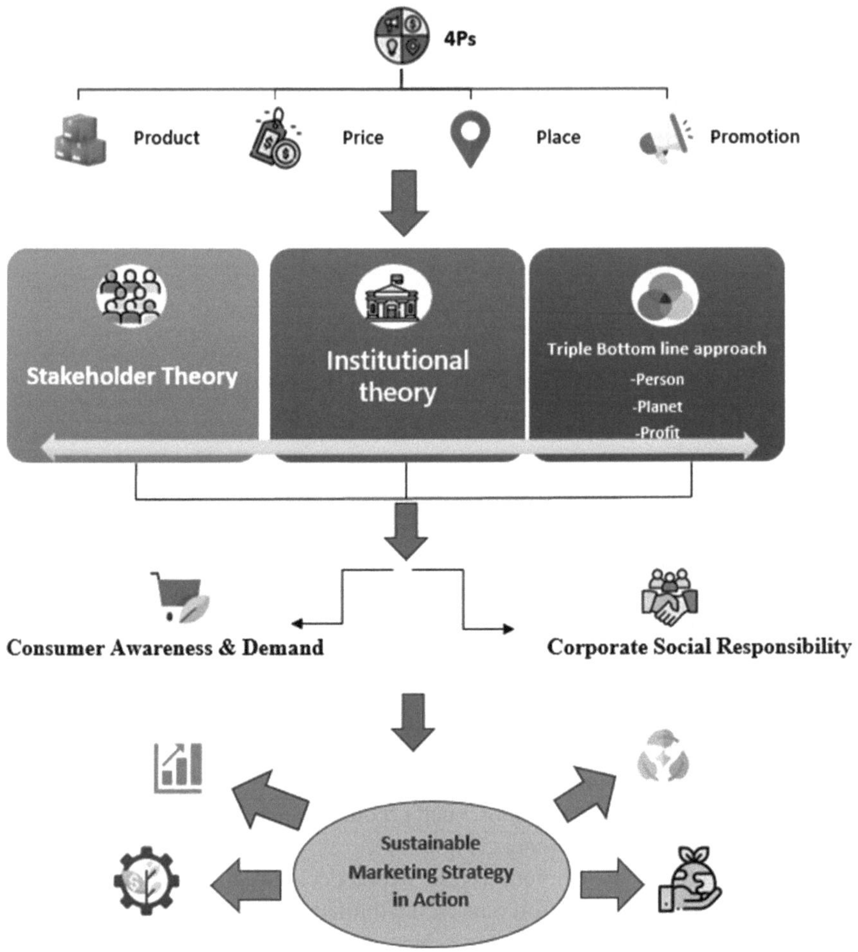

Fig. 19.1 Framework showing how marketing tools, theories, and drivers align to enable sustainable marketing strategies

19.5 Hybrid Models as a Transition

The blending of market and non-market strategies is increasingly considered an essential strategy for firms seeking sustainable growth, competitive edge, and legitimacy (Basco et al., 2021). Market strategies of cost-effectiveness, innovation, and environmental record are also reinforced with non-market actions like regulatory dialogue, stakeholder collaboration, and corporate social responsibility (Qian et al., 2024).

A few examples show how hybrid sustainability models i.e. the integration of market incentives with non-market assistance, can propel effective, inclusive, and scalable solutions. Amul's cooperative system, assisted by India's Operation Flood program, facilitated 3.6 million milk producers to enter formal markets via government-supported infrastructure, which contributed to increasing India's milk production from 20 million tons in 1970 to over 210 million tons in 2021 (Shimokado, 2021). Likewise, Google's 24/7 carbon-free energy operations are a hybrid model that combines internal technological innovation, like AI for grid optimization, with external collaborations with policymakers, utilities, and climate experts (Sharon, 2021). SELCO India is also a good example of this model, having served more than two million people through a combination of solar product sales, microfinance services, and coordination with public electrification targets (Pai & Hiremath, 2016). ITC's e-Choupal links four million farmers with real-time farm data, enhancing procurement efficiency by 10–15% by leveraging digital corporate solutions, government rural programs, and grassroots networks (Venugopal & Agrawal, 2023). Public–private partnerships are also apparent in sanitation, where the Swachh Bharat Mission has built 100 million toilets via public financing, whereas Unilever's Domex program educated 600 sanitation entrepreneurs, reaching a combined 600 million people (Iyer et al., 2023). Tesla's achievement in the electric vehicle market also demonstrates the resilience of hybrid models; the automaker sold more than 1.3 million EVs in 2022 by taking advantage of $2.8 billion in federal subsidies and carbon credits and its innovation-based business model (Cui & Zhao, 2024). Tata Group illustrates a company-wide sustainability agenda that encompasses Tata Power's 1.3 GW of renewable energy and Tata Steel's green production, backed by CSR mandates, government partnerships like Skill India, and its market leadership (Chaudhuri et al., 2022). Flipkart's pledge to transition its logistics fleet to 100% electric by 2030 under the Climate Group's EV100 initiative equally combines private investment with public EV policy and partnerships with domestic logistics companies (Manda et al., 2024). Internationally, business organizations such as Interface Inc. (USA), a carpet production company, have cut their emissions of greenhouse gases by 96% since the year 1996 through closed-loop manufacturing, bio-based products, and concordance with global climate initiatives and NGO approvals (Sim & Prabhu, 2018). On the policy side, Rwanda's cooperation with the United Nations to build Africa's first e-waste recycling plant, with an annual capacity to process 10,000 tons, is a textbook example of how multi-stakeholder collaborations can effectively catalyze the creation of green infrastructure in emerging economies (Twagirayezu et al., 2021). Such examples prove the success of hybrid approaches to sustainability that blend business-driven innovation, state support, and cooperation with civil society to build resilient and inclusive market systems.

19.6 Revisiting the Question—Is It Market Driven?

Today, Sustainability cannot be squeezed into market-driven versus non-driven solutions but exists through a systems-based, synergistic approach combining both paradigms. This hybrid model recognizes that while market mechanisms have scalability, innovation, and efficiency, non-market solutions have contextual relevance, inclusivity, and long-term community ownership (Tolliver et al., 2020). At the international level, the Paris Agreement also establishes this duality, even though it is essentially a state-led, non-market policy instrument based on nationally determined contributions (NDCs), it also includes market-based mechanisms such as international carbon trading under Article 6 (Li et al., 2025). Likewise, the United Nations Sustainable Development Goals (SDGs)- specifically SDG 7 (Affordable and Clean Energy) and SDG 13 (Climate Action)- promote partnerships cutting across public, private, and civil society players, regulatory and commercial endeavors (Tiwari et al., 2025; Zarghami, 2025). The global green technology and sustainability market, worth USD 13.76 billion in 2022, is expected to grow to USD 61.92 billion by 2030 at a compound annual growth rate of 21.6%, reflecting the fast growth of market-based solutions (Mertzanis & Tebourbi, 2025). However, United Nations Development Programme (UNDP) research shows that involvements that combine institutional commands with stakeholder engagement are 70% more likely to deliver lasting environmental and social outcomes, setting out the critical role of non-market engagement (Leal Filho et al., 2024) (Fig. 19.2).

In India, this hybridization is also visible. The National Action Plan on Climate Change (NAPCC) is an example of top-down state intervention in its eight missions, while promoting decentralized participation at local levels (Deshpande et al., 2025). The PM-KUSUM scheme, targeting to set up 30.8 GW of solar capacity by 2026, combines government incentives with rural stakeholder engagement, reflecting a combination of policy support and market adoption. Concurrently, India also saw a 30% year-over-year increase in ESG investment inflows in 2023, which is an indicator of increasing private sector investment in sustainable finance (Vishnoi et al., 2024). Nonetheless, non-market efforts like Jal Shakti Abhiyan, Mission Amrit Sarovar, and Zero Budget Natural Farming (ZBNF) remain active in ecological transformation and climate resilience (Ranjan, 2024). Around the world, Denmark and Costa Rica also better illustrate hybrid sustainability models, utilizing both sound regulatory systems and market openness to move toward clean energy economies. At the conceptual level, hybrid models illustrate systems thinking sustainable development not as an isolated effort but as an interdependent game. Such models bypass extreme limitations by arranging market forces, public policy, and community agency together as one concerted effort. Thus, on this evidence, sustainability becomes less a matter of being or not being market-driven, but an interdependent strategy of diverse parts, in which both forces evolve together to produce long-term influence.

Types	Market-Driven	Non-Market Driven	Hybrid Models
Criteria	$ Profit-Centric	Mission-Centric	Dual Purpose
Stakeholders	Consumers	Community/ Government	Multi-Stakeholder
Strategy	BRAND Branding/ Innovation	Policy/Social Campaigns	Long-term Trust + Impact
Benefits	Rapid Innovation due to market share	Targeted Impact	Enhanced Coordination
Challenges	Short term focus	Limited scalability	Coordination Complexity

Fig. 19.2 Comparative analysis of market-driven, non-market-driven, and hybrid sustainability models, highlighting their key drivers, benefits, challenges and structural dynamics

19.7 Addressing Challenges and Unfolding Future Prospects of Hybrid Sustainable Solutions

Hybrid sustainability models, involving public, private, and civil society actors, hold great potential for addressing dynamic global challenges, but are hampered by multiple systemic constraints that call for institutional and operational innovation. A primary concern is coordination complexity, wherein various stakeholders—governments, companies, NGOs, and communities—act with different priorities and cultures, leading to disjointed efforts and delays (Camarinha-Matos et al., 2024). New responses are co-design practices, participatory planning, and more explicit role articulation to facilitate collaboration (Hinrichs & Johnston, 2020). Policy-market misalignment is equally urgent, given that conventional regulatory frameworks rarely support hybrid logics and markets continue to reward immediate profitability over long-term sustainability efforts. Thus, regulatory sandboxes, adaptive licensing, and revised incentive structures are being deployed to narrow this institutional gap.(J. Li et al., 2022). The integrity of sustainability claims is also under threat from greenwashing, where companies exaggerate environmental or social pledges in order to earn reputational benefit (Santos et al., 2024). Accordingly, regulators are pushing third-party certification, disclosure requirements, and independent verification systems as a means to ensure accountability (Dempere et al., 2024). Hybrid models also have gaps in measurement and accountability because current evaluation systems tend to miss multidimensional results; digital monitoring tools, combined dashboards, and stacked assessment frameworks, which are increasingly improving impact visibility and traceability (Pérez-Durán, 2024; Zhang, 2024). Funding imbalances also add complexity to hybrid success, with for-profit segments attracting investment and community-based or nonprofit activities underfunded, leading to the emergence of blended finance, social bonds, and mission-aligned capital to address these imbalances (Al Anshori et al., 2023). On the demand side, consumer distrust and confusion—based on ambiguous messaging or lack of trust—are tackled through enhanced sustainability communication, participatory design, and increased transparency (Bhaduri & Copeland, 2021; Riva et al., 2024). Internally, weak governance and trust shortages can undermine hybrid cohesion and legitimacy, and thus, there has been the embracing of inclusive models of governance, e.g., advisory boards and stakeholder representation systems (Flew, 2021; Hinrichs & Johnston, 2020). A second enduring issue is corporate short-termism, in which companies value immediate returns ahead of sustainability in the longer term; nevertheless, increasing acknowledgment of ESG integration and forward-thinking planning exists among investors and leadership groups (Haessler, 2020). Moreover, global sustainability solutions often fail to account for localized socio-ecological realities, limiting their effectiveness; community-led and context-sensitive approaches are increasingly prioritized to tailor solutions more appropriately (Benz et al., 2024; Constantin et al., 2021). Finally, limitations that come with scalability continue to be a persistent problem, as successful scaling up of trial schemes to broader applications tends to be unfocused by institutional, political, or logistical limitations—thus the call for modular designs, platform technologies, and collaborations (Losa & Cossent, 2024; Makrygiorgou et al., 2023). All these practices combined are increasingly coming to represent a growing stress on overcoming universal restrictions and advancing the creation of powerful, inclusive, and scalable hybrid routes to sustainability (Fig. 19.3).

19.8 Conclusions

This chapter has illustrated that intricate sustainability challenges require a multifaceted solution irrespective of dependency on either market or non-market strategies. Instead, hybrid solutions purposefully combine market mechanisms' efficiency and innovative potential with non-market organizations' values, inclusiveness, and accountability to provide a more inclusive and robust foundation for sustainable

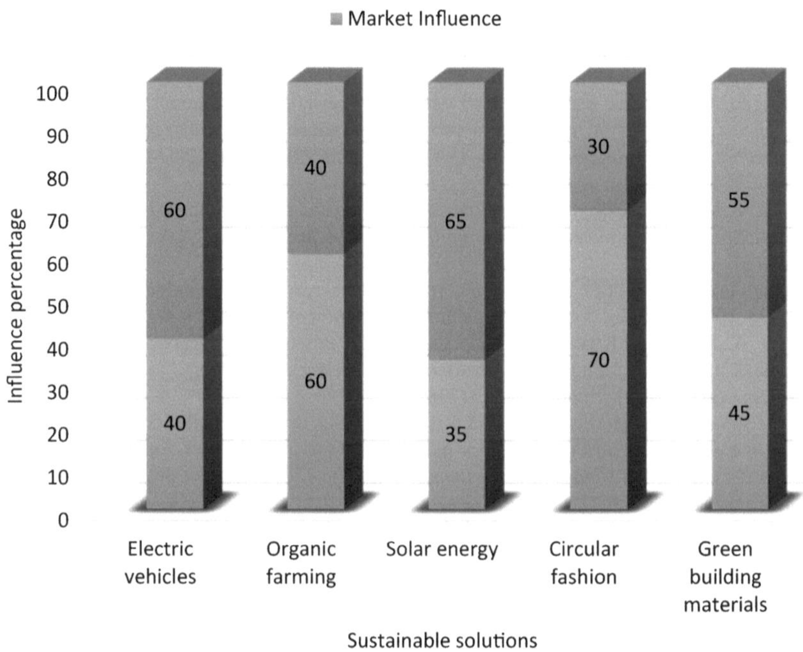

Fig. 19.3 Hybrid Models in marketing sustainable solutions across sectors. The graph depicts the proportional influence of market-driven and policy-driven forces in five key domains: electric vehicles, organic farming, solar energy, circular fashion, and green building materials

development. Based on evidence from a broad variety of global contexts and the Indian context, the study emphasizes that hybrid solutions are more likely to manage complexity in socio-environmental processes. Hence, sustainable marketing cannot be imagined as a market process irrespective of an overall system emphasizing integration, flexibility, and long-term outcomes. In conclusion, the future of sustainability is not in the either-or of selecting between market and non-market strategies, but in our capacity to bridge them meaningfully and to develop innovative and equitable solutions.

References

Ahmad, S., Wong, K. Y., Tseng, M. L., & Wong, W. P. (2018). Sustainable product design and development: A review of tools, applications, and research prospects. *Resources, Conservation and Recycling, 132*, 49–61. https://doi.org/10.1016/j.resconrec.2018.01.020

Al Anshori, F., Salomo, R. V., & Kusumastuti, R. (2023). Understanding blended finance: How different definitions of blended finance result in different inputs and outputs and what to expect. *Technium Social Sciences Journal, 44*, 15–27. https://doi.org/10.47577/tssj.v44i1.8928

Alić, M. B., & Antunica, N. (n.d.). *Ivona Milić-Beran system dynamic model of marketing in Hotel Company.*

Alziady, A. A. D. J., & Enayah, S. H. (2019). Studying the effect of institutional pressures on the intentions to continue green information technology usage. *Asian Journal of Sustainability and Social Responsibility, 4*(1), 4. https://doi.org/10.1186/s41180-018-0023-1

Ambili K. (2024). Strategic marketing interventions for sustainable economic development: A comprehensive analysis of innovative approaches and global case studies. *World Journal of Advanced Research and Reviews, 21*(1), 1520–1528. https://doi.org/10.30574/wjarr.2024.21.1.0046

Arora, N. K., & Mishra, I. (2023). Responsible consumption and production: A roadmap to sustainable development. *Environmental Sustainability, 6*(1), 1–6. https://doi.org/10.1007/s42398-023-00266-9

Arora, B., & Puranik, R. (2004). A review of corporate social responsibility in India. *Development, 47*(3), 93–100. https://doi.org/10.1057/palgrave.development.1100057

Arranz, C. F. A., Sena, V., & Kwong, C. (2022). Institutional pressures as drivers of circular economy in firms: A machine learning approach. *Journal of Cleaner Production, 355*, Article 131738. https://doi.org/10.1016/j.jclepro.2022.131738

Arribas, I., Espinós-Vañó, M. D., García, F., & Riley, N. (2021). Do irresponsible corporate activities prevent membership in sustainable stock indices? The case of the Dow Jones Sustainability Index world. *Journal of Cleaner Production, 298*, Article 126711. https://doi.org/10.1016/j.jclepro.2021.126711

Athreye, S., Saeed, A., & Baloch, M. S. (2021). Financial crisis of 2008 and outward foreign investments from China and India. *Journal of World Business, 56*(3), Article 101190. https://doi.org/10.1016/j.jwb.2021.101190

Awa, H. O., Ojiabo, O. U., & Emecheta, B. C. (2024). Sustainable marketing practices and consumer engagement: Evidence from emerging economies.*Journal of Sustainable Marketing, 15*(2), 101–118

Barrett, C. B., Islam, A., Mohammad Malek, A., Pakrashi, D., & Ruthbah, U. (2022). Experimental evidence on adoption and impact of the system of rice intensification. *American Journal of Agricultural Economics, 104*(1), 4–32. https://doi.org/10.1111/ajae.12245

Basco, R., Rodríguez-Escudero, A. I., Martin Cruz, N., & Barros-Contreras, I. (2021). The combinations of market and non-market strategies that facilitates family firm survival. *Entrepreneurship Research Journal, 11*(3), 245–286. https://doi.org/10.1515/erj-2019-0258

Belz, F.-M., & Peattie, K. (2012). *Sustainability marketing: A global perspective.* John Wiley & Sons.

Benz, C., Scott-Jeffs, W., McKercher, K. A., Welsh, M., Norman, R., Hendrie, D., Locantro, M., & Robinson, S. (2024). Community-based participatory-research through co-design: Supporting collaboration from all sides of disability. *Research Involvement and Engagement, 10*(1), 47. https://doi.org/10.1186/s40900-024-00573-3

Beumer, K., Maat, H., & Glover, D. (2022). It's not the market, stupid: On the importance of non-market economies in sustainability transitions. *Environmental Innovation and Societal Transitions, 42*, 429–441. https://doi.org/10.1016/j.eist.2022.02.001

Bhaduri, G., & Copeland, L. (2021). Going green? How skepticism and information transparency influence consumers' brand evaluations for familiar and unfamiliar brands. *Journal of Fashion Marketing and Management: An International Journal, 25*(1), 80–98. https://doi.org/10.1108/JFMM-08-2019-0175

Bhuiyan, F., Rana, T., Baird, K., & Munir, R. (2023). Strategic outcome of competitive advantage from corporate sustainability practices: Institutional theory perspective from an emerging economy. *Business Strategy and the Environment, 32*(7), 4217–4243. https://doi.org/10.1002/bse.3362

Bhusankar, S., & Kashyap, Prof. R. (2023). Green marketing practices by Wipro Infotech company and its impact on customer buying behavior. *International Journal of Scientific Research in Engineering and Management*, *07*(04). https://doi.org/10.55041/IJSREM18907

Bowie, N. E. (2012). *Corporate social responsibility in business.*

Camarinha-Matos, L. M., Rocha, A. D., & Graça, P. (2024). Collaborative approaches in sustainable and resilient manufacturing. *Journal of Intelligent Manufacturing, 35*(2), 499–519. https://doi.org/10.1007/s10845-022-02060-6

Carroll, A. B. (2015). Corporate social responsibility: The centerpiece of competing and complementary frameworks. *Organizational Dynamics, 44*(2), 87–96. https://doi.org/10.1016/j.orgdyn.2015.02.002

Carroll, A. B., & Laasch, O. (2020). *From managerial responsibility to CSR and back to responsible management*. Edward Elgar Publishing. https://doi.org/10.4337/9781788971966.00011

Carter, R. E., & Curry, D. J. (2010). Transparent pricing: Theory, tests, and implications for marketing practice. *Journal of the Academy of Marketing Science, 38*(6), 759–774. https://doi.org/10.1007/s11747-010-0189-2

Cătoiu, I., Vrânceanu, D., Maria & Filip, A. (2010). Setting fair prices-fundamental principle of sustainable marketing. In *Amfiteatru Economic Journal* (Vol. 12, Issue 27). http://creativecommons.org/licenses/by/4.0/

Charter, M., & Tischner, U. (2017). *Sustainable solutions: Developing products and services for the future*. Routledge.

Chaudhuri, B. R., George, P., Mattoo, N., & Shah, J. (2022). *Tata power CSR: The paradigm shift for sustainability*. SAGE Publications. https://doi.org/10.4135/9781529795257

Constantin, A., Alexandru, C., Korte, J., Wilson, C., Fails, J. A., Sim, G., Read, J. C., & Eriksson, E. (2021). Distributing participation in design: Addressing challenges of a global pandemic. *International Journal of Child-Computer Interaction, 28*, Article 100255. https://doi.org/10.1016/j.ijcci.2021.100255

Cosa, M. (2024). *Equity integration in corporate social responsibility: Analyzing stakeholder, legitimacy, and social activism dynamics* (pp. 133–154). https://doi.org/10.1007/978-981-97-4795-5_6

Cui, S., & Zhao, N. (2024). A study on the current status and future prospects of EV automotive market. *Journal of Social Science and Cultural Development, 1*(2). https://doi.org/10.70767/jsscd.v1i2.296

Danciu, V., & Marketing, M. &. (2013). The contribution of sustainable marketing to sustainable development. In *Challenges for the Knowledge Society* (Vol. 8, Issue 2).

Davies, I. A. (2003). Ethical decision making in fair trade companies. *Journal of Business Ethics, 45*(1/2), 79–92. https://doi.org/10.1023/A:1024124629399

Dempere, J., Alamash, E., & Mattos, P. (2024). Unveiling the truth: greenwashing in sustainable finance. *Frontiers in Sustainability, 5*. https://doi.org/10.3389/frsus.2024.1362051

Deshpande, T., Mukherji, R., & Sastry, M. (2025). Policy styles and India's national action plan on climate change (NAPCC). *Policy Studies, 46*(1), 46–63. https://doi.org/10.1080/01442872.2023.2261388

Dhawan, E., Goodman, E., Harris, S., & Mitchell, C. (2010). *Unilever and its supply chain: Embracing radical transparency to implement sustainability*. http://www.unilever.com/sustainability/introduction/ceo/index.aspx

Elkington, J. (1997). Cannibals with forks: The triple bottom line of 21st century business. Oxford: Capstone Publishing.

Flew, T. (2021). The global trust deficit disorder: A communications perspective on trust in the time of global pandemics. *Journal of Communication, 71*(2), 163–186. https://doi.org/10.1093/joc/jqab006

Freeman, R. E. (1984). Strategic management: A stakeholder approach. Boston, MA: Pitman.

Friedman, M. (1970). The social responsibility of business is to increase its profits. The New York Times magazine, september 13.

Ganatra, V., Sinha, R., Srishti, S., Pandey, R., Kadam, P., Ristiansyah, S. A., Sin, L. G., Yin, C. L., Kee, D. M. H., Jin, L. Y., Wei, O. Y., & Wei, L. P. (2021). The body shop "forever against animal testing". *International Journal of Applied Business and International Management, 6*(1), 90–100. https://doi.org/10.32535/ijabim.v6i1.1082

Glover, J. L., Champion, D., Daniels, K. J., & Dainty, A. J. D. (2014). An institutional theory perspective on sustainable practices across the dairy supply chain. *International Journal of Production Economics, 152*, 102–111. https://doi.org/10.1016/j.ijpe.2013.12.027

Gleim, M. R., Smith, J. S., Andrews, D., & Cronin, J. J. (2023). Against the green: A multi-method examination of the barriers to green consumption.*Journal of Retailing, 99*(1), 44–61.

Goh, C. S., Chong, H.-Y., Jack, L., & Mohd Faris, A. F. (2020). Revisiting triple bottom line within the context of sustainable construction: A systematic review. *Journal of Cleaner Production, 252*, Article 119884. https://doi.org/10.1016/j.jclepro.2019.119884

Haessler, P. (2020). Strategic decisions between short-term profit and sustainability. *Administrative Sciences, 10*(3), 63. https://doi.org/10.3390/admsci10030063

Hinrichs, M. M., & Johnston, E. W. (2020). The creation of inclusive governance infrastructures through participatory agenda-setting. *European Journal of Futures Research, 8*(1), 10. https://doi.org/10.1186/s40309-020-00169-6

Hong, Z., & Xiao, K. (2024). Digital economy structuring for sustainable development: The role of blockchain and artificial intelligence in improving supply chain and reducing negative environmental impacts. *Scientific Reports, 14*(1), 3912. https://doi.org/10.1038/s41598-024-53760-3

Hörisch, J., Freeman, R. E., & Schaltegger, S. (2014). Applying stakeholder theory in sustainability management. *Organization & Environment, 27*(4), 328–346. https://doi.org/10.1177/1086026614535786

Huang, L., Wang, C., Chin, T., Huang, J., & Cheng, X. (2022). Technological knowledge coupling and green innovation in manufacturing firms: Moderating roles of mimetic pressure and environmental identity. *International Journal of Production Economics, 248*, Article 108482. https://doi.org/10.1016/j.ijpe.2022.108482

Hult, G. T. M., Gonzalez-Perez, M. A., Morgeson, F. V., & Moonesar, I. A. (2023). A theory of market-based sustainability: Integrating economics-based supply and demand theory with doing good, warm glow, and price fairness. *Journal of Sustainable Marketing, 4*(2), 149–176. https://doi.org/10.51300/JSM-2023-115

Imperatives, S. (1987). Report of the world commission on environment and development: Our common future. *Accessed Feb, 10*(42), 427.

Ishak, S., & M. Zabil, N. F. (2012). Impact of consumer awareness and knowledge to consumer effective behavior. *Asian Social Science, 8*(13). https://doi.org/10.5539/ass.v8n13p108

Iyer, P., Pandey, A., Vashisht, M., & Smith, D. W. (2023). Swachh Bharat mission or the mission to make India clean: Addressing open defecation at massive scale (A). *Indian Institute of Management Ahmedabad*, 1–10. https://doi.org/10.1108/CASE.IIMA.2023.000041

Jadhav, S., & Zaware, N. (2024). An assessment of green practices in relation to the packaging of selected Indian FMCG companies. *SSRN Electronic Journal.* https://doi.org/10.2139/ssrn.4402449

Jerman, D., & Zavrsnik, B. (2012). Model of marketing communications effectiveness in the business-to-business markets. *Economic Research-Ekonomska Istraživanja, 25*(sup1), 364–388. https://doi.org/10.1080/1331677X.2012.11517569

John ORCID, K. L., Orcid, S. P., Orcid, J. T., Maxine ORCID, A. I., Orcid, R. C., Joyce ORCID, A., Guzman, D., & Denice ORCID, S. (n.d.). *Assessing the impact of environmental education on sustainable practices: A semi-systematic literature review.* www.ijassjournal.com

Kosovych, V., Kosovych, B., & Rym, O. (2022). Socialization of the economy as a component of the Anthropocene age: Economic and legal dimension. *Financial and Credit Activity Problems of Theory and Practice, 2*(43), 336–341. https://doi.org/10.55643/fcaptp.2.43.2022.3694

Kotler, P. (1994). Reconceptualizing marketing: An interview with Philip Kotler. *European Management Journal, 12*(4), 353–361. https://doi.org/10.1016/0263-2373(94)90021-3

Lagoudaki, G., Tsitskari, E., Karagiorgos, T., Yfantidou, G., Tzetzis, G., & Tsiotras, G. (2024). Corporate social responsibility and consumer behavior in sports: Exploring and adapting a participatory sports scale. *Sustainability, 16*(14), 5825. https://doi.org/10.3390/su16145825

Langsdorf, S., Löschke, S., Möller, V., Okem, A., Officer, S., Rama, B., Belling, D., Dieck, W., Götze, S., Kersher, T., Mangele, P., Maus, B., Mühle, A., Nabiyeva, K., Nicolai, M., Niebuhr, A., Petzold, J., Prentzler, E., Savolainen, J., Weyer, N. (2022). *Technical summary frequently asked questions part of the working group II contribution to the sixth assessment report of the intergovernmental panel on climate change.* www.environmentalgraphiti.org

Leal Filho, W., Dibbern, T., Pimenta Dinis, M. A., Coggo Cristofoletti, E., Mbah, M. F., Mishra, A., Clarke, A., Samuel, N., Castillo Apraiz, J., Rimi Abubakar, I., & Aina, Y. A. (2024). The added value of partnerships in implementing the UN sustainable development goals. *Journal of Cleaner Production, 438*, Article 140794. https://doi.org/10.1016/j.jclepro.2024.140794

Li, J., Sun, X., & Hu, C. (2022). The role of Skepticism and transparency in shaping green brand authenticity and green brand evangelism. *Sustainability, 14*(23), 16191. https://doi.org/10.3390/su142316191

Li, M., Pelz, S., Lamboll, R., Wang, C., & Rogelj, J. (2025). A principle-based framework to determine countries' fair warming contributions to the Paris agreement. *Nature Communications, 16*(1), 1043. https://doi.org/10.1038/s41467-025-56397-6

Lim, W. M., & Rasul, T. (2022). Customer engagement and social media: Revisiting the past to inform the future. *Journal of Business Research, 148*, 325–342. https://doi.org/10.1016/j.jbusres.2022.04.068

Losa, I., & Cossent, R. (2024). Scalability and replicability analysis in smart grid demonstration projects: Lessons learned and future needs. *Energies, 17*(21), 5312. https://doi.org/10.3390/en17215312

Majid, I. A., & Koe, W.-L. (2012). *Sustainable entrepreneurship (SE): A revised model based on triple bottom line (TBL).* www.hrmars.com/journals

Makrygiorgou, D. I., Andriopoulos, N., Georgantas, I., Rong, J., Moraitis, I., Calatayud, E. P., & Matoses, M. S. (2023). Scalability and replicability analysis of smart grid projects: Insights from the H2020 CROSSBOW project. *Frontiers in Energy Research, 11*. https://doi.org/10.3389/fenrg.2023.1167517

Manda, V. K., Mampilly, A. J., Gupta, V., & Nammi, L. (2024). *The rise of two-wheeler electric vehicles in India* (pp. 503–533). https://doi.org/10.4018/979-8-3693-3755-4.ch019

Mani, S. (2017). *Leadership in the automobile industry: The case of India's Tata Motors*. Edward Elgar Publishing. https://doi.org/10.4337/9781783476794.00010

Maradin, D., Malnar, A., & Kaštelan, A. (2022). Sustainable and clean energy: The case of Tesla Company. *Journal of Economics, Finance and Management Studies, 05*(12). https://doi.org/10.47191/jefms/v5-i12-10

Menon, A. S., Pillai, R., & Pai, Y. P. (2024). Customer engagement through transformational campaigns: A Netnographic exploration on the storytelling power of ' *Jaago Re*'. *Journal of Creative Communications*. https://doi.org/10.1177/09732586241276345

Mertzanis, C., & Tebourbi, I. (2025). Geopolitical risk and global green bond market growth. *European Financial Management, 31*(1), 26–71. https://doi.org/10.1111/eufm.12484

Michel, G. M., Feori, M., Damhorst, M. L., Lee, Y., & Niehm, L. S. (2019). Stories we wear: Promoting sustainability practices with the case of Patagonia. *Family and Consumer Sciences Research Journal, 48*(2), 165–180. https://doi.org/10.1111/fcsr.12340

Modreanu, A., Andrișan, G. N., Sârbu, A.-M., & Grădinaru, C. (2022). *Corporate social responsibility, a strategic tool for sustainable value creation: A case study of Unilever's sustainable living plan.* https://doi.org/10.24818/BASIQ/2022/08/076

Mohr, J., & Nevin, J. R. (1990). Communication strategies in marketing channels: A theoretical perspective. *Journal of Marketing, 54*(4), 36–51. https://doi.org/10.1177/002224299005400404

Mougenot, B., & Doussoulin, J.-P. (2023). A bibliometric analysis of the Global Reporting Initiative (GRI): Global trends in developed and developing countries. *Environment, Development and Sustainability, 26*(3), 6543–6560. https://doi.org/10.1007/s10668-023-02974-y

Nagano, A. (2023). Institutional values and CDR for green ITC: Transforming E-waste to ethical gems. In *2023 10th international conference on wireless networks and mobile communications (WINCOM)*, 1–6. https://doi.org/10.1109/WINCOM59760.2023.10322959

Nielsen. (2001). Global consumer attitudes toward sustainability. Nielsen Media Research.
Nzegwu, L., & Towolawi, D. (2024). Responsible pricing. In *Sustainable and responsible business in Africa* (pp. 125–140). Springer Nature Switzerland. https://doi.org/10.1007/978-3-031-35972-9_7
P.D., J. (2016). Business and society: Creating shared value: In conversation with N. R. Narayana Murthy, Founder, Infosys. *IIMB Management Review, 28*(1), 43–51. https://doi.org/10.1016/j.iimb.2016.02.003
Pai, V. S., & Hiremath, C. V. (2016). SELCO India: Solar energy for the underserved. *South Asian Journal of Business and Management Cases, 5*(2), 145–154. https://doi.org/10.1177/2277977916665929
Pareek, R. (2025). *Leveraging digital technologies for sustainable corporate practices in India* (pp. 67–100). https://doi.org/10.4018/979-8-3693-4373-9.ch004
Pérez-Durán, I. (2024). Twenty-five years of accountability research in public administration: Authorship, themes, methods, and future trends. *International Review of Administrative Sciences, 90*(3), 546–562. https://doi.org/10.1177/00208523231211751
Peterson, M. (2021). *Sustainable marketing: A holistic approach.*
Prakash, D., Bisla, M., & Arora, T. (2023). Role of environment dimensions to strive sustainable entrepreneurship: A triple bottom line approach. *International Journal of Professional Business Review, 8*(3). AOS-Estratagia and Inovacao. https://doi.org/10.26668/businessreview/2023.v8i3.698
Publication, S., & Monteiro, E. (2022). Google scholar citation: IJCSBE International Journal of Case Studies in Business, IT and education (IJCSBE) A Refereed International Journal of Srinivas University. *International Journal of Case Studies in Business, IT, and Education (IJCSBE), 6*(1), 2581–6942. https://doi.org/10.5281/zenodo.6556108
Qian, J., Ma, Y., & Tang, X. (2024). In the frontier zone of market transition: Economic possibilities across the market/non-market divide. *Environment and Planning a: Economy and Space, 56*(6), 1710–1730. https://doi.org/10.1177/0308518X241249859
Raj, B., Rahul, J., Singh, P. K., Rao, V. V. L. K., Kumar, J., Dwivedi, N., Kumar, P., Singh, D., & Strzałkowski, K. (2023). Advancements in PET packaging: Driving sustainable solutions for today's consumer demands. *Sustainability, 15*(16), 12269. https://doi.org/10.3390/su151612269
Ranjan, A. (2024). Environmental politics in India between 2014 and 2019: A critique of policies and projects. *Social Change, 54*(4), 526–542. https://doi.org/10.1177/00490857241277324
Rastegar, H., Eweje, G., & Sajjad, A. (2024). Sustainability-driven market impacts of climate change and firms' renewable energy innovation: A conceptual analysis. *Corporate Governance: The International Journal of Business in Society, 24*(6), 1337–1359. https://doi.org/10.1108/CG-07-2023-0298
Rhein, S., & Schmid, M. (2020). Consumers' awareness of plastic packaging: More than just environmental concerns. *Resources, Conservation and Recycling, 162*, Article 105063. https://doi.org/10.1016/j.resconrec.2020.105063
Riva, F., Magrizos, S., Rizomyliotis, I., & Uddin, M. R. (2024). Beyond the hype: Deciphering brand trust amid sustainability skepticism. *Business Strategy and the Environment, 33*(7), 6491–6506. https://doi.org/10.1002/bse.3829
Ruggerio, C. A. (2021). Sustainability and sustainable development: A review of principles and definitions. *Science of the Total Environment, 786*, Article 147481. https://doi.org/10.1016/j.scitotenv.2021.147481
Santos, C., Coelho, A., & Marques, A. (2024). A systematic literature review on greenwashing and its relationship to stakeholders: State of art and future research agenda. *Management Review Quarterly, 74*(3), 1397–1421. https://doi.org/10.1007/s11301-023-00337-5
Sarker, T., Ray, S., & Gazder, B. (2017). *Mahindra & Mahindra—mainstreaming sustainability through knowledge building* (pp. 145–165). https://doi.org/10.1007/978-3-319-45160-2_8
Sharma, S. (2024). *Fostering green product design and innovation for a sustainable future* (pp. 89–114). https://doi.org/10.4018/979-8-3693-2595-7.ch005

Sharon, T. (2021). Blind-sided by privacy? Digital contact tracing, the Apple/Google API and big tech's newfound role as global health policy makers. *Ethics and Information Technology, 23*(S1), 45–57. https://doi.org/10.1007/s10676-020-09547-x

Shimokado, N. (2021). Inclusive business and sustainable rural development in India: A case study of the AMUL community-based food chain. In *Management for sustainable and inclusive development in a transforming Asia* (pp. 59–71). Springer Singapore. https://doi.org/10.1007/978-981-15-8195-3_3

Sim, J., & Prabhu, V. (2018). The life cycle assessment of energy and carbon emissions on wool and nylon carpets in the United States. *Journal of Cleaner Production, 170*, 1231–1243. https://doi.org/10.1016/j.jclepro.2017.09.203

Skea, J., Slade, R., Khourdajie, A., Van Diemen, R., Mccollum, D., Pathak, M., Some, S., Vyas, P., Fradera, R., Belkacemi, M., Hasija, A., Lisboa, G., Luz, S., Malley, J., Schotanus, F., & Nicolas, R. (2023). *Coercive, mimetic and normative influences on the uptake of sustainable public procurement: An institutional perspective.* www.ekomatcentrum.se/wp-content/uploads/2019/06/Rapport-Marknadsrapport-

Sujanska, L., & Nadanyiova, M. (2023). Sustainable marketing and its impact on the image of the company. *Marketing and Management of Innovations, 14*(2), 51–57. https://doi.org/10.21272/mmi.2023.2-06

Svensson, G., Ferro, C., Høgevold, N., Padin, C., Carlos Sosa Varela, J., & Sarstedt, M. (2018). Framing the triple bottom line approach: Direct and mediation effects between economic, social and environmental elements. *Journal of Cleaner Production, 197*, 972–991. https://doi.org/10.1016/j.jclepro.2018.06.226

Takahashi, S., & Takahashi, V. P. (2022). Analysis of front end dynamic in the value co-creation with multiple stakeholders. *International Journal of Managing Projects in Business, 15*(5), 742–768. https://doi.org/10.1108/IJMPB-11-2021-0301

Tate, W. L., & Bals, L. (2018). Achieving shared triple bottom line (TBL) value creation: Toward a social resource-based view (SRBV) of the firm. *Journal of Business Ethics, 152*(3), 803–826. https://doi.org/10.1007/s10551-016-3344-y

Titumir, R. A. M., Afrin, T., & Islam, M. S. (2023). Managing natural resources sustainably: Market and non-market approaches. In *Natural resource degradation and human-nature wellbeing* (pp. 37–74). Springer Nature Singapore. https://doi.org/10.1007/978-981-19-8661-1_2

Tiwari, S., Sharif, A., Sofuoğlu, E., & Nuta, F. (2025). A step toward the attainment of carbon neutrality and SDG-13: Role of financial depth and green technology innovation. *Research in International Business and Finance, 73*, Article 102631. https://doi.org/10.1016/j.ribaf.2024.102631

Tolliver, C., Keeley, A. R., & Managi, S. (2020). Drivers of green bond market growth: The importance of nationally determined contributions to the Paris agreement and implications for sustainability. *Journal of Cleaner Production, 244*, Article 118643. https://doi.org/10.1016/j.jclepro.2019.118643

Trajkovska Petkoska, A., Daniloski, D., D'Cunha, N. M., Naumovski, N., & Broach, A. T. (2021). Edible packaging: Sustainable solutions and novel trends in food packaging. *Food Research International, 140*, Article 109981. https://doi.org/10.1016/j.foodres.2020.109981

Twagirayezu, G., Irumva, O., Uwimana, A., Nizeyimana, J. C., & Nkundabose, J. P. (2021). Current status of E-waste and future perspective in developing countries: Benchmark Rwanda. *Energy and Environmental Engineering, 8*(1), 1–12. https://doi.org/10.13189/eee.2021.080101

Venugopal, P., & Agrawal, D. (2023). *Can corporate social responsibility make business sense? Framework based on ITC e-Choupal* (pp. 69–81). https://doi.org/10.1108/S2043-905920230000016005

Vishnoi, G., Narang, R., & Ganguly, A. (2024). *Impact assessment of macroeconomic elements on India's ESG index* (pp. 27–50). https://doi.org/10.4018/979-8-3693-6617-2.ch002

Vishnubhatla, V., & Agashe, A. (2022). Is conscious consumerism a step towards society 5.0? A review paper. *ECS Transactions, 107*(1), 3267–3279. https://doi.org/10.1149/10701.3267ecst

Viti, M., Löwe, R., Sørup, H. J. D., Rasmussen, M., Arnbjerg-Nielsen, K., & McKnight, U. S. (2022). Knowledge gaps and future research needs for assessing the non-market benefits of nature-based solutions and nature-based solution-like strategies. *Science of the Total Environment, 841*, Article 156636. https://doi.org/10.1016/j.scitotenv.2022.156636

Yue, X., Huo, B., & Ye, Y. (2023). The impact of coercive pressure and ethical responsibility on cross-functional green management and firm performance. *Journal of Business & Industrial Marketing, 38*(5), 1015–1028. https://doi.org/10.1108/JBIM-09-2021-0446

Zaharia, R. M., & Zaharia, R. (2021). Triple bottom line. In *The Palgrave Handbook of corporate social responsibility* (pp. 75–101). Springer International Publishing. https://doi.org/10.1007/978-3-030-42465-7_2

Zaman, R., Jain, T., Samara, G., & Jamali, D. (2022). Corporate governance meets corporate social responsibility: Mapping the interface. *Business & Society, 61*(3), 690–752. https://doi.org/10.1177/0007650320973415

Zarghami, S. A. (2025). The role of economic policies in achieving sustainable development goal 7: Insights from OECD and European countries. *Applied Energy, 377*, Article 124558. https://doi.org/10.1016/j.apenergy.2024.124558

Zhang, Y. F. (2024). Too little or too much transparency? Influencing accountability in project management through the practices of using digital technologies. *International Journal of Project Management, 42*(6), Article 102636. https://doi.org/10.1016/j.ijproman.2024.102636

Chapter 20
Exploring the Production of Bioenergy and Biofuel from an Ethical and Socio-Economic Perspective

Deepshikha, Shreya Sharma, and Komal Agrawal

Abstract Biofuel and bioenergy production have emerged as a sustainable alternative for the establishment of a circular bioeconomy. However, their development and large-scale implementation are associated with significant social, ethical and policy-related challenges. The key concerns limiting their development are directed toward food security, land use, and environmental protection. Despite the growing number of studies focusing on the technical, economic and environmental impact of biofuel and bioenergy, the ethical perspective remains unexplored. This chapter contributes to bridging this knowledge gap by giving the latest ethical perspective focusing on land use change, social equity, and resource security, thereby incorporating ethical and social dimensions of biofuel and bioenergy development. Additionally, the chapter highlights the necessity of integrating ethical, social and environmental parameters into biofuel policy framework. A comprehensive approach that combines advanced technological innovation with sustainability and social justices is essential for ensuring positive contribution of biofuel and bioenergy toward circular economy.

Keywords Biofuels · Bioenergy · Ethical · Policies · Sustainability · Bioeconomy

20.1 Introduction

Bioenergy and biofuels are increasingly regarded as a key renewable energy source with the potential to mitigate the adverse environmental impacts associated with fossil fuel consumption (Zhi et al., 2023). Under specific conditions, these are considered to be carbon neutral, since the carbon dioxide released during combustion is balanced by the amount absorbed by plants during photosynthesis. Derived from

Deepshikha · S. Sharma · K. Agrawal (✉)
Department of Microbiology, School of Bio Engineering and Biosciences, Lovely Professional University, Phagwara, Punjab, India
e-mail: komalagarwal935@gmail.com

P. Verma (ed.), *Sustainable Practices in Biorefinery*,
https://doi.org/10.1007/978-981-95-6071-4_20

organic materials, biofuels encompass a wide range of sources including crops, agricultural residues, forestry by-products, animal waste and algae (Kafeel et al., 2025; Nair et al., 2022). Based on their form and processing requirements, these are categorized into primary and secondary biofuels. The primary biofuel resources, such as firewood, wood chips, and animal waste are used directly for heating, cooking, or power generation, particularly in developing regions. In contrast secondary biofuels undergo processing and can be employed as transport fuels either independently or blended with conventional fuels (Khan et al., 2021). These include bioethanol, biodiesel, bio-methanol, and synthetic fuels. First-generation biofuels are produced from edible crops such as sugar and starch-rich plants for ethanol or oilseeds for biodiesel. However, their dependence on food resources and agricultural land has raised concerns over food security and land use competition (Kumar et al., 2020; Malode et al., 2021). To address these challenges, research and policy increasingly shifted toward second-generation biofuels, which are derived from lignocellulosic biomass. In addition to these, third-generation biofuels are gaining attention, primarily derived from algae; these represent a significant advancement due to their higher yield and lower greenhouse gas (GHG) footprint compared to earlier feedstocks (Igwebuike et al., 2024). More recently, fourth-generation biofuels have entered the research landscape, incorporating synthetic biology approaches to further enhance efficiency, sustainability, and carbon capture potential (Zhang et al., 2025).

Various studies revealed that bioenergy adoption can enhance employment opportunities, generate income streams, and contribute to macroeconomic growth (Creutzig et al., 2015). It offers the potential for a stable, long-term energy supply at relatively constant prices. Importantly, bioenergy can provide additional revenue streams, rural development through sustainable and clean energy, while creating new employment opportunities (Welfle et al., 2023). Bioenergy constitutes a major component of the global energy portfolio, representing ~9.5% of total primary energy supply and nearly 70% of renewable energy utilization (Reid et al., 2020). A significant share of this energy is derived from traditional biomass application, primarily from household cooking and heating as well as small-scale industries (Chowdhury et al., 2025). Liquid biofuel production for transportation exhibited rapid expansion before 2010, with annual growth rates exceeding 10%, before moderating to approximately 4% between 2010 and 2016 (International Energy Agency, 2017). Similarly, bioenergy-based electricity capacity expanded at an average annual growth rate of 6.5% during the same period. Projections for 2018–2023 indicate that bioenergy, including liquid biofuels, will account for nearly 30% of the global increase in renewable energy production (International Energy Agency, 2018).

Sustainable energy, fair trade, food security, climate resilience, and social justice are all impacted by a social and ethical analysis of biofuels and bioenergy, which contributes to SDG 7 (Affordable and Clean Energy), SDG 12 (Responsible Consumption and Production), SDG 13 (Climate Action), and SDG 15 (Life on Land) by addressing land use change, biodiversity protection and ethical supply chains. This chapter highlights the ethical perspective on biofuels and bioenergy and their socio-economic impact. The ethical dimensions of biofuel and bioenergy development are discussed, along with the implementation of biofuel and bioenergy policies. The economic viability of Biofuel and Bioenergy development have been outlined in this chapter focusing on ethical based studies. The challenges and prospects of ethics in biofuel and bioenergy are also highlighted.

20.2 Socio-Economic Impact of Biofuel and Bioenergy Development

In transition from fossil-based economy toward a sustainable green economy, biofuels and bioenergy hold significant potential. The utilization of these biofuels such as bioethanol, can reduce GHG emission by ~65%, whereas biodiesel derived from waste cooking oil can achieve a reduction of up to 87% compared to petroleum diesel (Datta et al., 2024). In addition, to reduce carbon footprint biofuels exhibit lower flammability which can contribute to improved engine performance and operational efficiency (Rist et al., 2009). The social implications of biofuel production are both profound and multifaceted. A major advantage lies in the reduction of dependency on imported petroleum, providing economic benefits and enhancing energy security (Jeswani et al., 2020). The United States (Van der Horst and Vermeylen, 2011) and the European Commission (Vackeová and Noyon, 2022) have emphasized that biofuel contributes toward improving the energy security of supply while simultaneously mitigating the GHG emission and promoting economic stability.

The evaluation of bioenergy economic impacts on agricultural markets necessitates the use of various indicators and metrics that capture the changes in supply, demand, prices, and welfare (Brinkman et al., 2019). Variations in crop prices are central indicators of market dynamics and resource allocations. Tracking price trends, differences between bioenergy and food crops and price transmission mechanisms can provide insights and can influence the agricultural markets (Osuagwu et al., 2023). Another factor is land use attributing to bioenergy expansion and offering valuable information on the spatial redistribution of agricultural activities and environmental impacts. However, the effect of bioenergy economic welfare is often assessed through shifts in producers and consumer surplus, changes in income distribution, and overall societal welfare (Núñez-Regueiro et al., 2021). Analytical approaches such as cost–benefit analysis, welfare economics, and social matrices are frequently applied to capture the net profit and distributional outcomes of bioenergy development projects (Brinkman et al., 2019).

20.3 Ethical Dimensions in Bioenergy and Biofuel Development

From the mid-2000s onwards, the concept of bioeconomy gained increasing attention as a means of addressing fossil fuel dependence by utilizing biomass for sustainable energy. The bioeconomy encompasses both food and non-food related applications of biotechnology, including genetically modified microorganisms (Popp et al., 2021). Its prominence was reinforced through adoption by the European Union (EU) and the Organization of Economic Co-operation and Development (OECD), which established bioeconomy as policy agenda to promote the development of new products, markets, and applications based on biomass (Patermann & Aguilar, 2018). In earlier stages, bioenergy was primarily addressed for energy-related challenges with emphasis on enhancing energy security and reducing reliance on fossil fuels such as oil and coal (Rather et al., 2022). However, the social and environmental aspects of biofuel and bioenergy were given limited attention as it is considered sustainable energy for the future (Raman et al., 2025). Although being promoted as a contributor to a low-carbon future, the first-generation liquid biofuels have raised significant concerns due to their impacts on climate change, agriculture, and environment (Jeswani et al., 2020).

20.3.1 Environmental Impact of Bioenergy from an Ethical Perspective

During 2000 and 2010 biofuels received considerable public and political attention largely due to its prominent effect on GHG. This positioned biofuels like bioethanol and biodiesel as a strategy against climate mitigation (Hasan et al., 2023). Alongside, a particular emphasis was given to national and economic interest as it would reduce the dependency on imported petroleum. This narrative held significant importance in North America and Europe (Gomiero et al., 2010). Furthermore, the cultivation of biofuel feedstocks was promoted as a source of economic opportunity for farmers. In United States, this was framed as a means of supporting domestic agriculture, whereas in Europe it extended as creating income streams in low-income partner countries. However, this period also witnessed the emergence of critical perspectives that challenged the perceived benefits of biofuels (Buyx & Tail., 2011). The technical and environmental limitations of first-generation biofuels were increasingly highlighted, with some studies suggesting that these contributed to climate change and ecological degradation. Similarly social concerns were raised due to the implication of large-scale biofuel expansion in less industrialized regions, where increased use of land derived unjust appropriation against farming systems (Mohr & Raman., 2013). In response to this, the Nuffield Council of Bioethics in the United Kingdom undertook a comprehensive review of biofuels in 2009. The council reported a set of normative principles intended to guide the ethical assessment of biofuel technologies

(Mortimer, 2013). These principles encompass respect for human rights, assurance of environmental sustainability and adherence to standards of fair trade, in addition to broader imperative climate change mitigation.

One of the major concerns from the ethical perspective of biofuel is the food VS fuel debate. The redirection of edible crops for energy use was argued to threaten global food security by contributing to rising prices. In response to the ethical concerns surrounding biofuels, two major policies were directed (Chowdhury et al., 2025). The first involved the establishment of certification systems, in which an independent organization evaluated biofuel production against standards designed to translate ethical concerns into measurable supply chain criteria (Pols, 2015). These voluntary certification schemes are distinct from the regulatory mechanisms, such as the United States Renewable Fuel standard, which primarily enforces compliance with legislative mandates for incorporating biofuels into the liquid fuel supply. The second response is concerned with strategic investment in research on advanced biofuels (Škapa & Vochozka, 2020).

These concerns have directed the research trajectories toward addressing the food security, which is frequently treated as the most significant ethical challenge to biofuel and bioenergy development. Large-scale production programs have been concentrated on utilizing non-food crops as feedstock (Ahmed et al., 2021). These include using plants capable of growing on marginal or degraded lands and designing microbial and catalytic processes. Evaluating whether large-scale biofuel research has successfully engaged with global ethical concerns remains essential to assessing its long-term social implications (Osman et al., 2024). Such concerns have also influenced the incorporation of ethical principles in justice, equity, sustainability, and social responsibility into biofuel and bioenergy development processes.

20.3.2 Ethical Principles for Biofuel and Bioenergy Development

An ethical framework for biofuel and bioenergy development has been established, which shares moral values in comprising human rights, environmental stability, and promotes sustainability. These include-

Principle 1: Human rights

Although many nations have well-established social and labor regulations, concerns persist regarding the rapid expansion of biofuel industries in regions where legal practices safeguard for human rights are insufficient (Thompson, 2024). This issue has been recognized as a critical ethical boundary that must not be overlooked in favor of economic interests or policy driven pressures from industrial nations. The challenge becomes particularly significant when countries with strong biofuel policies are unable to meet domestic demand through internal production, leading to increased reliance on imports from developing nations with abundant resources and comparatively lower production cost (Pool, 2013). Thus, this principle incorporates that biofuel production should not compromise the fundamental human rights, including access to adequate food, clean water, healthcare, employment, and land use (Chowdhury et al., 2025).

Principle 2: Environmental sustainability

The key concern addressed under this principle is directly linked to ecological consequences of large-scale biofuel production in regions where environmental protection frameworks are weak (de Paula Leite et al., 2025). Similar to the risks associated with human rights, the primary factor driving localized threats to environmental integrity is the increasing demand for low-cost biofuel imports from developing nations, stimulated by policies in more industrialized countries (Singh & Clough, 2024). In particular, the allocation of extensive land areas for biofuel cultivation poses a significant risk, either as the primary cause or as a contributing factor to habitat degradation and ecosystem. Thus, biofuels production must adhere to principles of environmental sustainability, ensuring that expansion does not result in biodiversity loss (El-Araby, 2024).

Principle 3: Climate change

The biofuel generation is regarded as a credible measure for climate change mitigation. Thus, biofuel utilization must be demonstrated to result in net reduction of GHG emissions rather than contributing to global warming (Khanna et al., 2011). This criterion forms a fundamental basis for the justification and promotion of biofuel policies. The net reduction in GHG emissions are commonly assessed through life cycle assessment (LCA), which is an established methodology for quantifying environmental impacts across production and consumption stages (Usmani, 2023).

Principle 4: Just reward

The development of biofuels should be aligned with principles of fair trade that ensure equitable rewards, encompassing both labor rights and intellectual property rights. With respect to labor rights, a central concern is whether farmers and workers engaged in biofuel production receive adequate financial compensation for their contributions (Tsitrouli, 2021). Although this issue is often emphasized in relation to developing countries that serve as exporters of biofuels, similar considerations arises in nations implementing biofuel policies (Das & Gundimeda, 2022). The dimension of intellectual property rights pertains to the recognition and protection of innovations and resources that facilitate biofuel development, including the introduction of novel feedstocks, technological advancements, and capital investments in production infrastructure (Kanjilal & Saha, 2019).

Principle 5: Equitable distribution

The costs and benefits associated with biofuel development should be distributed in an equitable manner. Beyond the requirement of fair compensation in direct economic exchanges, biofuel production can exert broader impacts on society, which may be economic, environmental, social, political, or cultural in nature (Velenturf &

Purnell, 2021). Such impacts often emerge when new crops, accompanied by unfamiliar agricultural practices and altered social dynamics, are introduced into regions that lack sufficient preparation or institutional capacity to manage them. Particular concerns arise in the context of developing countries, where large-scale production intended for international biofuel markets may conflict with small-scale systems designed to address the immediate needs of local populations (Pols & Spahn, 2013).

Principle 6: An ethical duty

If the first five principles are followed and the biofuel production is able to make a significant contribution to climate change, then a moral obligation exists to pursue their development. In this context, the moral imperative to advance biofuel production as a strategy for achieving sustainable development within the global climate change agenda (Souza et al., 2017). It has been acknowledged that under appropriate conditions, biofuel policies can be designed to align fully with the five ethical principles. Where such alignment is achievable, the opportunities for practical implementation should not be disregarded, given the urgency of the challenges that biofuels are intended to address (Pools, 2013).

20.4 Biofuel and Bioenergy Policies

Policies, strategies, and programs that have been implemented to encourage and control the production and use of biofuels, including ethanol and biodiesel, are generally referred to as biofuel policies. Major nations, including Australia, Brazil, Canada, China, the EU, India, Japan, Malaysia, and the United States, produced 99% of the biofuel (Usmani et al., 2023). The biofuel polices for these countries are designed based on the six ethical principles discussed above (Tait et al., 2011).

20.4.1 Policy Implementation and Stakeholders in Biofuel and Bioenergy Generation

The geopolitical organization ASEAN has founding members such as Indonesia, Malaysia, Philippines, Singapore and Thailand that have developed policies, incentives, blending mandates and plans for the expansion of biofuel production in recent years (Kumar et al., 2013). The government organizations of different countries focus on revising the policies with evolving technologies and sustainability need to become world leaders (Wattana, 2014). Roadmaps of different countries, like Malaysia, Thailand, the United States of America (USA), and India, are discussed in detail in Table 20.1. Over the decades, the U.S. government has gradually shifted focus toward renewable and low-carbon energy. The Inflation Reduction Act (2022) focused on renewable diesel, biofuel incentives, CO_2 sequestration and financing, thereby integrating ethical considerations of social equity into bioenergy policy. The benefits of this act incorporated the Advanced Energy Project Credit extension, Clean Fuel Production Credit foundation, and financing rural economy for bioenergy establishments. Bioenergy and biofuel policies established by the USA, ASEAN, and India showed both convergence and divergence. A pattern of biofuel and bioenergy-focused policies can be observed being established and evolving over the last 30–50 years. Developed countries prioritize sustainability, whereas emerging countries focus on energy security and advancements. The importance of balanced policy frameworks is essential for consistency and evolution of biofuel production (Usmani et al., 2023). Biofuel policies have ethical significance in maintaining an equilibrium between the social construct, security, environmental sustainability, and mitigation of rural and urban society.

The policy framework of a country is one of the key factors for the overall development of biofuel and bioenergy on a global scale. Thus, some of the ethically significant policies and initiatives are the US Inflation Reduction Act (Bang, 2025), the EU's RED II (Webster, 2020), and India's National Bioenergy Programme (MNRE, 2022). In India, the Ethanol Blending Programme (EBP) was launched in 2002 to promote renewable fuels by blending ethanol with petrol (EBP) and diesel. It utilizes sugarcane and other crops from fields for ethanol production. This mandate was then revised due to the rise of ethical queries of food and water scarcity (Roy et al., 2019). Others are the National Biodiesel Mission, the National Policy on Biofuels, Revised Policy of Biofuels (2018), which aimed for ethanol 20% blending in petrol and biodiesel 5% in diesel by 2030 (Saravanan et al., 2020). A few of the Russian policies focusing on blending targets and mandates are the Energy Policy of 1992, the Authorized technical standard of 2002 (5% blending of ethanol with petrol), the Authorized 2004 (10% blending of ethanol with petrol), and the Authorized 2005 (5% of biodiesel with diesel).

Beyond their technical and environmental justifications, biofuel blending regulations have ethical implications in enhancing energy security, lowering oil imports, boosting rural incomes, and helping cut GHG emissions. The EU biofuel policies have been overtaken by blending mandates in recent years, which could lead to an increase in prices for consumers (Koster et al., 2023; Lundberg et al., 2023). Ethically, these blending targets result in excessive land stress and resource scarcity, like water demand for feedstocks (Lee et al., 2020). It is important to assess the policies and blending targets that focus on bioenergy and biofuel advancement which do not cause social inequality, injustice, economic stress, and environmental degradation to the vulnerable communities. Policies that are target-based are encouraged by nations to scale up biofuel production (Marin-Burgos et al., 2017). Blending fuels is being utilized in transport and industries and can establish an alternative pathway for replacing non-renewable oils in the transportation sector (Duo & Huijsmans, 2025).

Apart from blending mandates, government organizations also focus on research and development (R&D) for biofuel and bioenergy advancement. A few of these initiatives and funding plans formulated by government bodies are R&D grants which focus on funding and patents, loan guarantees, tax benefits, and long-term agreements of bioenergy development (IEA Bioenergy, 2023). The Indian government has made numerous investments and collaborations at both national and international

Table 20.1 Biofuel and bioenergy policies roadmap from different countries

Country	Policies/Blending mandates	Year	Aim	References
India	Oilfields (Regulation and Development) Act	1948	Regulation of oilfields and development of mineral oil resources	Fatima et al., 2025; National Policy on Biofuels – 2018
	Essential Commodities Act	1955	Production, supply, and distribution of necessary commodities (petroleum) to ensure availability at fair prices	
	Ethanol Blending Programme (EBP)	2002	5% blending mandate, which was later increased to 10% in 2008. Sugarcane, Molasses and non-edible oils were used to produce bioethanol and biodiesel.	
	National Biodiesel Mission	2003	Blending mandate at 5% from 2007, increasing to 20% in 2012	
	Strategic Petroleum Reserve Programme	2004	The emergency crude oil stockpile plan was designed for the regulation of energy security	
	Petroleum and Natural Gas Regulatory Board Act	2006	Regulation of downstream activities petroleum and natural gas sector	
	National Policy on Biofuels	2009 (revised 2018)	Biodiesel and bioethanol at 20% blending (by 2017)	
	Galvanizing Organic Bio-Agro Resources	2018	Establishing rural energy security by producing compressed biogas and organic manure	
	Pradhan Mantri JI-VAN Yojana	2020	Bioethanol production from lignocellulosic biomass. Target of 20% ethanol blending in fuel by 2025.	Roadmap for Ethanol blending in India 2021
	Scheme to enhance ethanol distillation capacity	2020	Financial assistance for ethanol production	
	Waste to Energy Programme	2021	Biogas, biomass, and waste-to-energy in implementing circular economy models.	
	National Bioenergy Programme	2022	Promote surplus biomass and waste for energy generation	

(continued)

Table 20.1 (continued)

Country	Policies/Blending mandates	Year	Aim	References
	National Hydrogen Mission	2023	Green hydrogen production, usage, and export by 2030	
Malaysia	Petroleum Development Act	1974	Governing the Malaysian oil and gas industry (export and import)	Abdul-Manan et al., 2015
	National Energy Policy	1979	Foundational policy to overcome oil crises by establishing strategies for efficient, and sustainable energy supply	
	Four-Fuel Diversification Policy	1981	Formulated to reduce oil dependency.	
	5th fuel diversification policy and renewable energy	2000	Established to promote biogas and other bioenergy's.	
	National Biofuel Policy	2006	Adopted for biofuel production and promotion	
	Malaysian Biofuel Act	2007	Mandates biofuel use, licensing associated with its production, storage, and trading.	
	Ninth Malaysian Plan	2006 – 2010	Established for further promotion of biofuels	
	Hydrogen Economy & Technology Roadmap	2023	Establish the country as a leader in the global hydrogen economy by 2050, focusing on green hydrogen production.	IEA, 2025
Thailand	Petroleum Act	1971	Regulates the exploration, production, and management of petroleum resources.	Wattana, 2014
	Emergency Decree of the Remedy and Prevention of Shortage of Fuel Oils (B.E. 2516)	1973	Regulation of fuel oil supply, pricing, and distribution during energy shortages.	
	Alternative Energy Development Plan (AEDP)	2004 – 2011	The renewable energy objective was set to reach 25% of the nation's total energy consumption by 2021	

(continued)

Table 20.1 (continued)

Country	Policies/Blending mandates	Year	Aim	References
	Second - followed by the AEDP	2008 – 2022	Increase biofuels and green technology, create communities, and increase the use of alternative energy to 20% of total consumption	
USA	The Higher Blends Infrastructure Incentive Program (HBIIP)	2020	Supports higher blends of ethanol and biodiesel, thereby advancing renewable fuel use, rural development, and environmental goals	IEA, 2025
	Biofuels Research to Reduce Transportation Emissions	2021	Supports biofuels research and deployment to reduce transportation emissions	
	ARPA-E Research Programme, Biofuels	2021	Provides funding for the development of biofuel technology to increase efficiency, lower emissions, and ensure energy security.	
	Investment in Direct Air Capture CO2	2021	Enhance carbon removal technologies through funding and incentives	
	Infrastructure and Jobs Act: Carbon capture, utilization, and storage investment	2021	Establishes funding for carbon capture, utilization, and storage projects	
	Energy awards for clean hydrogen technologies	2021	Enhance innovation, commercialization, and deployment of low-carbon hydrogen	
	Inflation Reduction Act	2022	Aims to expand green energy and regulatory support for sustainable fuels	

levels, funding 75 joint R&D projects (Department of Biotechnology and Department of Science and Technology) (Mission innovations, 2025). The EU launched the European Research Area (ERA) system to ensure unethical acts like plagiarism, manipulation, and duplication can be avoided in research (EC, 2000, 2014). Such initiatives ensure the technological development aligning with principles of justices, sustainability and social responsibility in bioenergy and biofuel sector.

20.4.2 Integration of Social, Economic and Ethical Parameters in Biofuel and Bioenergy Development

The expansion of biofuel production, particularly for the aviation and maritime sectors, is accompanied by a spectrum of social costs that require thorough assessment. However, a major concern with biofuel development is competition for resources (Kourkoumpas et al., 2024). The biofuel production utilizing non-food residues, including pellets, straw, vineyard, olive grove, and other organic waste are expected to have minimal social costs (Solarte-Toro & Cardona Alzate et al., 2023). Achieving an effective balance of economic growth, environmental stewardship, and social well-being remains critical for the successful large-scale implementation of biofuels. The social cost–benefit analysis represents a structural and comprehensive framework for assessing the overall efficiency of a project from a societal perspective (Popp et al., 2016). This entails the identification, quantification, and comparison of both costs and benefits. Social-Life Cycle Assessment (S-LCA) serves as a decision-making guide ensuring interventions are not only aligned with intended objectives but also yield optimal returns (Mattioda et al., 2020). Kostidi et al. (2024) analyzed biofuel production from the maritime and aviation sectors by performing S-LCA and S-CBA. The study enhanced the social responsibility and hazards in their supplier chains. This revealed social impact hotspots, economic costs, and provided detailed information regarding the sustainability of biofuel production. In a related study, the S-LCA was conducted on feedstock for biodiesel production. The findings of the study revealed unfair wages between the wealthier and the impoverished workers, social inequalities, and highlighted that the cooperative models contribute positively toward improving workers' conditions and social well-being (Costa & Oliveira, 2022). The findings give evidence to the social influence of bioprocess and help formulate plans and policies. Facilitating evidence-based decision-making enables policymakers and stakeholders to optimize resource allocation and enhance the effectiveness of public initiatives, particularly in addressing global challenges such as climate and sustainable development (Ncube et al., 2024).

The economic evaluation of a project through cost–benefit analysis is commonly employed to determine whether a project or policy should be implemented. Such evaluations can be enhanced by incorporating complementary methodologies that account for broader welfare outcomes. Within biofuel and bioenergy development (Zetterholm et al., 2020). Social Cost–benefit Analysis (S-CBA) serves as comprehensive tool to evaluate both direct and indirect impacts of alternative fuels. It identifies the affected population groups, distinguishing between beneficiaries and those potentially disadvantaged, and allocates benefits and costs across defined time horizons (Bouillass et al., 2021). Furthermore, by integrating social consideration into the evaluation process, S-CBA provides a structural approach for capturing well-being impacts thereby linking socio-economic benefits with the sustainability outcomes of biofuel adoption (Vance et al., 2022). These first-generation biofuels have been argued to contribute toward food scarcity by competing with agricultural land and resources while also driving deforestation in developing countries which in turn accelerates GHG emission (Kostidi & Lyridis., 2024).

20.5 Socio-Economic Viability of Biofuel and Bioenergy Development

Globally, ~3.6 million tons of certified biofuel was utilized in 2019, resulting in an estimated reduction of 9.7 million tons of CO_2. This is an average of achieving ~83% reduced GHG reduction compared to fossil fuels (Liepold et al., 2024). Second-generation biofuels are considered a key option for decarbonization of transport sectors. Their role is particularly significant in carriers' sectors such as aviation, maritime shipping, and heavy-duty road transport (Arias et al., 2024). Additionally, owing to the high demand for biofuels from these sectors, biofuel production in Germany was continued to expand, accompanied by increasing reliance on imported biogenic feedstock. As a result, the German bioeconomy is projected to depend on imports from regions outside the EU, including the global south (Wohlgemuth et al., 2021). However, sustainability criteria for such imports are not explicitly defined under Article 28 of the EU Renewable Energy Directive III (RED III), thereby externalizing a range of social impacts associated with feedstock production and trade (Zeug et al., 2023). Based on the sustainability criteria analysis and stakeholder criteria, the EU's Renewable Energy Directive II (RED II, 2021–2030) is a policy framework that acts to preserve biodiversity, sustainable bioenergy supply, resource efficiency, and Indirect Land Use Change (ILUC). RED II works in maintaining the ethical rights of workers and the local communities. Ethical drawbacks of the sustainable aspects of waste, like utilization of palm oil and soy for biodiesel, could lead to deforestation and risk to food security, and must be discussed with all parties involved (stakeholders) (Mai-Moulin et al., 2021).

Toward South America, the Brazilian biodiesel is often synthesized using feedstocks such as soybean, castor bean, jatropha, and palm tree. Biodiesel production is supported by the National Petroleum Agency and the Social Fuel Stamp program. These government organizations support the supply target, and tax exemptions aimed at regional areas are provided. In India, energy demand is projected to grow at an annual rate of 4–fivefold over the coming decade. Consequently, policy makers are increasingly considering biofuels as a viable option to enhance national energy security. Over the last two decades biofuels initiatives in India have influenced land use patterns, environmental sustainability and rural livelihoods, highlighting both opportunities and challenges associated with large-scale production. Sorghum and pearl millet both predominantly rain-fed crops have attracted attention as potential feedstock for bioethanol production. Life Cycle Assessment (LCA) of ethanol derived from sorghum and pearl millet revealed that farming activities contribute nearly 30% of total energy inputs, with fertilizers and pesticides being the largest sources of GHG emission. Although both crops are rain-fed, sorghum was found to be more energy intensive than pearl millet due to higher water requirements and lower fodder production. This case study demonstrated that sorghum and pearl millet offer considerable potential as bioethanol feedstock. With targeted investments in research and development, optimized water and fertilizer use, and active participation of smaller holder farmers, these crops could play a constructive role in reducing fossil fuel dependence, strengthening the rural economy, and contributing to long-term energy goals (Reddy & Reddy, 2021).

20.6 Future Prospects

Reducing dependence on fossil fuel and advancing the development of biofuels necessitate the integration of ethical, social, and environmental parameters in policy-making processes. The biofuel and bioenergy sector requires standardized rules in addition to country and category-specific policies, which would regulate the advances in a target-based strategy. The major contributing factor in this decision can be associated with LCA of bioprocesses, which would evaluate the environmental impact for biofuel production while promoting greater sustainability and supporting the circular economy. In terms of ethical perspective, advanced approaches such as S-LCA and Ethical LCA can extend this evaluation to broader dimensions, including land use, financial equity, food security, labor rights, etc. They can help provide clarity on mandates, grants, and indirect land use charges, resource scouring, and project analysis. These ethical prospects ensure the protection of justice, human rights, sustainability, social inclusion, and integrity in bioenergy development. The social and ethical perspective of biofuel and bioenergy dimensions, along with environmental and economic via S-LCA, helps achieve a green economy and sustainable future. Various sustainable studies focusing on Land Use Change (LUC) and resource extraction for bioenergy synthesis are a new trend in setting sustainable standards by evaluating biodiversity, water, soil, and air quality. Factors typically associated with assessing LUC include time, spatial, policy, and dimensional aspects (Austin et al., 2022).

Other advances in ethical considerations for biofuel and bioenergy bioprocesses are Artificial Intelligence and digital ethics. Blockchains such as the high-energy-consuming blockchain are data management technologies that can be utilized in the biomass supply chain and data storage for the biofuel, biogas, and hydrogen sector (Mould et al., 2022). The traceability, protection, and anonymity features of cryptocurrencies are essential for secure transactions (Yi, 2022). In terms of ethical considerations, blockchains facilitate efficient governance due to their trustworthiness, stability, and transparency for supply chains. Blockchains can also be utilized to ensure ethical conduct and enable legal rights (Koh et al., 2020). Issues with personalized and organized privacy are primarily attributed to the loss of privacy due to inadequate protection of workers' wages, identity, and transaction data, as well as the organization's expenses, grouped data, performance, and intellectual property (Feng et al., 2019). Apart from blockchains, AI-driven biomass supply chains are being utilized for their predictive capabilities, smart decision-making, accuracy, feedstock screening, and optimization of bioenergy/biofuel production (Anbarasu et al., 2025). Unfortunately, AI ethics raises concerns of responsibility, transparency, and security. AI relies on data collection, which can lead to hacking and privacy issues. Additionally, its lack of accountability during problem-solving can result in improper handling of issues. To oversee the AI and digital ethics and gaps involved in bioenergy production, it is important to establish standardized rules and expose the direct reasons made by AI (Naidu et al., 2024).

20.7 Conclusion

The development of biofuel and bioenergy represents an important step toward achieving a circular bioeconomy. Additionally, their ethical and social challenges such as food security, land use, and environmental protection continue to shape the trajectory toward research and policy making. These challenges reinforce the need to incorporate principles of human rights, justice, and sustainability in bioenergy development. For ensuring responsible deployment, future strategies must incorporate regulatory mechanisms, funding schemes, and tools which evaluate land use changes alongside resource governance and project assessment. The integration of digital ethics and AI-driven monitoring further strengthens the accountability and transparency of bioenergy system. Ultimately incorporating such principles will ensure the positive contribution of biofuel and bioenergy toward sustainable developmental goals and long-term energy transitions.

References

Abdul-Manan, A. F., Baharuddin, A., & Chang, L. W. (2015). Application of theory-based evaluation for the critical analysis of national biofuel policy: A case study in Malaysia. Evaluation and program planning, 52, 39-49. https://doi.org/10.1016/j.evalprogplan.2015.03.007

Ahmed, S., Warne, T., Smith, E., Goemann, H., Linse, G., Greenwood, M., Kedziora, J., Sapp, M., Kraner, D., Roemer, K., & Stoy, P. C. (2021). Systematic review on effects of bioenergy from edible versus inedible feedstocks on food security. *npj Science of Food*, *5*(1), 9. https://doi.org/10.1038/s41538-021-00091-6

Anbarasu, K., Thanigaivel, S., Sathishkumar, K., Alam, M. M., Al-Sehemi, A. G., & Devarajan, Y. (2025). Harnessing artificial intelligence for sustainable bioenergy: Revolutionizing optimization, waste reduction, and environmental sustainability. *Bioresource Technology, 418*, Article 131893. https://doi.org/10.1016/j.biortech.2024.131893

Arias, A., Nika, C. E., Vasilaki, V., Feijoo, G., Moreira, M. T., & Katsou, E. (2024). Assessing the future prospects of emerging technologies for shipping and aviation biofuels: A critical review. *Renewable and Sustainable Energy Reviews, 197*, Article 114427. https://doi.org/10.1016/j.rser.2024.114427

Austin, K., Jones, J., & Clark, C. (2022). A review of domestic land use change attributable to U.S. Biofuel policy. *Renewable and Sustainable Energy Reviews, 159*, 112181. https://doi.org/10.1016/j.rser.2022.112181.

Baharuddin, N. A. F. A., & Chang, L. W. (2015). Ex-post critical evaluations of energy policies in Malaysia from 1970 to 2010: A historical institutionalism perspective. *Energies*, *8*(3), 1936–1957. https://doi.org/10.3390/en8031936.

Bang, G. (2025). The US inflation reduction act: Climate policy as economic crisis response. *Environmental Politics*, 1–22. https://doi.org/10.1080/09644016.2024.2437886.

IES Bioenergy (2023). https://www.ieabioenergy.com/wp-content/uploads/2024/06/IEA-Bioenergy-Task-39-SAF-report.pdf.

Bouillass, G., Blanc, I., & Perez-Lopez, P. (2021). Step-by-step social life cycle assessment framework: A participatory approach for the identification and prioritization of impact subcategories applied to mobility scenarios. *The International Journal of Life Cycle Assessment, 26*(12), 2408–2435. https://doi.org/10.1007/s11367-021-01988-w

Brinkman, M. L., Wicke, B., Faaij, A. P., & Van der Hilst, F. (2019). Projecting socio-economic impacts of bioenergy: Current status and limitations of ex-ante quantification methods. *Renewable and Sustainable Energy Reviews, 115*, Article 109352. https://doi.org/10.1016/j.rser.2019.109352

Buyx, A., & Tait, J. (2011). Ethical framework for biofuels. *Science, 332*(6029), 540–541. https://doi.org/10.1126/science.1206064

Chowdhury, P., Mahi, N. A., Yeassin, R., Chowdhury, N., & Farrok, O. (2025). Biomass to biofuel: Impacts and mitigation of environmental, health, and socioeconomic challenges. *Energy Conversion and Management: X, 25*, Article 100889. https://doi.org/10.1016/j.ecmx.2025.100889

Creutzig, F., Ravindranath, N. H., Berndes, G., Bolwig, S., Bright, R., Cherubini, F., Chum, H., Corbera, E., Delucchi, M., Faaij, A., Fargione, J., Haber, H., Heath, G., Lucon, O., Plevin, R., Popp, A., Robledo-Abad, C, Rose, S., Smith, P., Stromman, A., Syh, S., & Masera, O. (2015). Bioenergy and climate change mitigation: An assessment. *Gcb Bioenergy, 7*(5), 916–944. https://doi.org/10.1111/gcbb.12205

Das, P., & Gundimeda, H. (2022). Is biofuel expansion in developing countries reasonable? A review of empirical evidence of food and land use impacts. *Journal of Cleaner Production, 372*, Article 133501. https://doi.org/10.1016/j.jclepro.2022.133501

Datta, D., Biswas, S., Barman, D., Mandal, E., & Das, B. (2024). Evolution, challenges and benefits of biofuel production and its potential role in meeting global energy demands. In *Emerging sustainable technologies for biofuel production* (pp. 595–632). Cham: Springer Nature Switzerland. https://doi.org/10.1007/978-3-031-52167-6_23

de Paula Leite, A. C., Pimentel, L. M., & de Almeida Monteiro, L. (2025). The impact of climate change policies on the biofuels sector: A stakeholder perspective. *Energy Sources, Part b: Economics, Planning, and Policy, 20*(1), 2477510. https://doi.org/10.1080/15567249.2025.2477510

Dou, K., & Huijsmans, J. (2025). Biofuels. In *Embracing the future, powering growth: An energy system renewed for China* (pp. 213–234). https://doi.org/10.1007/978-3-031-73075-7_10.

EC (2000). Towards a European research area, communication from the commission to the European parliament, the council, the European economic and social committee and the committee of the regions, COM, 6 Final.

EC (2014). *Research and innovation FP7*. http://ec.europa.eu/research/fp7/index_en.cfm.

El-Araby, R. (2024). Biofuel production: exploring renewable energy solutions for a greener future. Biotechnology for Biofuels and Bioproducts, 17(1), 129. https://doi.org/10.1186/s13068-024-02571-9

EU Biofuels Chain. (2022). *Five reasons Europe needs to do better on biofuels*. Politico. https://www.politico.eu/sponsored-content/five-reasons-europe-needs-to-do-better-on-biofuels/.

Fatima, N., Khanam, N., Kumari, R., Joshi, V. C., & Bhattacharya, S. (2025). Biofuels in India: Policies, reviews, and strategic analysis. *BioEnergy Research, 18*(1), 40. https://doi.org/10.1007/s12155-025-10843-x

Feng, Q., He, D., Zeadally, S., Khan, M. K., & Kumar, N. (2019). A survey on privacy protection in blockchain system. *Journal of Network and Computer Applications, 126*, 45–58. https://doi.org/10.1016/j.jnca.2018.10.020

Gomiero, T., Paoletti, M. G., & Pimentel, D. (2010). Biofuels: Efficiency, ethics, and limits to human appropriation of ecosystem services. *Journal of Agricultural and Environmental Ethics, 23*(5), 403–434. https://doi.org/10.1007/s10806-009-9218-x

Hasan, M., Abedin, M. Z., Amin, M. B., Nekmahmud, M., & Oláh, J. (2023). Sustainable biofuel economy: A mapping through bibliometric research. *Journal of Environmental Management, 336*, Article 117644. https://doi.org/10.1016/j.jenvman.2023.117644

Igwebuike, C. M., Awad, S., & Andrès, Y. (2024). Renewable energy potential: Second-generation biomass as feedstock for bioethanol production. *Molecules, 29*(7), 1619. https://doi.org/10.3390/molecules29071619

International Energy Agency. (2017). *Technology roadmap—Delivering sustainable bioenergy*. https://webstore.iea.org/technology-roadmap-delivering-sustainable-bioenergy.

International Energy Agency. (2018). *Market report series: Renewables 2018*. https://webstore.iea.org/market-report-series-renewables-2018.

Jeswani, H. K., Chilvers, A., & Azapagic, A. (2020). Environmental sustainability of biofuels: A review. *Proceedings of the Royal Society a, 476*(2243), 20200351. https://doi.org/10.1098/rspa.2020.0351

Kafeel, K., Zhou, J., Khan, S., Hronec, M., & Suplata, M. (2025). Exploring the environmental impacts of biofuels: Do affluence, green technological innovation, and green finance matter for top biofuel abundant economies? *Regional Science Policy & Practice, 17*(9), Article 100211. https://doi.org/10.1016/j.rspp.2025.100211

Kanjilal, B., & Saha, S. (2019). Ethical implications of biofuel production and use and its relationship with environment and society. *Ethics in Biology, Engineering and Medicine: An International Journal, 10*(1). https://doi.org/10.1615/EthicsBiologyEngMed.2020033930.

Khan, N., Sudhakar, K., & Mamat, R. (2021). Role of biofuels in energy transition, green economy and carbon neutrality. *Sustainability, 13*(22), 12374. https://doi.org/10.3390/su132212374

Khanna, M., Crago, C. L., & Black, M. (2011). Can biofuels be a solution to climate change? The implications of land use change-related emissions for policy. *Interface Focus, 1*(2), 233–247. https://doi.org/10.1098/rsfs.2010.0016

Koh, L., Dolgui, A., & Sarkis, J. (2020). Blockchain in transport and logistics—paradigms and transitions. *International Journal of Production Research, 58*(7), 2054–2062. https://doi.org/10.1080/00207543.2020.1736428

Koster, M., De Simone, F., & Saint-Supéry, M. V. (2023). Overview of biofuels policies and markets across the EU. Tech. rep. Brussels: The European renewable ethanol association, Oct. 2022. https://www.epure.org/wpcontent/uploads/2022/10/221011-DEF-REP-Overview-of-biofuelspolicies-and-markets-across-the-EU-October-2022.pdf.

Kostidi, E., & Lyridis, D. (2024). Social impact assessment of biofuel production for maritime and aviation sectors: A case study of a pilot biorefinery project. *Frontiers in Energy Research, 12*, 1454862. https://doi.org/10.3389/fenrg.2024.1454862

Kourkoumpas, D., Bon, A., Sagani, A., Atsonios, K., Grammelis, P., Karellas, S., & Kakaras, E. (2024). Life cycle assessment of novel thermochemical—biochemical biomass-to-liquid pathways for sustainable aviation and maritime fuel production. *Bioresource Technology, 393*, Article 130115. https://doi.org/10.1016/j.biortech.2023.130115

Kumar, B., Bhardwaj, N., Agrawal, K., Chaturvedi, V., & Verma, P. (2020). Current perspective on pretreatment technologies using lignocellulosic biomass: An emerging biorefinery concept. *Fuel Processing Technology*, 199. https://doi.org/10.1016/j.fuproc.2019.106244.

Lee, J. Y., Naylor, R. L., Figueroa, A. J., & Gorelick, S. M. (2020). Water-food-energy challenges in India: Political economy of the sugar industry. *Environmental Research Letters, 15*(8), Article 084020. https://doi.org/10.1088/1748-9326/ab9925

Liepold, C., Fabianek, P., & Madlener, R. (2024). A critical evaluation of the 2022 greenhouse gas mitigation quota in Germany from an environmental economics and policy perspective. *Energy Policy, 191*, Article 114200. https://doi.org/10.1016/j.enpol.2024.114200

Lundberg, L., Cintas Sanchez, O., & Zetterholm, J. (2023). The impact of blending mandates on biofuel consumption, production, emission reductions and fuel prices. *Energy Policy, 183*, Article 113835. https://doi.org/10.1016/j.enpol.2023.113835

Mai-Moulin, T., Hoefnagels, R., Grundmann, P., & Junginger, M. (2021). Effective sustainability criteria for bioenergy: Towards the implementation of the European renewable directive II. *Renewable and Sustainable Energy Reviews, 138*, Article 110645. https://doi.org/10.1016/j.rser.2020.110645

Malode, S. J., Prabhu, K. K., Mascarenhas, R. J., Shetti, N. P., & Aminabhavi, T. M. (2021). Recent advances and viability in biofuel production. *Energy Conversion and Management: X, 10*, Article 100070. https://doi.org/10.1016/j.ecmx.2020.100070

Marin-Burgos, V., & Clancy, J. S. (2017). Understanding the expansion of energy crops beyond the global biofuel boom: Evidence from oil palm expansion in Colombia. *Energy, Sustainability and Society, 7*(1), 21. https://doi.org/10.1186/s13705-017-0123-

Mattioda, R. A., Tavares, D. R., Casela, J. L., & Junior, O. C. (2020). Social life cycle assessment of biofuel production. *Biofuels for a More Sustainable Future*, 255–271. https://doi.org/10.1016/B978-0-12-815581-3.00009-9.

Mission Innovations (2025). https://mission-innovation.net/our-members/india/investments/#:~:text=Under%20the%20collaborative%20R&D%20programme,plant%20as%20viability%20gap%20funding.

MNRE (2022). https://mnre.gov.in/en/bio-energy/.

Mohr, A., & Raman, S. (2013). Lessons from first generation biofuels and implications for the sustainability appraisal of second generation biofuels. *Energy Policy, 63*, 114–122. https://doi.org/10.1016/j.enpol.2013.08.033

Mortimer, N. D. (2013). The ethics of biofuels: A review within the framework of the Nuffield Council on bioethics report. *Biofuels, 4*(5), 501–509. https://doi.org/10.4155/bfs.13.40

Mould, K., Silva, F., Knott, S. F., & O'Regan, B. (2022). A comparative analysis of biogas and hydrogen, and the impact of the certificates and blockchain new paradigms. *International Journal of Hydrogen Energy, 47*(93), 39303–39318. https://doi.org/10.1016/j.ijhydene.2022.09.107

Naidu, G., Narkhede, U., Shahare, P., Wankhede, P., Deshkar, R., & Gudadhe, A. (2024). Ethical considerations in AI-driven supply chain management: A review of emerging trends and challenges. In *2024 2nd DMIHER international conference on artificial intelligence in healthcare, education and industry (IDICAIEI)* (pp. 1–7). IEEE. https://doi.org/10.1109/IDICAIEI61867.2024.10842944.

Nair, L. G., Agrawal, K., & Verma, P. (2022). An overview of sustainable approaches for bioenergy production from agro-industrial wastes. *Energy Nexus, 6*(March), Article 100086. https://doi.org/10.1016/j.nexus.2022.100086

National Policy on Biofuels (2018). Press Information Bureau, Government of India, Ministry of Petroleum & Natural Gas. https://www.pib.gov.in/Pressreleaseshare.aspx?PRID=1532265#:~:text=The%20Policy%20encourages%20setting%20up,Policy%20document%20to%20synergise%20efforts.

Ncube, M. M., & Ngulube, P. (2024). Enhancing environmental decision-making: A systematic review of data analytics applications in monitoring and management. *Discover Sustainability, 5*(1), 290. https://doi.org/10.1007/s43621-024-00510-0

Núñez-Regueiro, M. M., Siddiqui, S. F., & Fletcher, R. J., Jr. (2021). Effects of bioenergy on biodiversity arising from land-use change and crop type. *Conservation Biology, 35*(1), 77–87. https://doi.org/10.1111/cobi.13452

Osman, A. I., Fang, B., Zhang, Y., Liu, Y., Yu, J., Farghali, M., Rashwan, A.K., Chen. Z., Chen, L., Ihara, I., Rooney, D. W., & Yap, P. S. (2024). Life cycle assessment and techno-economic analysis of sustainable bioenergy production: A review. *Environmental Chemistry Letters, 22*(3), 1115–1154. https://doi.org/10.1007/s10311-023-01694-z

Osuagwu, E. C., Uwaga, A. M., & Inemeawaji, H. P. (2023). Effects of leachate from osisioma open dumpsite in aba, Abia State, Nigeria on Surrounding Borehole Water Quality. In *Water resources management and sustainability: Solutions for arid regions* (pp. 319–333). Cham: Springer Nature Switzerland. https://doi.org/10.1007/978-3-031-24506-0_21.

Patermann, C., & Aguilar, A. (2018). The origins of the bioeconomy in the European Union. *New Biotechnology, 40*, 20–24. https://doi.org/10.1016/j.nbt.2017.04.002

IEA Policies (2025). https://www.iea.org/policies?country%5B0%5D=United%20States&topic%5B0%5D=Fuels.

Pols, A. J. K. (2015). The rationality of biofuel certification: A critical examination of EU biofuel policy. *Journal of Agricultural and Environmental Ethics, 28*(4), 667–681. https://doi.org/10.1007/s10806-015-9550-2

Pols, A., & Spahn, A. (2013). Biofuels: Ethical aspects. In *Encyclopedia of food and agricultural ethics* (pp. 1–8). Springer, Dordrecht.

Pool, R. (2013). *The Nexus of biofuels, climate change, and human health: Workshop summary.*

Popp, J., Harangi-Rákos, M., Gabnai, Z., Balogh, P., Antal, G., & Bai, A. (2016). Biofuels and their co-products as livestock feed: Global economic and environmental implications. *Molecules, 21*(3), 285. https://doi.org/10.3390/molecules21030285

Popp, J., Kovács, S., Oláh, J., Divéki, Z., & Balázs, E. (2021). Bioeconomy: Biomass and biomass-based energy supply and demand. *New Biotechnology, 60*, 76–84. https://doi.org/10.1016/j.nbt.2020.10.004

Raman, R., Sreenivasan, A., Kulkarni, N. V., Suresh, M., & Nedungadi, P. (2025). Analyzing the contributions of biofuels, biomass, and bioenergy to sustainable development goals. *iScience, 28*(4). https://doi.org/10.1016/j.isci.2025.112157.

Rather, R. A., Wani, A. W., Mumtaz, S., Padder, S. A., Khan, A. H., Almohana, A. I., Almojil, S. F., Alam, S. S., & Baba, T. R. (2022). Bioenergy: A foundation to environmental sustainability in a changing global climate scenario. *Journal of King Saud University-Science, 34*(1), Article 101734. https://doi.org/10.1016/j.jksus.2021.101734

Reddy, M. G., & Reddy, B. S. (2021). Economics of biofuel production: A case of sorghum and pearl millet in India. *Biofuels and Biodiesel*, 287–316. https://doi.org/10.1007/978-1-0716-1323-8_19.

Reid, W. V., Ali, M. K., & Field, C. B. (2020). The future of bioenergy. *Global Change Biology, 26*(1), 274–286. https://doi.org/10.1111/gcb.14883

Rist, L., Lee, J. S. H., & Koh, L. P. (2009). Biofuels: Social benefits. *Science, 326*(5958), 1344–1344. https://doi.org/10.1126/science.326.5958.1344-a

Roadmap for Ethanol blending in India 2020-25 (2021). Niti Aayog, Ministry of Petroleum and Natural Gas. https://www.niti.gov.in/sites/default/files/2025-07/Roadmap-For-Ethanol-Blending-In-India-2020-25.pdf

Roy, M. M., & Chandra, A. (2019). Promoting biofuels: The case of ethanol blending initiative in India. *Clean Technologies and Environmental Policy, 21*(5), 953–965. https://doi.org/10.1007/s10098-019-01687-z

Saravanan, A. P., Pugazhendhi, A., & Mathimani, T. (2020). A comprehensive assessment of biofuel policies in the BRICS nations: Implementation, blending target and gaps. *Fuel, 272*, Article 117635. https://doi.org/10.1016/j.fuel.2020.117635

Singh, J., & Clough, Y. (2024). Challenges and opportunities to a sustainable bioenergy utilization in climate mitigation: A global perspective. *Frontiers in Sustainable Energy Policy, 3*, 1460370. https://doi.org/10.3389/fsuep.2024.1460370

Škapa, S., & Vochozka, M. (2020). Towards higher moral and economic goals in renewable energy. *Science and Engineering Ethics, 26*(3), 1149–1158. https://doi.org/10.1007/s11948-019-00109-z

Solarte-Toro, J. C., & Cardona Alzate, C. A. (2023). Sustainability of biorefineries: Challenges and perspectives. *Energies, 16*(9), 3786. https://doi.org/10.3390/en16093786

Souza, G. M., Ballester, M. V. R., De Brito Cruz, C. H., Chum, H., Dale, B., Dale, V, H., Fernandes, E. C. M., Foust, T., Karp, A., Lynd, L., Osseweijer, P., & Van der Wielen, L. (2017). The role

of bioenergy in a climate-changing world. *Environmental Development*, *23*, 57–64. https://doi.org/10.1016/j.envdev.2017.02.008
TAIT, J. (2011). The ethics of biofuels. *GCB Bioenergy*, *3*(3), 271–275. https://doi.org/10.1111/j.1757-1707.2011.01107.x.
Thompson, P. B. (2012). The Agricultural Ethics of Biofuels: The Food vs Fuel Debate. *Agriculture*, *2*(4), 339–358. https://doi.org/10.3390/agriculture2040339
Tsitrouli, Z. (2021). Sustainable Biofuel Policies: Challenges and ethical considerations. *Bioethica*, *7*(1), 46–63. https://doi.org/10.12681/bioeth.26541.
Usmani, R. A., Mohammad, A. S., & Ansari, S. S. (2023). Comprehensive biofuel policy analysis framework: A novel approach evaluating the policy influences. *Renewable and Sustainable Energy Reviews, 183*, Article 113403. https://doi.org/10.1016/j.rser.2023.113403
Usmani, R. A. (2023). Biofuel consumption and global climate change: Solutions and challenges. *Environmental Sustainability of Biofuels*, 183–200. https://doi.org/10.1016/B978-0-323-91159-7.00019-9.
Vackeová, S., & Noyon, X. (2022). *RePowerEU: Biofuels play a strategic role in boosting Europe's energy independence.* Euractiv. https://www.euractiv.com/section/biofuels/opinion/repowereu-biofuels-play-a-strategic-role-in-boosting-europes-energy-independence.
Van der Horst, D., & Vermeylen, S. (2011). Spatial scale and social impacts of biofuel production. *Biomass and Bioenergy, 35*(6), 2435–2443. https://doi.org/10.1016/j.biombioe.2010.11.029
Vance, C., Sweeney, J., & Murphy, F. (2022). Space, time, and sustainability: The status and future of life cycle assessment frameworks for novel biorefinery systems. *Renewable and Sustainable Energy Reviews, 159*, Article 112259. https://doi.org/10.1016/j.rser.2022.112259
Velenturf, A. P., & Purnell, P. (2021). Principles for a sustainable circular economy. *Sustainable Production and Consumption, 27*, 1437–1457. https://doi.org/10.1016/j.spc.2021.02.018
Wattana, S. (2014). Bioenergy Development in Thailand: Challenges and Strategies. Energy Procedia, 52, 506-515. https://doi.org/10.1016/j.egypro.2014.07.104
Webster, E. (2020). Transnational legal processes, the EU and RED II: Strengthening the global governance of bioenergy. *Review of European, Comparative & International Environmental Law, 29*(1), 86–94. https://doi.org/10.1111/reel.12315
Welfle, A. J., Almena, A., Arshad, M. N., Banks, S. W., Butnar, I., Chong, K. J., Cooper. S. G., Daly, H., Freites. S. G., Gulec, F., Hardacre, C., Holland, R., Lan. L., Lee, C. S., Robertson, P., Rowe, R., Shepherd, A., Skillen, N., Tedesco, S., Thornley, P., & Röder, M. (2023). Sustainability of bioenergy–Mapping the risks & benefits to inform future bioenergy systems. *Biomass and Bioenergy, 177*, Article 106919. https://doi.org/10.1016/j.biombioe.2023.106919
Wohlgemuth, R., Twardowski, T., & Aguilar, A. (2021). Bioeconomy moving forward step by step–A global journey. *New Biotechnology, 61*, 22–28. https://doi.org/10.1016/j.nbt.2020.11.006
Yi, H. (2022). A traceability method of biofuel production and utilization based on blockchain. *Fuel, 310*, Article 122350. https://doi.org/10.1016/j.fuel.2021.122350
Zetterholm, J., Bryngemark, E., Ahlström, J., Söderholm, P., Harvey, S., & Wetterlund, E. (2020). Economic evaluation of large-scale biorefinery deployment: A framework integrating dynamic biomass market and techno-economic models. *Sustainability, 12*(17), 7126. https://doi.org/10.3390/su12177126
Zeug, W., Yupanqui, K. R. G., Bezama, A., & Thrän, D. (2023). Holistic and integrated life cycle sustainability assessment of prospective biomass to liquid production in Germany. *Journal of Cleaner Production, 418*, Article 138046. https://doi.org/10.1016/j.jclepro.2023.138046
Zhang, C., Singh, R. P., Yadav, P., Kumar, I., Kaushik, A., Roychowdhury, R., Mubeen, M., Singh, S. K., Kumar, A., & Wang, J. (2025). Recent advances in biotechnology and bioengineering for efficient microalgal biofuel production. *Fuel Processing Technology, 270*, Article 108199. https://doi.org/10.1016/j.fuproc.2025.108199
Zhi, L., He, Z., Li, P., & Cao, X. (2023). In the direction of a sustainable future: A comprehensive review of evolution, environmental impacts, and future prospects of bioenergy. In *E3S web of conferences* (Vol. 466, p. 02005). EDP Sciences. https://doi.org/10.1051/e3sconf/202346602005.

Index

P. Verma (ed.), *Sustainable Practices in Biorefinery*,
https://doi.org/10.1007/978-981-95-6071-4

FSC
www.fsc.org
MIX
Papier aus verantwortungsvollen Quellen
Paper from responsible sources
FSC® C105338

If you have any concerns about our products,
you can contact us on
ProductSafety@springernature.com

In case Publisher is established outside the EU,
the EU authorized representative is:
Springer Nature Customer Service Center GmbH
Europaplatz 3, 69115 Heidelberg, Germany

Printed by Libri Plureos GmbH
in Hamburg, Germany